THE MOLECULAR BASIS OF NEOPLASIA

THE MOLECULAR BASIS OF NEOPLASIA

A Collection of Papers Presented at the Fifteenth Annual Symposium on Fundamental Cancer Research, 1961

PUBLISHED FOR

THE UNIVERSITY OF TEXAS M. D. ANDERSON

HOSPITAL AND TUMOR INSTITUTE

UNIVERSITY OF TEXAS PRESS, AUSTIN

Library of Congress Catalog Card No. 62–14609

Manufactured in the United States of America
by the Printing Division of The University of Texas

Acknowledgment

The staff of The University of Texas M. D. Anderson Hospital and Tumor Institute gratefully acknowledges the assistance of the National Science Foundation; the American Cancer Society, Texas Division; the Bertner Foundation; the Heuermann Foundation; and the State of Texas Department of Health, for providing funds for support and publication of this symposium.

Gratitude is expressed also to the members of the 1961 symposium committee for their efforts in arranging the program. Members of the committee were Saul Kit, Chairman, Daniel Billen, Joe E. Boyd, Jr., Felix L. Haas, T. C. Hsu, Bruno Jirgensons, and David Trkula.

This symposium volume was edited and arranged for publication by the following members of the Publications Department: Russell W. Cumley, Marilyn Abbott, Dorothy M. Aldridge, Judith Haroz, Elaine Heinsohn, Joan McCay, and Barbara Troller.

The book was produced by Joan McCay and Hester Finke.

Finally, the staff acknowledges The University of Texas Press and the Printing Division of The University of Texas for their fine cooperation in the publication of this volume.

Table of Contents

Controlling Mechanisms and Biochemical Alterations Induced by Viral Nucleic Acids

Ribosomes and Protein Synthesis

MOLECULAR BASIS
OF
NEOPLASIA

Introduction

R. Lee Clark, M.D., M.Sc., D.Sc. (Hon.)

Director and Surgeon-in-Chief
The University of Texas M. D. Anderson Hospital
and Tumor Institute,
Houston, Texas

That a full and extensive symposium can be held on the subject, "The Molecular Basis of Neoplasia," is in itself an illustration of the degree of sophistication that cancer research has attained. Credit for this may be given impartially to both the quality and the quantity of research carried on by workers in cellular biochemistry and physiology.

Boveri's proposal in 1912 that an abnormal chromatin complement is a characteristic of a neoplastic cell may be regarded as the first step toward the results which will be discussed here. This general concept embraces all the manifold processes of abnormalities at the molecular level.

Much of the current work in cancer research is based on research in pure biochemistry and in pure biophysics. The brilliant elaboration of nucleic acid structure proposed by Watson and Crick provides the framework upon which to base our theories and test them for physical feasibility. The molar base ratio studies of our symposium chairman, Saul Kit, and of others, and the infinitely detailed and group analysis techniques provide methods to justify our suppositions chemically.

A further indication of the intellectual maturity being achieved in cancer research is the extensive material coming available with regard to viruses, and the role of these molecular-sized particles in tumor etiology. Not surprisingly, the models and techniques of pure biochemical research have led to outstanding developments in virology. Many years ago, the early geneticists hinted at the close relationship between viruses and genes. It now appears that their speculations may bear abundant fruit.

The integrated, fully correlated sessions of this Fifteenth Annual Symposium on Fundamental Cancer Research are a tribute to the hard work and enduring interest of the 1961 symposium committee: Dr. Saul Kit, chairman, and committee members, Mr. Joe E. Boyd, Jr., Drs. Daniel Billen, Felix L. Haas, T. C. Hsu, Bruno Jirgensons, and David Trkula.

Gratitude is expressed to the co-sponsors, the National Science Foundation, the State of Texas Department of Health, and The University of Texas Postgraduate School of Medicine, who have helped to make this symposium possible.

The Place of the Symposium in Scientific Communication

HARRY H. RANSOM, PH.D., LITT.D., LL.D.

President, Main University,
The University of Texas, Austin, Texas

There was a time when the term *science* was related to man's broadest concern for both knowledge and wisdom. Popular usage may have restricted some of the connotations of the word; our human condition has broadened the relationships of science to all aspects of our culture and has vastly increased the scientist's obligation.

More than any previous generation, we rely upon the scientific method for advancement of knowledge. More than any previous society, we look to science for the relief of ailment and the correction of evil—individual and social, physical and mental, economic and intellectual.

This excessive reliance has produced in the popular press and in millions of untrained minds many wistful notions. One is that if mankind could garb enough intelligent men and women in laboratory coats and provide them with enough equipment, all the world's problems would be solved and the future secured to happiness.

Another notion, equally wistful and almost equally erroneous, is that scientists, however wise, may have confronted the foolhardy with a choice between giving up the search for truth, or of destroying the world by the perversion of truth.

This modern scientific melodrama, in which the scientists themselves have played no part, is based on the false assumption that man's existence must depend upon a clear-cut choice between blind fear and blind hope. It neglects the function of truth. It underestimates the power of intelligent men to exchange ideas.

The exchange of ideas, sharing of knowledge, and social uses of wisdom have been the steady occupation of many intelligent men since the foundation of the Royal Society. Much earlier than that association of courageous intellects, every nation civilized enough to be remembered offered opportunities for the common practice of the mind. In ancient times, the Greek symposium was only one means by which men of intellect were brought together and through which they could put together what they had learned separately.

Today the symposium as an institution brings us up against the modern world's most pressing need: men of science who are capable of communicating with one another. It is ironic that in our advancement of learning the proliferation of knowledge is almost as great an obstacle to scientific progress as are the prejudices of politics.

It is specially appropriate, therefore, that a great research hospital and scientific center designed to cure man's physical ills should periodically bring together scholars bent on curing man's ignorance. In such company and on such occasions, there is no temptation to substitute shoddy optimism for truth. There is no inclination to trade the necessary and the difficult for the pleasures of self-comfort or delusions of mere expediency.

The University of Texas has no policy about truth. Truth makes its own policies. But the University does take the stand that in this Institute and all institutions like it, this meeting of scientists and all that it undertakes must be considered as a proper function of a university. The University of Texas therefore feels privileged to sponsor this symposium, and we are grateful for the sense of obligation that brings you together.

What will be presented will not be immediately intelligible to the majority of men. However, there is a conviction everywhere that although men do not live in a world of scientists, they do live in a scientific world, and in that scientific world there is a figurative symposium of all men. Their need of application of scientific knowledge is painfully manifest. That need will be met only by the refinement of such knowledge as will be exchanged at this symposium and by its broadest possible communication.

To the extent that this symposium gathers and tests knowledge, it does generate truth. That generation of truth is our most important duty and, really, the only hope for man's future.

NUCLEIC ACIDS

Biological and Physical Chemical Aspects of Reversible Denaturation of Deoxyribonucleic Acids

J. Marmur, C. L. Schildkraut,* and P. Doty

Graduate Department of Biochemistry, Brandeis University, Waltham, Massachusetts; and Department of Chemistry, Harvard University, Cambridge, Massachusetts

The Watson-Crick model for the structure of deoxyribonucleic acid (DNA) has provided a basis for many studies of its genetic role and its physical chemical properties. The implication that the complementary strands separate and that each serves as a template for the synthesis of new complementary strands has been supported by the experiments of Levinthal and Thomas (1957) and Meselson and Stahl (1958). The latter workers did not define the basic replicating unit of DNA. However, subsequent work by Marmur and Lane (1960), Doty, Marmur, Eigner, and Schildkraut (1960), and Schildkraut, Marmur, and Doty (1961) on the reversible denaturation of DNA has presented further data consistent with the notion that the replicating units are indeed the complementary DNA strands themselves.

Reversible denaturation of DNA has provided a unique tool for studying some of its physical chemical properties and a new vehicle for investigation of the molecular basis of some aspects of genetics.

Experiments and Results

DNA strand separation and subsequent renaturation by exposure to elevated temperatures below the melting temperature (T_m) can

* Present address: Department of Biochemistry, Stanford University, Palo Alto, California.

be studied by biological means as well as by physical chemical techniques. The thermally induced denaturation of DNA, which can be compared to the melting of a crystal, occurs within a narrow temperature range. The helix-to-coil transition of the DNA can be followed in a number of ways: the loss of transforming activity, the increase in immunological reactivity (Levine, Murakami, Van Vunakis, and Grossman, 1960), an increase in relative absorbance at 260 mμ, an increase in the buoyant density in a cesium chloride gradient, the separation of the strands of hybrid N^{14}–N^{15} labeled DNA in density gradient ultracentrifugation, the fall in molecular weight by a factor of two (measured by sedimentation and viscosity) and changes in shape observed by the electron microscope (Doty, Marmur, Eigner, and Schildkraut, 1960). The renaturation also can be followed by each or all of the above techniques.

The denaturation and renaturation of DNA is readily followed by assaying the transforming activity of *Diplococcus pneumoniae* DNA after the various thermal exposures, since the helical form is necessary for activity. The transforming activity is plotted in Figure 1 for quickly cooled aliquots taken from a solution held at 100°C, and then at various times during the slow cooling (shown at the right of the vertical dashed line in Figure 1) as the temperature of

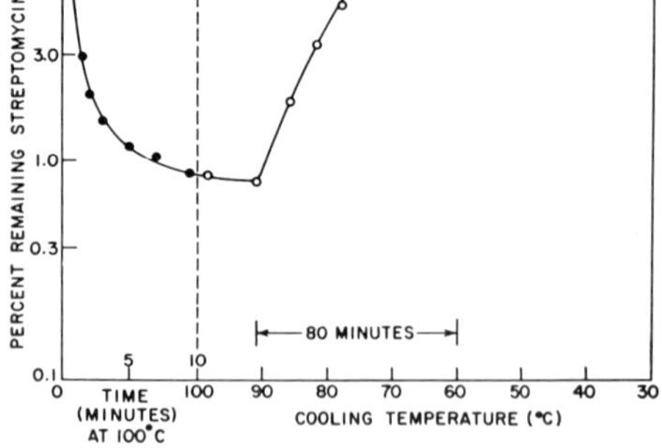

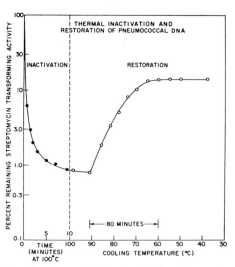

FIG. 1. Thermal inactivation and restoration of the transforming activity of *D. pneumoniae* DNA. Pneumococcal DNA at 20 μg/ml. in 0.15 M NaCl plus 0.015 M Na citrate was preheated for one and one-half minutes at 85.5°C (no loss in biological activity), then transferred to a boiling water bath at 0 minutes. At the times shown, samples were removed to an equal volume of 1.5 M NaCl plus 0.15 M Na citrate in an ice-water bath. After 10 minutes', exposure at 100°C, an equal volume of hot (100°C) 1.5 M NaCl plus 0.15 M Na citrate was mixed with the DNA solution, the mixture transferred to a large water bath and then cooled slowly. During the gradual descent of the temperature, samples were removed (shown at the right of the dashed vertical line) to prechilled tubes in an ice-water bath and then assayed for the ability to transform with respect to the streptomycin resistance marker.

the bath decreased. Thus, it is seen that restoration of the biological activity begins when the temperature of the slow cooling is about 90°C and continues until about 65°C. While in this experiment the recovery of the biological activity is approximately 15 per cent, values as high as 50 to 60 per cent have been attained using improved conditions (Marmur and Doty, 1961).

The remainder of this presentation will be devoted to (1) some factors which influence strand separation, (2) those influencing renaturation, (3) the thermal stability of renatured DNA, (4) studies on the formation of molecular hybrids between homologous and heterologous DNA, and (5) the genetic and taxonomic aspects of renatured hybrid formation.

Some Factors Influencing Strand Separation of DNA

The most useful methods in following strand separation have been the observation of the hyperchromic effect at 260 mμ, the buoyant density in ultracentrifugation and the loss of transforming activity.

Effect of Temperature and Time of Exposure

When native DNA is exposed to temperatures several degrees above the T_m, strand separation ensues. Using hybrid N^{14}–N^{15} DNA preparations isolated from *Escherichia coli* (grown for many generations in $N^{15}H_4Cl$ as the sole nitrogen source, followed by one generation in $N^{14}H_4Cl$ as described by Meselson and Stahl (1958), strand separation is readily demonstrated (Figure 2) using the density gradient technique. By carefully controlling the time and temperature of exposure, it is possible to denature part of the population of DNA molecules. These denatured, single strands, each containing N^{14} or N^{15}, have an increased buoyant density in cesium chloride and are readily recognized. By varying the time of exposure to a constant temperature above the T_m, increasing proportions of the DNA molecules become denatured. These experiments not only demonstrate strand separation, but also confirm the contention that denaturation by heating and fast cooling is an all-or-none phenomenon. Furthermore, they also clearly demonstrate DNA heterogeneity. By partially denaturing the DNA at 93.8°C for 20 minutes, the adenine plus thymine rich molecules are the first to melt out, leaving behind relatively richer guanine plus cytosine containing DNA molecules that can be recognized by their higher buoyant density.

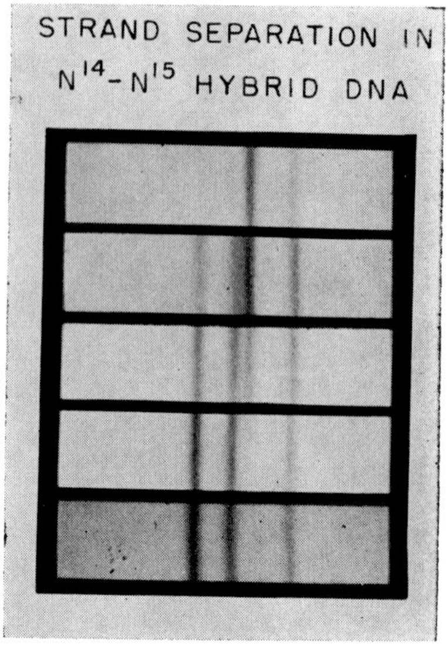

FIG. 2. Thermally induced strand separation of hybrid N^{14}–N^{15} *E. coli* B DNA. The hybrid DNA was prepared from *E. coli* grown for many generations in a synthetic medium with $N^{15}H_4Cl$ as the sole nitrogen source followed by one generation in $N^{14}H_4Cl$ containing medium, according to the method described by Meselson and Stahl, 1958. The ultraviolet absorption photographs, taken after centrifugation to equilibrium in CsCl at 44,770 rpm, show different stages of the thermally induced strand separation. In each strip, the band at the far right, which was introduced into the centrifuge cell as a standard, is DNA from *D. pneumoniae.* In the top photograph, the other band is native, biologically formed hybrid N^{14}–N^{15} *E. coli* DNA. The second photograph shows the stability of the hybrid to a 20 minute exposure in 0.15 M NaCl plus 0.015 M Na citrate at 93.8°C. At 100°C the number of molecules separating increases with time of exposure, as shown in the next three photographs. The samples were heated in the same solvent at 20 μg./ml. for 30 seconds, one, and 10 minutes, respectively.

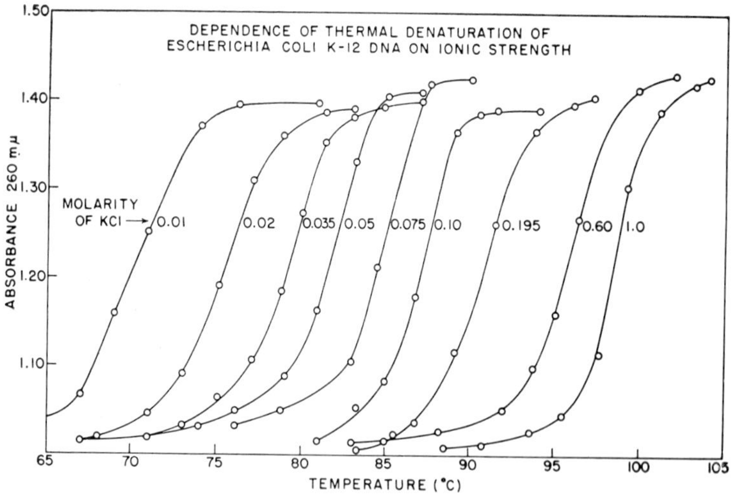

FIG. 3. Dependence of thermal denaturation of *E. coli* K-12 DNA on ionic strength. *E. coli* DNA, suspended in various concentrations of KCl in glass stoppered quartz cuvettes, was heated in the Beckman spectrophotometer chamber and the relative absorbance (corrected for thermal expansion) was measured at the elevated temperatures.

Effect of Ionic Strength

It would be expected that raising the salt concentration of the suspending medium would produce a shielding of the repulsive forces of the charged phosphate groups of the DNA molecule which require higher temperatures for denaturation. This is shown to be the case for *E. coli* K-12 DNA heated in various concentrations of KCl (Figure 3). The increase in relative absorbance (measured at the elevated temperatures) of DNA at various ionic strengths was followed as a function of the temperature to which it was exposed in the chamber of the Beckman spectrophotometer. The T_m (temperature after 50 per cent of the total increase in relative absorbance) for DNA dissolved in 0.01 M KCl is approximately 70°C and increases to approximately 98°C in 1.0 M KCl. The T_m is also dependent on the guanine plus cytosine content of the DNA (see *Effect of Base Composition*, below), on the pH of the solvent, and has recently been shown to be increased by the presence of certain polyamines (Mahler, Mehrotra, and Sharp, 1961). Small amounts of protein associated with purified DNA preparations or the presence of small quantities of divalent ions (when the denaturation is carried out in the presence of saline-citrate) have little or no detectable effect on the T_m. DNA degraded by sonic vibration to molecular weights of 300,000 has the same T_m as high molecular weight DNA ($10\text{–}20 \times 10^6$).

Effect of Base Composition

The T_m for the thermal denaturation of DNA from various sources, varying in base composition, has been found to be proportional to its guanine plus cytosine (or hydroxymethylcytosine) content (Figure 4). This can be explained in part by the presence of an extra hydrogen bond between the guanine and cytosine (Pauling and Corey, 1956). The curve obtained at the lower ionic strength is parallel to that in 0.15 M NaCl plus 0.015 M Na citrate, and has been used to determine the T_m values of DNA whose denaturation cannot be estimated in the latter solvent because of their high guanine plus cytosine contents (e.g., poly d-GC and *Streptomyces viridochromogenes*).

The base compositions of the DNA samples shown in Figure 4 were obtained from published reports (Belozersky and Spirin, 1960; Chargaff, 1955). However, with the relation well established, it can be used to estimate the base compositions of the new DNA

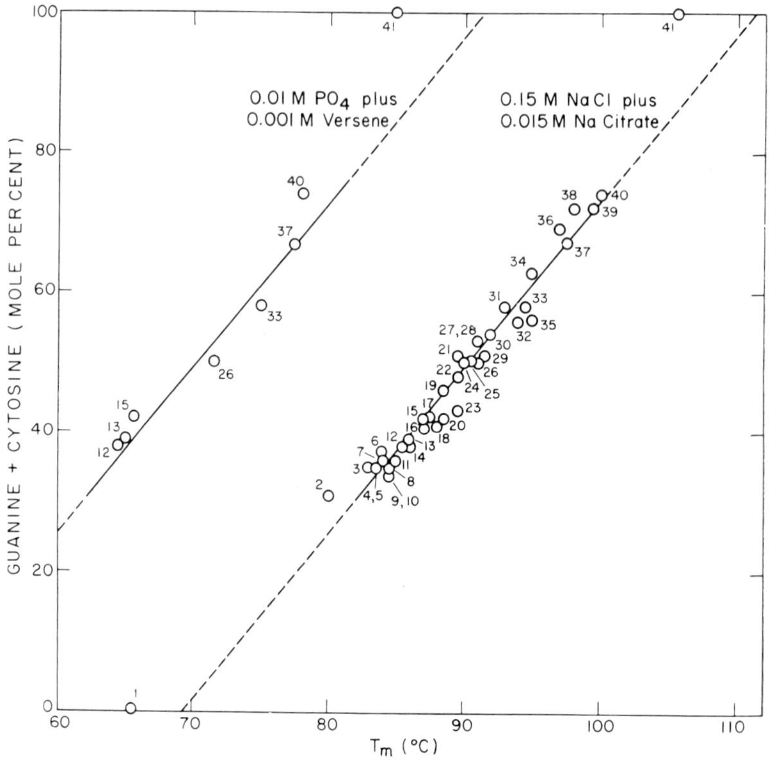

FIG. 4. Dependence of the denaturation temperature, T_m, on the guanine plus cytosine content of various samples of DNA. Native DNA samples (isolated by the method of Marmur, 1961) were dissolved in either of the two solvents shown in the figure. The T_m represents the midpoint of the thermal transition curve (carried out and plotted as shown in Figure 3) and has been plotted as a function of the guanine plus cytosine content (determined chemically and obtained from published reports). The numbers next to each T_m value in the figure refer to the DNA extracted from the following organisms: 1, poly d-GC; 2, *Streptomyces viridochromogenes*; 3, *Micrococcus lysodeikticus*; 4, *Pseudomonas aeruginosa*; 5, *Mycobacterium phlei*; 6, *Aerobacter aerogenes*; 6a, *Azotobacter vinelandii*; 7, *Serratia marcescens*; 8, *Brucella abortus*; 9, *Salmonella typhimurium*; 10, *Shigella dysenteriae*; 11, *Escherichia coli*; 11a, phage T_3; 12, *Bacillus licheniformis*; 13, phage T_7; 13a, *Vibrio cholerae*; 14, *Bacillus subtilis*; 15, salmon sperm; 16, calf thymus; 17, *Hemophilus influenzae*; 18, *Diplococcus pneumoniae*; 19, *Bacillus megaterium;* 20, bakers' yeast; 21, phage T_2r+; 22, phage T_4r+; 23, phage T_6r+; 24, *Bacillus thuringiensis;* 25, *Micrococcus pyogenes* var. *aureus;* 26, *Bacillus cereus;* 27, *Clostridium perfringens;* 28, poly d-AT. The first and last samples, the enzymatically prepared polymers, were obtained through the generosity of A. Kornberg, J. Josse, and J. Adler. The curve on the right was fitted to the points by the method of least squares.

samples simply from measuring their T_m (Marmur and Doty, in preparation). Extrapolation of the T_m curve beyond 25 and 75 per cent G + C remains uncertain at the moment.

Substitution of cytosine by glucosylated hydroxymethylcytosine (in bacteriophages T_2, T_4 and T_6) has no influence on the T_m. Denaturation temperature of DNA isolated from a thermophile, *B. stearothermophilus*, grown at an elevated temperature, is not abnormal and can be predicted from its base composition (Marmur, 1960). Genetically related organisms yield DNA with similar T_m values; taxonomically related microorganisms do not always.

Effect of pH

When DNA is exposed to increasingly acid conditions, the T_m

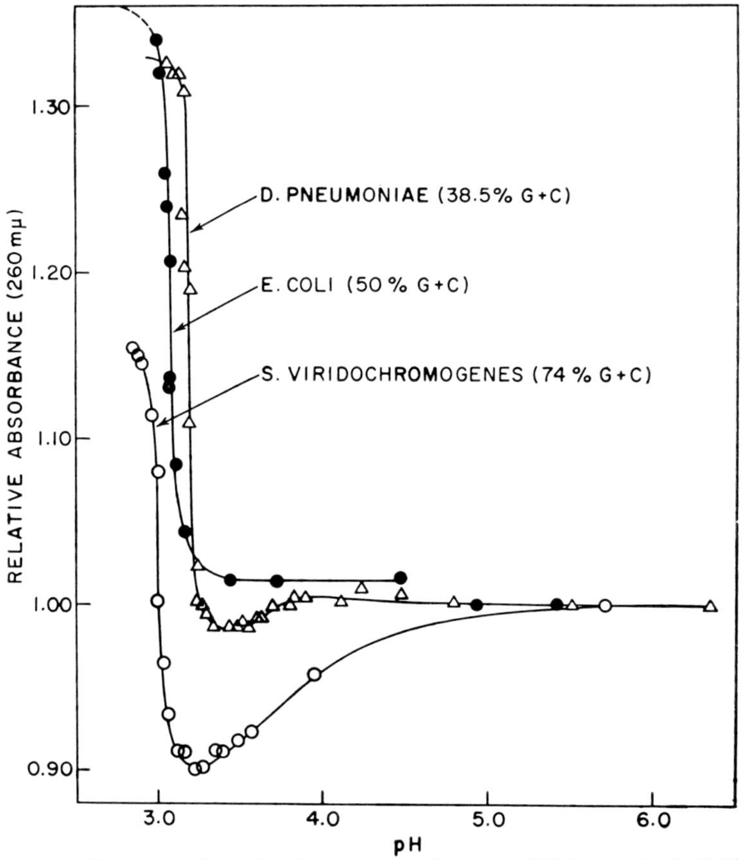

FIG. 5. Effects of acid on the denaturation of various DNA samples in 0.05 M NaCl at 25°C. Samples of DNA dissolved in 0.05 M NaCl were titrated with HCl at 25°C and the pH and relative absorbance measured after each addition.

is lowered until it passes below room temperature. Denaturation can be detected by changes in optical density (Figure 5) or the separation of the strands of hybrid N^{14}–N^{15} DNA (Figure 6). Figure 5 clearly shows that if the DNA has a higher composition of guanine plus cytosine, lower pH values must be reached in order to cause denaturation. The most acid (and temperature) resistant naturally occurring DNA thus far encountered has been isolated from the actinomycetes *Streptomyces viridochromogenes* and *Streptomyces albus*, each possessing approximately 74 per cent guanine plus cytosine (Belozersky and Spirin, 1960).

When hybrid N^{14}–N^{15} *E. coli* DNA was exposed to pH 2.8 (in 0.05 M NaCl at room temperature), neutralized and then centrifuged in a CsCl gradient, two bands were obtained with buoyant densities corresponding to that expected for N^{14} and N^{15} single-stranded *E. coli* DNA (Figure 6). The same situation was found true for native hybrid *E. coli* DNA exposed to high pH values, e.g., 11.5, in experiments carried out in collaboration with R. Cox.

Effect of Formamide

High concentrations of formamide have been shown to denature DNA (Helmkamp and Ts'o, 1961; Marmur and Ts'o, 1961). By increasing the concentration of formamide to which *D. pneumoniae* DNA is exposed, a concentration range is reached (55 to 65 per cent, in 0.02 M NaCl plus 0.002 M Na citrate at 37°C) where the transforming activity abruptly decreases. These conditions provide a mild method for the denaturation of DNA and may be found useful where little or no degradation or depurination (induced, in part, by heat treatments) is desired.

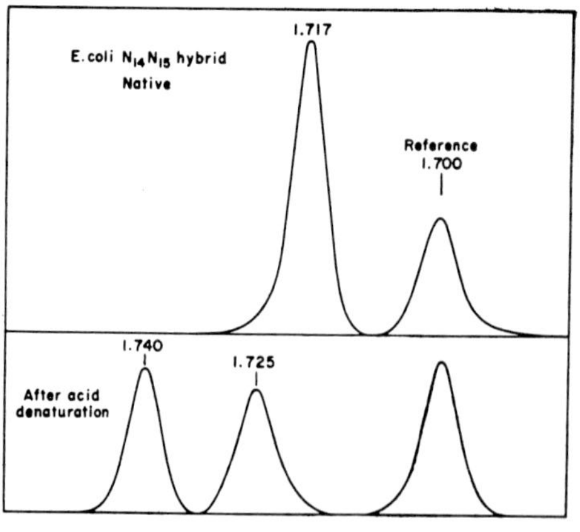

FIG. 6. Acid-induced strand separation of *E. coli* DNA. Hybrid N^{14}—N^{15} *E. coli* B DNA was exposed to pH 2.8 in 0.05 M NaCl at 25°C, re-neutralized and centrifuged for 24 hours at 44,770 rpm in a CsCl gradient in the Spinco ultracentrifuge. The microdensitometer tracings represent the DNA concentration (ordinate) as a function of distance from the axis of rotation. The native reference DNA is *D. pneumoniae* which has a density of 1.700 g./cm.[3]

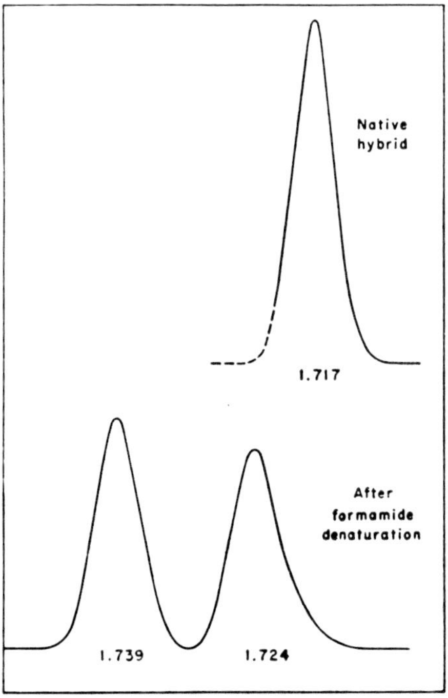

FIG. 7. Formamide-induced strand separation of *E. coli* DNA. Hybrid N^{14}—N^{15} *E. coli* B DNA was exposed to 95 per cent formamide in 0.02 M NaCl plus 0.002 M Na citrate at 37°C for 10 minutes, dialyzed free of formamide, and centrifuged for 24 hours at 44,770 rpm in a CsCl gradient in the Spinco ultracentrifuge. The microdensitometer tracings represent the DNA concentration (ordinate) as a function of the distance from the axis of rotation.

Denaturation is also detectable by treating hybrid N^{14}–N^{15} *E. coli* DNA with formamide, dialyzing out the denaturing agent and centrifuging the treated DNA in a CsCl gradient. Strand separation is again detected by the presence of two bands (Figure 7) whose buoyant densities correspond to denatured N^{14} and N^{15} *E. coli* DNA (Marmur and Ts'o, 1961).

Maximal Thermal Inactivation of Transforming Activity

If the transforming activity of *D. pneumoniae* DNA necessitates its presence in the double-strand helical form, then it should be possible to destroy completely the biological activity by selecting proper conditions of DNA concentration, ionic strength, temperature, and quick cooling. Thus, *D. pneumoniae* DNA was heated in 0.01 M phosphate plus 0.001 M ethylenediaminetetra aceate (EDTA), pH 6.8, at 100°C and, at varying times, aliquots were removed with prechilled pipettes and diluted into solvent of the same composition kept at ice-bath temperature. The loss of transforming activity for the streptomycin marker is seen in Figure 8. The initial sharp drop in biological activity within the first few minutes can be related to

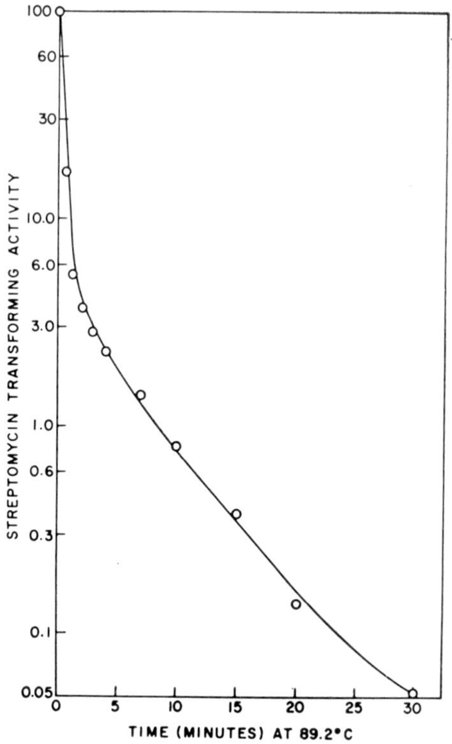

FIG. 8. Maximal thermal inactivation of *D. pneumoniae* transforming DNA. Conditions described in text.

strand separation; the slower component is in all likelihood due to inactivation by depurination and/or strand scission which have been shown to take place at elevated temperatures (Greer and Zamenhof, 1959; Doty, Marmur, Eigner, and Schildkraut, 1960). Since the T_m values of *D. pneumoniae* DNA and poly d-GC in this solvent are 65°C and 84°C, respectively (Figure 4), then all base pairs should have separated by exposing the transforming DNA to 100°C. The residual activities exhibited beyond the stage of base pair separation are unlikely to be due to renaturation, since little or no effect is noted if the same experiment is repeated at various DNA concentrations. They are also unlikely to be due to any extraordinarily resistant DNA, since DNA isolated from cells which have been transformed by this residual activity exhibits the same sensitivity to heat as the original DNA.

The most likely reason for the small residual activity is the probability that a small portion of the denatured DNA possesses transforming activity. Residual activities have been noted when strand separation has been induced by acid or alkali (Marmur and Lane, unpublished data) or formamide (Marmur and Ts'o, 1961). Since denaturation by formamide is performed under mild conditions, the residual activities are higher than by thermal denaturation, as no depurination and/or strand scission would be expected to take place. If the residual activity is indeed due to single-strand DNA, it is not clear at this time whether this may be due to the presence of some transforming molecules which have folded back on themselves to mimic the double-strand structure enough to satisfy the minimal requirements for cell entry. It is also possible that some of the transformable cells are in a certain physiological state (e.g., spheroplasts or L-forms, Madoff and Dienes, 1958) that can adsorb and be transformed by single-strand DNA.

Some Factors Influencing Renaturation

In studying the renaturation of denatured DNA, it has been found useful to employ the techniques of transformation of genetic markers and to follow the changes in optical density after various thermal exposures.

Effect of DNA Source

Although the T_m for strand separation of DNA samples having similar base compositions is independent of their source (except for the breadth of the transition), the extent to which renaturation proceeds is found to be greatly influenced by the type of DNA being studied. This is explicable by the observation that renaturation is dependent upon the concentration of specific complementary strands during the renaturation (Marmur and Lane, 1960). Thus, since there are about 5,000 times more molecules of DNA per cell in mammalian cells than in bacteria (Vendreley, 1958; Crampton, Lipshitz, and Chargaff, 1954; Brown and Brown, 1958), it is to be expected that at the same DNA concentration, renaturation will hardly take place in mammalian DNA, while it proceeds far toward completion in the case of bacterial DNA. Under similar conditions, it would be expected to proceed faster and farther in the case of even simpler sources, e.g., bacteriophage.

In order to explore this matter, renaturation was studied by following the optical density at 260 mμ. This was done by denaturing and quickly cooling the appropriate samples. In this denatured form, about 60 per cent of the hydrogen bonds have reformed in a nonspecific manner, determined from the optical density change.

When the temperature is raised again, to about 65°C, these non-specific bonds dissociate and the strands are free to renature. If renaturation occurs, the optical density at 260 mμ will fall. Results of experiments of this type are shown in Figure 9. It can be seen that after the melting of the weak, intramolecular hydrogen bonds of the denatured, fast-cooled DNA, renaturation of some of the DNA sample occurs. The rate and extent of renaturation of DNA is seen to be dependent upon its source. Calf thymus DNA (as well as DNA from salmon sperm and tobacco leaves) does not renature; *D. pneumoniae* DNA (as DNA from most bacterial sources) readily renatures; whereas T_6r+ (as well as T_2 and T_4) and *Mycoplasma gallisepticum* (avian PPLO) whose DNA is more homogeneous

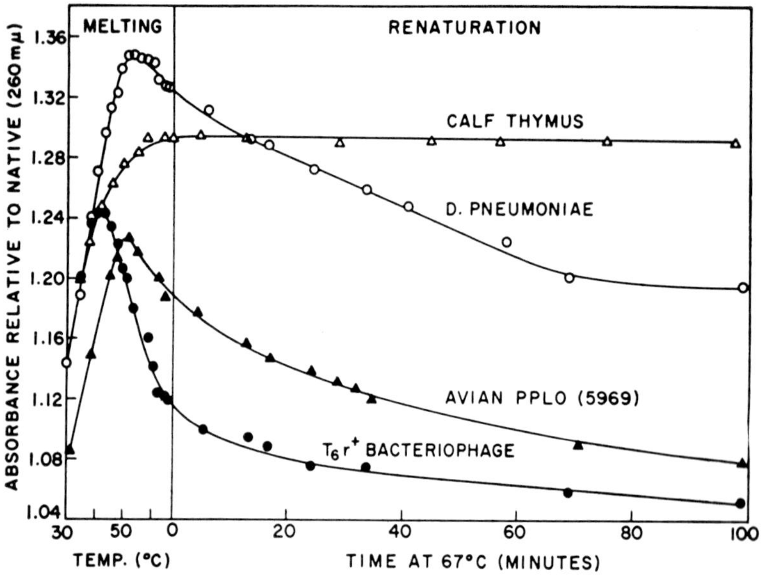

FIG. 9. Effect of source on the renaturation of thermally denatured DNA. DNA at 20 μg./ml. was heated at 100°C for 10 minutes in 0.3 M NaCl plus 0.03 M Na citrate and quickly cooled in an ice bath. The samples of DNA (in ground glass stoppered cuvettes) at the same concentration and in the same solvent, were then placed in the Beckman spectrophotometer which was prewarmed at 67°C. The initial part of the graph represents the *increase* in optical density at 260 mμ (melting) as the denatured DNA samples reach temperature equilibrium. The curves to the right of the vertical line (renaturation) represent the *decrease* in optical density of the temperature equilibrated, renaturing samples as a function of time of exposure at 67°C. The DNA samples employed were isolated from the organisms shown in the figure.

(Burgi and Hershey, 1960; Guild, Morowitz, and Castro, 1960; Guild, 1961), renature the most readily.

Effect of Temperature

Renaturation of DNA by slowly cooling a sample in a large water bath has led to somewhat varying results due to the difficulty of controlling accurately the rate of cooling. In order to find the optimal renaturation temperature of *D. pneumoniae*, denatured samples were exposed at different constant temperatures for varying periods of time. The rate and extent of renaturation was followed by either the decrease in optical density or the recovery of transforming activity.

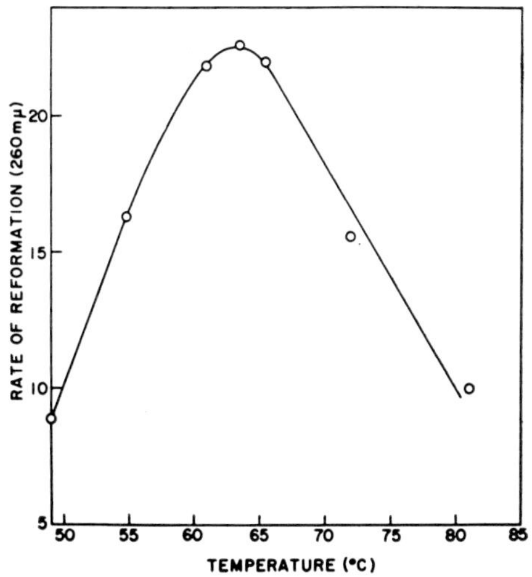

FIG. 10. Effect of temperature on the renaturation rate of denatured *D. pneumoniae* DNA in 0.3 M NaCl plus 0.03 M Na citrate, by optical density study. Conditions are similar to those described under Figure 9. The initial rates of *decrease* in optical density after temperature equilibrium is reached are plotted against the renaturation temperature.

It has been shown above that the renaturation of DNA can be followed by the decrease in optical density after the intramolecular hydrogen bonds of denatured, fast-cooled DNA are melted out. When the initial rate of decrease in the optical density is plotted against the renaturation temperature, the curve shown in Figure 10 is obtained. The optimum renaturation temperature for *D. pneumoniae* DNA is approximately 65°C and is dependent on the base composition of the DNA, increasing gradually for DNA samples with higher guanine plus cytosine contents (Marmur and Doty, 1961).

When the course of renaturation of *D. pneumoniae* DNA is followed by the restoration of the ability to transform with respect to the streptomycin resistance marker, the results are found to depend very much on the temperature. As shown in Figure 11, the recovery of biological activity displays an initial rapid rate, followed by a slower one. At the optimum temperature, the slow increase continues for at least five hours. When a plateau is reached in the

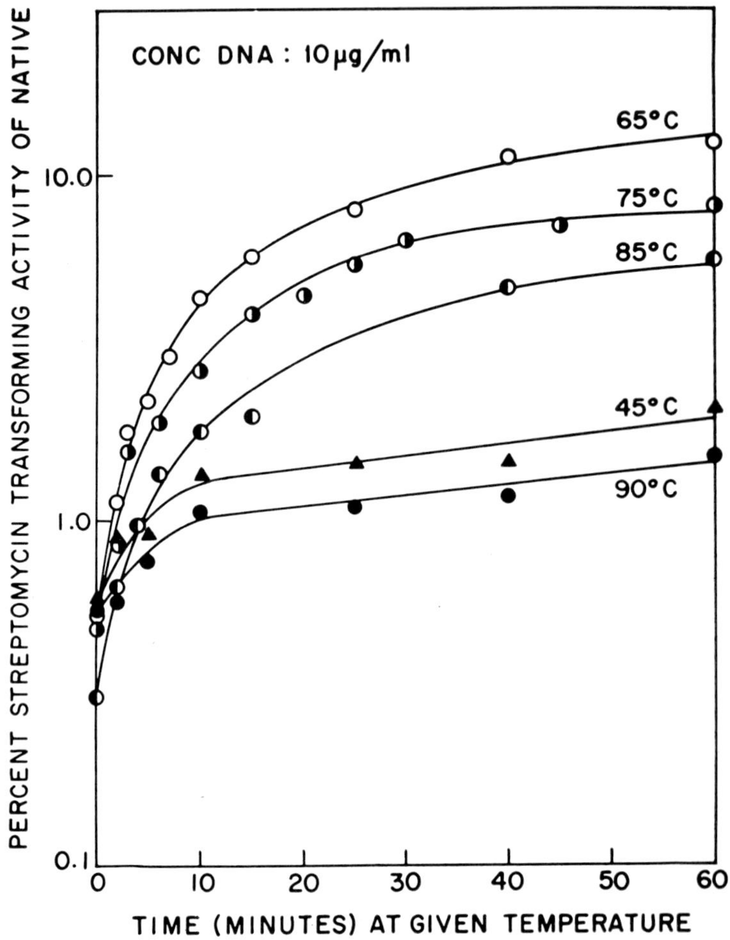

FIG. 11. Effect of temperature on the recovery of streptomycin-transforming activity of thermally denatured *D. pneumoniae* DNA. DNA from streptomycin-resistant cells of *D. pneumoniae* was denatured at 10 μg per ml. by heating for 10 minutes at 100°C in 0.3 M NaCl plus 0.03 M Na citrate. Aliquots, at the same DNA concentration and in the same solvent, were then distributed and exposed to various temperatures. Samples were removed and quickly cooled at different times and assayed for streptomycin-transforming activity.

restoration of the biological activity, subsequent cooling to room temperature results in an additional increment in transforming activity (10 to 50 per cent), depending on the previous temperature. By exposing denatured DNA to the optimum renaturation temperature for two to three hours, as well as a subsequent slow cooling to room temperature, restoration of 40 to 50 per cent of the original biological activity is generally obtained for *D. pneumoniae* DNA (Marmur and Doty, 1961). These conditions may readily be used for the renaturation of DNA which has suffered denaturation by means other than thermal exposure, such as formamide (see *Effect of Formamide*, above); thus, a mild method for renaturation which avoids exposure to relatively high temperatures is available.

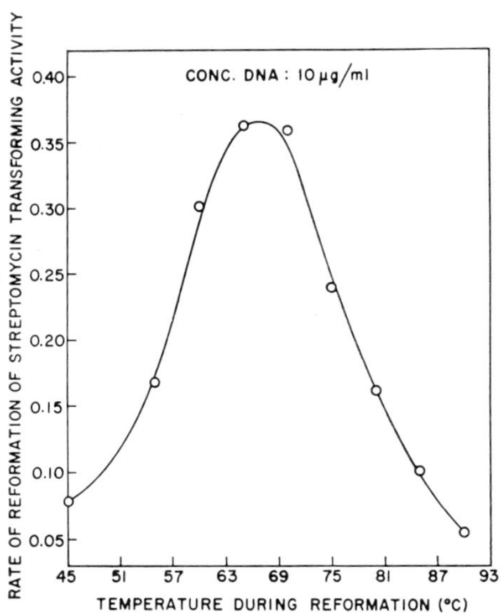

FIG. 12. Effect of temperature on the recovery of transforming activity of denatured *D. pneumoniae* DNA in 0.3M NaCl plus 0.03M Na citrate. The initial rates of recovery of the biological activity of the DNA shown in Figure 11 are plotted against the renaturation temperature.

In order to find the optimum temperature for the restoration of the transforming activity of *D. pneumoniae* DNA at the ionic strength employed, the initial rates of recovery of the biological activity were plotted against the renaturation temperature (Figure 12). The optimum temperature lies within the range of 65 to 70°C. The slightly higher value obtained by this method than that obtained by the optical density method may be a reflection of the observation that the streptomycin resistance marker (used in the biological assay for the renaturation) is probably associated with a DNA molecule which has a higher guanine plus cytosine content than the average composition of the total DNA population (Marmur and Lane, 1960).

Effect of Molecular Weight

In order to compare the rate and extent of the renaturation of denatured DNA as a function of the molecular weight, *D. pneumoniae* DNA was sonically degraded, in the presence of 2 aminoethylisothiuronium bromide hydrogen bromide (AET) to prevent free radical damage (Litt, Marmur, Ephrussi-Taylor, and Doty, 1958), from a molecular weight of 10×10^6 to 0.55×10^6. The degraded material retained 0.24 per cent of its transforming activity with respect to the streptomycin resistance marker. The renaturation of thermally denatured samples of both the undegraded and sonically treated DNA samples was studied by the restoration of the biological activity under optimum conditions of temperature and ionic strength.

In Figure 13 is shown the difference in the rate and extent of renaturation of the two samples. The transforming DNA was first denatured by heating the samples in 0.3 M NaCl plus 0.03 M Na citrate at 100°C for 10 minutes and then incubated at 65°C at 15 μg/ml. in the same solvent. Aliquots, removed at various times and quickly cooled, were assayed for the ability to transform sensitive cells of *D. pneumoniae* to streptomycin resistance. It can readily be seen that both the rate and extent of the recovery of biological activity are dependent on the molecular weight. Similar results are obtained when renaturation is followed by the optical density method (Marmur and Doty, 1961).

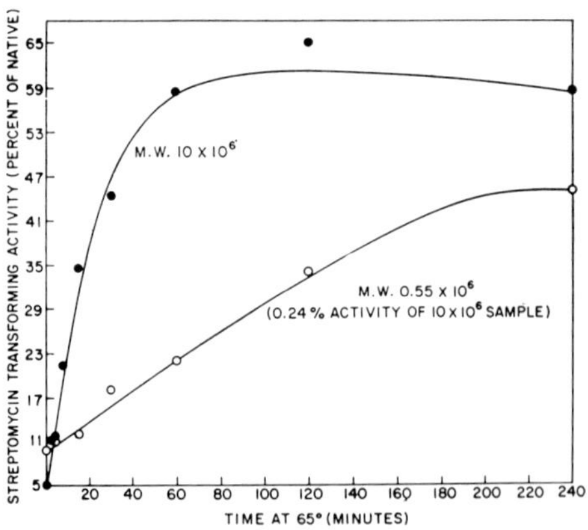

FIG. 13. Effect of molecular weight on the recovery of streptomycin-transforming activity of denatured *D. pneumoniae* DNA in 0.3 M NaCl plus 0.03 M citrate. Conditions are described in the text and are similar to those employed for Figure 11.

Thermal Stability of Renatured DNA

If renaturation is indeed the restoration of hydrogen bonding between complementary strands whose bases are in register, then the thermal stability of renatured DNA should mimic that of native DNA. This was tested by exposing both renatured and native DNA to a temperature several degrees above the T_m and following their transforming activity as a function of time. This has been shown previously (Doty, Marmur, and Sueoka, 1959) to result in an easily measurable, time-dependent loss of transforming activity due to denaturation of the molecules carrying the genetic marker.

Renatured DNA was prepared as follows: *D. pneumoniae* was heated at 100°C for 10 minutes in 0.3 M NaCl plus 0.03 M Na citrate and then exposed to 65°C at 20μg/ml. in the same solvent for varying periods of time. Samples were removed at several times, quickly cooled, and dialyzed against 0.15 M NaCl plus 0.015 M Na citrate.

The thermal inactivation curves at 89.2°C in 0.15 M NaCl plus 0.015 M Na citrate of the native and renatured, dialyzed samples are shown in Figure 14. DNA renatured for three hours (41 per cent restoration of biological activity) as well as those renatured for 25 minutes (33 per cent restoration) and 60 minutes (36 per cent restoration) showed the same thermal stability as native DNA. Data for the latter two renatured samples are not shown in the figure. DNA renatured for four minutes (7 per cent restoration of biological activity) shows an abnormally higher thermal resistance

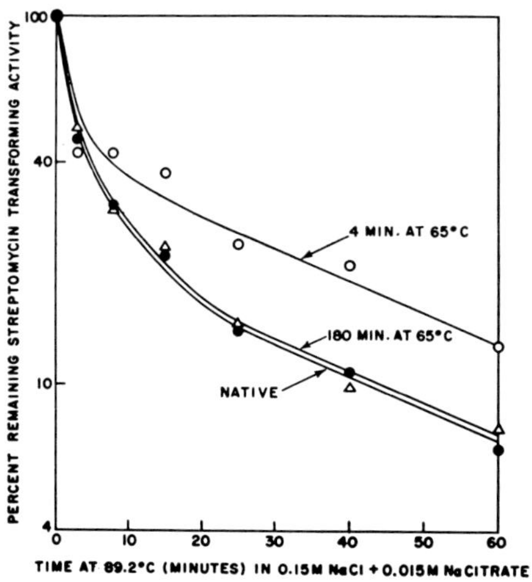

FIG. 14. Stability of renatured and native *D. pneumoniae* DNA to thermal inactivation of streptomycin transforming activity. Samples were exposed to 0.15 M NaCl plus 0.015 M Na citrate for various times at 89.2°C and aliquots removed and quickly cooled for biological activity at various times. Conditions are described in text.

which may be a reflection of the presence of a resistant component selected during the initial (100°C) thermal exposure.

It is suggested that this (or the optical density-temperature profile) criterion of the thermal stability of the material should be used as a test of its nativelike structure to rule out the possibility of nonspecific aggregation.

The optical density-temperature profile can also be employed as a criterion to check the structure of renatured DNA. The profiles of native and denatured DNA differ significantly (Doty *et al.*, 1959). Whereas native DNA melts very sharply, resulting in a steep rise in optical density in the T_m region, denatured DNA gives rise to a broad profile.

Because of the high degree of homogeneity of the DNA from phage and PPLO, an attempt was made to see to what extent DNA from these sources could be renatured and to examine their thermal stability. T_6r+ DNA and avian PPLO DNA were denatured and then renatured under optimum conditions in 0.3 M NaCl plus 0.03 M Na citrate. Each was then compared to its corresponding native preparations for thermal stability in the same solvent. From Figures 15a and 15b it is seen that a large portion of each pair of curves may be superimposed in the T_m region and can be readily accounted for if one assumes that 70 to 80 per cent of the denatured molecules have renatured when exposed to the optimum renaturation conditions. We have recently found (Cordes, Epstein, and Marmur, 1961) that denatured DNA from phage α can be renatured to the extent of approximately 90 per cent by using the criterion

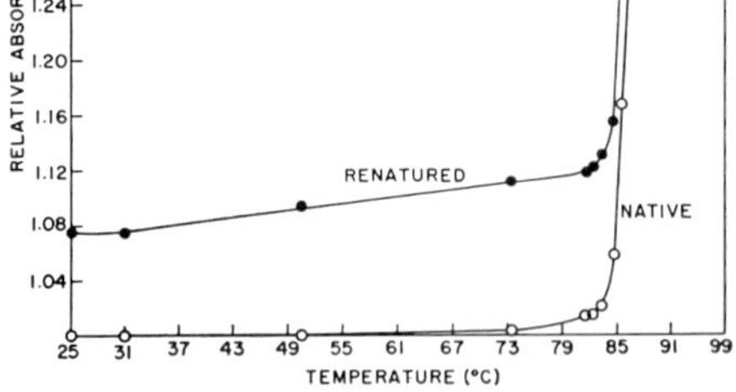

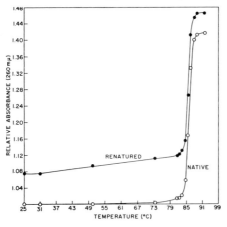

FIG. 15a. Thermal stability of renatured and native T_6r+ DNA in 0.3 M NaCl plus 0.03 M Na citrate. Conditions are described in text.

of the extent of the superimposing of the optical density-temperature curves in the T_m region.

Studies on Molecular Hybrid Formation

The preceding work has demonstrated two reliable routine methods for studying renaturation. It has shown that as the degree of renaturation of a given sample increases there is a continuous decrease in absorbance as well as a parallel increase in transforming activity. A third, very clear way to follow strand separation and recombination is by the buoyant density of the DNA in the CsCl gradient.

Renaturation of Denatured DNA

When a solution of bacterial DNA in 0.30 M NaCl and 0.030 M Na citrate is heated and quickly cooled, and then adjusted to 5.7 M in CsCl and centrifuged, it is found that the buoyant density has increased about 0.015 g./cm.^{3} (Sueoka, Marmur, and Doty, 1959). If, before centrifugation, an aliquot of the cooled solution is placed at 68°C for two hours and then slowly cooled to room temperature at about 5°C every 15 minutes, the renatured DNA band is only 0.004 g./cm.^{3} heavier than the native sample. In addition, some material whose density corresponds to that of the fast-cooled sample still remains. It is believed that the slight difference in density between the native and renatured molecules is due to the latter having unpaired ends. This should be expected as a direct consequence of the thermal depolymerization that unavoidably occurs during

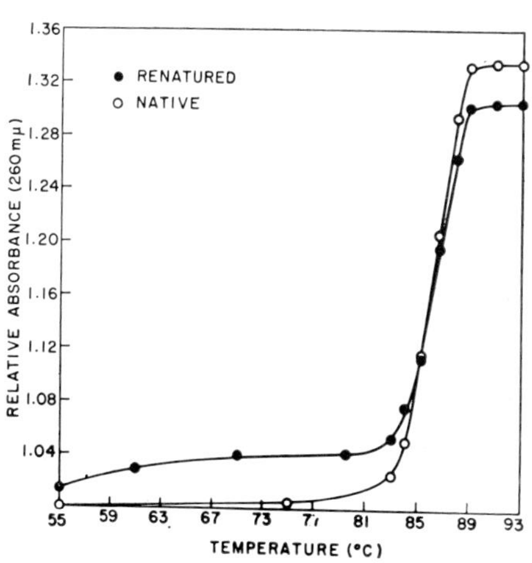

FIG. 15b. Thermal stability of renatured and native *Mycoplasma gallisepticum* (avian PPLO 5969) DNA in 0.3 M NaCl plus 0.03 M Na citrate. Conditions are described in text.

strand separation and renaturation and/or the random breakage of the double-strand DNA in its isolation from the cell. Single strands broken at somewhat different places would be produced during thermal exposure and these would not match completely during

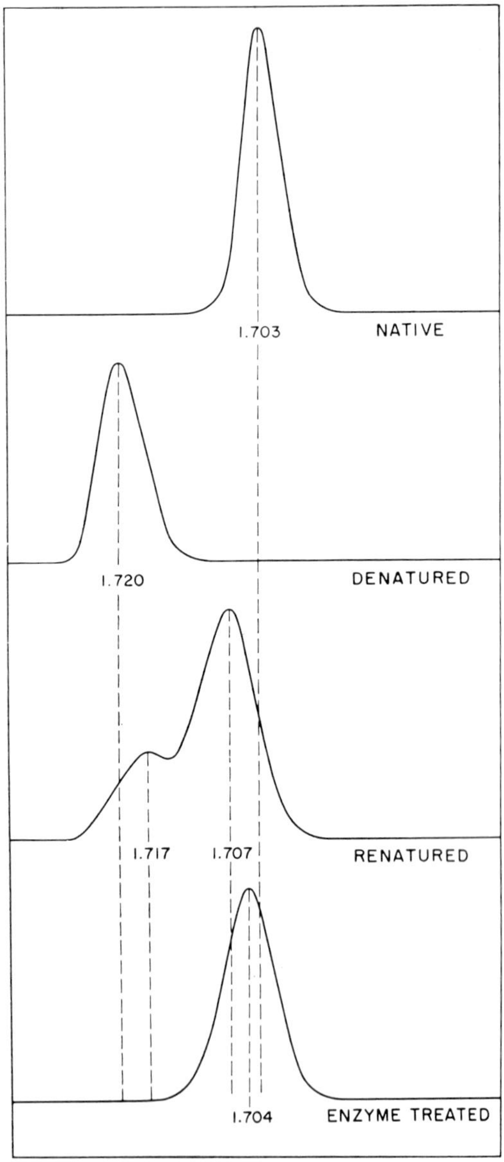

FIG. 16. Renaturation of *B. subtilis* DNA. When a solution of native DNA (band profile shown in top tracing) is heated for 10 minutes at 10 μg per ml. at 100°C in 0.285 M NaCl plus 0.0258 M Na citrate and quickly cooled, the density increases 0.017 g./cm.^{3} (second tracing). An aliquot of this solution was slowly cooled and, as is evident from the third tracing from the top, about 80 per cent of the DNA renatures. Treatment with the *E. coli* phosphodiesterase (Lehman, 1960) causes the complete disappearance of the denatured band and a decrease in the buoyant density of the renatured band (bottom tracing).

renaturation. These overlapping regions at the ends are thought to be responsible for the slightly higher densities. Results for *Bacillus subtilis* DNA are shown in Figure 16.

Recently, an enzyme that appears to have single-strand DNA as its optimum substrate has been isolated from *E. coli* (Lehman, 1960). Further evidence that this enzyme attacks only single-strand DNA has been obtained by incubation with the slowly cooled *B. subtilis* mixture whose band profile is shown in Figure 16. The resultant band profile strongly indicates that there remains only one component which is very similar to native *B. subtilis* DNA. This is also shown in Figure 16 where an additional change is evident: the density of the renatured material has decreased. This confirms the hypothesis that single-strand ends were present in the renatured DNA. The only change observed as a result of the action of the phosphodiesterase on the renatured DNA is the removal of these unpaired ends.

Molecular Hybrid Formation

It is possible, by means of density gradient centrifugation, to show that renaturation does take place by the union of two complementary single strands that were not previously paired together. This is done by using heavy-labeled N^{15}-deuterated DNA which can be distinguished clearly from the corresponding unlabeled material. These two native samples are separated by a sufficient distance to allow unambiguous detection of hybrid double helical molecules, each consisting of one heavy-labeled and one unlabeled strand.

The heating and slow cooling (after two hours at 68°C) of a mixture of 5 μg./ml. each of heavy-labeled and unlabeled *B. subtilis* DNA should result in the labeled and unlabeled forms each giving rise to denatured and renatured DNA as well as a hybrid whose density is the average of the two renatured samples. Thus, centrifugation of this solution in CsCl should produce five bands. A typical tracing is shown in Figure 17 (upper). The bands, in order of increasing density are: renatured normal, denatured normal, hybrid, renatured heavy-labeled, and denatured heavy-labeled *B. subtilis* DNA.

An aliquot of this same slow-cooled mixture was dialyzed against the buffer (0.067 M glycine, pH 9.2) in which the *E. coli* phosphodiesterase treatment is carried out. Incubation with this single-strand attacking enzyme eliminated two bands, as expected, leaving

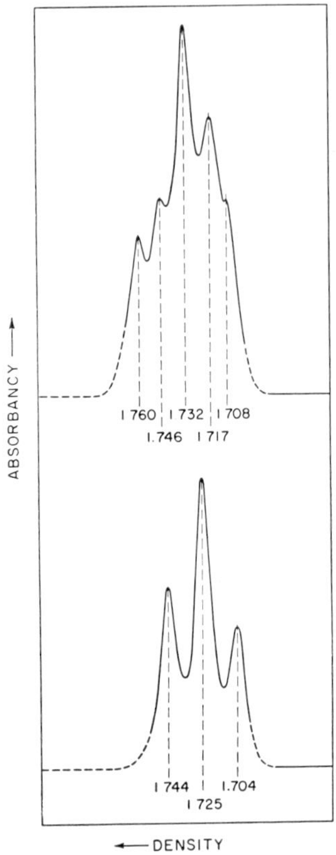

FIG. 17. Effect of *E. coli* phosphodiesterase on a slowly cooled mixture of heavy-labeled and normal *B. subtilis* DNA. Treatment with the phosphodiesterase eliminates the two denatured bands, decreases the density of the renatured bands so as to approach the buoyant densities of native material and greatly increases the resolution of the CsCl density gradient technique. Since the area of each band is proportional to the amount of DNA it contains, it is clear that there is approximately twice as much hybrid as either of the uniformly labeled components.

the three types of double helical molecules: both strands unlabeled, density 1.704 g./cm.^{3}; both strands heavy-labeled, density 1.744 g./cm.^{3}; and one strand unlabeled, one heavy-labeled, density 1.725 g./cm.^{3}. These results are shown in the lower tracing of Figure 17. Moreover, the density of these renatured and "cleaned up" molecules matches that of the native material instead of being about 0.004 units heavier as heretofore. The same studies were repeated using labeled and normal DNA isolated from *E. coli* B and these results were similar to those just described for *B. subtilis*.

Test of Homologies

It is to be expected from their close taxonomic, physiological and, in some cases, genetic (*E. coli* B recombines with strain K-12) relationships that all strains identified as *E. coli* should have DNA whose base sequences are for the most part similar. Thus, any *E. coli* strain should yield DNA which will form a five-band pattern in CsCl after heating and slow cooling with an equal amount of N^{15}

deuterated *E. coli* B DNA. The results of such an investigation are shown in Figure 18. All strains except the "alkali-producing-form" mutant (II–IV–4) of *E. coli* I formed five bands. The position of the hybrid band varies somewhat; however, this may not be significant. Ideally, each five-component mixture should have been treated with *E. coli* phosphodiesterase before banding. Only strains K-12, B and W have been checked so far, and each gives the expected three-band pattern after enzyme digestion.

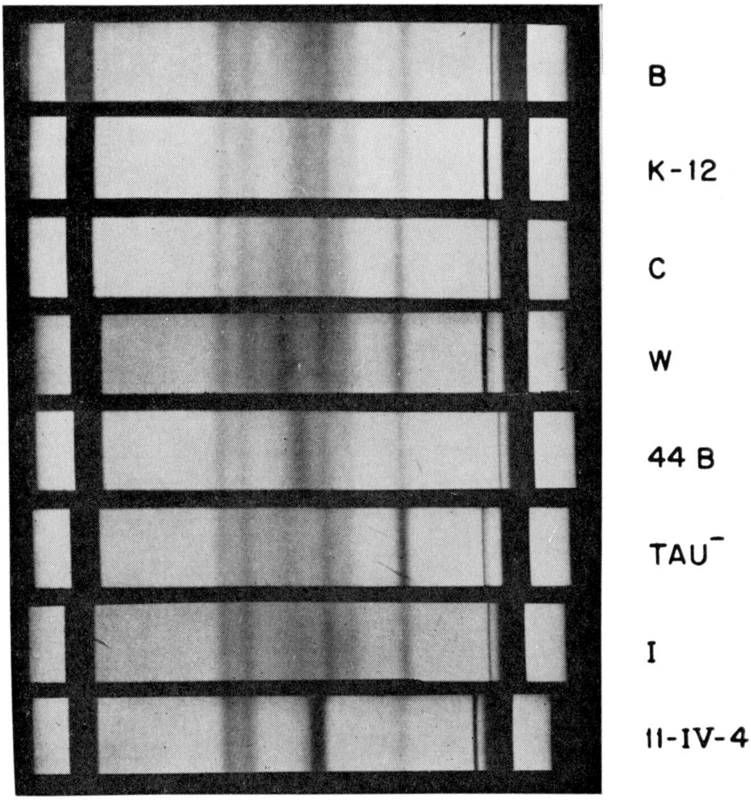

FIG. 18. Hybrid formation between *E. coli* B and other *E. coli* strains. *E. coli* DNA labeled with N^{15} and deuterium was mixed with DNA from each of the strains listed above and heated and slowly cooled in separate experiments. The concentrations were 5 μg./ml. each and the denaturation and renaturation conditions were the same as those described in Figure 20. Each of the eight different ultracentrifuge runs is represented in the above figure by a typical ultraviolet absorption photograph. Six DNA bands appear in all but the last experiment. The photographs have been lined up according to the position of the standard at the far right which is DNA from *Cl. perfringens.*

Detection of Nonspecific Aggregates

Many investigators have reported effects with DNA that can best be explained by the hypothesis that the molecules under observation are entangled or connected by some type of nonchemical bond such as hydrogen or hydrophobic bonds. A vivid example is gel formation observed after heating and slowly cooling salmon sperm DNA at concentrations as low as 260 μg./ml. (Eigner, 1960). Since aggregation is a reality, it should be asked why it does not occur during hybrid formation. How is it possible to distinguish a native-like, hybrid, double helical structure from an aggregate of renatured or denatured normal and heavy-labeled DNA?

It seemed likely that any nonhelical aggregate would be degraded by the *E. coli* phosphodiesterase. With this in mind, equal amounts of DNA from organisms having significantly different GC contents were heated together at high concentration and slowly cooled. When examined in the CsCl gradient, bands of intermediate density and high diffusion coefficients were observed. When aliquots of these mixtures were treated with the phosphodiesterase and centrifuged again, the intermediate band disappeared. Examples of some of these aggregates, formed at high concentrations and banding at intermediate densities, and their elimination are seen in Figure 19.

It was also possible to form aggregates between *Bacillus subtilis* DNA and *Bacillus brevis* or *Bacillus macerans* DNA using concentrations of 40 and 50 μg./ml., respectively. The GC base composition of *B. subtilis* DNA is similar to that of *B. brevis*, while that of *B. macerans* is somewhat higher. The density of the aggregates was considerably higher than the average of the two renatured "parent" samples, as expected if renaturation was not complete. Again, the intermediate bands were eliminated by the *E. coli* phosphodiesterase treatment. When *B. subtilis* and calf thymus DNA were heated together and slowly cooled at a total concentration of 100 μg./ml., the heavy-labeled *B. subtilis* DNA reformed completely, while the calf thymus DNA maintained at the denatured density. No intermediate bands were visible. Thus, the conditions under which false intermediate bands can form have been clarified. The use of low concentrations and checks with *E. coli* phosphodiesterase will avoid artifacts.

Interspecies Hybridization

The minimal requirement for molecular hybrid formation appears to be close similarity in base composition. When DNA samples of quite different base composition are heated and slowly cooled, even at double the usual concentration, no hybrid is formed. In addition, the results of slow cooling DNA from two genetically unrelated species of *Bacillus* having very similar base compositions show

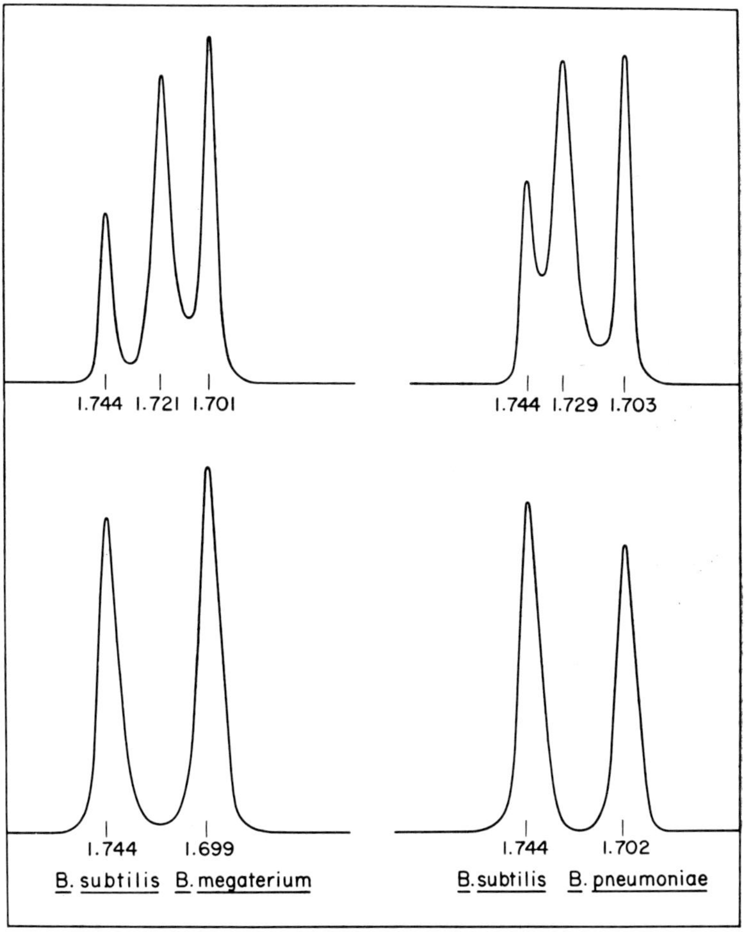

FIG. 19. Nonspecific aggregation in the renaturation of high concentrations of denatured DNA. N^{15}–deuterated DNA from *B. subtilis* was heated with either DNA from *B. megaterium* or *D. pneumoniae* at a concentration of 50 µg./ml. each in 0.285 M NaCl plus 0.025 M Na citrate. The mixtures were then slowly cooled under the usual conditions. Aliquots were centrifuged in CsCl before (upper tracings) and after (bottom tracings) treatment with the *E. coli* phosphodiesterase. Microdensitometer tracings were made on the ultraviolet photos of the bands when equilibrium had been reached in the density gradient centrifugations using the Spinco ultracentrifuge at 44,770 rpm.

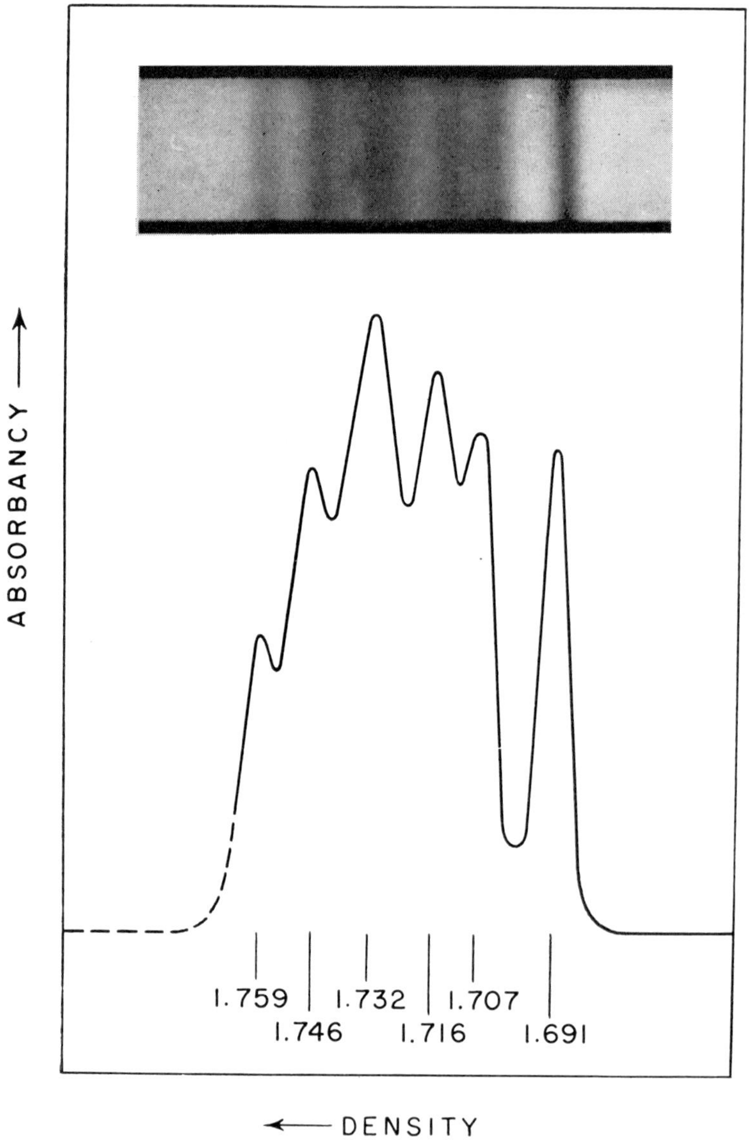

FIG. 20. Hybrid formation between the DNA of *B. subtilis* and *B. natto.* A mixture of 5 μg./ml. of each DNA was denatured (10 minutes at 100°C) and renatured (two hours at 68°C, then cooled to 25°C over a period of two hours) in 0.285 M NaCl plus 0.285 M Na citrate. The material was then centrifuged at 44,770 rpm in a CsCl gradient. The ordinate of the microdensitometer tracings represents the concentration of DNA in the centrifuge cell. Buoyant densities

no hybrid formation. Hybrid formation was possible, however, when two species of *Bacillus* had the same base composition and were related by the ability of one to transform the other. This is shown for the DNA of *B. subtilis* and *B. natto* in Figure 20.

Three members of the family *Enterobacteriaceae* having similar base compositions (Lee, Wahl, and Barbu, 1956) and which are genetically related have also been examined. *E. coli* K-12 shows a high degree of genetic exchange by conjugation and transduction with *E. coli* B and *Shigella dysenteriae* (Lennox, 1955; Luria, Adams, and Ting, 1960; Luria and Burrous, 1957), whereas *Salmonella typhimurium* mates fairly well with K-12 but is transduced only to a very limited extent, if at all (Zinder, 1960).

In an effort to see if there are any major base sequence homologies between the DNA of *E. coli* B and that of either *Shigella* or *Salmonella,* attempts to form hybrid molecules were begun. Unlabeled DNA isolated from *Sh. dysenteriae* was substituted for the unlabeled *E. coli* DNA in the procedure discussed in *Molecular Hybrid Formation,* above, and after the slowly cooled mixture was treated with *E. coli* phosphodiesterase, three bands were observed. The hybrid band was less than either of the renatured parental bands, indicating that the extent of homology between the heterologous strains is less than that between two DNA preparations from the same strain of *E. coli* B.

Similar studies were carried out with DNA isolated from different species and strains of *Salmonella.* Heating heavy *E. coli* B DNA at 100°C and slow cooling with DNA isolated from each of the *Salmonella* species, *typhosa, typhimurium, ballerup,* and *arizona* was carried out. The results for all the *Salmonella* samples were similar. The *Sal. typhimurium* and the heavy-labeled *E. coli* DNA concentrations were at 10 and also at 20 μg./ml. each. In the latter case, an intermediate band appeared; however, this did not remain after digestion with the phosphodiesterase. No intermediate band at all formed in the former case. Thus, there seems to be little, if any, sequence complementary between the DNA of *Salmonella* and *E. coli* B as measured by hybrid formation. The experiments were also repeated using the *Sal. typhimurium* DNA and the

---

(expressed in g./cm.^{3}) correspond to the following DNA molecular species: 1.691–*Cl. perfringens* (used as a standard); 1.707 and 1.716–renatured and denatured *B. natto* DNA, respectively; 1.732–hybrid *B. natto–B. subtilis* DNA; 1.746 and 1.759–renatured and denatured N^{15}–deuterated *B. subtilis* DNA, respectively.

heavy-labeled DNA from *E. coli* K-12. The latter behaved exactly like *E. coli* B DNA.

It should be noted that these results do not rule out the possibility of close homology only between several molecules of the heterologous total DNA populations, or between small sequences within their molecules. This might be enough to satisfy the minimal requirement for genetic exchange by conjugation. Very low concentrations of hybrids would not be observable in the analytical ultracentrifuge, but could be isolated by using larger amounts of interacting DNA and working with the preparative swinging-bucket rotor.

Genetic and Taxonomic Aspects of Molecular Hybrid Formation

It has recently been pointed out that there is a relationship between the taxonomic and genetic relationships of microorganisms and the base compositions of their DNA (Lee, Wahl, and Barbu, 1956; Belozersky and Spirin, 1960; Lanni, 1960). Those organisms which are genetically related most likely possess homologous base sequences; a minimum requirement is that they have similar base compositions. The question can now be asked, how molecular hybrid formation is related to the taxonomy and genetics of microorganisms as well as to their DNA base compositions. Which is a better test of homology, the extent of molecular hybrid formation or of genetic exchange? At a more practical level, we can ask if molecular hybrid formation can be used as a tool in studying the taxonomic and genetic relationship of microorganisms.

It has already been pointed out in the previous section that molecular hybrid formation takes place only between organisms possessing similar base compositions. Table 1 summarizes the results to date where such genetic exchanges have been observed; in each case where molecular hybrid formation takes place, the organisms are related taxonomically and genetically. Wherever the base compositions of the DNA differ (e.g., *E. coli* and *Serratia marcescens* or *Aerobacter aerogenes*), even though the organisms belong to the same taxonomic group, or if they belong to the same taxonomic group but are genetically unrelated (*B. subtilis and B. brevis*), no molecular hybrid formation can be detected.

In order to compare molecular hybrid formation and genetic compatibility as a measure of homology, it is first necessary to mention briefly the various methods of genetic exchange in bacteria.

The four main routes of genetic transfer are: F-duction, conjugation, transduction, and transformation (Ravin, 1958). F-duction (Jacob, Schaeffer, and Wollman, 1960) is mediated by an episomal element, and since this method of genetic exchange can take place between bacteria with dissimilar base composition (Falkow *et al.*, 1961; Nakaya, Nakahura, and Murata, 1961) it would appear to be the poorest test of DNA homologies. This is borne out by the fact that the transferred material may or may not be integrated even between closely related organisms (Jacob, Schaeffer, and Wollman, 1960) and, in the case of F-duction between *E. coli* and *S. marcescens*, the incoming material can be detected as a separate band in CsCl density gradient centrifugation of the DNA isolated from the hybrid and thus presumed not to be integrated into the host chromosome (Marmur *et al.*, 1961).

The second method of genetic exchange, conjugation, would appear to be less demanding than molecular hybrid formation (or transduction) for sequence homologies. Thus, Zinder (1960) found that whereas genetic exchange between *Sal. typhimurium* and *E. coli* K-12 can take place by conjugation, little or no exchange of certain markers is achieved by transduction. It should be possible however to transduce the markers in the regions where the homologies exist that satisfy the criteria for genetic exchange by conjugation. As seen in Table 1, no molecular hybrid formation is noted between the DNA of *E. coli* B and of various *Salmonella* species indicating that very little homology exists.

It would appear that transformation, transduction, and molecular hybrid formation are the best criteria for homology, and it remains to be shown which is the most demanding. This question might be answered by studying the extent of interspecific molecular hybrid formation among the DNA's isolated from various *Hemophilus* species (Table 1). Since they transform one another with varying degrees of efficiency (Schaeffer, 1958), it would be of great interest to see whether the extent of hybrid formation can be predicted by the transformation efficiency. This has not yet been accomplished because of the difficulty of obtaining heavy isotope labeled *Hemophilus* DNA, but can probably be carried out with *B. subtilis* (Spizizen, 1959). Preliminary experiments (Marmur, Seaman, and Levine, in preparation) with two *Bacillus* species may be of interest in this connection. *Bacillus polymyxa* and *Bacillus niger* DNA transforms *B. subtilis* at very low efficiencies with respect to the indole marker, yet the extent of molecular hybrid formation

TABLE 1

Genetic, Taxonomic, and DNA Composition Relationships of Several Groups of Microorganisms

Taxonomic group	Per cent G+C† of DNA of related organisms	Representative organism	Genetically related to representative organism	DNA molecular hybrid formation with representative organism
Lactobacillaceae	*D. pneumoniae* 39 *Str. salivarius* 39 *L. acidophilus* 39	*D. pneumoniae*	*Streptococcus*	Not examined
Brucellaceae	*H. influenzae* 38 *H. parainfluenzae* 38 *H. suis* 38 *H. aegyptius* 39	*H. influenzae*	*H. parainfluenzae* *H. aegyptius* *H. suis*	Not examined
Enterobacteriaceae	*E. coli* B, C, W, K-12, TAU⁻, 44-B, I 50 *E. freundii* (17) 50 *Sh. dysenteriae* 50 *Sal. arizona* 50 *Sal. ballerup* 51.5 *Sal. typhosa* 50 *Sal. typhimurium* 51.5 *Erwinia carotovora* 51.5	*E. coli* B	*E. coli* K-12 *Sh. dysenteriae* *Sal. typhosa* *Sal. typhimurium*	*E. coli* B, C, W, K-12, TAU⁻, 44-B, I *E. freundii* (17) *Sh. dysenteriae*
Bacillaceae	*B. subtilis* 43 *B. natto* 43 *B. subtilis* var. *atterimus* 43 *B. macerans* 50 *B. licheniformis* 46 *B. polymyxa* 44 *B. stearothermophilus* 44 *B. brevis* 43 *B. firmus* 41 *B. laterosporus* 40 *B. pumilus* 40 *B. sphaericus* 37	*B. subtilis*	*B. natto* *B. subtilis* var. *atterimus*	*B. subtilis* *B. natto* *B. subtilis* var. *atterimus*

(Continued on next page.)

Table 1. Continued from preceding page.

Taxonomic group	Per cent G+C† of DNA of related organisms		Representative organism	Genetically related to representative organism	DNA molecular hybrid formation with representative organism
Bacillaceae	*B. megaterium*	37		*B. polymyxa***	
	B. circulans	35			*B. polymyxa***
	B. megaterium-cereus	34			
	B. thuringiensis	34			
	B. cereus	33			
	B. cereus var. *mycoides*	33			
	B. alvei	33			
E. coli viruses	T_2	34.8*			
	T_4	34.8*			
	T_6	34.8*	T_4 bacteriophage	T_2, T_6	T_2, T_6
	T_7	48			
	T_3	49.6*			
	T_5	39*			

† The guanine plus cytosine content of the DNA was estimated from the T_m (melting temperature) since it was found to give more self-consistent values for the strains of bacteria used in this study (Figure 4).
* Value obtained from the literature (Sinsheimer, 1960).
** Interacts at reduced levels.

between their DNA and that of *B. subtilis,* while not equal to the amount formed between homologous strains, is greater than would be expected from the transformation efficiencies. From this preliminary result one might conclude that transformation is a better test of homology, within certain limited regions of the DNA molecule, than is hybrid formation. Molecular hybrid formation is of course a measure of the entire population of DNA molecules. When the interspecific transformation efficiency of *B. subtilis* by DNA from heterologous species (e.g., *B. natto* and *B. subtilis* var. *atterimus*) is high, the extent of molecular hybrid formation (Table 1) is also high.

Since there is a close relationship between *in vitro* molecule hybrid formation, taxonomy, and genetic compatibility of microorganisms, it is proposed that organisms yielding DNA that form hybrids should belong to the same taxonomic group. Thus, if one wishes to utilize this technique to examine taxonomic (and possibly the genetic) relationship among a group of microrganisms, its

DNA should first be examined for the identity of base composition; and if this minimal criterion is met, heterologous pairs of DNA samples should be examined for their ability to form molecular hybrids.

It should be pointed out that since unfractionated samples of DNA's of higher plants and animals do not renature (see *Effect of DNA Source*) under conditions in which microbial nucleic acids will renature, the principles discussed above are applicable only to microorganisms. It is possible, however, that homogeneous fractions of the DNA of one higher species might hybridize with the corresponding fraction of the DNA of a closely related species, employing the techniques described for DNA from microorganisms.

Summary

The complementary strands of the DNA molecule which are held together by lateral hydrogen bonds between the base pairs adenine-thymine and guanine-cytosine can be separated by heat, acid, base, and formamide. The factors influencing the thermally induced transition from the native double-stranded form to the denatured single-stranded state as well as the renaturation of complementary strands have been studied by a number of techniques, such as the measurement of the biological activity of transforming factor DNA, the variation of ultraviolet absorption and cesium chloride density gradient centrifugation.

The separation of the DNA strands and their specific renaturation on subsequent cooling at temperatures below the melting temperature have made it possible to form "hybrid" molecules between the DNA of closely related strains of microorganisms. The molecular hybrids are recognized by their buoyant density in CsCl which is intermediate between the two "reactants": heavy (labeled with N^{15} and deuterium) and light, normal DNA. Minimum requirements for hybrid formation to occur are that the base compositions of the DNA samples be similar and that they have relatively little composition heterogeneity. Thus far it has been found that only microorganisms which are genetically related possess DNA which yields molecular hybrids *in vitro* on thermal denaturation and subsequent slow cooling. It is proposed that genetic compatibility and *in vitro* hybrid formation are dependent on homologous base sequences and that hybrid formation is indicative of and should predict close genetic and taxonomic relationships.

ACKNOWLEDGMENTS

The authors are grateful for the valuable discussions and suggestions offered by Drs. N. Sueoka, S. Falkow, E. Seaman and D. Green, as well as Mr. R. Rownd. The technical assistance of Miss D. Lane, Mr. W. Torrey and Miss M. Cahoon is gratefully acknowledged. The experiments on hybrid formation with the *E. coli* bacteriophages were carried out in collaboration with Dr. K. L. Wierzchowski and Dr. D. Green. The authors are also grateful to Dr. L. Grossman for his generous gift of the *E. coli* phosphodiesterase.

This work was supported by Grant C-2170 from the U.S. Public Health Service.

REFERENCES

Belorzersky, A. N., and A. S. Spirin. 1960. "Chemistry of the Nucleic Acids of Microorganisms," *The Nucleic Acids*, E. Chargaff and J. N. Davidson, Eds., Vol. 3, pp. 147–185. New York, New York: Academic Press, Inc.

Brown, G. L., and A. V. Brown. 1958. Fractionation of Deoxyribonucleic Acids and Reproduction of T2 Bacteriophage. *Symposia of the Society for Experimental Biology*, 12:6–30.

Chargaff, E. 1955. "Base Composition of Deoxypentose and Pentose Nucleic Acids in Various Species," *The Nucleic Acids*, E. Chargaff and J. N. Davidson, Eds., Vol. 1, pp. 521–531. New York, New York: Academic Press, Inc.

Cordes, S. A., H. Epstein, and J. Marmur. 1961. Some Properties of the Deoxyribonucleic Acid of Phage Alpha. *Nature, London*, 191: 1097–1098.

Crampton, C. W., R. Lipshitz, and E. Chargaff. 1954. Studies on Nucleoproteins. II. Fractionation of Deoxyribonucleic Acids Through Fractional Dissociation of their Complexes with Basic Proteins. *Journal of Biological Chemistry*, 211:125–142.

Doty, P., H. Boedtker, J. R. Fresco, R. Haselkorn, and M. Litt. 1959. Secondary Structure in Ribonucleic Acids. *Proceedings of the National Academy of Sciences of the U.S.A.*, 45:482–499.

Doty, P., J. Marmur, J. Eigner, and C. Schildkraut. 1960. Strand Separation and Specific Recombination in Deoxyribonucleic Acids: Physical Chemical Studies. *Proceedings of the National Academy of Sciences of the U.S.A.*, 46:461–476.

Eigner, J. 1960. *The Native, Denatured and Renatured States of Deoxyribonucleic Acid.* Ph.D. Dissertation. Harvard University, Cambridge, Massachusetts.

Falkow, S., J. Marmur, W. F. Carey, W. M. Spilman, and L. S. Baron. 1961. Episomic Transfer Between *Salmonella typhosa* and *Serratia marcescens. Genetics*, 46:703–706.

Greer, S., and S. Zamenhof. 1959. Loss of Purines from DNA Heated in Mutagenic Conditions at Physiological pH. (Abstract) *Federation Proceedings*, 18:939.

Guild, W. R. 1961. Fractionation of Microbial DNA by Density. (Abstract) *Fifth Annual Meeting of the Biophysical Society*, FB9.

Guild, W. R., H. J. Morowitz, and E. Castro. 1960. Some Properties of DNA from PPLO. (Abstract) *Fourth Annual Meeting of the Biophysical Society*, p. 19.

Helmkamp, G. K., and P. O. P. Ts'o. 1961. The Secondary Structures of Nucleic Acids in Organic Solvents. *Journal of the American Chemical Society*, 83:138–142.

Hershey, A. D., and E. Burgi. 1960. Molecular Homogeneity of the Deoxyribonucleic Acid of Phage T2. *Journal of Molecular Biology*, 2:143–152.

Jacob, F., P. Schaeffer, and E. L. Wollman. 1960. Episomic Elements in Bacteria. *Microbial Genetics* (Tenth Symposium of the Society for General Microbiology at the Royal Institution, London) pp. 67–91. London, England: Cambridge University Press.

Lanni, F. 1960. Genetic Significance of Microbial DNA Composition. *Perspectives in Biology and Medicine*, 3:418–432.

Lee, K. Y., R. Wahl, and E. Barbu. 1956. Contenu en bases puriques et pyrimidiques des acides desoxyribonucleiques des bacteries. *Annales de l'Institut Pasteur*, 91:212–224.

Lehman, I. R. 1960. The Deoxyribonucleases of *Escherichia coli*. I. Purification and Properties of a Phosphodiesterase. *Journal of Biological Chemistry*, 235:1479–1487.

Lennox, E. S. 1955. Transduction of Linked Genetic Characters of the Host by Bacteriophage P1. *Virology*, 1:190–206.

Levine, L., W. T. Murakami, H. Van Vunakis, and L. Grossman. 1960. Specific Antibodies to Thermally Denatured Deoxyribonucleic Acid of Phage T4. *Proceedings of the National Academy of Sciences of the U.S.A.*, 46:1038–1043.

Levinthal, C., and C. A. Thomas, Jr. 1957. Molecular Autoradiography: The β-Ray Counting from Single Virus Particles and DNA Molecules in Nuclear Emulsions. *Biochimica et biophysica acta*, 23:453–465.

Litt, M., J. Marmur, H. Ephrussi-Taylor, and P. Doty. 1958. The Dependence of Pneumococcal Transformation on the Molecular Weight of Deoxyribose Nucleic Acid. *Proceedings of the National Academy of Sciences of the U.S.A.*, 44:144–152.

Luria, S. E., J. N. Adams, and R. C. Ting. 1960. Transduction of Lactose-Utilizing Ability Among Strains of *E. coli* and *S. dysenteriae* and the Properties of the Transducting Phage Particles. *Virology*, 12:348–390.

Luria, S. E., and J. N. Burrous. 1957. Hybridization Between *Escherichia coli* and *Shigella*. *Journal of Bacteriology*, 74:461–476.

Madoff, S., and L. Dienes. 1958. L Forms from Pneumococci. *Journal of Bacteriology*, 76:245–250.

Mahler, H. R., B. D. Mehrotra, and C. W. Sharp. 1961. Effects of Diamines on the Thermal Transition of DNA. *Biochemical and Biophysical Research Communications*, 4:79–82.

Marmur, J. 1960. Thermal Denaturation of Deoxyribonucleic Acid Isolated from a Thermophile. *Biochimica et biophysica acta*, 38:342–343.

———. 1961. A Procedure for the Isolation of Deoxyribonucleic Acid from Micro-organisms. *Journal of Molecular Biology*. 3:208–218.

Marmur, J., and P. Doty. 1959. Heterogeneity in Deoxyribonucleic Acids. I.

Dependence on Composition of the Configurational Stability of Deoxyribonucleic Acids. *Nature, London*, 183:1427–1429.

———. 1961. Thermal Renaturation of Deoxyribonucleic Acids. *Journal of Molecular Biology*. 3:585–594.

———. Determination of the Base Composition of Deoxyribonucleic Acid from its Thermal Denaturation Temperature. (In preparation).

Marmur, J. R. Rownd, S. Falkow, L. S. Baron, C. Schildkraut, and P. Doty. 1961. The Nature of Intergenus Episomal Infection. *Proceedings of the National Academy of Science of the U.S.A.*, 47:972–979.

Marmur, J., and D. Lane. 1960. Strand Separation and Specific Recombination in Deoxyribonucleic Acids: Biological Studies. *Proceedings of the National Academy of Sciences of the U.S.A.*, 46:453–461.

———. Unpublished data.

Marmur, J., E. Seaman, and J. Levine. Interspecific Transformation in *Bacillus*. (In preparation).

Marmur, J., and P. O. P. Ts'o. 1961. Denaturation of Deoxyribonucleic Acid by Formamide. *Biochimica et biophysica acta*, 51:32–36.

Meselson, M., and F. Stahl. 1958. The Replication of DNA in *Escherichia coli. Proceedings of the National Academy of Sciences of the U.S.A.*, 44:671–682.

Nakaya, R., A. Nakahura, and Y. Murata. 1960. Resistance Transfer Agents in *Shigella. Biochemical and Biophysical Research Communications*, 3:654–659.

Pauling, L., and R. B. Corey. 1956. Specific Hydrogen-Bond Formation Between Pyrimidines and Purines in Deoxyribonucleic Acids. *Archives of Biochemistry and Biophysics*, 65:164–181.

Ravin, A. W. 1958. Bacterial Genetics. *Annual Review of Microbiology*, 12: 309–364.

Schaeffer, P. 1958. Interspecific Reactions in Bacterial Transformation. *Symposia of the Society for Experimental Biology*, 12:60–74.

Schildkraut, C. L., J. Marmur, and P. Doty. 1961. The Formation of Hybrid DNA Molecules and Their Use in Studies on DNA Homologies. *Journal of Molecular Biology*, 3:595–617.

Sinsheimer, R. L. 1960. "The Nucleic Acids of Bacterial Viruses," *The Nucleic Acids*. E. Chargaff and J. N. Davidson, Eds., Vol. 3, pp. 187–244. New York, New York: Academic Press, Inc.

Spizizen, J. 1959. Genetic Activity of Deoxyribonucleic Acid in the Reconstitution of Biosynthetic Pathways. *Federation Proceedings*, 18:957–965.

Sueoka, N., J. Marmur, and P. Doty. 1959. Heterogeneity in Deoxyribonucleic Acids. II. Dependence of the Density of Deoxyribonucleic Acids on Guanine-Cytosine. *Nature, London*, 183:1429–1431.

Vendreley, R. 1958. La Notion d'espece à travers quelques données biochimiques recentes et le cycle L. *Annales de l'Institut Pasteur*, 94:142–166.

Zinder, N. D. 1960. Hybrids of *Escherichia* and *Salmonella*. *Science*, 131: 813–815.

Observations on the Replication of DNA

LIEBE F. CAVALIERI AND BARBARA HATCH ROSENBERG

Sloan-Kettering Division, Graduate School of Medical Sciences, Cornell University Medical College, New York, New York

We have recently carried out a series of investigations which have demonstrated a new complexity in the structure of the deoxyribonucleic acid (DNA) molecule and have led us to a revised concept of DNA replication in the cell. Our view represents a fundamental departure from the quasi-accepted scheme of Watson and Crick, without, however, altering the basic concept of information storage in the nucleotide sequence. Our replication scheme will be outlined, and some of the evidence supporting it surveyed.

One of the major problems which concerns modern biologists is the manner in which the genetic information contained in DNA is transferred faithfully to progeny molecules. Since the question is asked in molecular terms, the answer immediately requires that DNA molecules be described in precise physical terms. This, in turn, requires that the molecules in bulk solution *in vitro* bear some definable relation to the molecules *in vivo*. The DNA must be extracted from the nucleoprotein without degradation. Furthermore, the particles in solution must be the smallest possible, commensurate with full biological integrity; they should not be aggregated. While this is a mere technical problem, it has been the greatest stumbling block in the molecular biology of DNA simply because it is the first step in any investigation. In another communication (Cavalieri, Deutsch, and Rosenberg, 1961) we have presented a detailed investigation which deals with the general problem of disaggregation and molecular weight determination. The molecular weights we obtained after disaggregation of DNA from diverse sources were in the range of 0.6 to 2.4 million. These are much lower than those generally reported; we were able to show, however, that they were not due to enzymatic or shear degradation.

Having determined that the physical state of the DNA molecules we were investigating was meaningful, we set out to study the structure of the self-replicating unit of DNA. The work of Meselson and Stahl (1958) demonstrated that DNA in *Escherichia coli* B replicates through a semiconservative mechanism. They isolated hybrid (N^{15}–N^{14}) DNA molecules after one replication cycle in labeled medium, and were able to separate them into the biologically conserved N^{15} and N^{14} moieties by heating in concentrated cesium chloride. The nature of these conserved units was ambiguous. We prepared DNA in an identical manner and confirmed their discovery that *E. coli* DNA contains two units separable upon heating in cesium chloride. This was shown by two different techniques: gradient equilibrium centrifugation, and light scattering. Upon examining DNA samples from many sources, we found that they fall into two classes: those, like *E. coli* DNA, whose molecular weight halves upon heating in concentrated cesium chloride, and those whose molecular weight remains constant. DNA of the former class has been called biunial, by analogy with *E. coli* DNA (which contains two separately conserved units per molecule). DNA of the latter class, apparently containing only one conserved unit, has been called unitary (Cavalieri and Rosenberg, 1961a).

The problem was to determine the structural distinction between unitary and biunial DNA, since an answer to this question might clarify the nature of the conserved unit. The fact that neither calf thymus nor salmon sperm DNA, both believed to be two-stranded, split in hot concentrated cesium chloride, whereas *E. coli*, *Pneumococcus*, and mouse sarcoma-180 DNA did split, led us to examine in critical fashion the number of polynucleotide strands per molecule of each type.

If one wishes to determine the number of strands in a DNA molecule, a method must be used which actually permits the counting of the strands. We have accomplished this by three different experimental approaches. First, the kinetics of enzymatic degradation were investigated. Deoxyribonuclease (DNase) II was used because it requires no divalent metal ions, which are known to cause aggregation under some conditions. Briefly, one relates the number of molecular cleavages to the number of internucleotide bonds hydrolyzed. The former is calculated from the molecular weight decay observed by either light scattering or viscometry—the latter, from the titer. If a molecule possesses only one strand, its molecular weight will start to decay as soon as it comes in contact with the enzyme; if it possesses two or more strands, there will be an initial lag until all the strands have been cleaved at or near the same place. One can thus calculate the number of strands per molecule, and, in addition, obtain information as to the strengths of the hydrogen and other bonds which hold the strands together. In another communication (Cavalieri and Rosenberg, 1961b), the equations for the process were derived and it was shown that the enzyme attacks the DNA in a random fashion. The final working equation for random degradation is

$$\log \frac{1\text{-}R}{R} = \log(m\pi B)_N + n \log p_t$$

where R is the ratio of the weight-average molecular weight after a time *t* to the initial molecular weight; m is the number of nucleotides per strand; πB is a function which takes into account the fact that molecular cleavage may occur even when scissions of the internucleotide bonds in the various strands do not occur directly opposite one another; $(m\pi B)_N$ is a number-average quantity; p_t is the cumulative probability of cleavage of a given internucleotide bond in time *t*; n is the number of strands per molecule. The probability p_t is initially proportional to time, but it can also be evaluated more exactly as T_t/m_o, where the titer T_t is the number of internucleotide bonds cleaved in a given sample during time *t* and m_o is the total number of internucleotide bonds initially present in the sample. It should be noted that $\frac{1\text{-}R}{R}$ is the number of molecular cleavages which have occurred in time *t*.

The kinetics of degradation of undenatured *E. coli* 15_{T-} DNA as observed by both light scattering and viscometry are shown in Figure 1; the values of the molecular weight ratio obtained by the two methods are in close agreement. The degradation of denatured *Pneumococcus* DNA, observed by light scattering, is also included. In Figure 2, the fraction of internucleotide bonds cleaved, obtained by titration, is plotted against time. This fraction is equivalent to p_t, the cumulative probability of cleavage of any given bond. In order to calculate the number of strands per molecule one must plot log

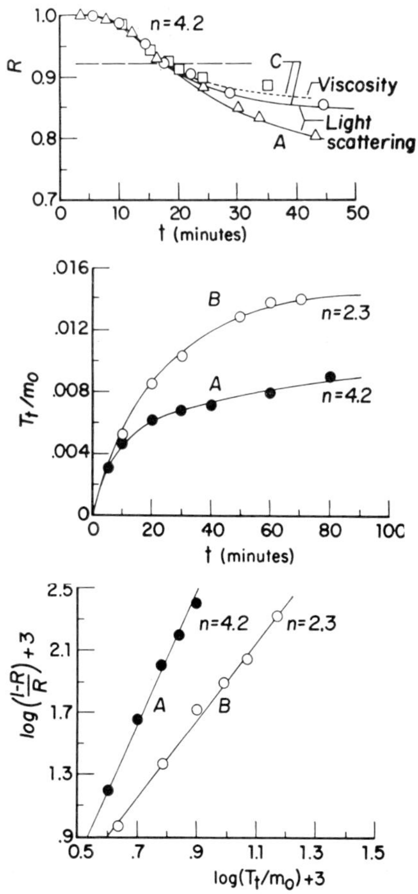

FIGS. 1 to 3. Curves A and B: *Pneumococcus* DNA; A(n = 4.2) has been heated without cesium chloride, B(n = 2.3) has been heated in cesium chloride. Curve C: *E. coli* 15_{T-} DNA undenatured.. T_t/m_0 is the fraction of bonds hydrolyzed by the enzyme in time *t*, and is equivalent to the probability of hydrolysis, p_t; R is the ratio of the molecular weight at time *t* to that at time 0; $\frac{1\text{-R}}{\text{R}}$ is the number of molecular cleavages at time *t;* n is the number of strands/molecule.

Figure 1. The molecular weight decay during enzymatic degradation, as determined by light scattering (unbroken curves) and by viscometry (broken curve).

Figure 2. The fraction of bonds hydrolyzed versus time.

Figure 3. Logarithmic plots of the number of molecular cleavages versus the fraction of individual bonds cleaved. The slopes of the curves give the number of strands/molecule.

p_t versus log $\frac{1\text{-R}}{\text{R}}$. Accordingly, time in Figure 1 can be converted to T_t/m_o, or p_t, from the data in Figure 2. Then a plot of log $\frac{1\text{-R}}{\text{R}}$ versus log T_t/m_o, as in Figure 3, gives the number of strands per molecule directly from the slope.

The results are shown in Table 1. It can be seen that biunial molecules (those which are cleaved by heating in cesium chloride) have approximately four strands, while unitary molecules are two-stranded. Essentially the same results were obtained by the two experimentally independent methods of light scattering and viscometry.

TABLE 1

The Number of Strands (n) in Various DNA Molecules

				n by enzyme method		n by X-ray method
Source	Class	Treatment	Molecular weight	Light scattering	Viscosity	Light scattering
E. coli B	Biunial	Heat-denatured	2.4×10^6	3.9	..	..
E. coli B		Heated in CsCl	1.3×10^6	2.2	..	..
E. coli 15_{T-}	Biunial	Undenatured	1.2×10^6	4.2	4.1	..
E. coli 15_{T-}	Biunial	Heat-denatured	1.1×10^6	3.7	..	..
Pneumococcus	Biunial	Heat-denatured	1.5×10^6	4.2	..	..
Pneumococcus	Biunial	Undenatured	1.6×10^6	..	..	3.2
Pneumococcus		Heated in CsCl	0.84×10^6	2.3	..	..
Mouse sarcoma-180	Biunial	Heat-denatured	1.3×10^6	3.8	..	..
Mouse sarcoma-180		Heated in CsCl	0.61×10^6	2.2	..	..
Calf thymus	Unitary	Acid-denatured	1.7×10^6	2.3	..	..
Calf thymus	Unitary	Undenatured		1.7	1.5	1.6
Sea urchin	Unitary	Undenatured	2.2×10^6	..	..	1.5

The second method of strand counting involved the utilization of a degrading agent which is entirely different from the enzyme—X-irradiation (Cavalieri, Finston, and Rosenberg, 1961). By this method, scission of the polynucleotide strands is caused by free radicals, formed by the action of X rays on water. Since free radicals are formed in clusters which have an initial diameter of about 20 Å, whenever such a cluster forms in the immediate vicinity of a molecule, it is possible that more than one strand could be attacked at once. This would make the degradation, to some extent, nonrandom, indicating that the equation previously used would no longer apply. However, it has been shown elsewhere (Cavalieri and Rosenberg, 1961b) that if the random equation is used when degradation is nonrandom, a minimum value of n will be obtained. Therefore, the equation for random degradation was employed, and, since the probability of internucleotide bond cleavage (p_t) is proportional to radiation dose, $\log \frac{1\text{-R}}{\text{R}}$ was plotted against log[dose]. The decay in molecular weight was followed by light scattering. The results are contained in Table 1 and Figure 4, where it can be seen that, as expected, the values for n were somewhat lower than those obtained with enzyme kinetics. The salient point is that the apparent number of strands per molecule for *Pneumococcus* DNA was twice that for calf thymus or sea urchin sperm DNA, all of which were undenatured and had the physical properties of stiff chains or double helices. Thus, these results support those obtained from enzyme kinetics.

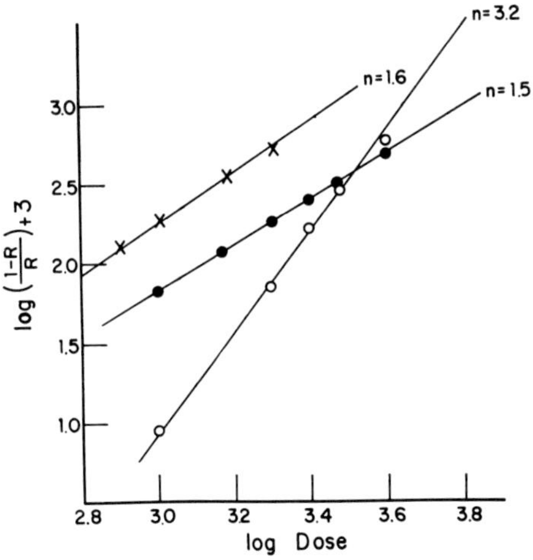

FIG. 4. Plot of log [molecular cleavages] versus log [dose], where the dose is given in rads. The slopes of the lines give n values of 1.5, 1.6, 3.2 for calf thymus, sea urchin sperm, and *Pneumococcus* DNA, respectively.

The third approach to strand counting had an entirely different experimental basis. Instead of degradation kinetics, the average mass per unit length of the molecules was determined (in collaboration with Cecil Hall), by electron microscopy and light scattering, (Hall and Cavalieri, 1961). Certain significant morphological features of individual molecules were also observed. The same *Pneumococcus* DNA used in the kinetic experiments was used.

The lengths of 587 particles were measured in the micrographs. A typical low magnification field is shown in Figure 5. Most of the particles were relatively stiff, separate, unbranched rods resembling those that have been previously interpreted as Watson-Crick double helices. Some of these particles, as in Figure 6, show a thickening that suggests partial separation of two elements lying side by side. A smaller number of particles (66) were branched at one or both ends as shown in Figure 7. We do not believe that the branches could be interpreted as the partially separated single strands of a double helix, since they are too thick and too rigid. Single strands would assume a random coil configuration, like denatured DNA, appearing as flattened patches (Hall and Litt, 1958).

All of the particles, both branched and unbranched, had approximately the same height, 20 to 30 Å, as calculated from shadow lengths. There was no appreciable change in shadow length where the two branches came together into one structure, i.e., their height perpendicular to the grid surface was unchanged by their association. This indicates that the two elements lie side by side rather than twisted about one another.

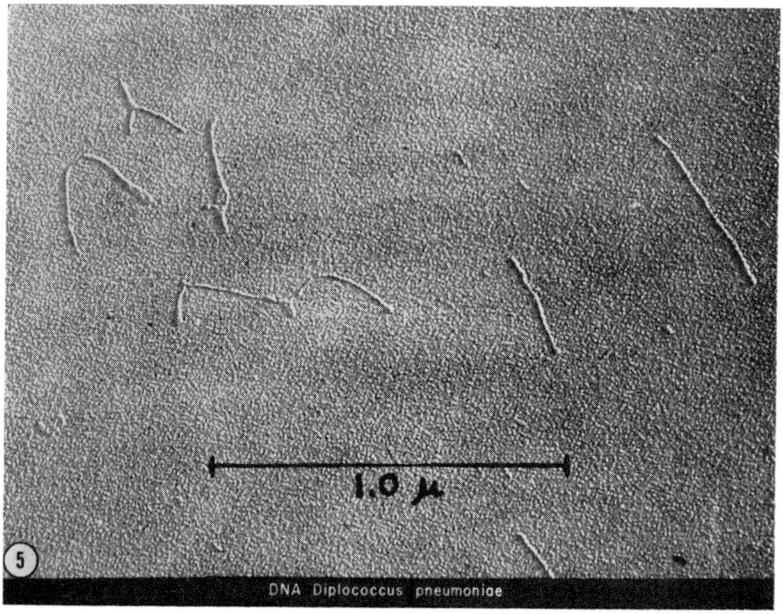

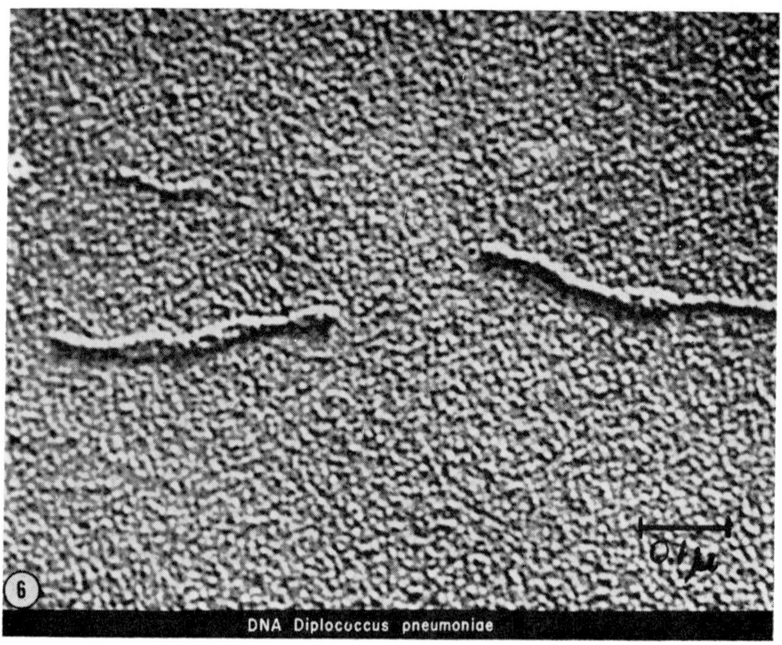

See legends on page 51.

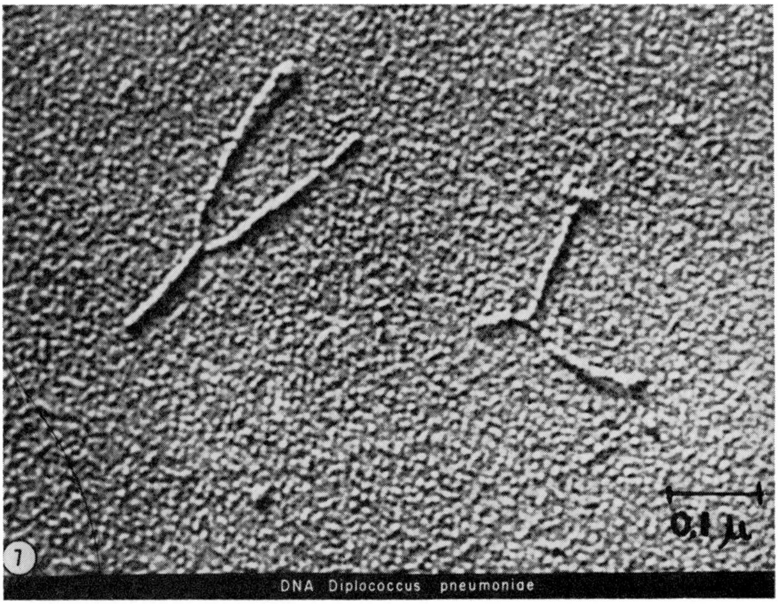

The number-average and weight-average lengths of the particles are summarized in Table 2. Because the weight averages for branched and unbranched particles are closely similar, the calculated mass per unit length of the particles is relatively insensitive to morphological considerations. The unbranched particles do have a significantly shorter number-average length, due to the fact that in this class we have included everything, even that which must be small debris. This small material has less effect on the weight average. If one divides the weight-average molecular weight from light scattering, 1.6 million, by the weight-average length, 4,300 Å, one obtains 370 molecular-weight units/Å, or approximately twice the value of 208 expected for a Watson-Crick double helix. This is equivalent to 3.6 strands/molecule.

On the basis of morphology alone, one can conclude that all the branched particles are at least four-stranded, and all the unbranched

---

FIG. 5. *Pneumococcus* DNA particles in a typical low magnification field. The specimens were shadow-cast with platinum and later stripped as described elsewhere (Hall and Litt, 1958).

FIG. 6. Rodlike *Pneumococcus* DNA particles showing bulges that suggest local separation of two lateral elements.

FIG. 7. Branched particles of *Pneumococcus* DNA. The shadow length does not change where the two branches come together.

particles are at least two-stranded. Consequently, at least 30 per cent of the material by weight must have four or more strands. If the branched particles are no more than four-stranded, the average mass per unit length requires that most of the unbranched particles be four-stranded as well. There is no reason to assume that there is any difference between branched and unbranched particles, especially since branched particles have nearly the same weighted length as the rest of the population.

TABLE 2

Electron Microscopy of Pneumococcus DNA

	Number of particles counted	Number-average length	Weight-average length
	N	$\frac{\Sigma NL}{\Sigma N}$	$\frac{\Sigma NL^2}{\Sigma NL}$
Unbranched	521	2,568 Å	4,220 Å
Branched	66	4,300 Å	4,650 Å
Both, combined	587	2,740 Å	4,300 Å

Electron microscopy, like DNase and X-ray degradation kinetics, has thus demonstrated that biunial DNA has an average of close to four strands/molecule; these appear to be organized as a pair of loosely linked double helices. In addition, these experiments have shown that the units into which biunial DNA is split by hot cesium chloride are two-stranded, as is undenatured unitary DNA. Since the former are the biologically conserved units in *E. coli*, we concluded that genetic information is passed on by means of a two-stranded DNA structure, probably a double helix.

To confirm this hypothesis, we sought a direct demonstration of the changes in the DNA molecule which would be predicted to occur during the replication cycle of the cell. Theoretically, it may be shown that even for a random population of cells there will be fluctuations with time for any given property, e.g., the molecular weight of DNA. However, the changes will be small and hence difficult to observe. For this reason we chose to study the thymineless mutant *E. coli* 15_{T-}, which can be synchronized with respect to DNA synthesis and cell division (Barner and Cohen, 1956). DNA prepared from this organism before and after synchronization was found to be biunial, until the period of DNA synthesis was reached. At this time the DNA became unitary; it possessed two strands rather than four, its molecular weight was half that of DNA prepared but a short time earlier, but the molecular length remained unchanged and the hydrogen bonds between bases remained intact (Cavalieri and Rosenberg, 1961c).

This evidence, together with other findings, indicates that in *E. coli,* and probably other organisms as well, the conserved unit of DNA is a stiff double helix such as the unitary DNA isolated at the start of DNA synthesis. At first the unit is laterally attached to a similar unit, then separates, replicates without loss of integrity, and eventually passes (as part of a biunial molecule containing one old and one new double helical unit) to one of the daughter cells. The demonstration by electron microscopy that the two double helices of the biunial molecule lie side by side rather than intertwined suggests that the replication mechanism involves the transfer of information from the parental double helix to a nascent structure forming in an adjacent rather than concentric position.

At the beginning of its replication cycle, the *E. coli* DNA molecule consists of two double-helical units laterally attached to one another. This molecule, inherited from the parent cell, eventually splits into two parts, each of which then synthesizes a new partner. Thus, just before cell division, there are two biunial molecules identical with the original one. At cell division, each goes to a different daughter cell. Replication of the parental molecule is therefore semiconservative, but replication of the double helix is conservative. The unitary stage appears to be brief, relative to the generation time, in proliferating cells, such as bacteria and sarcoma-180, which ordinarily yield biunial DNA. But in cells not destined to divide again, such as calf thymus or salmon sperm, the DNA is arrested permanently in the unitary state. This generalization is based on a study of DNA from seven sources, ranging from bacteria to mammals. However, just as the order and timing of the replication of chromosomal segments is a species characteristic (Taylor, 1960), so may be the order and timing of unit separation. That is, in some cells all DNA molecules may become unitary at once, whereas in other cells the molecules split in sequence. It is also possible that there are species in which the unitary stage is more extended, or in which the nondividing cell is arrested after DNA synthesis, making the molecules biunial; no such species have been encountered.

This replication scheme (Figure 8) differs in a major respect from that suggested by Watson and Crick (1953). According to their hypothesis, the two strands of the double helix untwist while, simultaneously, new complementary strands form along the free parts of the parental strands. The mechanism by which parental strands act as templates is the specific pairing of complementary bases. When the original strands have completely separated there are two identical double-helical molecules, each composed of one new and one old strand. This hypothesis, based solely on the proposed complementary double-helical structure of DNA and the fact that the hereditary material must replicate itself somehow, is appealing because of its directness and simplicity. However, apparent

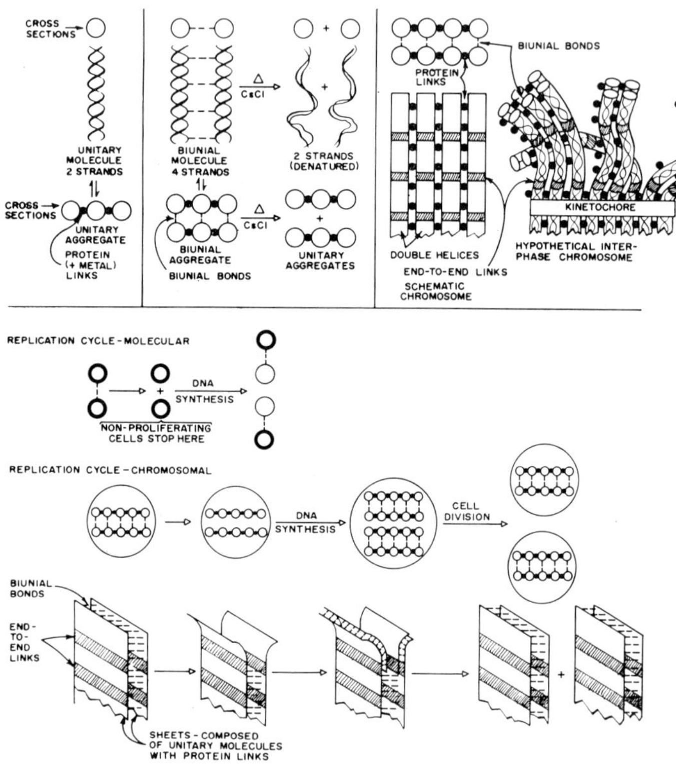

FIG. 8. Outline of the results discussed in this chapter. Top: unitary and biunial molecules and aggregates, showing the effects of disaggregation and of heating in cesium chloride. Protein is indicated schematically by black dots, biunial bonds by dashed lines; the cross-section of a double helix is represented by a circle. The cross-section of the schematic chromosome is supported by the data, while the end-to-end arrangement of the sheets of molecules is one of several possible arrangements. The hypothetical interphase chromosome, shown before separation of the units, illustrates a possible configuration in which the "sheet" structure would not be morphologically apparent. Bottom: the molecular (DNA) and chromosomal replication cycles are diagramed in cross-section, and the replication behavior of the schematic chromosome above is suggested.

simplicity is not a sufficient guarantee of truth, especially in view of our extensive ignorance of the structure and function of genetic material as a whole.

Most of the evidence that has been adduced in support of the Watson-Crick replication hypothesis has shown that the replication of DNA (Meselson and Stahl, 1958) and chromosomes (Taylor, Woods, and Hughes, 1957) is semi-conservative. This is, of course, indirect evidence and applies equally well to the scheme presented here. Other evidence, also indirect, is related to specific base pairing; for example, in Kornberg's synthetic system, base analogs replace only those natural bases that have the same hydrogen-bonding properties (Bessman *et al.*, 1958). While there might be other ways of interpreting these data, it is not necessary to invoke them here since there is at this time no compelling evidence contradictory to the mode of template action suggested by Watson and Crick. Even though the two strands of the double helix do not separate, the hydrogen bonds between them may break, all at once or in sequential groups, to allow the bases to make contact with precursor bases. Such a mechanism has been proposed by Bloch (1955). Its essential feature is that, once the new strands have been synthesized, the old strands rejoin. There is no reason to assume that the exact dimensions of the molecular structure, as determined by X-ray diffraction, would have to be maintained during replication.

Since both chromosomes and the DNA molecules composing them replicate semiconservatively, there is no doubt that the anaphase chromosome is double and that each conserved half contains one conserved unit (or double helix) of each DNA molecule. Furthermore, we have shown that DNA molecules are laterally associated in small groups until most or all protein has been removed (Cavalieri, Deutsch, and Rosenberg, 1961). At least in the case of *E. coli* DNA, such aggregates are not artifacts. They appear to be held together by small amounts of protein, perhaps with the aid of divalent metal ions. These observations fit a double sheet model of the anaphase chromosome, in which each sheet is composed of a row of double helices (each combined with protein) and the two sheets are held together by biunial bonds. In this model, the DNA could be oriented either perpendicular or parallel to the length of the chromosome; if perpendicular, the model would be consistent with a central protein core structure (Taylor, 1957) or with a sharply-folded single nucleoprotein strand structure in which the nucleoprotein molecules are joined end-to-end at the fold-points

(Freese, 1958). However, we prefer to think of the DNA as parallel to the length of the chromosome, because of the data on birefringence, dichroism of adsorbed vital stains, and anisotropic swelling in unfixed salivary gland chromosomes (Ambrose and Gopal-Ayengar, 1952; Ambrose, 1956). In the parallel cases there would have to be labile end-to-end connections that are mostly ruptured during isolation.

During replication, the biunial bonds break and the two sheets must separate, perhaps one segment at a time in the order in which the DNA molecules replicate (Taylor, 1960). Each sheet produces a new sheet, attached to itself by biunial bonds. At the completion of DNA synthesis there will be two double sheets, constituting the two daughter chromatids. These are attached to one another only at the kinetochore, and separate completely at the next anaphase. In cells not destined to synthesize DNA or divide, the two sheets of the chromosome apparently separate and remain in that condition. This behavior of the chromosome, outlined in Figure 8, is deduced entirely from what we have learned about the DNA replication cycle.

Mazia (1960; Mazia, Harris, and Bibring, 1960) has recently made an observation which is very revealing of the basic structure of chromosome and DNA. He found that if dividing sand dollar eggs were blocked at metaphase with β-mercaptoethanol, and the block removed after a certain interval (during which no DNA synthesis occurred), the eggs divided four ways. Since the quadruplet daughter cells continued to proliferate, each must have received a complete set of genetic information, and therefore each metaphase chromosome must have contained four such sets. If β-mercaptoethanol had not been added, these chromosomes would have divided two ways at anaphase. This, then, is direct cytological proof that the normal anaphase chromosome consists of two sets of information which can separate and still remain functional and complete in terms of information. These parts must of course be the two conserved halves of the anaphase chromosome, which apparently can be caused to separate prematurely under unusual conditions. If each chromosome half had been composed of single strands from double helices, as necessitated by the Watson-Crick hypothesis, it would, first, have been a formidable problem to untwist each DNA molecule and its protein in the condensed chromosome; and second, it is doubtful whether a complex chromosome made up of single polynucleotide strands would behave normally. However,

Mazia's observations are fully consistent with the chromosome structure presented here, in which the anaphase chromosome has two parts, each composed of one double helix from each biunial DNA molecule. Premature rupture of the biunial bonds (i.e., at anaphase rather than the following interphase) would produce two easily separable and completely stable chromatids, identical in information content, from each anaphase chromosome, or four in all from each metaphase chromosome. These chromatids could act as chromosomes in the quadripartitioning egg, without requiring any change in the normal mechanisms of function and replication.

REFERENCES

Ambrose, E. J. 1956. The Structure of Chromosomes. *Progress in Biophysics and Biophysical Chemistry*, 6:25–55.

Ambrose, E. J., and A. R. Gopal-Ayengar. 1952. Molecular Organization in Giant Chromosomes. *Nature, London*, 169:652–653.

Barner, H. D., and S. S. Cohen. 1956. Synchronization of Division of a Thymineless Mutant of *Escherichia coli*. *Journal of Bacteriology*, 72:115–125.

Bessman, M. J., I. R. Lehman, J. Adler, S. B. Zimmerman, E. S. Simms, and A. Kornberg. 1958. Enzymic Synthesis of Deoxyribonucleic Acid. III. The Incorporation of Pyrimidine and Purine Analogs into Deoxyribonucleic Acid. *Proceedings of the National Academy of Sciences of the U.S.A.*, 44:633–640.

Bloch, D. P. 1955. A Possible Mechanism for the Replication of the Helical Structure of Desoxyribonucleic Acid. *Proceedings of the National Academy of Sciences of the U.S.A.*, 41:1058–1064.

Cavalieri, L. F., J. F. Deutsch, and B. H. Rosenberg. 1961. The Molecular Weight and Aggregation of DNA. *Biophysical Journal*, 1:301.

Cavalieri, L. F., R. Finston, and B. H. Rosenberg. 1961. Multi-Stranded DNA as Determined by X-Irradiation. *Nature, London*, 189:833.

Cavalieri, L. F., and B. H. Rosenberg. 1961a. The Replication of DNA. I. Two Molecular Classes of DNA. *Biophysical Journal*, 1:317.

———. 1961b. The Replication of DNA. II. The Number of Polynucleotide Strands in the Conserved Unit of DNA. *Biophysical Journal*, 1:323.

———. 1961c. The Replication of DNA. III. Changes in the Number of Strands in *E. coli* DNA During Its Replication Cycle. *Biophysical Journal*, 1:337.

Freese, E. 1958. "The Arrangement of DNA in the Chromosome," *Exchange of Genetic Material: Mechanisms and Consequences* (Cold Spring Harbor Symposia on Quantitative Biology, Vol. 23), pp. 13–18. Cold Spring Harbor, New York: Long Island Biological Association.

Hall, C. E., and L. F. Cavalieri. 1961. Four-Stranded DNA as Determined by Electron Microscopy. *The Journal of Biophysical and Biochemical Cytology*, 10:347.

Hall, C. E., and M. Litt. 1958. Morphological Features of DNA Macromolecules as Seen with the Electron Microscope. *The Journal of Biophysical and Biochemical Cytology*, 4:1–4.

Mazia, D. 1960. The Analysis of Cell Reproduction. *Annals of the New York Academy of Sciences*, 90:455–469.

Mazia, D., P. J. Harris, and T. Bibring. 1960. The Multiplicity of the Mitotic Centers and the Time-Course of their Duplication and Separation. *The Journal of Biophysical and Biochemical Cytology*, 7:1–20.

Meselson, M., and F. W. Stahl. 1958. The Replication of DNA in *Escherichia coli*. *Proceedings of the National Academy of Sciences of the U.S.A.*, 44:671–682.

Taylor, J. H. 1957. The Time and Mode of Duplication of Chromosomes. *American Naturalist*, 91:209–221.

———. 1960. Asynchronous Duplication of Chromosomes in Cultural Cells of Chinese Hamster. *The Journal of Biophysical and Biochemical Cytology*, 7:455–464.

Taylor, J. H., P. S. Woods, and W. L. Hughes. 1957. The Organization and Duplication of Chromosomes as Revealed by Autoradiographic Studies Using Tritium-Labeled Thymidine. *Proceedings of the National Academy of Sciences of the U.S.A.*, 43:122–128.

Watson, J. D., and F. H. C. Crick. 1953. "The Structure of DNA," *Viruses* (Cold Spring Harbor Symposia on Quantitative Biology, Vol. 18), pp. 123–131. Cold Spring Harbor, New York: Long Island Biological Association.

Fractionation of Nucleic Acids in Relation to Cancer

K. S. Kirby, B.Sc., M.Sc., Ph.D.

Chester Beatty Research Institute, Institute of Cancer Research, London, England

Ribonucleic Acids

The various methods used for the isolation of ribonucleic acids (RNA) have been discussed by Magasanik (1955). In order to compare RNA from normal and tumor tissues, it was essential to have a method that combined a good yield with an undegraded product.

Preparation

With this in mind, an adaptation of the phenol extraction method described by Westphal, Lüderitz, and Bister (1952) was investigated utilizing mammalian tissues. These authors found that extraction of acetone-dried bacteria with a phenol-water mixture yielded a two phase system in which RNA and polysaccharides were present in the aqueous phase, and protein was denatured or dissolved in the phenol, while deoxyribonucleic acid (DNA) remained insoluble. Application of this method to rat liver (Kirby, 1956) yielded a similar distribution of components, and as the DNA remained insoluble, it was not necessary to separate cell nuclei before the extraction. RNA was separated from polysaccharides by extraction into 2-methoxyethanol or dimethylsulphoxide from 1.25 M phosphate (pH 7.5).

Gierer and Schramm (1956) prepared RNA from tobacco mosaic

virus by extraction with phenol and, more important, showed that the nucleic acid so prepared retained some infectivity. The method has been used to isolate RNA from several viruses.

While the phenol and water extraction gave a reasonable yield of RNA (~ 500 mg. RNA/100 Gm. liver), difficulties were sometimes experienced by emulsification and an improvement resulted when 0.015 M naphthalene-1, 5-disulphonate (NDS) (pH 6.5) was used. The yield and base composition of the RNA remained the same but the fractionation proceeded differently (see below).

The latest modification we have adopted is to break down the tissue in 0.015 M NDS and to extract the tissue with phenol containing 0.1 per cent 8-hydroxyquinoline. This method has resulted in an improved yield of RNA (~ 750 mg./100 Gm. rat liver), which appears to be less degraded than RNA prepared by the previous methods.

Littauer and Eisenberg (1959) also found that RNA prepared by the phenol method from *Escherichia coli* was degraded if ethylene diamine tetra-acetate was not present during the preparation, and Laskov, Margoliash, Littauer, and Eisenberg (1959) have applied this method to the isolation of RNA from rat liver and separated a fraction of high molecular weight by precipitation with M sodium chloride.

Sibatani, Yamana, Kimura, and Okagaki (1959) made the important observation that the rate of uptake of radioactive phosphorus was much greater for the fraction of RNA which remained in the phenol layer and Georgiev, Mantieva, and Zbarsky (1960) found that treatment of tissues with phenol at pH 6.0 led to separation of "phenolic nuclei" which contain DNA and RNA. Presumably this insoluble RNA was the same as that which incorporated radioactive phosphorus at a greater rate.

Heterogeneity of RNA

The previous results indicated that most preparations are heterogeneous and various methods of fractionating RNA have been discussed before (Kirby, 1960a). Solvent fractionation and countercurrent distribution (C.C.D.) have been used in the present study to investigate the different molecular species in a given preparation of RNA.

Addition of either 2-butoxyethanol or 2-ethoxyethanol to solutions of RNA resulted in fractional precipitation and the fraction with the highest proportion of guanine always separated first. The

TABLE 1

Base Compositions of Fractions Obtained by Fractional Precipitation of Rat Liver RNA (Phenol-Water) with 2-Butoxyethanol

Fraction	Guanine	Adenine	Cytosine	Uracil
1	38.5	11.5	36.5	13.5
2	35.1	17.6	31.4	15.9
3	32.2	21.9	28.6	17.1

results of the fractionation of rat liver RNA (phenol-water preparation) with 2-butoxyethanol are shown in Table 1. The amount which precipitated as fraction 1 varied with the method of preparation and the yields and base compositions of fraction 1 and residual amino acids associated with rat liver RNA prepared by different methods are shown in Table 2. Mouse liver RNA behaved in a similar way, but nearly 80 per cent of chicken liver RNA was precipitated as fraction 1 when prepared by the phenol-NDS method.

The greater proportions of fractions 2 and 3, the decreased adenine content of fraction 1, and the solubility characteristics indicated that RNA prepared by the phenol-water method was somewhat degraded, in agreement with the suggestion of Laskov, Margoliash, Littauer, and Eisenberg (1959), and studies with C.C.D. confirmed this.

Countercurrent Distribution of RNA

This technique, which was developed by Craig (cf. Craig and Craig, 1950), involves the distribution of a substance between organic and aqueous phases, and from the distribution it is possible to assess the purity of a component or the complexity of a mixture. It could therefore be a particularly useful method for a characterizing RNA, where the number of components is unknown.

The choice of solvent systems was based on ability of 2-ethoxy- and 2-butoxy-ethanol to fractionate RNA and satisfactory systems

TABLE 2

Comparison of RNA and Fraction 1 Prepared by Different Methods

Method	Amino acids associated with RNA (per cent)	Yield fraction 1	Guanine/ adenine
Phenol-H_2O	1.5	30	38.5/11.5
Phenol-NDS	0.5	50	36.0/17.5
HQ-Phenol-NDS	0.2	75	34.5/18.0

Abbreviations:
HQ, 8-hydroxyquinoline; NDS naphthalene-1, 5-disulphonate.

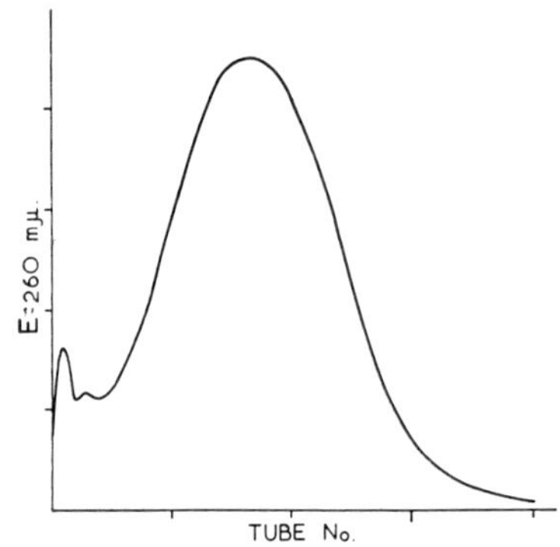

Fig. 1. C.C.D. curve for rat liver RNA (phenol-water preparation) 96 transfers.

for RNA prepared by the phenol-water method were mixtures of ethylene glycol monoethers and either phosphate solutions (pH 7.5) or ammonium sulphate solution (Kirby, 1960a). The C.C.D. curves of rat liver RNA prepared by the phenol-water and phenol-NDS methods are shown in Figures 1 and 2, respectively. The C.C.D. curve of RNA prepared by the phenol-NDS method showed a greater quantity of material remaining in the aqueous phase and the height of the peak in tubes 0 to 10 was associated with the amount of material precipitated as fraction 1 by 2 butoxyethanol. Examination of the C.C.D. curves of the fractions obtained by precipitation of RNA (phenol-water preparation) showed that the values of the curves could not be summed to that of the original material. Obviously some interaction occurs between the various components, and this interaction is almost certainly due to hydrogen-bonding between adenine-uracil (A-U) and between guanine-cytosine (G-C) units. Examination of synthetic polynucleotides (provided by A. M. Michelson [Micheloson, 1959]) showed that poly A was the most soluble in the organic phase, while poly G had

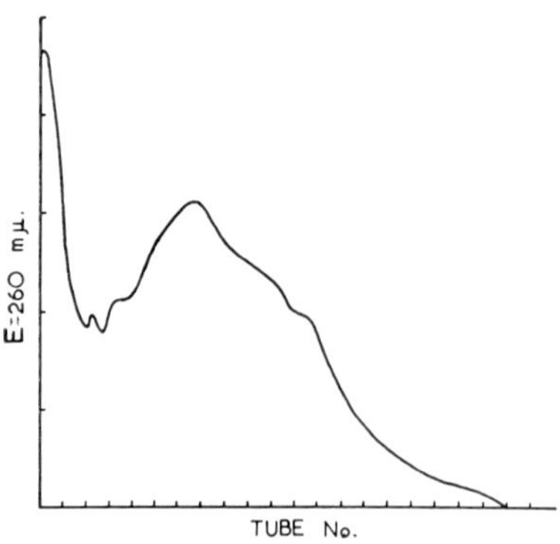

Fig. 2. C.C.D. curve for rat liver RNA (phenol-NDS preparation) 96 transfers.

greater affinity for the aqueous phase; there was less interaction between poly A and poly U in the solvent than between poly G and poly C.

Evidence that RNA prepared by the phenol-water method was somewhat degraded was obtained by limited action of ribonuclease on fraction 1. No change in the base composition occurred during the reaction, but the C.C.D. curves were considerably modified (indicating the sensitivity of the method). After reaction for one hour, the curve had changed from one in which most of the material remained in the first 10 tubes to one similar to that obtained by distributing rat liver RNA prepared by the phenol-water method (Figure 1).

If the material which traveled in the organic phase had a high adenine content, as suggested by the partition values of the synthetic polynucleotides, then such a fragment must have been cleaved during the isolation and also by the limited reaction of ribonuclease on fraction 1. The presence of such a fragment was detected after recovery of the RNA fractions after C.C.D.

The original solvent systems were not completely satisfactory for distribution of RNA, but addition of 2 to 5 per cent NN-dibutylaminoethanol to the organic solvent mixtures improved the partition in favor of the organic phase and, it is believed, reduced the interaction between the components. Distribution of fraction 3 from rat liver RNA (phenol-water preparation) has been reported (Kirby, 1960b) and nine fractions were recovered. C.C.D. curves of the different fractions were evidence that the fractionation achieved was not due to cleavage during partition in the two-phase system. Fraction 3 was probably of smallest molecular weight and further distributions with fractions 1 and 2 from rat liver RNA showed that C.C.D. can be generally used and the separation again obviously depends upon the base composition (Table 3). Fractions

TABLE 3

Base Compositions of Some Fractions Obtained by C.C.D. of RNA (Phenol-NDS and Phenol-Water)

Guanine	Adenine	Cytosine	Uracil
41.6	5.5	39.7	13.2
42.0	8.0	37.4	12.6
38.2	14.8	31.7	15.3
36.7	19.6	28.2	15.5
34.2	21.6	27.0	17.2
30.5	26.3	24.4	15.8
28.8	34.6	21.0	15.6

richer in adenine are being separated from those richer in guanine and there is little variation in the uracil content of the different fractions.

The C.C.D. curve of one fraction from rat liver RNA (phenol-NDS) is shown in Figure 3, and after recovery of the fractions their redistribution in the same solvent system is shown in Figure 4. The curve of the fraction is more complex than that of whole RNA, indicating improved separation of the components, and the curves of some of the fractional material indicate that some components are beginning to approach homogeneity by this method.

The fraction containing the greatest proportion of adenine was found only in fraction 3 from preparations made by the phenol-water method; obviously this fraction is a segment of a larger molecule. Since the fraction with the highest adenine content was the result of degradation, it is possible that the fraction with the lowest

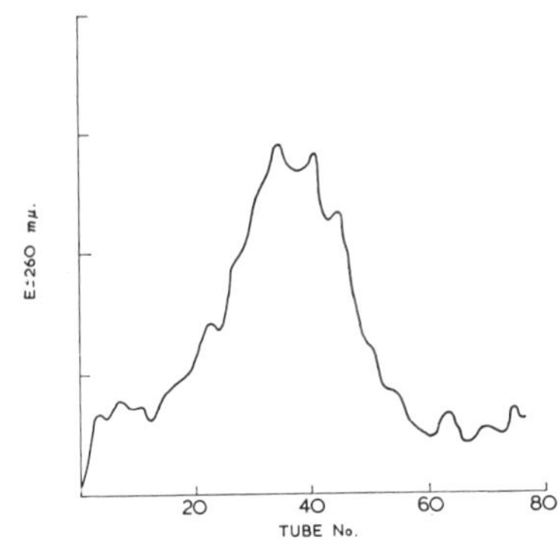

Fig. 3. C.C.D. curve of fraction of rat liver RNA (phenol-NDS preparation) using NN-dibutylaminoethanol in solvent system. 80 transfers.

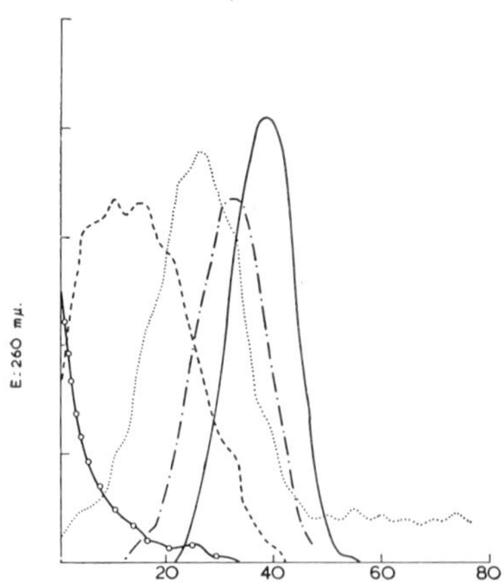

Fig. 4. C.C.D. curves of the individual fractions after recovery from C.C.D. shown in Figure 3.

adenine content also came from a similar cleavage. If this should prove to be the case it would show that the distribution of adenine and guanine along the chain of RNA is far from random.

Fractionation of RNA by C.C.D. appears to depend largely on the base composition, while fractionation by ion-exchange chromatography depends on the molecular weight of the species. A combination of both methods may therefore lead to the preparation of RNA fractions of reasonable purity for further chemical studies.

C.C.D. has also been applied to the fractionation of soluble RNA (S RNA) and Holley, Apgar, and Doctor (1960) have succeeded in separating S RNA's which transfer valine, threonine, leucine, and tyrosine after relatively few transfers.

Countercurrent Distribution of DNA

Since the separation of RNA by C.C.D. depends upon interaction of the bases with the organic solvent, it was not surprising to find that undenatured DNA remained largely in the aqueous phase. However, since a solution to the coding sequences in DNA and RNA demands a study of the base sequences in both compounds, a preliminary study of the fractionation of commercial calf thymus DNA has been initiated.

TABLE 4

Base Compositions of Some Fractions Obtained by C.C.D. of DNA (Commercial Preparation)

	Guanine	Adenine	Cytosine	Thymine
Original	23.2	22.6	15.9	38.3
	30.3	21.7	13.0	35.0
	27.9	21.8	13.5	36.8
	22.9	23.3	13.8	40.0
	16.9	24.7	16.2	42.2
	13.6	24.8	15.4	46.4
	12.1	25.8	16.5	45.6

The commercial material is degraded and has higher partitions in the organic phase than fractions from RNA. The base compositions of some fractions recovered after C.C.D. are shown in Table 4. Contrary to RNA, the fractionation depends much more upon the guanine than the adenine content and a comparison of the G/C and A/U ratios of RNA with the G/C and A/T (thymine) ratios of DNA (Table 5) shows that relative constancy of G/C in RNA is matched by that of A/T in DNA, while variations in A/U in RNA

TABLE 5

Composition of the Base Ratios of Fractions Obtained by C.C.D. of RNA and DNA

RNA		DNA	
Guanine/ Cytosine	Adenine/ Uracil	Guanine/ Cytosine	Adenine/ Thymine
1.05	0.42	0.73	0.56
1.12	0.63	0.90	0.54
1.20	0.97	1.03	0.59
1.30	1.27	1.66	0.58
1.27	1.27	1.78	0.57
1.25	1.66	2.07	0.59
1.37	2.22	2.33	0.62

are matched by those of G/C in DNA. It would be premature to draw conclusions from a comparison of fractions of rat liver RNA with fractions of a commercial preparation of calf thymus DNA, but the results indicate the power of the C.C.D. technique in fractionating polyribonucleotides and polydeoxyribonucleotides, and this should be of value in determining what relationship exists between base sequences in the two types of nucleic acid.

Deoxyribonucleic Acid

No standard method exists for the isolation of DNA from tissues and organisms, and a feature of the problem has been the varying degree of difficulty with which DNA is separated from the protein. DNA in herring sperm was easily dissociated from the protamine by M NaCl but this method is not generally applicable.

Preparation

A DNA-protein complex was released from calf thymus tissue by extraction with strong salt solution (Fisher, Anderson, and Wilbur, 1959) and DNA could be isolated after removing the protein with sodium dodecylsulphate (Chargaff, 1955). Dounce and Monty (1955) have pointed out the necessity to stir this gel produced by the action of salt on the tissue for some hours before adding the dodecysulphate; otherwise very little DNA is obtained. It was assumed that some enzyme reactions have degraded the gel during this time and cleaved the protein which then could be removed with dodecylsulphate, leaving the DNA in solution.

The method based on dodecysulphate gave very satisfactory yields of DNA from calf thymus gland, but the separation did not proceed so smoothly with rat liver. A method for the preparation of DNA.

free from protein and in good yield, was discovered during an investigation of the release of nucleic acids from mammalian tissues by the action of different salts and phenol (Kirby, 1957). After testing a large number of salts, it became clear that many organic anions with a lipophilic grouping and in combination with phenol could release DNA to which some residual protein was attached. Trichloroacetate, benzoate, *p*-toluenesulphonate, and phenylphosphate all acted in a similar way in this respect. Salts with hydrophilic groups (e.g., citrate, glycerophosphate or *p*-hydroxybenzoate) released no DNA from rat liver into the aqueous phase after extraction with phenol.

DNA with no protein attached was obtained from rat liver only when the salt concerned had lipophilic and chelating properties; or when two salts were used, each having one of the two required properties. On the basis of these results, it was suggested that some of the DNA in the chromosome was bound to protein by metal linkages.

A comparison of the effect of some different anions which have been used to study the lability of the DNA-protein complex in rat liver is shown in Table 6.

TABLE 6

Comparison of the Effects of Different Anions on the Release of DNA from Rat Liver

Molarity	Anion	Product
0.3	Chloride	....
0.3	Fluoride, azide	DNA, 1% protein
0.15	*p*-Hydroxybenzoate	....
0.15	Salicylate	DNA
0.3	Diethylacetate	DNA, 4% protein
0.3	Diethyldithiocarbamate	DNA
0.03	1-Naphthol-4-sulphonate	....
0.03	2-Nitroso-1-naphthol-4-sulphonate	DNA, 2% protein

p-Aminosalicylate was found empirically to be the most satisfactory for the preparation of DNA from rat liver. Application of this method to other tissues resulted in release of a good yield of DNA, but the amount of residual protein associated with DNA isolated from different tissues varied as shown in Table 7 (Kirby, 1959). The results with mouse liver show quite clearly that a choice of other salts may be more effective than *p*-aminosalicylate for the isolation of DNA with the minimum amount of protein. While DNA from normal and regenerating rat liver were isolated free from protein, the DNA from a transplantable hepatoma was

TABLE 7

Amount of Residual Protein Associated with DNA Prepared by PAS-Phenol Method from Different Tissues

Tissue	Residual protein
Mouse liver 1	1.0
Mouse liver 2*	0.4
Mouse spleen	0.45
Mouse hepatoma	0.5
Chicken liver	0.5
Chick embryo liver	0.65
Chick spleen	1.6
Rat spleen	2.7
Rat hepatoma	0.8
Rat liver	0.0

* Mouse liver 2 prepared with 0.15 M naphthalene-2-sulphonate + 0.05 M ethylenediaminetetra-acetate.
PAS = *p*-aminosalicylate.

isolated with 0.8 per cent residual protein. DNA from a spontaneous mouse hepatoma differed from normal mouse liver DNA in having less residual protein.

The results showed that the bindings between DNA and protein varied in each tissue and this variation explained the differences found in the facility with which DNA was released from the tissues.

While the *p*-aminosalicylate-phenol method gave a good yield of DNA, it was necessary to use ribonuclease for the final removal of small amounts of RNA associated with the preparation. It would be useful to have a method capable of separating DNA from RNA without the use of this enzyme in order to show that ribonuclease had no degradative effect on the DNA.

Such an effect was achieved by using phenolphthalein diphosphate (0.15 M, pH 6.0) to break down the tissue and then to extract the mixture with phenol (Kirby, 1961a). After centrifuging, all the DNA was present as a white, insoluble precipitate, from which the DNA could be brought into solution by extracting with 20 per cent sodium acetate or sodium benzoate and isolated in good yield and with little residual protein. A similar qualitative separation was obtained when either 2-methyl-1, 4-dihydroxynaphthalene diphosphate (Synkavit) or diethylstilbestrol diphosphate was used, but only 50 to 60 per cent yield of DNA was obtained when fructose-1, 6-diphosphate or pyrophosphate were used, again emphasizing the different effects of hydrophilic salts.

DNA-Protein

While the *p*-aminosalicylate-phenol method yielded DNA with very little residual protein, it was noted that when other salts were used the proportions of the amino acids in the residual protein were not typical of a histone. There were high contents of aspartic and glutamic acids and cystine and tryptophan were also present.

In order to examine this protein more carefully, rat liver was broken down in 0.07 M benzoate, and after extraction with phenol, a viscous mixture was obtained from which a DNA protein could be separated and which could be dispersed again to form an opalescent solution (Kirby, 1958). Extraction of other tissues with 0.07 M benzoate phenol showed that there was a range in the amount of residual protein, again emphasizing the difference in the DNA-protein binding in different tissues (Frearson, unpublished data). The results are summarized in Table 8. Acidic proteins have been extracted from nuclei by Stedman and Stedman (1947), and by Wang, Mayer, and Thomas (1953). Mirsky and Ris (1951) made chromosome preparations from different tissues and showed that, after removing DNA and histone, a residual protein fraction remained, the amount of which varied with the tissue.

The DNA-protein obtained from rat liver with 0.07 M benzoate and phenol was a mixture, since, after drying, it could be redispersed and fractionated by centrifugation at 20,000 rpm into a clear supernatant solution from which DNA with about 3 per cent residual protein could be obtained and a sediment which could be dispersed again in water to form a swollen gel and which contained the bulk of the protein. When DNA was broken in benzoate of greater molarity (0.21 M or 0.28 M) none of the gel-type material was isolated, and a clear solution of DNA resulted with about 1 to 3 per cent residual protein.

These results indicate that there are at least two types of acidic protein associated with the DNA structure and it seems possible that the two types of salts (lipophilic and chelating) required for

TABLE 8

Amount of Residual Protein Associated with DNA Extracted from Tissues with 0.07 M Benzoate-Phenol

Tissue	DNA (per cent)	Protein (per cent)
Rat liver	66	34
Rat spleen	96	4
Mouse liver	75	25
Mouse spleen	85	15
MA tumor	66	34

the removal of most of the residual protein may be associated with separation of these different proteins. Further details of this suggestion have been discussed previously (Kirby and Frearson, 1960; Kirby, in press) and provisionally one protein, residual protein A, is presumed to link the DNA chains end to end and amounts to about 3 per cent of the DNA. This protein was removed by chelating agents and may be bound to some extent by metal linkages. The other protein, residual protein B, is the basis of the gels which were isolated, is more variable in amount and is removed by lipophilic anions such as benzoate. It probably forms cross links with residual protein A, partly perhaps through salt and partly through lipophilic linkages. A possible means of uniting DNA, residual protein A and residual protein B is shown in Figure 5.

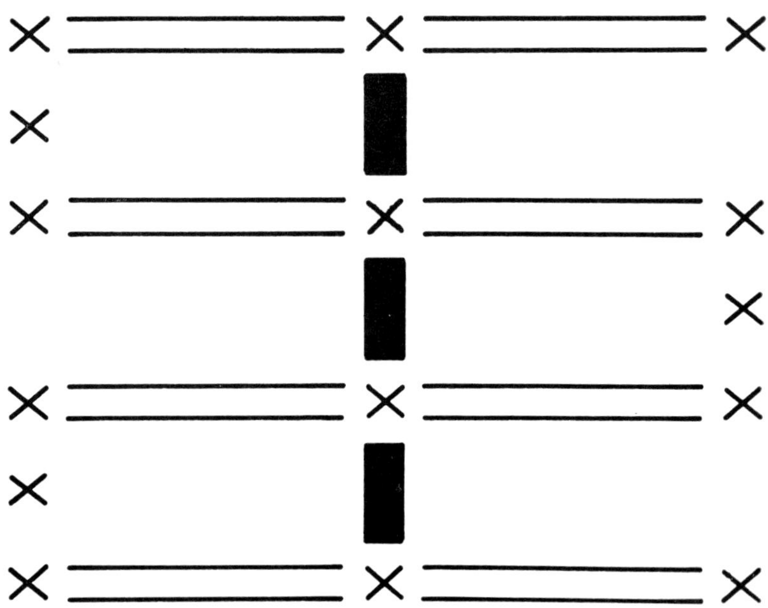

FIG. 5. Possible means of linking DNA by residual proteins A and B. DNA ==, Residual Protein A ×, Residual Protein B, ■.

Three proteins would be present in the whole structure as it is presumed that histones would function to cross link the DNA chains.

It should be emphasized that the structure proposed has arisen mainly from results obtained by dissociation of the DNA protein complex from rat liver and the variation in the type of bonding between the units and the relative amounts of the different units may well occur in other tissues.

Relation to Other Structures

The structure proposed for DNA in the chromosomes is similar to those already suggested by Taylor (1958), Freese (1958), and Kellenberger (1960). All these authors suggested DNA molecules were linked end to end by some subunit which was presumed to be protein. Genetic evidence or studies of the bacterial chromosome in the electron microscope provided the experimental bases for these suggestions.

Dounce, O'Connell, and Monty (1957) and Monty and Dounce (1957, 1958) have pointed out the importance of residual protein in maintaining the structure of DNA in the chromosome and also have suggested that this protein may be bound at the end of the DNA chains. The inability of dodecylsulphate to release DNA until some enzymatic hydrolysis had taken place could be explained by the proposed structure and the polydispersity of the preparations would follow if different DNA molecules were released with small amounts of residual protein A or B or A and B attached. Dounce and Monty (1955) also showed that the bonds between DNA and residual protein could be broken by relatively low doses (1,000 r) of X rays, and such a cleavage would be expected between the weaker links in the structure.

Relation to the Induction of Cancer

A possible correlation between the structure suggested for DNA and protein in the chromosome and the induction of cancer has been discussed previously (Kirby, in press). If it is assumed that the code for RNA resides in the sequence of nucleotides in DNA, while the code for amino acids in proteins resides in the sequence of nucleotides in RNA, and also that the enzymes DN-polymerase (Kornberg, 1960) and RN-polymerase (Weiss, 1960) are associated with the chromosome structure, possibly with residual protein B, then it is clear that the DNA-DN-polymerase system is cyclic:

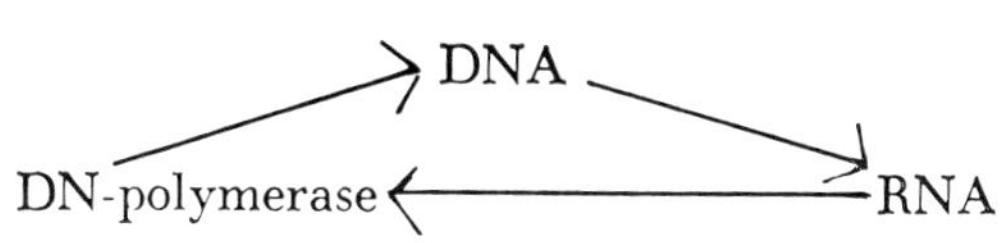

If this system could be isolated from the chromosome and given the necessary precursors, energy, and means of splitting the double helices of the DNA formed, it could, theoretically, continue to produce all its components. This type of action is probably the basis of the reproduction of a DNA virus and the system RNA ⇆ RN-polymerase probably plays a similar role for RNA viruses.

The sensitivity of DNA-protein linkages to radiation appears to be well founded, and it is possible that random damage to a chromosome may release a segment containing DNA which codes for DN-polymerase. If this system remained intact, it could produce more of this enzyme than required for normal duplication of the cell. The excess DN-polymerase would tend to associate itself with the chromosome structure and gradually either replace the RN-polymerase or prevent it from acting effectively. This situation would result in production of less RNA than normal and because of the excess DN-polymerase lead to an increased mitotic rate or polyploidy.

The replacement of RN-polymerase may well be slow, probably random, but could increase over a series of cell divisions. This process could continue until the enzymes concerned with the function of the cell were largely lost and the energy and metabolites were channeled into the production of enzymes concerned with reproduction.

The result of this process is identical with that envisaged by Potter (1958) from a study of the enzymes of normal and tumor tissues and which he has elaborated as the "enzyme deletion hypothesis." Mitchell (1960) has also suggested that the point of attack of radiation is the enzyme system attached at the end of the DNA molecules, and his studies on Synkavit are relevant here because of the remarkable activity of the diphenolic diphosphates in splitting DNA-protein links.

The enzyme systems of cells in relation to the cancer problem have been reviewed by Bergel (1960) and deletions in cells from the point of view of carcinogenesis have been discussed by Haddow (1955) and Burnet (1957). The present hypothesis is useful mainly as a basis for further experimental work. It has been pointed out that differences have been found in the DNA-protein relationships of normal liver and of hepatoma tissue, but much more understanding of this change is required before it can be related to carcinogenesis. Further fractionations of DNA and RNA are required before we can comprehend the types of RNA present in a cell and their relationship to DNA and the enzymes which are present. Greater understanding of the manner in which DNA, RNA, and their polymerase enzymes interact could lead, it is hoped, to new methods of attacking the cancer problem.

ACKNOWLEDGMENTS

I wish to thank Mr. P. M. Frearson for permission to include some of his results prior to publication and for helpful discussions, and Professor A. Haddow, F.R.S., for his interest. I also wish to thank the Elsevier Publishing Company for permission to include two figures and one table from *Biochimica et biophysica acta* 40:193–205, 1760.

This investigation has been supported by grants to the Chester Beatty Research Institute (Institute of Cancer Research: Royal Cancer Hospital) from the Medical Research Council, the British Empire Cancer Campaign, the Jane Coffin Childs Memorial Fund for Medical Research, the Anna Fuller Fund, and the National Cancer Institute of the National Institutes of Health, United States Public Health Service.

REFERENCES

Bergel, F. 1960. *Chemistry of Enzymes in Cancer*. 84 pp. Springfield, Illinois: Charles C Thomas.

Burnet, M. 1957. Cancer—A Biological Approach. *British Medical Journal*, 1:779–786, 841–846.

Chargaff, E. 1955. "Isolation and Composition of DNA and of Corresponding Nucleoproteins," *The Nucleic Acids*, E. Chargaff, and J. N. Davidson, Eds., Vol. 1, pp. 307–371. New York, New York: Academic Press, Inc.

Craig, D., and L. C. Craig. 1950. "Countercurrent Distribution," *Techniques in Organic Chemistry*, A. Weissburger, Ed., Vol. 3, Part 1, pp. 149–332. New York, New York: Interscience Publishers, Inc.

Dounce, A. L., and K. J. Monty. 1955. Factors Influencing the Ability of Isolated Cell Nucleic to Form Gels in Dilute Alkali. *The Journal of Biophysical and Biochemical Cytology*, 1:155–160.

Dounce, A. L., M. P. O'Connell, and K. J. Monty. 1957. Action of Mitochondrial DNAse I in Destroying the Capacity of Isolated Nuclei to Form Gels. *The Journal of Biophysical and Biochemical Cytology*, 3:649–662.

Fisher, W. D., N. G. Anderson, and K. M. Wilbur. 1959. Physical Properties of Deoxyribonucleoproteins from Rat Thymus in 1M NaCl. *Experimental Cell Research*, 18:100–111.

Frearson, P. M. Unpublished data.

Freese, E. 1958. "Arrangements of DNA in the Chromosomes," *Exchange of Genetic Material: Mechanisms and Consequences* (Cold Spring Harbor Symposia on Quantitative Biology, Vol. 23), pp. 13–18. Cold Spring Harbor, New York: Long Island Biological Association.

Georgiev, G. P., V. L. Mantieva, and I. B. Zbarsky. 1960. RNA Fractions in Cell Nuclei Isolated by Phenol and by Sucrose-Glycerophosphate. *Biochimica et biophysica acta*, 37:373–374.

Gierer, A., and G. Schramm. 1956. Die Infektiösität der Nucleinsäure aus Tabakmosaikvirus. *Zeitschrift für Naturforschung,* 11b:138–142.

Haddow, A. 1955. Biochemistry of Cancer. *Annual Review of Biochemistry,* 24:689–742.

Holley, R. W., J. Apgar, and B. P. Doctor. 1960. Separation of Aminoacid Specific "Soluble"-Fraction RNA. *Annals of the New York Academy of Sciences,* 88:745–751.

Kellenberger, E. 1960. "The Physical State of the Bacterial Nucleus," *Microbial Genetics* (Tenth Symposium of the Society for General Microbiology), pp. 39–66. Cambridge, Massachusetts: Harvard University Press.

Kirby, K. S. 1956. New Method for the Preparation of RNA. *Biochemical Journal,* 64:405–408.

———. 1957. New Method for the Isolation of DNA: Evidence on the Nature of Bonds Between DNA and Protein. *Biochemical Journal,* 66:495–504.

———. 1958. Preparation of Some DNA-protein Complexes from Rat Liver Homogenates. *Biochemical Journal,* 70:260–265.

———. 1959. Preparation of DNA by the *p*-Aminosalicylate-Phenol Method. *Biochimica et biophysica acta,* 36:117–124.

———. 1960a. Fractionation and Countercurrent Distribution of RNA. *Biochimica et biophysica acta,* 40:193–205.

———. 1960b. Fractionation of RNA by Countercurrent Distribution. *Biochimica et biophysica acta,* 41:338–340.

———. 1961a. Separation of DNA from RNA Without the Use of Enzymes. *Biochimica et biophysica acta,* 47:18–26.

———. (in press b). "Nucleic Acids and Cancer," *Progress in Experimental Tumor Research,* F. Homburger, Ed., Vol. 2. Basel, Switzerland: S. Kargar.

Kirby, K. S., and P. M. Frearson. 1960. "Investigations on the Bonding Between DNA and Protein," *The Cell Nucleus,* J. S. Mitchell, Ed., pp. 211–213. London: Butterworth & Co.

Kornberg, A. 1960. Die biologische Synthese von Desoxyribonucleinsäure. *Angewandte Chemie,* 72:231–236.

Laskov, R., E. Margoliash, U. Z. Littauer, and H. Eisenberg. 1959. High Molecular Weight RNA from Rat Liver. *Biochimca et biophysica acta,* 33:247–248.

Littauer, U. Z., and E. Eisenberg. 1959. RNA from *E. coli. Biochimica et biophysica acta,* 32:320–337.

Magasanik, B. 1955. "Isolation and Composition of Pentose Nucleic Acids and of Their Corresponding Nucleoproteins," *The Nucleic Acids,* E. Chargaff and J. N. Davidson, Eds., Vol. 1, pp. 373–407. New York, New York: Academic Press, Inc.

Michelson, A. 1959. Polynucleotides. II. *Journal of the Chemical Society,* December: 3655–3669.

Mirsky, A. E., and H. Ris. 1951. Composition and Structure of Isolated Chromosomes. *Journal of General Physiology,* 34:475–492.

Mitchell, J. S. 1960. *Studies in Radiotherapeutics.* Oxford, England: B. Blackwell, 274 pp.

Monty, K. J., and A. L. Dounce. 1957. "Discussion," *Symposium on the Chemical Basis of Heredity*, W. D. McElroy and B. Glass, Eds., pp. 546–550. Baltimore, Maryland: Johns Hopkins Press.

———. 1958. The Properties and Enzymatic Degradation of Desoxyribonucleoprotein from Liver Cell Nuclei. *Journal of General Physiology*, 41:595–608.

Potter, V. R. 1958. Biochemical Approaches to the Cancer Problem. *Federation Proceedings*, 17:691–697.

Sibatani, A., K. Yamana, K. Kimura, and H. Okagaki. 1959. Fractionation with Phenol of RNA of Animal Cells. *Biochimica et biophysica acta*, 33:590–591.

Stedman, E., and E. Stedman. 1947. Chemical Nature and Functions of Components of Cell Nuclei. *Cold Spring Harbor Symposia on Quantitative Biology*, 12:224–236.

Taylor, J. H. 1958. The Duplication of Chromosomes. *Scientific American*, 198:37–42.

Wang, T. Y., D. T. Mayer, and L. E. Thomas. 1953. A Liver Protein of Rat Liver Nuclei. *Experimental Cell Research*, 34:102–106.

Weiss, S. B. 1960. Enzymatic Incorporation of Ribonucleoside Triphosphates into Interpolynucleotide Linkages of RNA. *Proceedings of The National Academy of Sciences of the U.S.A.*, 46:1020–1030.

Westphal, O., O. Lüderitz, and F. Bister. 1952. Reindarstellung eines Polysaccharid-Pyrogens aus *Bacterium coli. Zeitschrift für Naturforschung*, 7b:536–542.

Studies on the Incorporation of Ribonucleotides into Terminal Positions of Ribonucleic and Deoxyribonucleic Acids

E. S. Canellakis, Ph.D.

Senior Fellow of the United States Public Health Service, and Department of Pharmacology, Yale University School of Medicine, New Haven, Connecticut

The elucidation of the mechanism of the biosynthesis of ribonucleic acid (RNA), as well as the mechanism which determines the specificity of the ribonucleotide sequence in the RNA has received much attention. About three years ago (Canellakis, 1959) knowledge in this field was a reflection primarily of studies of (1) a bacterial enzyme system (Grunberg-Manago and Ochoa, 1955) which polymerized ribonucleoside diphosphates to yield increased amounts of ribonucleic acid polymer, and (2) a mammalian enzyme system which incorporated ribonucleotides from ribonucleoside triphosphate precursors into terminal positions of a low molecular weight RNA called S RNA (Heidelberger, *et al.*, 1956; Canellakis, 1957; Herbert, 1958; Hecht, Zamecnik, Stephenson, and Scott, 1958). The former system provided the prerequisite for net synthesis of RNA, but the product lacked the specificity in nucleotide sequence which is to be expected of a biological polymer, while the latter enzyme system showed an apparent specificity in the type of reaction it could catalyze, but lacked the ability to provide any net synthesis of polymer. It appeared reasonable to expect that some other enzyme system might exist which, under some conditions, would combine the major characteristics of these two enzyme systems.

With this in mind, we pursued the problem of RNA synthesis from two parallel paths. The first approach was purifying from the cytoplasmic fraction of rat liver the enzymes associated with the terminal incorporation of ribonucleotides into S RNA, in order that we could better understand the details of this reaction.

In our second approach, we attempted to identify enzymes associated with the synthesis of ribonucleic acid from other sources. Basing our work on the results obtained by Allfrey and Mirsky (1957) with isolated calf thymus nuclei, we assayed extracts of this cell fraction in the hope that we could identify some enzyme system with the combined properties outlined above. However, we became deeply involved in a study of incorporation of ribonucleotides into terminal positions of a nucleic acid; in this case, the ribonucleotide was incorporated into the terminal positions of deoxyribonucleic acid (DNA).

In this presentation some of the results obtained in the course of our studies on these two enzyme systems associated with the terminal addition of ribonucleotides on nucleic acids will be outlined.

Rat Liver Cytoplasmic Enzymes Which Incorporate Ribonucleotides into Terminal Positions of S RNA

We have pursued the study of this reaction in association with Dr. Edward Herbert of the Massachusetts Institute of Technology. The results of these studies have been published (Canellakis and Herbert, 1960a), and I shall attempt only to outline the main conclusions which may be derived from these studies.

The Main Characteristics of the Reaction

The enzymes present in the soluble cytoplasmic fraction of rat liver are capable of incorporating ribonucleotides into terminal positions of S RNA (Canellakis, 1957; Herbert, 1958; Hecht, Zamecnik, Stephenson, and Scott, 1958). This may be exemplified by the reaction:

$$\text{ATP} + \text{CMP-(S RNA)} \rightarrow \text{AMP-CMP-(S RNA)} + \text{P-P}$$

The characteristics of this reaction are that (1) the triphosphates serve as precursors, (2) the enzyme shows a unique specificity of action by attaching only adenylic acid to the exposed cytidylic acid of the S RNA molecule, and (3) the reaction ends after this addition has been made.

TABLE 1

Composition of S RNA-β and S RNA-γ

	Ribonucleosides*				
Component	Adenosine	Uridine	Guanosine	Cytidine	Guanosine Diphosphate*
S RNA-β	0.60	...	0.24	0.10	1.02
S RNA-γ	0.23	0.10	0.51	0.14	0.95

	2′,3′-Ribonucleotides*						
	AMP	UMP	UMP	GMP	CMP	Number of nuclei/ chain	Weight of chain
S RNA-β	7.2	6.0	1.01	13.0	13.2	42	15,000
S RNA-γ	6.0	5.0	1.21	11.1	11.0	36	13,800

* Molar composition calculated by assuming that one terminal ribonucleoside residue corresponds to one polynucleotide chain.

Abbreviations: AMP, adenosine monophosphate; CMP, cytosine monophosphate; GMP, guanosine monophosphate; UMP, uridine monophosphate.

(After Herbert and Canellakis, 1960.)

Analytical Data on S RNA-β and S RNA-γ

We have separated, from the soluble cytoplasmic fraction of rat liver, two fractions of S RNA which we have called S RNA-β and S RNA-γ (Canellakis and Herbert, 1960a,b). The analysis of these two fractions is given in Table 1. The data on the end-group analysis (Herbert and Canellakis, 1960) presented in this table permit us to distinguish four varieties of S RNA molecules which have been schematically presented in Figure 1. These have in common a guanylic acid unit in the nucleoside diphosphate end and a variety of nucleotides at the nucleoside end. The predominant forms of S RNA are two: one has adenylic acid at the nucleoside end, while the other has guanylic acid in the nucleoside end. Nucleotide analyses indicate that there is one residue of pseudouridylic acid per chain, and that the total adenylic acid content approximates the sum of the uridylic acid and the pseudouridylic acid components, while the guanylic acid content approximates the cytidylic acid content. Some of the main points of this analysis are in agreement with the analyses presented by Zillig, Schachtsabel, and Krone (1960) and by Singer and Cantoni (1960).

Pyrophosphorolysis of the S RNA

The enzymes associated with the incorporation of ribonucleotides

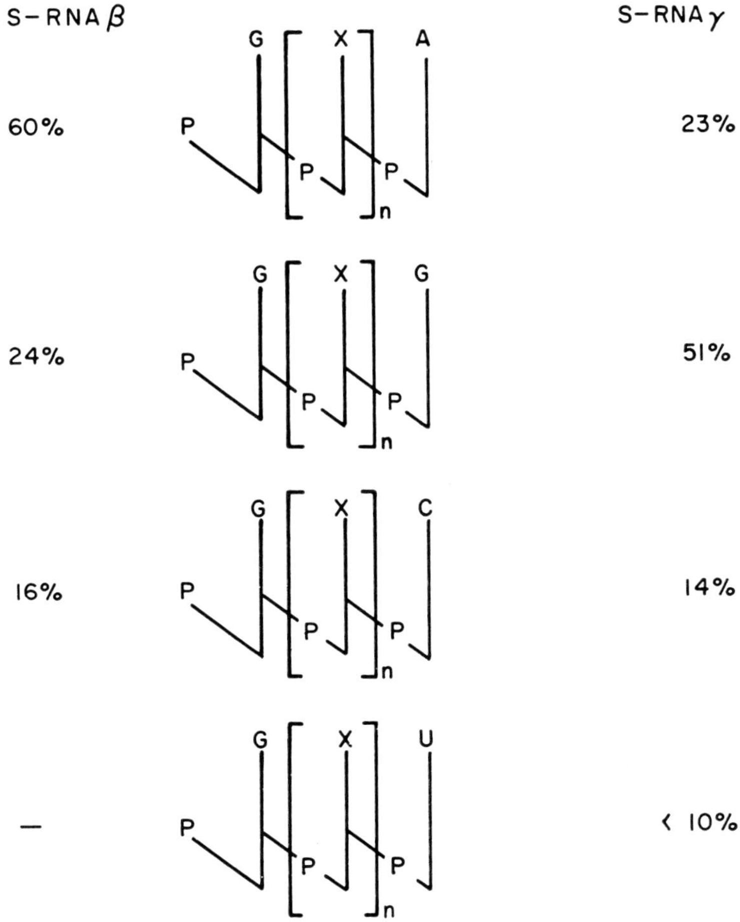

FIG. 1. Schematic presentation of the four varieties of S RNA molecules as derived from the analytical date of Table 1.

into S RNA will pyrophosphorylize the S RNA in the presence of pyrophosphate (Canellakis and Herbert, 1961), according to the equation:

$$\text{P-P} + \text{AMP-CMP-CMP-AMP-(S RNA)} \rightarrow \text{ATP} + 2\ \text{CTP} + \text{AMP-(S RNA)}$$

The pyrophosphorolysis leads to the removal of the last three ribonucleotide units and exposure of the fourth ribonucleotide, which has been identified as adenylic acid. This has been shown by the incorporation of P^{32}-cytidylic acid into pyrophosphorylized S RNA and localizing the site of attachment of the P^{32} after alkaline hydrolysis of the radioactive S RNA.

After such an experiment, we find the P^{32} equivalently distributed between cytidylic acid and adenylic acid, as would be expected from the formulation presented in Figure 2 if adenylic acid was the fourth ribonucleotide of the terminal sequence.

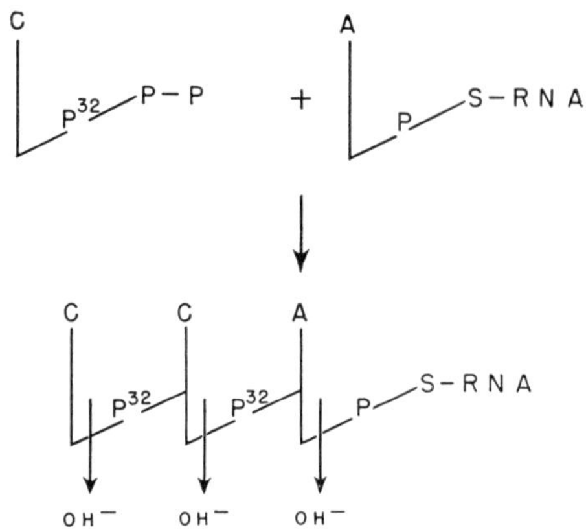

FIG. 2. Incorporation of CTP(P^{32}-P-P-) into pyrophosphorylized S RNA followed by alkaline hydrolysis of the product leads to equivalent distribution of the P^{32} between cytidylic acid and adenylic acid. (After Canellakis and Herbert, 1961.)

The Effect of Snake Venom Phosphodiesterase on the Incorporation of Ribonucleoside 5′-Monophosphates into S RNA

S RNA-β and -γ were treated with snake venom phosphodiesterase and the resultant S RNA was isolated. This S RNA was then incubated with C^{14}-labeled ATP, CTP, or UTP in the presence and absence of the complementary nonradioactive ribonucleoside 5′-triphosphates. The results obtained are presented in Table 2, together with results of control experiments performed with S RNA which had not been treated with snake venom phosphodiesterase.

The phosphodiesterase-treated S RNA had a decreased ability to accept adenylic acid, but an enhanced capacity to accept cytidylic acid and uridylic acid. When the three complementary nonradioactive ribonucleoside 5′-triphosphates were added to the various incubation mixtures, the incorporation of adenylic acid and of cytidylic acid were actually enhanced, whereas that of uridylic acid was inhibited.

These results indicate that, after the S RNA is degraded with snake venom phosphodiesterase, the composition of the incubation mixture with respect to ribonucleoside 5′-triphosphates affects the extent of incorporation of individual ribonucleotides into S RNA.

TABLE 2

Effect of Phosphodiesterase on the Incorporation of ^{14}C-ATP, CTP, and UTP into S RNA-β and S RNA-γ

	Ribonucleotide additions		Radioactive ribonucleotide incorporated* mμ moles/ mg. S RNA
	Radioactive	Nonradioactive	
(1) Normal S RNA	^{14}C-ATP	None	2.0
	^{14}C-ATP	CTP, UTP, GTP	2.68
Diesterase S RNA	^{14}C-ATP	None	0.99
	^{14}C-ATP	CTP, UTP, GTP	13.68
(2) Normal S RNA	^{14}C-CTP	None	2.2
	^{14}C-CTP	ATP, UTP, GTP	2.2
Diesterase S RNA	^{14}C-CTP	None	38.7
	^{14}C-CTP	ATP, UTP, GTP	46.0
(3) Normal S RNA	^{14}C-UTP	None	0.26
	^{14}C-UTP	CTP, GTP, ATP	0.11
Diesterase S RNA	^{14}C-UTP	None	1.8
	^{14}C-UTP	CTP, GTP, ATP	0.17

* Results recalculated on the basis of mμ moles/mg. S RNA.
Abbreviations: ATP, adenosine triphosphate; CTP, cytosine triphosphate; GTP, guanosine triphosphate; UTP, uridine triphosphate.
(After Herbert and Canellakis, 1961.)

Reconstitution of Diesterase-Treated S RNA

From the work of Zachau, Acs, and Lipmann (1958), as well as from that of Hecht, Stephenson, and Zamecnik (1959), we know that the S RNA has the unique characteristic of binding amino acids at the adenylic acid end of the molecule. This is not a random reaction, but one which is specific in that a given S RNA molecule binds specifically a certain amino acid and not others, as shown by Preiss *et al.* (1959). This specificity of S RNA for a given amino acid has been thought to reside in the nucleotide sequence of the S RNA, as has been suggested by Holley and Merrill (1959).

Previous experiments by Hecht, Stephenson, and Zamecnik (1959) had established that the pyrophosphorylized S RNA, from which the terminal nucleotides had been removed, cannot attach amino acids. In addition, these workers had shown that upon the reincorporation of AMP and CMP (from the corresponding triphosphates) into S RNA the capacity of this S RNA to accept amino acids was re-established.

The question which we tried to answer was whether we could further degrade the S RNA and still be able to reconstitute its ability to accept amino acids (Herbert and Canellakis, 1961). For this purpose we treated S RNA with snake venom phosphodiesterase, under conditions which led to the degradation of approximately 10 per cent of the S RNA; from end-group analysis of this S RNA we could confirm that a random degradation had taken place.

The results of such an experiment, shown in Table 3, indicate that degradation of the S RNA with phosphodiesterase results in a significant decrease in its capacity to accept threonine. If the degraded S RNA is pretreated with ATP its capacity to accept threonine is further decreased. But pretreatment in the presence of CTP, as well as of ATP, led to the recovery of more than 50 per cent of the original capacity to accept threonine. If the pretreatment included exposure to CTP and UTP, as well as ATP, an additional enhancement in its ability to accept threonine was noted, while pretreatment with all four ribonucleoside triphosphates resulted in almost complete reconstitution of the capacity of this partially degraded S RNA to accept threonine (93 per cent of control).

These results indicate that all four ribonucleotides are required for the reconstitution of the ability of S RNA to accept threonine. They imply that the nucleotides are incorporated into a defined sequence; this interpretation is based on the assumption that the specificity of amino acid attachment to S RNA is defined by the ribonucleotide sequence in the S RNA molecule. The results are

TABLE 3

Reconstitution of the Capacity of S RNA-β and S RNA-γ to Accept Threonine

	Pretreatment Ribonucleotide incorporating enzyme plus:	mμmoles of threonine incorporated /mg. S RNA*
Normal S RNA	0	0.17
	ATP, CTP, UTP, GTP	0.22
Diesterase-treated S RNA	0	0.058
	ATP	0.020
	ATP, CTP	0.11
	ATP, CTP, UTP	0.13
	ATP, CTP, UTP, GTP	0.197

* The results recalculated on the basis of mμmoles of threonine/mg. S RNA.

The phosphodiesterase-treated S RNA was prepared by treatment of the S RNA with snake venom phosphodiesterase, and was then isolated free of the phosphodiesterase. The pretreatment of the S RNA was carried out as follows: 0.15 ml. of S RNA-β and -γ ($E_{260}=40$) were incubated with the equivalent amount of ribonucleotide-incorporating enzyme (0.15 ml.), 1 μmole of $MgCl_2$, 0.25 μmoles of the indicated ribonucleoside 5′-triphosphate in 0.08 M potassium phosphate buffer, pH 7.2; the total volume was 0.5 ml. After incubation for 15 minutes at 37°, 0.5 ml. of a mixture containing 0.2 ml. of the amino acid-activating enzyme fractions, 0.05 μmoles of C^{14}-threonine (3.5×10^6 c.p.m. /μmole), 4 μmoles of ATP and 2 μmoles $MgCl_2$, all in the 0.08 M potassium phosphate buffer, were added to each tube and the incubation was continued for 10 minutes more at 37° C. The S RNA was then isolated, freed of contaminant radioactivity and counted.

Abbreviations: ATP, adenosine triphosphate; CTP, cytosine triphosphate; GTP, guanosine triphosphate; UTP, uridine triphosphate.

(After Herbert and Canellakis, 1961.)

unduly complicated in that we are not using a single species of S RNA as a substrate, but that we are using a preparation in which the particular S RNA molecule for which we are assaying (threonine acceptor S RNA) does not constitute more than 2 per cent of the total S RNA.

These results indicate that this approach may be a feasible one to use in the study of the biosynthesis of an S RNA molecule with a specific ribonucleotide sequence. At present, further implementation of this approach is severely limited by the impurity of our S RNA preparations.

One corollary to be drawn from these results is that the enzymes which incorporate ribonucleotides into S RNA may not be limited to the ability of incorporating these ribonucleotides into terminal positions, but may also be capable of more extensive contributions to the synthesis of S RNA. This remains to be fully established.

Nuclear Enzymes Which Incorporate Ribonucleotides into Terminal Positions of DNA

Our work on calf thymus nuclei, done in collaboration with Drs. J. S. Krakow and H. O. Kammen (Krakow and Kammen, 1960), was directed to uncovering nuclear enzyme systems associated with ribonucleic acid synthesis. During the course of these investigations, we came across a number of nuclear enzyme fractions capable of incorporating ribonucleotides into RNA, but most of these appeared to have the characteristics of the terminal ribonucleotide-incorporating enzymes which, as mentioned previously, are present in the cytoplasmic fraction. We decided to concentrate on one type of incorporation which showed some correlation to DNA.

Characteristics of the Reaction

The requirements of the reaction are as shown in Table 4. It can be seen that, in the presence of an ATP-generating system, CTP-C^{14} was incorporated optimally into an acid-insoluble form. The presence of ribonuclease (RNase) did not inhibit the reaction; however, the reaction was inhibited by the addition of deoxyribonuclease (DNase). If the acid-insoluble material into which the cytidylic acid was incorporated was treated with RNase or with alkali no radioactivity could be labilized; however, treatment of this material with DNase rendered the radioactive ribonucleotide acid-soluble.

When CTP-(P^{32}-P-P) was used as the precursor (Table 5) and the labeled DNA isolated and treated with alkali to remove any

TABLE 4

Characteristics of the Ribonucleotide-Incorporating System

Additions	mμmoles of C^{14}-CMP fixed
Complete system	0.14
Omit Mg^{++}	0.01
Omit ATP	0.02
Omit creatine kinase	0.01
Omit creatine phosphate	0.01
Plus 20 μg. RNase	0.14
Plus 20 μg. DNase	0.01
Incubate the C^{14}-acid-insoluble material with 0.3 N NaOH overnight and reisolate	0.14

The complete system contained: 20 μmoles potassium phosphate buffer, pH 7.3; 10 μmoles $MgCl_2$; 30 mμmoles ATP; 7.7 μmoles creatine phosphate; 60 μg. creatine kinase; 30 mμmoles C^{14}-CTP (2.6×10^6 c.p.m./μmole); and 0.5 ml. of the nuclear pellet, in a total of 0.9–1.0 ml. Incubation was carried out for 40 minutes at 37° C.

RNA, and this alkali-treated DNA was further hydrolyzed with pancreatic DNase and snake venom phosphodiesterase (Koerner and Sinsheimer, 1957), the radioactivity was shown to be primarily associated with 5′-CMP-P^{32}, and not with cytidine 3′,5′-diphosphate or with deoxycytidylic acid. If, instead, this radioactive DNA was treated with micrococcal nuclease (Cunningham, Catlin, and de Garilbe, 1956) and spleen diesterase (Hilmoe, 1960) according to the method of Adler *et al.* (1958), the P^{32} was found associated with all four deoxyribonucleoside 3′-phosphates.

If CTP-C^{14} was used as the precursor (Table 6) and the product, after alkali treatment, was hydrolyzed with micrococcal nuclease and spleen diesterase, the C^{14} was found associated with the cytidine.

TABLE 5

*Distribution of the Radioactivity after Hydrolysis of (CMP^{32})-DNA**

(1) Pancreatic DNase and snake venom diesterase	
	Per cent
dCMP	0
5′-CMP	80
Unidentified	
3′,5′-CDP	0
(2) With micrococcal nuclease and spleen diesterase	
	Per cent
3′-dAMP	28
3′-dGMP	33
3′-dCMP	19
3′-dTMP	20

* The CMP^{32}-DNA was incubated with 0.3 N NaOH at 37° C overnight prior to isolation and enzymatic degradation.

Abbreviations: CMP, cytosine monophosphate; dAMP, deoxyadenosine monophosphate; dCMP, deoxycytosine monophosphate; dGMP, deoxyguanosine monophosphate; dTMP, deoxylhymidine monophosphate.

TABLE 6

*Distribution of Radioactivity after Hydrolysis of (C^{14}-CMP)-DNA with Micrococcal DNase and Spleen Diesterase**

	Per cent
Cytidine	95
3′-d CMP	5
3′-d TMP	1
3′-d GMP	1
3′-d AMP	1

* The (C^{14}-CMP)-DNA was incubated with 0.3 N NaOH at 37° C overnight prior to isolation and enzymatic degradation.
Abbreviations: AMP, adenosine monophosphate; CMP, cytosine monophosphate; GMP, guanosine monophosphate; TMP, thymidine monophosphate.

We shall now interpret these results in order to establish the type of incorporation with which we had been dealing. If the cytidylic acid is incorporated into a nonterminal position of the DNA chain (Figure 3), then regardless of the type of sugar substituent on the nucleotide attached adjacently, treatment with alkali would cleave along the arrow (because of the free 2′-OH group of the cytidylic acid), leaving an exposed 3′-terminal phosphate on the exposed radioactive cytidylic acid. Treatment of this with snake venom phosphodiesterase would yield C^{14} 3′,5′-cytidine diphosphate, whereas treatment with spleen diesterase would yield the C^{14}-

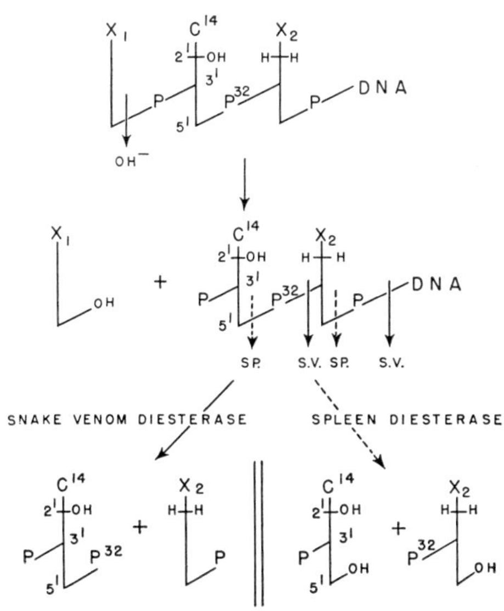

FIG. 3. The type of degradation products that would be expected if the radioactive ribonucleotide were incorporated into nonterminal postions of DNA. Sp. = Spleen diesterase; S.V. = Snake venom phosphodiesterase.

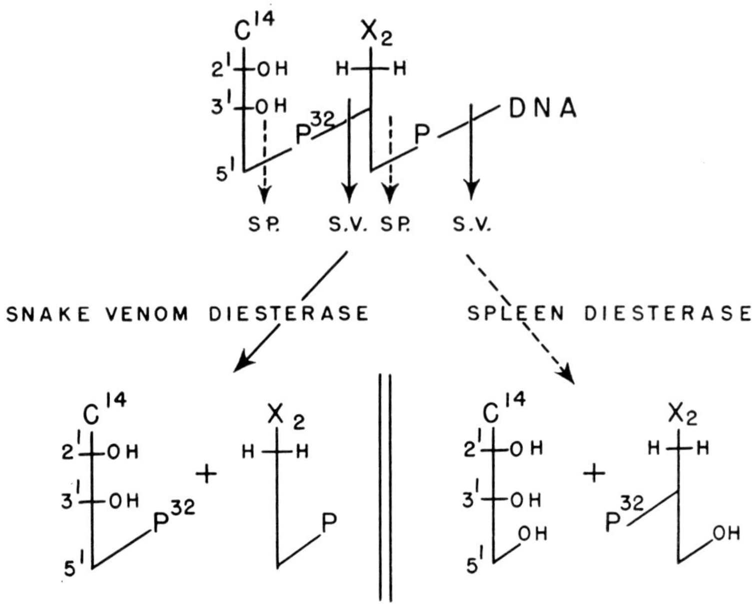

FIG. 4. The type of degradation products that would be expected if the ribonucleotides were incorporated into terminal positions of DNA. Sp. = Spleen diesterase; S. V. = Snake venom phosphodiesterase.

labeled cytidine 3′-phosphate. Since these results were not obtained experimentally, we may conclude that the incorporation of the cytidylic acid did not occur in the inner portion of the DNA chain.

If the ribonucleotide was incorporated in a terminal position, the results indicated in Figure 4 would have been obtained. The incorporated radioactive cytidylic acid would be stable to alkali, as in the previous case, snake venom phosphodiesterase would yield 5′-cytidylic acid (C^{14}- or P^{32}-labeled), while spleen diesterase would yield C^{14}-cytidine and the P^{32} attached to the neighboring deoxyribonucleotide. Since the mechanism shown in Figure 4 is in agreement with our experimental findings, it can be concluded that the cytidylic acid is incorporated in the DNA in a terminal position.

Requirements of the Reaction

This terminal labeling of the DNA can be modified only slightly (Table 7). When the complementary ribonucleoside triphosphates are added to the incubation mixture, only 2 per cent of the ribonucleotide incorporated into DNA becomes nonterminal. However, if the complementary deoxyribonucleoside triphosphates are added,

TABLE 7

Effect of the Complementary Nucleoside-Triphosphates on the Terminal Incorporation of C^{14}-GTP into DNA

Substrate	Terminal per cent	Nonterminal per cent
C^{14}-GTP	100	0
C^{14}-GTP plus ATP, UTP, CTP	98	2
C^{14}-GTP plus dATP, dUTP, dCTP	87	13

Abbreviations: ATP, adenosine triphosphate; CTP, cytosine triphosphate; dATP, deoxyadenosine triphosphate; dCTP, deoxycytosine monophosphate; dUTP, deoxyuridine triphosphate; GTP, guanosine triphosphate; UTP, uridine triphosphate.

13 per cent of the incorporated ribonucleotide becomes nonterminal.

The enzyme has been freed of nuclear DNA and the reaction can be shown to be dependent upon the presence of added DNA. All four ribonucleoside triphosphates will serve as precursors in this reaction; GTP appears to be incorporated most extensively and UTP the least. The purification procedure followed indicates that it is possible to remove DNA polymerase activity, while maintaining intact the ribonucleotide-incorporating activity.

Comparison to Other Enzyme Systems

This reaction, observed in extracts of calf thymus nuclei, bears the obvious similarity to that observed by Hurwitz (1959) in *Escherichia coli* extracts in that a ribonucleotide is incorporated into DNA; however, it differs in certain significant respects.

The thymus enzyme does not require the presence of the complementary deoxyribonucleoside triphosphates, as does the *E. coli* enzyme; in effect, it is inhibited in their presence. In addition, our results indicate that the extent of incorporation is not affected by the removal of a large portion of the DNA polymerase activity; in contrast, the *E. coli* enzyme is dependent upon the presence of the DNA polymerase. Finally, the thymus enzyme seems to incorporate ribonucleotides predominantly into terminal positions of the DNA; this does not appear to be a characteristic of the *E. coli* enzyme because the product synthesized by the *E. coli* enzyme is partially labile to RNase and to alkali, circumstances which imply that more than one ribonucleotide-diester linkage is formed on the same DNA chain.

These results are also reminiscent of the previously described terminal incorporation of ribonucleotides into S RNA, although there are certain obvious differences. It is hoped that we can now establish whether the similarities are more than superficial.

SUMMARY

An enzyme preparation from rat liver is described which catalyzes the incorporation of ribonucleotides into terminal positions of S RNA. The main features of this reaction are outlined. From this study it has become apparent that the fourth ribonucleotide in the S RNA of rat liver is adenylic acid. In addition, it is indicated that this enzyme preparation will reconstitute the ability of diesterase-degraded S RNA to accept amino acids.

An enzyme preparation from calf thymus nuclei is described which incorporates single ribonucleotides into terminal positions of DNA. Evidence is presented which permits us to establish unequivocally that single ribonucleotides are incorporated. The relationship of this reaction to others described in the literature is discussed.

ABBREVIATIONS

Abbreviations used in this paper are as follows: ADP, adenosine diphosphate; AMP, adenosine monophosphate; ATP, adenosine triphosphate; CDP, cytosine diphosphate; CMP, cytosine monophosphate; CTP, cytosine triphosphate; dAMP, deoxyadenosine monophosphate; dATP, deoxyadenosine triphosphate; dCMP, deoxycytosine monophosphate; dCTP, deoxycytosine triphosphate; DNA, deoxyribonucleic acid; DNase, deoxyribonuclease; dGMP, deoxyguanosine monophosphate; dTMP, deoxythymidine monophosphate; dUTP, deoxyuridine triphosphate; GMP, guanosine monophosphate; GTP, guanosine triphosphate; RNA, ribonucleic acid; RNase, ribonuclease; S RNA, soluble RNA; UMP; uridine monophosphate; UTP, uridine triphosphate.

REFERENCES

Adler, J., I. R. Lehman, M. J. Bessman, E. S. Simms, and A. Kornberg. 1958. Enzymatic Synthesis of Deoxyribonucleic Acid. IV. Linkage of Single Deoxynucleotides to the Deoxynucleoside Ends of Deoxyribonucleic Acid. *Proceedings of the National Academy of Sciences in the U.S.A.*, 44:641–647.

Allfrey, V. G., and A. E. Mirsky. 1957. Some Aspects of Ribonucleic Acid Synthesis in Isolated Cell Nuclei. *Proceedings of the National Academy of Sciences of the U.S.A.*, 43:821–826.

Canellakis, E. S. 1957. On the Mechanism of Incorporation of Adenylic Acid from Adenosine Triphosphate into Ribonucleic Acid by Soluble Mammalian Enzymes. *Biochimica et biophysica acta*, 25:217–218.

———. 1959. Mechanisms Involved in the Biosynthesis of Ribonucleic Acids. *Annals of the New York Academy of Sciences*, 81:675–678.

Canellakis, E. S., and E. Herbert. 1960a. Studies on S-RNA Synthesis. I. Purification and General Characteristics of the RNA-Enzyme Complex. *Proceedings of the National Academy of Sciences of the U.S.A.*, 46:170–178.

———. 1960b. Studies on S-RNA Synthesis. II. Assay and Method of

Purification of S-RNA α, β, and γ. *Biochimica et biophysica acta*, 45:133.

———. 1961. S-RNA Synthesis. IV. The Effect of Inorganic Pyrophosphate and a Method of Extraction of S-RNA. *Biochimica et biophysica acta*, 47:78–85.

Cunningham, L., B. W. Catlin, and M. P. de Garilbe. 1956. A Deoxyribonuclease of *Micrococcus pyogenes*. *Journal of the American Chemical Society*, 78:4642–4645.

Grunberg-Manago, M., and S. Ochoa. 1955. Enzymatic Synthesis and Breakdown of Polynucleotides; Polynucleotide Phosphorylase. *Journal of the American Chemical Society*, 77:3165–3166.

Hecht, L. I., M. L. Stephenson, and P. C. Zamecnik. 1959. Binding of Amino Acids to the End Group of a Soluble Ribonucleic Acid. *Proceedings of the National Academy of Sciences of the U.S.A.*, 45:505–518.

Hecht, L. I., P. C. Zamecnik, M. L. Stephenson, and J. F. Scott. 1958. Nucleoside Triphosphates as Precursors of Ribonucleic Acid End Groups in a Mammalian System. *Journal of Biological Chemistry*, 233:954–963.

Heidelberger, C., E. Harbers, K. C. Leibman, Y. Takagi, and V. R. Potter. 1956. Specific Incorporation of Adenosine-5′-Phosphate-^{32}P into Ribonucleic Acid of Rat Liver Homogenates. *Biochimica et biophysica acta*, 20:445–446.

Herbert, E. 1958. The Incorporation of Adenine Nucleotides into Ribonucleic Acid of Cell-Free Systems from Liver. *Journal of Biological Chemistry*, 231:975–986.

Herbert, E., and E. S. Canellakis. 1960. Studies on Synthesis of Soluble Ribonucleic Acid. III. Analytical Studies on Soluble Ribonucleic Acid of Rat Liver. *Biochimica et biophysica acta*, 42:363–364.

———. 1961. S-RNA Synthesis. V. Reconstruction of a Biological Property of Phosphodiesterase-Treated Soluble Ribonucleic Acid. *Biochimica et biophysica acta*, 47:85–92.

Hilmoe, R. J. 1960. Purification and Properties of Spleen Phosphodiesterase. *Journal of Biological Chemistry*, 235:2117–2121.

Holley, R. W., and S. H. Merrill. 1959. Countercurrent Distribution of an Active Ribonucleic Acid. *Journal of the American Chemical Society*, 81:753.

Hurwitz, J. 1959. The Enzymatic Incorporation of Ribonucleotides into Polydeoxyribonucleotide Material. *Journal of Biological Chemistry*, 234:2351–2358.

Koerner, J. F., and R. L. Sinsheimer. 1957. A Deoxyribonuclease from Calf Spleen. II. Mode of Action. *Journal of Biological Chemistry*, 228:1049–1062.

Krakow, J. S., and H. O. Kammen. 1960. The Incorporation of Ribonucleotides and Deoxyribonucleotides into Fractions of Calf Thymus Nuclei. (Abstract) *Federation Proceedings*, 19:307.

Preiss, J., P. Berg, E. J. Ofengand, F. H. Bergman, and M. Dieckmann. 1959. The Chemical Nature of the RNA-Amino Acid Compound Formed by Amino-Acid Activating Enzymes. *Proceedings of the National Academmy of Sciences of the U.S.A.*, 45:319–328.

Singer, M. F., and G. L. Cantoni. 1960. Studies on Soluble Ribonucleic Acid of Rabbit Liver. Terminal Groups and Nucleotide Composition. *Biochimica et biophysica acta*, 39:182–183.

Zachau, H. G., G. Acs, and F. Lipmann. 1958. Isolation of Adenosine Amino Acid Esters From a Ribonuclease Digest of Soluble Liver Ribonucleic Acid.

Proceedings of the National Academy of Sciences of the U.S.A., 44:885–889.

Zillig, W., D. Schachtsabel and W. Krone. 1960. Untersuchungen zur Biosynthese der Proteine. IV. Zusammensetzung, Funktion und Spezifität der Loslichen Ribonucleinsaure aus *Escherichia coli*. *Zeitschrift für Physiologische Chemie*, 318:100–114.

Nucleotide Sequences in Enzymatically Synthesized Deoxyribonucleic Acid

JOHN JOSSE, M.D.

Department of Biochemistry, Stanford University School of Medicine, Palo Alto, California

A body of convincing evidence has now accumulated which indicates that, except in certain of the viruses, deoxyribonucleic acid (DNA) is the genetic substance (Avery, MacLeod, and McCarty, 1944; Hotchkiss, 1957; Hershey, 1953). If this is the case, there must be means within the cell not only for the precise replication of DNA but also for the specific direction of protein synthesis by information carried in the DNA molecules, presumably in the sequences of nucleotides in the polynucleotide chains. An enzymatic mechanism for the replication of DNA has been described and characterized by Kornberg and associates (Kornberg, 1960). The problem of how DNA directs the synthesis of proteins remains unsolved. One approach to this problem presents the question, "How do the arrangements of the four (or more) bases in a polynucleotide chain of DNA determine or code the arrangements of the 20 amino acids in a peptide chain of protein?" This question, known as the coding problem, has been considered in its theoretical aspects by several workers (Gamow, Rich, and Ycas, 1956; Crick, 1958, 1959; Brenner, 1957; Golomb, Welch, and Delbrück, 1958; Sinsheimer, 1959). A direct and empirical attack on the coding problem is difficult for several reasons, the most obvious of which is the lack of an analytic method for determining nucleotide sequences in DNA. A genetic method which bypasses this chemical difficulty is correlation of genetic fine structure with protein amino acid sequences; investigations of this sort are being carried out in several laboratories on bacterial and bacteriophage systems (Yanofsky, 1960; Levinthal, 1959; Garen, 1960; Brenner and Barnett, 1959; Dreyer, unpublished material. However, for the ultimate solution to the coding problem in terms of nucleotides and amino acids, some form of chemical definition of nucleotide sequences in DNA would seem necessary.

At the present time little is known about sequences of nucleotides in DNA. One approach to this problem is that of partially degrading DNA, either by enzymatic or chemical means, and then studying the nature of the degradation products. Sinsheimer (1954, 1955) has identified several of the products of the digestion of calf thymus and wheat germ DNA's by pancreatic deoxyribonuclease (DNase); the average size of the limit product in these cases is a tetranucleotide. Laskowski and associates have carried out similar studies on the digestion of calf thymus DNA by pancreatic DNase and by streptococcal DNase (de Garilhe, Cunningham, Laurila, and Laskowski, 1957; Potter and Laskowski, 1959). Using micrococcal DNase, Rushizky and coworkers have studied the digestion of calf thymus DNA and have recovered 95 per cent of the material in the form of mono-, di-, and trinucleotides (Rushizky, Knight, Roberts, and Dekker, 1960). In studies of this sort, the nature of the degradative product obtained is a function of the specificity of the enzyme employed as well as of the structure of the DNA being digested. Acid degradation studies of various DNA's have been carried out by Shapiro and Chargaff, and by Burton and Peterson; these studies have given information on the relative frequencies of a pyrimidine nucleotide flanked on both sides by purine nucleotides and on the frequencies of short runs of pyrimidine nucleotides in the polynucleotide chains. These workers were able to deduce that there is a nonrandom arrangement of pyrimidine nucleotides in all of the DNA samples examined (Shapiro and Chargaff, 1957, 1960; Burton and Peterson, 1960; Burton, 1960).

By use of a technique of enzymatic degradation of P^{32}-labeled, enzymatically synthesized DNA into 3′-nucleotides we have been able to determine the relative frequencies with which one nucleotide locates next to another in the DNA chains and in this way study the patterns of the 16 possible nearest neighbor or dinucleotide sequences in a variety of DNA's. The results not only give information about the positioning of nucleotides in the DNA chains, but offer experimental support for certain aspects of the Watson-Crick model of DNA and the mechanism of replication of such a model during the enzymatic synthesis of DNA by the polymerase of *Escherichia coli* (Watson and Crick, 1953; Kornberg, 1960).

METHODS

The experiments were designed in the following way. DNA was synthesized using a purified fraction of *E. coli* polymerase, a particular primer DNA, and all four deoxynucleoside-5′-triphosphates, one of which was labeled with P^{32} in the phosphate esterified to the sugar. As shown in Figure 1, during the synthetic reaction this P^{32} atom becomes the bridge between the nucleoside of that labeled triphosphate (Y) and the nearest neighbor nucleotide (X) at the growing end of the polynucleotide chain with which it has reacted. After synthesis, during which of the order of 10^{15} such linkages were formed, the DNA was isolated and then enzymatically hydrolyzed by the consecutive actions of micrococcal DNase and calf

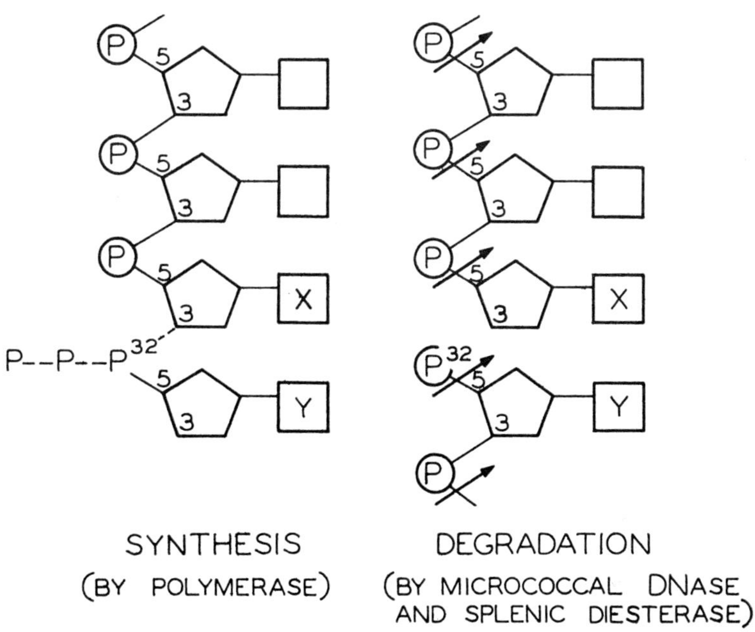

FIG. 1. Synthesis of a P^{32}-labeled deoxyribonucleic acid chain and its subsequent enzymatic degradation to 3′-deoxyribonucleotides. The arrows indicate the linkages split by micrococcal deoxyribonuclease and calf spleen phosphodiesterase, yielding a digest composed exclusively of 3′-deoxyribonucleotides.

TABLE 1

Nearest Neighbor Frequencies of Mycobacterium phlei *Deoxyribonucleic Acid*

Reaction no.	Labeled triphosphate	Isolated 3′-deoxyribonucleotide			
		Tp	Ap	Cp	Gp
1	$dATP^{32}$	a TpA .012	b ApA .024 I	c CpA .063 II	d GpA .065 III
2	$dTTP^{32}$	b TpT .026 I	a ApT .031	d CpT .045 IV	c GpT .060 V
3	$dGTP^{32}$	e TpG .063 II	f ApG .045 IV	g CpG .139	h GpG .090 VI
4	$dCTP^{32}$	f TpC .061 III	e ApC .064 V	h CpC .090 VI	g GpC .122
	Sums	.162	.164	.337	.337

These data: Ap + Tp/Gp + Cp=0.48.
Chemical analysis of primer: A + T/G + C=0.49.
As described in the text, identical Roman numerals designate those sequence frequencies which should be equivalent in a Watson-Crick DNA model with strands of opposite polarity; identical lower case letters designate sequence frequencies which should be equivalent in a model with strands of similar polarity.

spleen phosphodiesterase. These enzymes hydrolyze the bonds between phosphate and the 5-carbon of deoxyribose, leaving as products 3′-mononucleotides (Figure 1). Thus the P^{32} now labels the deoxyribose 3-carbon of that nucleotide in the chains with which the labeled triphosphate substrate reacted. The P^{32} content of each of the four 3′-mononucleotides, isolated by paper electrophoresis of the digest, is then a measure of the relative frequency with which the nucleotide, originally labeled in the 5′ position (as a deoxynucleoside-5′-triphosphate), locates next to another nucleotide in the synthesized polynucleotide chains. It is essential that the digestion to 3′-mononucleotides be complete and that the electrophoretic separations and subsequent recoveries be quantitative. This procedure may be carried out four times for each type DNA primer, using a different labeled triphosphate each time; in this way one may determine the relative frequencies of all 16 possible nearest neighbor or dinucleotide sequences in the synthesized DNA. This experimental procedure is described in detail elsewhere (Josse, Kaiser, and Kornberg, 1961).

Results

Nearest Neighbor Frequency Patterns

The data from such a series of four experiments can be assembled as illustrated in Table 1, which lists the results obtained when the primer DNA was derived from *Mycobacterium phlei*. In the first row, for example, are indicated the relative frequencies with which the P^{32} label originally 5′ to deoxyadenosine in $dATP^{32}$ distributes to each of the four 3′-mononucleotides after digestion. These numbers, therefore, represent the relative frequencies of the designated dinucleotide sequences in the enzymatically synthesized *M. phlei* DNA. It can be seen at once that all 16 of the possible nearest neighbor sequences are present in this DNA, and, further, that they occur with widely varying frequencies. Other nearest neighbor frequencies obtained with a variety of DNA primers are listed in Tables 2, 3, and 4.

Nonrandom Nature of Nearest Neighbor Frequencies in Enzymatically Synthesized DNA

The nearest neighbor frequencies obtained for all of the DNA's examined by this method, including those listed in Tables 1 to 4, are not those predicted by random ordering of the nucleotides in the DNA chains. For example, in *M. phlei* DNA (Table 1) the

TABLE 2

Nearest Neighbor Frequencies of Calf Thymus Deoxyribonucleic Acids

Nearest neighbor sequence	Native calf thymus DNA	Enzymatically synthesized "calf thymus" DNA*
ApA, TpT	.089, .087	.088, .083
CpA, TpG	.080, .076	.078, .076
GpA, TpC	.064, .067	.063, .064
CpT, ApG	.067, .072	.068, .074
GpT, ApC	.056, .052	.056, .051
GpG, CpC	.050, .054	.057, .055
TpA	.053	.059
ApT	.073	.075
CpG	.016	.011
GpC	.044	.042

* Only 5 per cent of this DNA is the native calf thymus primer; its synthesis is described in the text.

TABLE 3

Nearest Neighbor Frequencies of Bacterial Deoxyribonucleic Acids

Nearest neighbor sequence	*M. lysodeikticus* DNA (0.41)*	*M. phlei* DNA (0.48)	*A. aerogenes* DNA (0.80)	*E. coli* DNA (1.01)	*B. subtilis* DNA (1.26)	*H. influenzae* DNA (1.62)
ApA, TpT	.019, .017	.024, .026	.059, .061	.071, .076	.092, .095	.116, .116
CpA, TpG	.052, .054	.063, .063	.067, .069	.071, .071	.067, .068	.067, .067
GpA, TpC	.065, .063	.065, .061	.058, .057	.055, .056	.067, .065	.054, .052
CpT, ApG	.050, .049	.045, .045	.057, .056	.055, .055	.057, .058	.049, .050
GpT, ApC	.056, .057	.060, .064	.052, .052	.055, .054	.048, .048	.048, .049
GpG, CpC	.112, .113	.090, .090	.067, .065	.056, .056	.046, .046	.036, .037
TpA	.011	.012	.036	.051	.052	.073
ApT	.022	.031	.053	.068	.080	.095
CpG	.139	.139	.088	.067	.050	.038
GpC	.121	.122	.103	.083	.061	.053

* The numbers in parentheses are the $\frac{Ap + Tp}{Gp + Cp}$ ratios for each DNA.

TABLE 4

Nearest Neighbor Frequencies of Bacteriophage Deoxyribonucleic Acids

Nearest neighbor sequence	λ^+ DNA (1.00)*	λ dg DNA (1.00)	T2 DNA (1.74)	T4 DNA (1.80)	T6 DNA (1.74)
ApA, TpT	.069, .073	.072, .074	.111, .106	.109, .109	.106, .108
CpA, TpG	.070, .069	.070, .070	.061, .063	.061, .063	.062, .062
GpA, TpC	.060, .064	.059, .061	.059, .057	.059, .059	.059, .058
CpT, ApG	.056, .053	.056, .053	.054, .057	.056, .057	.058, .060
GpT, ApC	.054, .054	.054, .055	.051, .048	.052, .049	.051, .050
GpG, CpC	.062, .063	.057, .056	.036, .034	.035, .032	.034, .033
TpA	.047	.047	.089	.091	.090
ApT	.070	.068	.104	.105	.101
CpG	.064	.069	.030	.027	.028
GpC	.072	.079	.040	.036	.040

* The numbers in parentheses are the $\frac{Ap + Tp}{Gp + Cp}$ ratios for each DNA.

frequency of TpA in the first row (0.012) is less than one-half that of sequence ApT in the second row (0.031). A random assembly of nucleotides in the chains would dictate that these two sequences have identical frequencies. The data of each experiment have been statistically analyzed, and in every case there is significant and in some cases very striking deviation from the nearest neighbor frequencies predicted by random arrangement of the mononucleotides (Josse, Kaiser, and Kornberg, 1961). Some general conformity to arrangements expected from the nucleotide composition of the DNA is observed and is more marked in certain of the DNA's, e.g., in the T-even bacteriophages (Table 4); yet sequence frequencies for each DNA sample tested are unique and distinctly nonrandom in character.

Nearest Neighbor Sequence Data and Its Bearing on the Structure and Replication Mechanism of DNA

It can be seen in the sums of the nucleotide columns of Table 1 that there is an equivalence of deoxyadenylate and deoxythymidylate and also of deoxyguanylate and deoxycytidylate as expected in DNA and, furthermore, that the Ap + Tp/Gp + Cp ratio obtained from these data (0.48) is very similar to the A + T/G + C ratio obtained from independent base analysis of the native primer DNA (0.49) (Lehman *et al.*, 1958).

According to the Watson-Crick model of DNA, two polynucleotide chains of opposite polarity are wound about a central axis and held together by hydrogen bonds between adenine and thymine and between guanine and cytosine (Watson and Crick, 1953). In replication of such a model it was proposed that each of the two strands could serve as a template for the formation of new polynucleotide chains, the alignment of the bases in the new chains being mediated by the same hydrogen-bonding forces (Figure 2). This

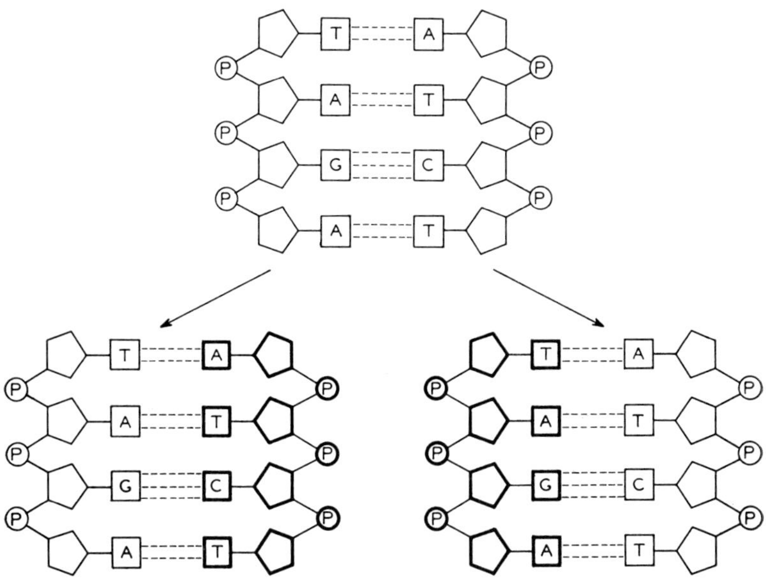

FIG. 2. Proposed scheme of replication of a Watson-Crick deoxyribonucleic acid model. Bold-lined polynucleotide chains of the two daughter molecules represent newly synthesized strands.

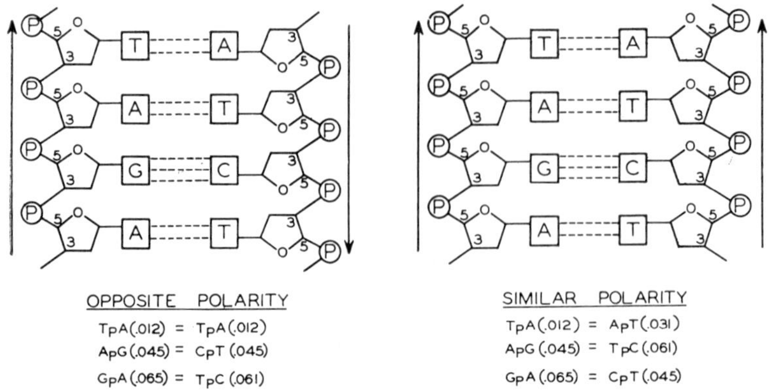

FIG. 3. Contrast of a Watson-Crick deoxyribonucleic acid (DNA) model with strands of opposite polarity, with a model with strands of similar polarity. The predicted matching nearest neighbor sequence frequencies are different. Values in parentheses are sequence frequencies from the experiment using *Mycobacterium phlei* DNA. (The strands represented here are the newly synthesized strands of Figure 2; for ease of comparison they are aligned as though complementary strands of the same double helix.)

postulated scheme allows for precise replication since one parent helix gives rise to two daughter helices identical to one another and to the parent molecule. This replication scheme, however, makes definite predictions about the pattern of nearest neighbor sequences found in DNA.

For example, the frequencies of ApA and TpT sequences should be equivalent, and so should the frequencies of GpG and CpC sequences; the data in Table 1 agree with this predicted equivalence. In examining the pairing of other sequences, it is essential to recognize that the results expected are distinctly different, depending upon whether the strands of the double helix are of similar or opposite polarity. The short strands illustrated in Figure 3 contrast strands of opposite polarity with strands of similar polarity. The matching sequences predicted by the two models are different.

In the model with opposite polarity, six matching sequences are predicted; they are indicated in Table 1 by the same Roman numeral. In each instance the agreement is good. The four values along the diagonal, which separates the data into two symmetrical halves, are independent and cannot be checked. In other words, every TpA sequence would be matched by a TpA sequence in the complementary strand of opposite polarity; the same constraint would apply to ApT, CpG, and GpC sequences.

In the model with strands of similar polarity, the 16 nearest neighbor sequence frequencies would fall into eight pairs of matching values, indicated in Table 1 by the same lower case letter. Excluding the ApA, TpT, CpC, and GpG sequences, which match similarly in both models, it is evident that in only two out of six instances are the values reasonably close. Statistical analysis of the data confirms good fit to the model of opposite polarity but significant deviation from the model of similar polarity (Josse, Kaiser, and Kornberg, 1961).

Nearest Neighbor Sequence Frequencies of DNA Synthesized Using a Native Versus an Enzymatically Prepared Primer

The sequence frequencies measured by this technique are those of the newly synthesized DNA. That they reflect an identical pattern in the native DNA used to prime in the synthetic reaction was tested in the following way. Enzymatically synthesized calf thymus DNA primer was prepared by the incubation of polymerase, native calf thymus DNA, and a large amount of the four deoxynucleoside-5′-triphosphates, all unlabeled. After an interval of six hours, the product isolated represented a twentyfold net synthesis over the amount of native calf thymus DNA originally added. A small portion of this product, in which only 5 per cent of the DNA consisted of the native calf thymus primer, was used as primer in a typical sequence analysis procedure. The results are compared with those obtained using the native calf thymus DNA as primer (Table 2). It may be seen that the nearest neighbor frequency patterns of the two DNA's are virtually identical. Whether enzymatically synthesized strands or native strands prime the reaction, the pattern of sequences found is the same. These results support the conclusion that the sequence frequencies observed in enzymatically synthesized DNA are the same as those in the native DNA primer.

Nearest Neighbor Frequencies of Bacterial and Bacteriophage DNA's

Table 3 lists the sequence frequencies obtained with six bacterial DNA's of differing base composition; Table 4 lists the sequence frequencies of the DNA's of five different coliphages. Like the data in Tables 1 and 2, these results agree closely with the base-pairing and opposite polarity of strands demanded by the Watson-Crick model. The results, while showing an over-all influence by the nucleotide composition, are not predictable by random arrangements of the nucleotides. It may be seen at once that the frequencies for the DNA's of the closely related temperate λ phages and their lysogenic host are very similar. Also it is apparent that the values for the T-even phages are virtually indistinguishable from one another, as might be expected from their intimate genetic relationship, and further that the values for these virulent phages are strikingly different from those of the host cell DNA.

Discussion

The current results on the nearest neighbor frequencies provide the clearest evidence for a mechanism of enzymatic synthesis of DNA involving the sequential ordering of nucleotides along a DNA template on the basis of hydrogen bonding of adenine to thymine and of guanine to cytosine. In addition, these results provide the first proof that the strands of the double helix have the opposite polarity postulated in the Watson-Crick model.

It should be pointed out, however, that this technique has definite limitations which restrict its general applicability to the problem of nucleotide sequence analysis. First, the method, as currently employed yields information only on dinucleotide sequence frequencies. Adaptations of the technique, substituting partial rather than total degradation of the P^{32}-labeled, enzymatically synthesized DNA, might allow some probing at trinucleotide or longer sequences, providing that adequate methods for separating and identifying these larger fragments become available. Second, the method fails to distinguish sequences involving the uncommon nucleotides, such as 5-methyldeoxycytidylate in calf thymus DNA. Finally, there are limitations in the accuracy of the analyses. An analytic error of as little as 1 per cent in the method would permit a relatively large number of errors to be made. For example, even the small chromosome of λ phage, containing about 10^5 nearest neighbor sequences, could differ from a related DNA in 1,000 nucleotide sequences without any difference being detectable by this technique.

Some of the differences and likenesses of nearest neighbor frequency patterns of different DNA's are quite striking. The genetically closely related T-even bacteriophages have virtually identical patterns which, in turn, are markedly different from that of the host cell *E. coli* DNA. Conversely, the sequence patterns of DNA's of the temperate phages λ and λdg are not readily distinguishable from that of *E. coli* DNA. The closely associated chromosomes of a prophage and its host cell might be expected to exhibit certain similarities in the structure of their DNA's. It is of interest that the DNA's of calf thymus and *Bacillus subtilis*, while indistinguishable on the basis of over-all nucleotide composition (similar Ap + Tp/Gp + Cp ratios), have grossly dissimilar nearest neighbor frequency patterns; this difference is not surprising in view of the lack of genetic similarity between the widely differing bovine and *Bacillus* species.

Just how do these data bear upon the coding problem? While we have learned something about the way nucleotides tend to locate next to one another in the chains of different DNA's, this information has thus far shed no light on the relationship between nucleotide sequences in nucleic acid and amino acid alignments in protein, if, indeed, such a relationship does exist. We are hopeful that the development of more refined enzymatic and chemical means of systematically degrading nucleic acids will allow a more complete analysis of nucleotide sequences in these polymers.

Summary

The technique of nearest neighbor sequence analysis has yielded the frequencies of the 16 possible nearest neighbor arrangements of the four deoxyribonucleotides in the chains of DNA. Samples of DNA from viral, bacterial, and animal sources were used as primers and led to the synthesis of products which in each case had a unique and nonrandom pattern of all 16 nearest neighbor sequence frequencies. The pattern of sequence frequencies was the same in DNA synthesized with native calf thymus DNA or with enzymatically prepared primer containing only traces of the original native DNA, indicating that the sequence frequencies observed in enzymatically synthesized DNA are a true reflection of identical sequences in the native DNA primer. The distribution of sequence frequencies in all DNA samples examined indicates that the mechanism of enzymatic synthesis, and, by inference, the native DNA structure, is based upon base-pairing of adenine to thymine and of guanine to cytosine; the results also furnish experimental evidence for opposite polarity of the two strands of the double helix as suggested by Watson and Crick in their model of DNA.

Acknowledgments

The work reported here was done with the guidance and help of Drs. Arthur Kornberg and A. D. Kaiser.

I am grateful for a fellowship from the National Foundation and for current support as a Scholar of the American Cancer Society. The work of this laboratory was made possible by Grants 2G 196 and E 3100 from the United States Public Health Service.

ABBREVIATIONS

Abbreviations used in this paper are as follows: A, T, G, C for the bases adenine, thymine, guanine, and cytosine, respectively; $dATP^{32}$, $dTTP^{32}$, $dGTP^{32}$, and $dCTP^{32}$ for triphosphates containing P^{32} at the phosphate esterified to the sugar; DNA for deoxyribonucleic acid; DNase for deoxyribonuclease; nucleotide for deoxyribonucleotide.

The notation employed for the structure of nucleotides and polynucleotides is that recommended by the Journal of Biological Chemistry.

REFERENCES

Avery, O. T., C. M. MacLeod, and M. McCarty. 1944. Studies on the Chemical Nature of the Substance Inducing Transformation of Pnuemococcal Types. Induction of Transformation by a Desoxyribonucleic Acid Fraction Isolated from Pneumococcus Type III. *Journal of Experimental Medicine*, 79:137–158.

Brenner, S. 1957. On the Impossibility of All Overlapping Triplet Codes in Information Transfer from Nucleic Acid to Proteins. *Proceedings of the National Academy of Sciences of the U.S.A.*, 43:687–694.

Brenner, S., and L. Barnett. 1959. "Genetic and Chemical Studies on the Head Protein of Bacteriophages T2 and T4," *Structure and Function of Genetic Elements* (Brookhaven Symposia in Biology, No. 12), pp. 86–94. Upton, New York: Brookhaven National Laboratory.

Burton, K. 1960. Frequencies of Nucleotide Sequences in Deoxyribonucleic Acids. *Biochemical Journal*, 77:547–552.

Burton, K., and G. B. Peterson. 1960. The Frequencies of Certain Sequences of Nucleotides in Deoxyribonucleic Acid. *Biochemical Journal*, 75:17–27.

Crick, F. H. C. 1958. "On Protein Synthesis," *The Biological Replication of Macromolecules* (Symposia of the Society for Experimental Biology, No. 12), pp. 138–163. New York, New York: Academic Press, Inc.

———. 1959. "The Present Position of the Coding Problem," *Structure and Function of Genetic Elements* (Brookhaven Symposia in Biology, No. 12), pp. 35–39. Upton, New York: Brookhaven National Laboratory.

de Garilhe, M. P., L. Cunningham, U. Laurila, and M. Laskowski. 1957. Studies on Isomeric Dinucleotides Derived from Deoxyribonucleic Acid. *Journal of Biological Chemistry*, 224:751–758.

Gamow, G., A. Rich, and M. Ycas. 1956. "The Problem of Information Transfer from the Nucleic Acids to Proteins," *Advances in Biological and Medical Physics*, J. H. Lawrence and C. A. Tobias, Eds., Vol. 4, pp. 23–68. New York, New York: Academic Press, Inc.

Garen, A. 1960. "Genetic Control of the Specificity of the Bacterial Enzyme Alkaline Phosphatase," *Microbial Genetics*, W. Hayes and R. C. Clowes, Eds., (Tenth Symposium of the Society for General Microbiology), pp. 239–247. Cambridge, England: Cambridge University Press.

Golomb, S. W., L. R. Welch, and M. Delbrück. 1958. Construction and

Properties of Comma-Free Codes. *Biologiske Meddelelser udgivet af Det Kongelige Danske Videnskabernes Selskab*, 23(9):1–34.

Hershey, A. D. 1953. "Functional Differentiation Within Particles of Bacteriophage T2," *Viruses* (Cold Spring Harbor Symposia on Quantitative Biology, Vol. 18), pp. 135–139. Cold Spring Harbor, New York: Long Island Biological Association.

Hotchkiss, R. D. 1957. "Criteria for Quantitative Genetic Transformation of Bacteria," *Symposium on the Chemical Basis of Heredity*, W. D. McElroy and B. Glass, Eds., pp. 321–335. Baltimore, Maryland: Johns Hopkins Press.

Josse, J., A. D. Kaiser, and A. Kornberg. 1961. Enzymatic Synthesis of Deoxyribonucleic Acid. VIII. Frequencies of Nearest Neighbor Base Sequences in Deoxyribonucleic Acid. *Journal of Biological Chemistry*, 236:864–875.

Kornberg, A. 1960. Biologic Synthesis of Deoxyribonucleic Acid. *Science*, 131:1503–1508.

Lehman, I. R., S. B. Zimmerman, J. Adler, M. J. Bessman, E. S. Simms, and A. Kornberg. 1958. Enzymatic Synthesis of Deoxyribonucleic Acid. V. Chemical Composition of Enzymatically Synthesized Deoxyribonucleic Acid. *Proceedings of the National Academy of Sciences of the U.S.A.*, 44:1191–1196.

Levinthal, C. 1959. "Genetic and Chemical Studies with Alkaline Phosphatase of *E. coli*," *Structure and Function of Genetic Elements* (Brookhaven Symposia in Biology, No. 12), pp. 76–85. Upton, New York: Brookhaven National Laboratory.

Potter, J. L., and M. Laskowski. 1959. Concerning the Specificity of Streptococcal Deoxyribonuclease (Streptodornase). *Journal of Biological Chemistry*, 234:1263–1267.

Rushizky, G. W., C. A. Knight, W. K. Roberts, and C. A. Dekker. 1960. A map of the Products Resulting from the Action of Micrococcal Nuclease on Thymus Deoxyribonucleic Acid and Its Use as a Guide to Specificity. *Biochemical and Biophysical Research Communications*, 2:153–158.

Shapiro, H. S., and E. Chargaff. 1957. Studies on the Nucleotide Arrangement in Deoxyribonucleic Acids. II. Differential Analysis of Pyrimidine Nucleotide Distribution as a Method of Characterization. *Biochimica et biophysica acta*, 26:608–623.

———. 1960. Studies on the Nucleotide Arrangement in Deoxyribonucleic Acids. IV. Patterns of Nucleotide Sequence in the Deoxyribonucleic Acid of Rye Germ and Its Fractions. *Biochimica et biophysica acta*, 39:68–82.

Sinsheimer, R. L. 1954. The Action of Pancreatic Desoxyribonuclease. I. Isolation of Mono- and Dinucleotides. *Journal of Biological Chemistry*, 208:445–459.

———. 1955. The Action of Pancreatic Desoxyribonuclease. II. Isomeric Dinucleotides. *Journal of Biological Chemistry*, 215:579–583.

———. 1959. Is the Nucleic Acid Message in a Two-Symbol Code? *Journal of Molecular Biology*, 1:218–220.

Watson, J. D., and F. H. C. Crick. 1953. "The Structure of DNA," *Viruses* (Cold Spring Harbor Symposia on Quantitative Biology, Vol. 18), pp. 123–131. Cold Spring Harbor, New York: Long Island Biological Association.

Yanofsky, C. 1960. The Tryptophan Synthetase System. *Bacteriological Reviews*, 24:221–245.

Interaction of Nucleic Acids with Cationic Substances

GARY FELSENFELD, PH.D.*

Department of Biophysics, University of Pittsburgh, Pittsburgh, Pennsylvania

The chemical individuality of nucleic acids is expressed largely though variation in the kind and order of the purine and pyrimidine bases. Conversely, a great many of the chemical properties which all nucleic acids have in common arise, not from the bases, but from the charged phosphodiester groups of the ribose- or deoxyribose-phosphate backbone. This paper is concerned with chemical properties arising from the presence of the charged backbone, and particularly with the strong interaction between nucleic acids and positively charged ions or molecules.

Many cations interact with the bases as well as the phosphate backbone of nucleic acids. There has been much recent interest in such metallic ions as Ni^{++}, Pb^{++} and Hg^{++} (Fuwa *et al.*, 1960; Stevens and Duggan, 1957; Yamane and Davidson, 1961), which appear to react in this manner. This paper will be restricted, however, to cations which appear to react principally with the phosphate groups. The literature contains many studies of cation-nucleic acid interactions of this kind. It is impossible to present a comprehensive review of this material here, but some representative papers may be cited. The binding of dyes and of certain divalent cations to deoxyribonucleic acid (DNA) has been investigated by a number of workers, including Cavalieri, Angelos, and Balis (1951), Cava-

* Present address: Laboratory of Molecular Biology, National Institute of Arthritis and Metabolic Diseases, N.I.H., Bethesda, Md.

lieri (1952), and Lawley (1956). Conductimetric titration methods were first applied some years ago to the study of DNA interactions with alkaline earth ions by Shack, Jenkins, and Thompsett (1953). The same authors (1952) have used membrane potential methods to study DNA-sodium ion interactions, a technique also employed by Creeth and Jordan (1949). A review mentioning much of this work has been written by Jordan (1955). More recent investigations have introduced new techniques or studied new cations (Jardetzky, 1958; Wiberg and Neuman, 1957; Inman and Jordan, 1960; Bradley and Wolf, 1959) or extended the studies to ribonucleic acid (RNA), better preparations of DNA (Boedtker, 1960; Zubay and Doty, 1958), and synthetic polyribonucleotides (Felsenfeld and Rich, 1957; Felsenfeld and Huang, 1959, 1960).

This paper is not concerned solely with the determination of the strength or extent of interaction between polynucleotides and cations. The studies which will be described are intended to demonstrate that the interaction between cations and the charged phosphate backbone can be modified both by the nature of the bases and the configuration of the nucleic acid. It will be shown that by proper choice of techniques, conditions, and reacting cations, it is possible to obtain information about configuration and base charge, as well as gain some understanding of the role of the backbone charges (and their counterions) in the formation and stabilization of ordered polynucleotide structures.

The Relationship Between Charge and Structure Formation: Synthetic Polyribonucleotides

The synthetic polyribonucleotides (Grunberg-Manago, Ortiz, and Ochoa, 1955) have proven ideal molecules for study of relationship between charge and structure. These polymers, which can be synthesized with any desired over-all base composition, form a variety of ordered structures. Of particular interest are the two-stranded, 1:1 complexes formed by the interaction of polyadenylic (poly A) and polyuridylic (poly U) acids (Warner, 1956, 1957; Rich and Davies, 1956; Felsenfeld and Rich, 1957) and by the interaction of polyinosinic (poly I) and polycytidylic (poly C) acids (Davies and Rich, 1958; Davies, 1960). The fiber X-ray diffraction patterns of these complexes are indicative of a high degree of order, the poly (A + U) pattern bearing many resemblances to that of DNA.

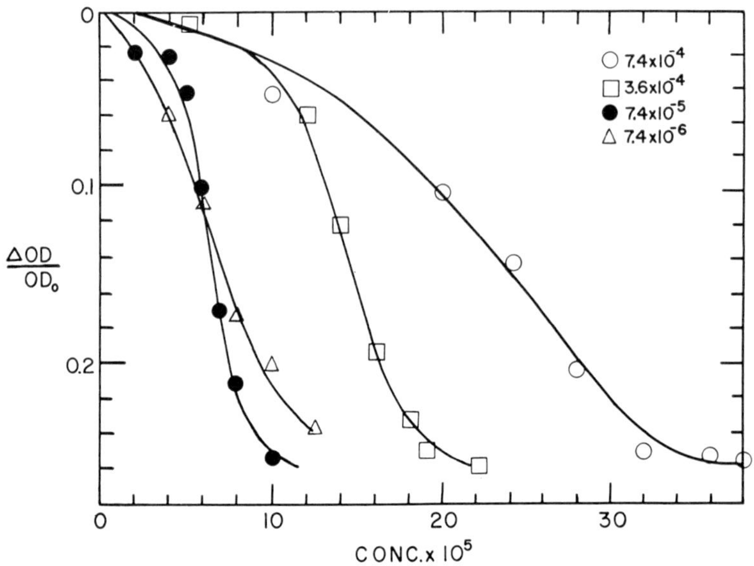

FIG. 1. Fractional optical density change (relative to separate poly A and poly U solutions at the same Mg^{++} concentration) of a series of 1:1 poly A — poly U mixtures as a function of Mg^{++} concentration. Polymer concentrations in monomoles are shown at the upper right. (Redrawn from Felsenfeld and Huang, 1960.)

Interactions between poly A and poly U or between poly I and poly C in 10^{-4} monomolar concentration proceed rapidly in 0.1 M NaCl at pH 7 (Felsenfeld and Rich, 1957; Ross and Sturtevant, 1960; Davies and Rich, 1958); in solutions of low ionic strength the reactions are slower, and if the polymers are mixed in distilled water there is no reaction. If various cations are now added to the distilled water mixed polymer solution, it is possible to study their effects upon the interaction between the polynucleotides (Warner, 1957; Felsenfeld and Rich, 1957; Felsenfeld and Huang, 1960). It is found that the divalent ions Mg^{++}, Ca^{++}, Ba^{++}, and Mn^{++} permit the formation of poly (A + U) when present in small concentration, while much larger concentrations of Na^{+} are required to produce the same effect. The results obtained with Mg^{++} are shown in Figure 1, in which the poly A + poly U interaction is followed by observing the decrease in optical density at 259 mμ which accompanies the interaction. At polymer concentrations of 10^{-4} M or above, an equivalent of Mg^{++}/mole of polymer phosphorus is sufficient to cause complete combination. Recent studies of the poly I – poly C interaction (Huang, 1961; Huang and Felsen-

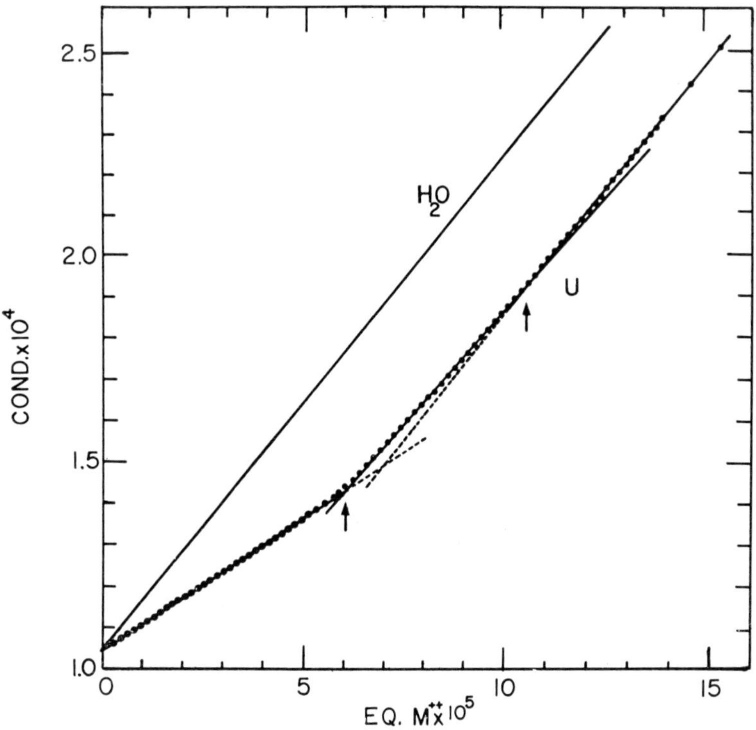

FIG. 2. The conductometric titration of 1.00×10^{-4} M poly U with 2×10^{-3} M $MnCl_2$. The arrow (right) shows the point at which the titration curve becomes approximately parallel to the curve for titration of water with $MnCl_2$ (shown by the line marked "H_2O"). (Redrawn from Felsenfeld and Huang, 1959.)

feld, in preparation) show a similar stoichiometric requirement for Mg^{++}.

These results suggest that divalent ions such as Mg^{++} react strongly with polynucleotides, and the stoichiometry of the reaction, as well as the known chemical behavior of Mg^{++}, makes it likely that the polymer phosphate groups are responsible for the interaction. Confirmation of this fact has been obtained by conductimetric titration of distilled water solutions of poly A or poly U with Mg^{++}, Mn^{++}, or Ba^{++}. Figures 2 and 3 show the results of such a titration (Felsenfeld and Huang, 1959). Though, for reasons discussed in the paper cited, the shape of the curve is not that of a classical titration, the interaction between polynucleotide and divalent ion is always complete at about one equivalent of divalent ion/mole of phosphorus. Furthermore, the polycation, polylysine,

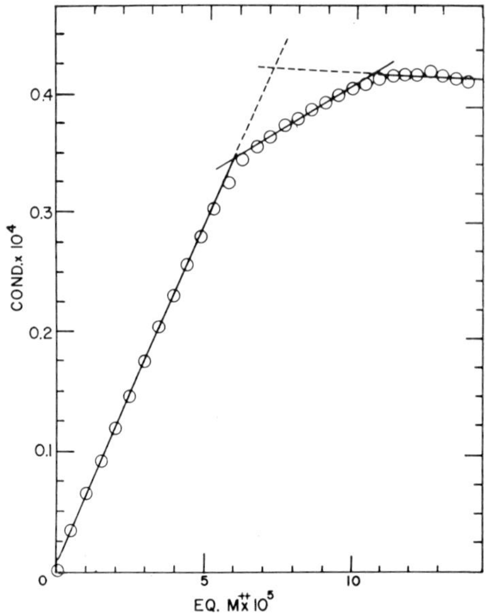

Fig. 3. The difference between the curve marked "H_2O" and the curve marked "U" in Figure 2. (Redrawn from Felsenfeld and Huang, 1959.)

which displaces divalent ions from polynucleotides, is found to displace about one equivalent of Mn^{++} from Mn^{++} — poly U when added in excess. All of these results are identical for poly A and for poly U. Thus, the bases do not appear to play a major role in this interaction. If they did, poly A would presumably be a much stronger binding agent than poly U.

There is a marked contrast between the behavior of the divalent ions and that of such monovalent ions as Na^+, or the positively charged amino acids (Figure 4). Polynucleotide combination in the presence of these ions requires large excesses of the ion, and the degree of combination is a function only of the small ion concentration, not of the polymer concentration, in a manner characteristic of "weak" interactions (Felsenfeld and Huang, 1960). Though most monovalent ions which do not react with the bases behave like Na^+, the dye acridine orange (AO) is an exception (Bradley and Wolf, 1959). The interaction between adjacent dye molecules stabilizes the dye bound to the polymer phosphate groups. Spectrophotometric titration of polynucleotides with AO reveals a 1:1 stoichiometry in dilute salt solution, and conductimetric titration of denatured DNA with AO in distilled water gives a titration curve very much like those shown in Figures 2 and 3.

The findings described in this section lead to the conclusions that certain ions, notably divalent ions such as Mg^{++}, are capable of

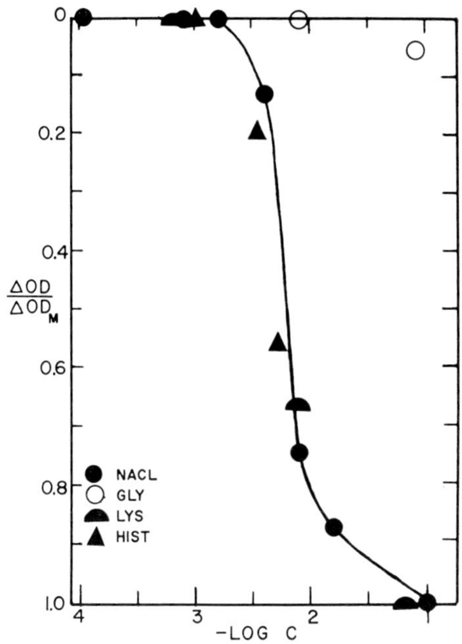

FIG. 4. Decrease in optical density of a 1:1 poly A — poly U mixture divided by maximum decrease in optical density (relative to the separate polymers in distilled water) plotted against the negative logarithm of the molar concentration of sodium chloride and glycine, and the molar concentration of the positively charged species of lysine and histidine. Polymer monomolar concentration = 7.2×10^{-5}. (Redrawn from Felsenfeld and Huang, 1960.)

interacting strongly with the polymer phosphate groups of synthetic polynucleotides, that in low ionic strength solutions the reaction involves complete neutralization of the polymer charge with stoichiometric quantities of cation, and that at low ionic strength such neutralization is a prerequisite for the formation of the ordered poly (A + U) and poly (I + C) structures. There is also ample evidence (Cavalieri, Rosoff, and Rosenberg, 1956; Inman and Jordan, 1960) that high counterion concentrations stabilize the ordered DNA structure, so that it may be stated as a general rule that stabilization of ordered polynucleotide structures requires that much of the phosphate backbone charge be neutralized or screened.

The Effect of Base Protonation Upon Backbone Reactivity

The cation-polynucleotide interactions discussed thus far have been chosen so that they may be treated entirely as cation-polyanion interactions, since the bases play little or no role in the "binding" of the cation. There has been some discussion in the literature (e.g., Zubay and Doty, 1958) of the possible contribution of the bases to binding of Mg^{++} and similar cations by direct complex formation. Several aspects of the evidence already presented

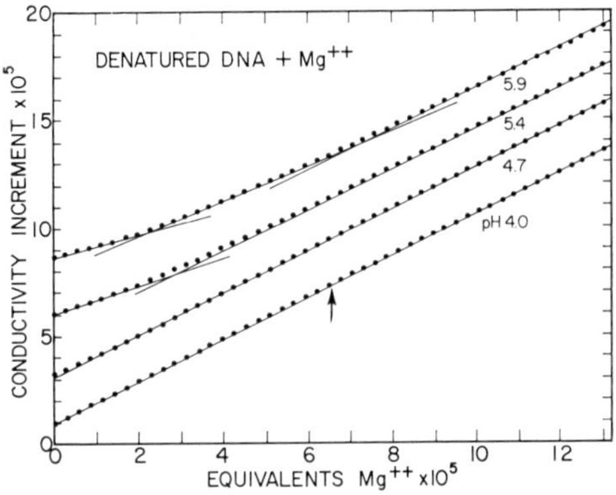

FIG. 5. Conductimetric titrations of denatured calf thymus DNA in distilled water with 2.5×10^{-3} M $MgCl_2$ at different values of pH. (Felsenfeld and Huang, in press.)
In this figure, the arrow shows the theoretical equivalence point.

show that the contribution, if it exists at all, is not a major factor in binding. Among the evidence are the identical shape of the conductimetric titration curves of poly A and poly U with Mg^{++}, and the similarity of the titration curves of polynucleotides titrated with Mg^{++} to curves obtained using AO as a titrant. Simple diamines such as putrescine and cadaverine, which cannot form complexes with bases, also give similar titration curves. Furthermore, it will be shown in a subsequent section that native DNA combines strongly and stoichiometrically with Mg^{++}, even though the bases of native DNA are not available for complex formation.

Although this evidence suggests that the bases are not directly involved in the binding of the class of cations considered here, there is now also good evidence for an important indirect effect of the bases upon the interaction. For example, in Figure 5 are shown the results of a series of conductimetric titrations of heat-denatured calf thymus DNA with Mg^{++} in which both the DNA and the titrant are adjusted to the same initial pH. If the titration is performed at pH 5.9 or above, a curve similar to that shown in Figure 2 for poly U is obtained, but at lower pH values the apparent end point of the titration shifts downward, and at pH 4.7 or below the evidence of interaction is almost indetectable by conductimetric methods. An even more dramatic demonstration of the effect of pH is obtained if the tetraamine, spermine, is substituted for Mg^{++} (Figure 6). In this case, the stoichiometry is maintained as the pH is lowered, but the shape of the titration curve is inverted at low pH.

All of this behavior is the result of protonation of the bases, which commences between pH 5 and pH 6 in distilled water solutions of denatured DNA (Cavalieri, Rosoff, and Rosenberg, 1956). That the effect is not the result of some direct action of H^+ upon phosphate

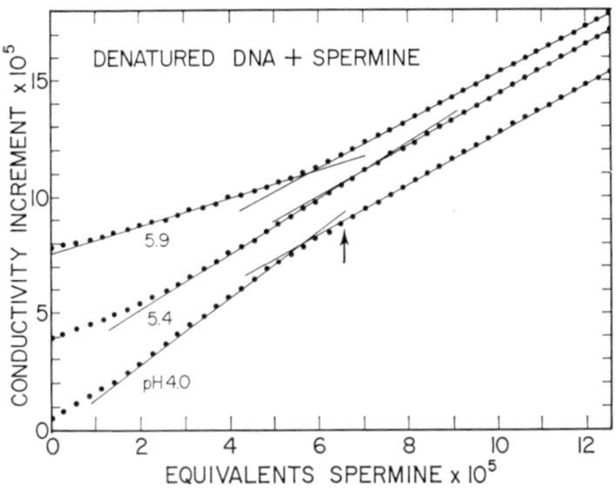

FIG. 6. Conductimetric titrations of denatured calf thymus DNA in distilled water with 1.25×10^{-3} M spermine tetrahydrochloride at different values of pH. (Felsenfeld and Huang, 1961.) Arrow shows the theoretical equivalence point.

groups is demonstrated by the fact that the poly U, which has no pK between pH 4 and 7, shows no variation in the shape of the Mg^{++} or spermine titration curves in that pH region. If the titration of denatured DNA with spermine is repeated while measuring pH rather than conductivity, it is found that the hydrogen ion activity rises until one equivalent of spermine per mole of phosphate has been added. There is no further increase in H^+ activity beyond the equivalence point, and the total increment in H^+ activity increases with decreasing starting pH, amounting to about 25 per cent of the polymer base concentration when the starting pH is 4.7 (Felsenfeld and Huang, 1961). The reaction of spermine with the phosphate groups of the backbone causes a decrease in the pK of the bases, resulting in the release of the base-bound protons into the solution. This displacement of high-conductivity protons explains the inversion of the low pH conductimetric titration curves shown in Figure 6. The effect of spermine clearly involves the phosphate groups and does not involve chemical reaction with the bases. The behavior of the Mg^{++} conductimetric titrations may be explained similarly, except that the affinity of Mg^{++} for the polymer is somewhat weaker than that of spermine. Cavalieri (1952) first reported that the pH of DNA solutions decreases when Mg^{++} is added, and he also observed the related decreased affinity of DNA for Mg^{++} at low pH, though he ascribed this effect to the direct involvement of the bases in Mg^{++} binding. A quantitative measurement of pH variation, as Mg^{++} is added, shows that a given equivalent concentration of Mg^{++} displaces only about half as many protons as the same concentration of spermine at the same starting pH, and that displacement continues after the equivalence point is reached. The reduction in affinity for divalent ion does not appear to be stoichiometrically related to the number of protons bound to the bases.

These experiments show that the state of charge of the bases affects the interaction of polynucleotides, even with those cations which do not react chemically with the bases, and it follows that the condition of charge of the backbone affects the degree of ionization of the bases.

The Relationship Between Structure And Cationic Interactions

Native DNA

In a preceding part of this paper it was shown that the formation of ordered polynucleotide structures depends upon neutralization of backbone charge. It is also true that the presence or absence of structure will affect the way in which cations react with polynucleotides. Figure 7 shows the titration of a solution of native DNA (sufficiently concentrated to prevent spontaneous denaturation) with Mg^{++}, in comparison with a titration of heat-denatured DNA at the same concentration. Shack, Jenkins, and Thompsett (1952) and Zubay and Doty (1958) pointed out considerable shape differences in the two curves, which differ by a factor of 1.5 in slope early in the titration. The titration curve shape will depend upon the effect of charge neutralization by titrant on the flexibility of the polymer (Felsenfeld and Huang, 1961). Without detailed analysis it is readily seen that a difference between the shapes of the

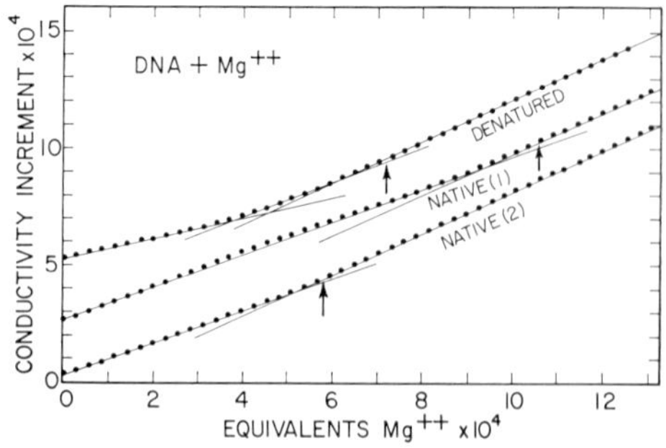

FIG. 7. Conductimetric titration of native calf thymus DNA in distilled water with $MgCl_2$, compared with the titration of denatured DNA at about the same concentration. Native (1) and native (2) refer to two different preparations of DNA. In curve (2) the values of Mg^{++} and the theoretical equivalence point have been plotted as one half the actual values in order to permit presentation on the same scale. The titrant $MgCl_2$ concentration was 2.5×10^{-2} M in the denatured and native (1) titrations, and 5×10^{-2} M in native (2). In native (1), the pH of the DNA solution was never permitted to drop below 6.8 while the material was dissolving, and the titration was performed at this pH. Native DNA (2) was dissolved in distilled water without pH adjustment, giving a pH of about 6.3. (Felsenfeld and Huang, 1961.) Arrows show the theoretical equivalence point.

two titration curves is to be expected, since we are examining the variation with titrant addition of a complex function dependent upon the polymer mobility and charge. These are, in turn, dependent upon the way in which reaction with titrant affects the degree of extension of polymer and the ability of its remaining charges to transport sodium counterions, some of which always move with the charged polyanion (Inman and Jordan, 1960). The difference in titration curve shape is related to the observation (Eisenberg, 1957) that the viscosity of native DNA, possessing inherent structural rigidity, is much less affected by the addition of excess ions than is denatured DNA, which collapses when the electrostatic repulsions within the polyion are reduced.

A more direct measure of some of the changes in mobility and sodium ion transport accompanying denaturation is obtained by a study of the change in conductivity which occurs when a solution of native DNA in dilute NaCl is heated. In order to make accurate measurements, it is necessary to compensate for the large dependence of the solvent's conductivity upon temperature. One way in which this can be done is to place a second conductivity cell, filled with solvent only, in an arm of the conductivity bridge adjacent to that containing the DNA solution. Both cells are placed in the same thermostatic bath, so that as the temperature is raised the ratio of their conductivities is measured. The percentage change in this ratio is plotted as a function of temperature in Figure 8. It coincides reasonably well with the familiar optical density denaturation curve for calf thymus DNA (Doty *et al.*, 1959). It is interesting to note that if $MgCl_2$ is used instead of NaCl, there is practically no variation in the conductivity ratio with temperature, since the DNA, whether native or denatured, is essentially neutral and contributes nothing to the conductivity (Felsenfeld and Huang, 1961).

Synthetic Polynucleotides

A demonstration of the relationship between structure and cationic interactions is provided by some recent studies of the effect upon the poly I — poly C interaction of the addition of polyamines (Huang and Felsenfeld, 1960, 1961). It has already been pointed out that divalent ions such as Mg^{++} affect the poly I — poly C reaction in the same way that they affect the poly A — poly U reaction. The same is true of diamines of the $^{+}NH_3(CH_2)_nNH_3^{+}$ group which includes putrescine and cadaverine. However, when the cation used is the tetraamine, spermine, a major difference

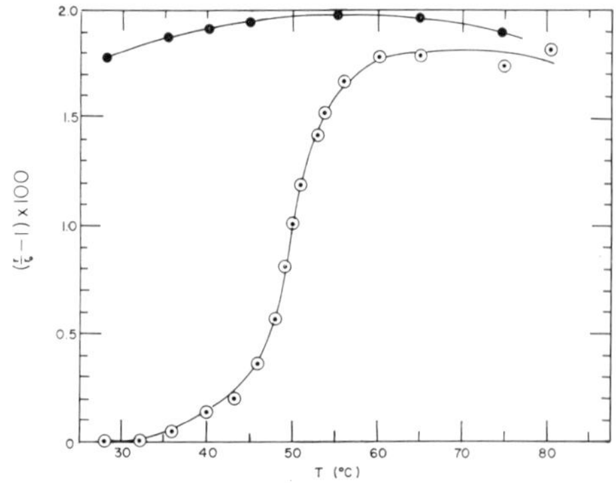

FIG. 8. Per cent change in the ratio of conductivities in a cell containing a solution of native calf thymus DNA and one containing solvent only, as a function of temperature. The solvent was 9.75×10^{-4} M NaCl, 1.87×10^{-4} M ethylenediamine tetraacetic acid, pH 7.0. The DNA concentration was about 2.0×10^{-4} M (polymer phosphate). The open circles show the results of the first heating, the closed circles the result of reheating the same solution. The variable r is the ratio of the conductivities of the two cells at temperature T, and r_0 is the value of r at room temperature. To facilitate comparison of the two curves, the same value of r_0 (that for undenatured DNA) has been used in plotting both.

appears between the poly I — poly C and poly A — poly U reactions. If spermine is added to any one of these polymers in excess, a precipitate will usually form in solutions of low ionic strength. When precipitated poly A and poly U are mixed, no further interaction occurs; when the precipitated poly I and poly C are mixed, the precipitate slowly redissolves (under appropriate conditions) and the spectrum of the ordered poly (I + C) structure appears. If less than equivalent quantities of spermine are used, no precipitate forms with poly I or poly C at pH 6.8 to 7.0, and the effect of spermine on the combination can be studied directly (Figure 9). The reaction requires stoichiometric concentrations of spermine. (Spermine carries four positive charges throughout the pH range used.) Another way of showing the relationship between solubility and structure is to add excess spermine to a series of solutions of already formed poly (I + C), in which each solution is buffered at a different pH. It is found (Huang and Felsenfeld, 1960) that the complex formed with spermine is soluble at every pH between 6.8 and 4.5. At pH 4.5 and below, where cytosine is being titrated and the poly (I + C) structure is probably altered, precipitation occurs. However, poly (A + U) precipitates completely with spermine at every pH between 6.8 and 4.5, and this can be used to separate poly (I + C) from poly (A + U). Cantoni (1960) has found that the

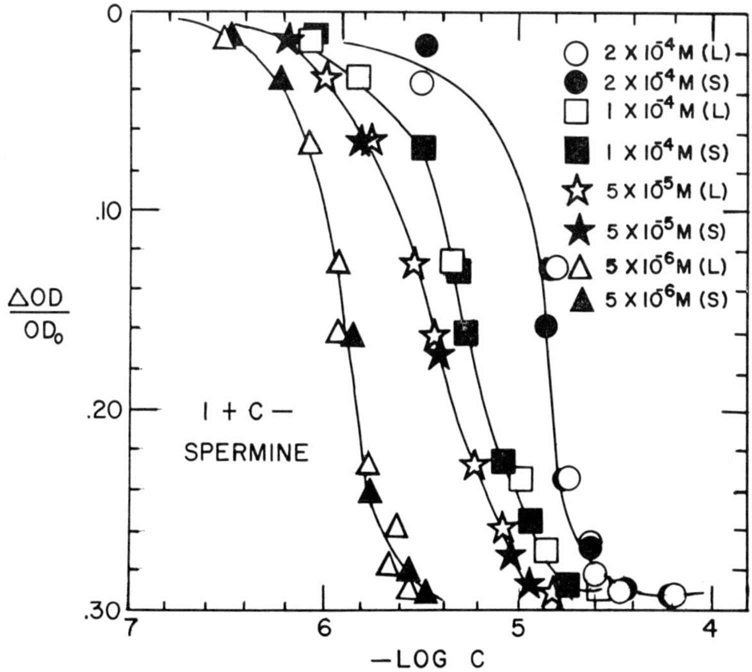

FIG. 9. The effect of addition of spermine tetrahydrochloride upon the combination of poly I with poly C. Optical density was measured at 248 mμ, and the fractional change is relative to separate poly I and poly C solutions at the same spermine concentration. The pH was adjusted to 6.8 to 7.0 with NaOH in all cases, and under these conditions, if the spermine is not in excess, no precipitation of poly I or poly C occurs. Polymer monomolar concentrations are given in the upper right. (L) and (S) refer to different preparations of polymer, with different sedimentation coefficients. (Huang, 1961; Huang and Felsenfeld, in preparation.)

"soluble" RNA, which has a high percentage of guanine and cytosine, shows a solubility dependence of the spermine complex on pH which resembles that of poly (I + C), except that there is a pH region of partial precipitation in which separation according to amino acid acceptor specificity is possible.

The formation of soluble ordered structures with poly (I + C) is not limited to spermine alone. In Figure 10 is shown the effect of adding polylysine (degree of polymerization about 50) to a distilled water mixture of poly I and poly C. To avoid precipitation, the reaction must be started at pH 7 or above, so that some of the polylysine groups are initially uncharged, although the stoichiometry of the interaction suggests that most of the amino groups of the

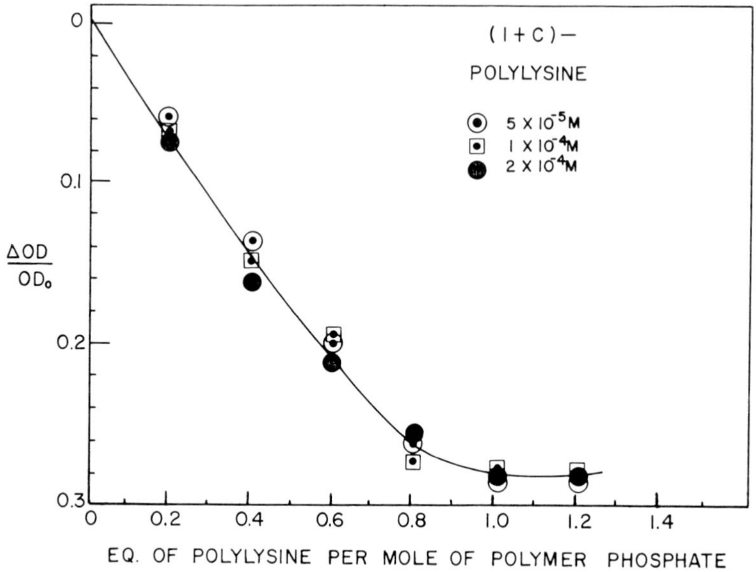

FIG. 10. The effect of addition of polylysine hydrobromide upon the poly I — poly C combination. The pH was adjusted to about 7.3 with NaOH. (Huang, 1961; Huang and Felsenfeld, in preparation.)

combined polylysine are positively charged. It should be noted that polylysine in excess causes precipitation of native and denatured DNA and of poly (A + U).

The ability of poly (I + C) to form soluble complexes with spermine or polylysine, while all of the other kinds of polynucleotides are precipitated, is an indication of the way in which structure modifies cationic interaction. It appears that only the ordered poly (I + C) structure is capable of accommodating the polycation in such a way as to avoid formation of matted, cross-linked aggregates, and to permit sufficient hydration to keep the molecule in solution.

Discussion

The experimental results presented here are intended to give some indication of the great variety of information concerning nucleic acids which can be obtained by studies of their interactions with cations. To a certain extent, the behavior of nucleic acids resembles that of synthetic polyelectrolytes such as polyacrylic acid, and though no mention has been made of the vast literature concerned with the behavior of polyelectrolytes, certain aspects of the ion-binding properties of polynucleotides can be discussed in these terms. One important distinction made in polyelectrolyte studies is that between "site binding" and "nonspecific interaction" (Lifson, 1957), the latter term denoting the general tendency of counterions to be concentrated in the neighborhood of the polyion because of the large value of the electrostatic potential there. With the exception of the sodium ion, for which the mode of interaction is not yet determined, all of the cations discussed in this paper probably belong to the class of "site bound" ions so far as nucleic acids are concerned.

Despite these fundamental similarities, most of the studies presented here have dealt with properties which distinguish nucleic acids from other polyelectrolytes. It has been shown that the polyelectrolyte character of nucleic acids is modified by the unique structures and charge distributions made possible by the presence of the bases. The results thus present two major possible points of approach to further investigation. Either the interactions between cations and phosphate backbone may be used to study indirectly the changes in configuration and base charge, or they may be used to study directly the role of the negatively charged backbone in nucleic acid chemistry. The first approach is exemplified by the conductivity-denaturation curve of Figure 8. Careful investigations of these curves as a new and perhaps unique tool for the study of DNA denaturation are being carried out in our laboratories. The second and more direct question of the role of the charged backbone is also being considered. Attention is now being given to such problems as the measurement of polynucleotide shape as a function of charge, the kinetics of DNA denaturation as a function of ionic composition, and the role played by the polyamines and other polycations in formation of structure. Though these are primarily questions of physical chemistry, their answers are likely to have bearing upon the biological functions of nucleic acids.

ACKNOWLEDGMENTS

Most of the investigations described here were supported by Grant C-3883 from the United States Public Health Service.

The technical assistance of Miss Joan Orris in some of the recent conductometric studies is gratefully acknowledged.

ABBREVIATIONS

Abbreviations in this paper are as follows: poly (A + U), 1:1 complex of poly A and poly U; poly (I + C), 1:1 complex of poly I and poly C.

REFERENCES

Boedtker, H. 1960. Configurational Properties of Tobacco Mosaic Virus Ribonucleic Acid. *Journal of Molecular Biology*, 2:171–188.

Bradley, D. F., and M. K. Wolf. 1959. Aggregation of Dyes Bound to Polyanions. *Proceedings of the National Academy of Sciences of the U.S.A.*, 45:944–952.

Cantoni, G. L. 1960. Spermine Fractionation of Soluble Ribonucleic Acid of Rabbit Liver. *Nature, London*, 188:300–301.

Cavalieri, L. F. 1952. Studies on the Structure of Nucleic Acids. V. On the Mechanism of Metal and Enzyme Interactions. *Journal of the American Chemical Society*, 74:1242–1247.

Cavalieri,L. F., A. Angelos, and M. E. Balis. 1951. Studies on the Structure of Nucleic Acids. IV. Investigation of Dye Interactions by Partition Analysis. *Journal of the American Chemical Society*, 73:4902–4906.

Cavalieri, L. F., M. Rosoff, and B. H. Rosenberg. 1956. Studies on the Structure of Nucleic Acids. X. On the Mechanism of Denaturation. *Journal of the American Chemical Society*, 78:5239–5247.

Creeth, J. M., and D. O. Jordan. 1949. Deoxypentose Nucleic Acids. Part V. An Attempted Interpretation of the Electrophoretic Mobilities of the Deoxypentose Nucleic Acid of Calf Thymus. *Journal of the Chemical Society*, 1949:1409–1413.

Davies, D. R. 1960. Polyinosinic Plus Polycytidylic Acid: A Crystalline Polynucleotide Complex. *Nature, London*, 186:1030–1031.

Davies, D. R., and A. Rich. 1958. The Formation of a Helical Complex Between Polyinosinic Acid and Polycytidylic Acid. *Journal of the American Chemical Society*, 80:1003.

Doty, P., H. Boedtker, J. R. Fresco, R. Haselkorn, and M. Litt. 1959. Secondary Structure in Ribonucleic Acids. *Proceedings of the National Academy of Sciences of the U.S.A.*, 45:482–499.

Eisenberg, H. 1957. Viscosity of Dilute Solutions of Preparations of Deoxyribonucleic Acid at Low and Medium Rates of Shear. *Journal of Polymer Science*, 25:257–271.

Felsenfeld, G., and S. Huang. 1959. The Interaction of Polynucleotides with Cations. *Biochimica et biophysica acta*, 24:234–242.

———. 1960. The Interaction of Polynucleotides with Metal Ions, Amino Acids, and Polyamines. *Biochimica et biophysica acta*, 37:425–433.

Felsenfeld, G., and S. L. Huang. 1961. Some Effects of Charge and Structure upon Ionic Interactions of Nucleic Acids. *Biochimica et biophysica acta*, 51:19–32.

Felsenfeld, G., and A. Rich. 1957. Studies on the Formation of Two- and Three-Stranded Polyribonucleotides. *Biochimica et biophysica acta*, 26:457–468.

Fuwa, K., W. E. C. Wacker, R. Bruyan, A. F. Bartholomay, and B. L. Vallee. 1960. Nucleic Acids and Metals. II. Transition Metals as Determinants of the Conformation of Ribonucleic Acids. *Proceedings of the National Academy of Sciences of the U.S.A.*, 46:1298–1307.

Grunberg-Manago, M., P. J. Ortiz, and S. Ochoa. 1955. Enzymatic Synthesis of Nucleic Acidlike Polynucleotides. *Science*, 122:907–910.

Huang, S. L. 1961. *The Studies of the Interaction of Synthetic Polynucleotides with Cations and the Electrolytic Properties of Nucleic Acids.* Ph.D. Dissertation. University of Pittsburgh, Pittsburgh, Pennsylvania.

Huang, S. L., and G. Felsenfeld. 1960. Solubility of Complexes of Polynucleotides with Spermine. *Nature, London,* 188:301–302.

Huang, S. L., and G. Felsenfeld. The Effect of Cations on the Interaction Between Polyinosinic and Polycytidylic Acids. (In preparation).

Inman, R. B., and D. O. Jordan. 1960. Deoxypentose Nucleic Acids. XI. The Denaturation of Deoxyribonuleic Acid in Aqueous Solution: Conductivity and Mobility Measurements. *Biochimica et biophysica acta,* 43:421–426.

Jardetzky, C. D. 1958. Interactions of Amino Acids with Deoxyribonucleic Acid. *Journal of the American Chemical Society,* 80:1125–1127.

Jordan, D. O. 1955. "The Physical Properties of Nucleic Acids," *The Nucleic Acids.* E. Chargaff and J. N. Davidson, Eds., Vol. 1, pp. 447–492. New York, New York: Academic Press, Inc.

Lawley, P.D. 1956. Interaction Studies with Deoxyribonucleic Acid. I. Binding of Rosaniline at Low Ratio of Concentrations Rosaniline: DNA, and Competitive Effect of Sodium and Other Metal Cations. *Biochimica et biophysica acta,* 19:160–167.

Lifson, S. 1957. Potentiometric Titration, Association Phenomena, and Interaction of Neighboring Groups in Polyelectrolytes. *Journal of Chemical Physics,* 26:727–734.

Rich, A., and D. R. Davies. 1956. A New Two-Stranded Helical Structure: Polyadenylic and Polyuridylic Acid. *Journal of the American Chemical Society,* 78:3548.

Ross, P. D., and J. M. Sturtevant. 1960. The Kinetics of Double Helix Formation from Polyriboadenylic Acid and Polyribouridylic Acid. *Proceedings of the National Academy of Sciences of the U.S.A.,* 46:1360–1365.

Shack, J., R. J. Jenkins, and J. M. Thompsett. 1952. The Binding of Sodium Chloride and Calf Thymus Deoxypentose Nucleic Acid. *Journal of Biological Chemistry,* 198:85–92.

———. 1953. The Interaction of Ions and Desoxypentose Nucleic Acid of Calf Thymus. *Journal of Biological Chemistry,* 203:373–387.

Stevens, V. L., and E. L. Duggan. 1957. Deformation of Deoxyribonucleate. II. Precipitation of Heat-Deformed DNA with Millimolar Lead Ion. *Journal of the American Chemical Society,* 79:5703–5706.

Warner, R. C. 1956. Ultraviolet Spectra of Enzymatically Synthesized Polynucleotides. *Federation Proceedings,* 15:379.

———. 1957. Studies on Polynucleotides Synthesized by Polynucleotide Phosphorylase. III. Interaction and Ultraviolet Absorption. *Journal of Biological Chemistry,* 229:711–724.

Wiberg, J. S., and W. F. Neuman. 1957. The Binding of Bivalent Metals by Deoxyribonucleic and Ribonucleic Acids. *Archives of Biochemistry and Biophysics,* 72:66–83.

Yamane, T., and N. Davidson. 1961. On the Complexing of DNA by Mer-Mercuric Ion. *Journal of the American Chemical Society,* 83:2599–2607.

Zubay, G., and P. Doty. 1958. Nucleic Acid Interactions with Metal Ions and Amino Acids. *Biochimica et biophysica acta,* 29:47–58.

NUCLEIC ACIDS AND PROTEINS

Effects of Alkylating Agents on Nucleic Acids and Their Relation to Other Mutagens

P. D. Lawley, B.A., Ph.D.

The Chester Beatty Research Institute, Institute of Cancer Research, Royal Cancer Hospital, London, England

The alkylating agents are a group of chemically simple substances some of which exert a variety of biological effects, including mutagenesis, carcinogenesis, and tumor-growth inhibition. The close relationship between biological (tumor-growth inhibitory) activity and chemical reactivity, particularly for a series of aromatic nitrogen mustards, suggested that the biological activity is due to the chemical action of alkylation and not to purely physical effects (Haddow, Kon, and Ross, 1948). Further correlations of importance are, first, the resemblance with regard to biological effects of alkylating agents and ionizing radiation, hence the designation of these agents as "radiomimetic"; second, that the two-armed or difunctional alkylating agents are more effective as tumor-growth inhibitors than the one-armed or monofunctional type (Loveless and Ross, 1950). Differences are also found when comparing the mutagenic properties of these two types of alkylating agent (Fahmy and Fahmy, 1961). The difunctional agents are not necessarily more effective as mutagens but they do produce a different mutational spectrum. The difunctional agents yield a higher proportion of complete relative to mosaic mutants; lethal to visible mutants; chromosome breaks; and gene inactivation resulting in small deficiencies.

The mutagenic properties of the alkylating agents, first shown

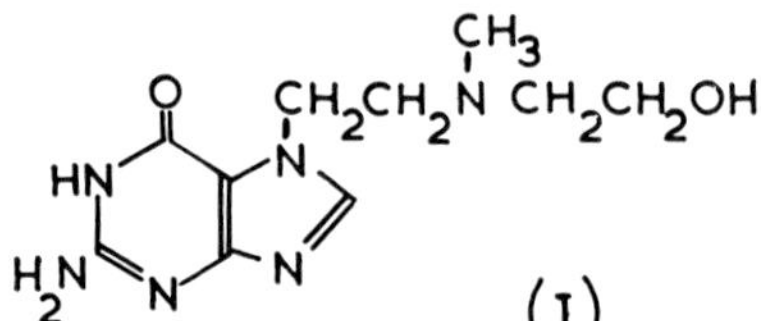

(I)

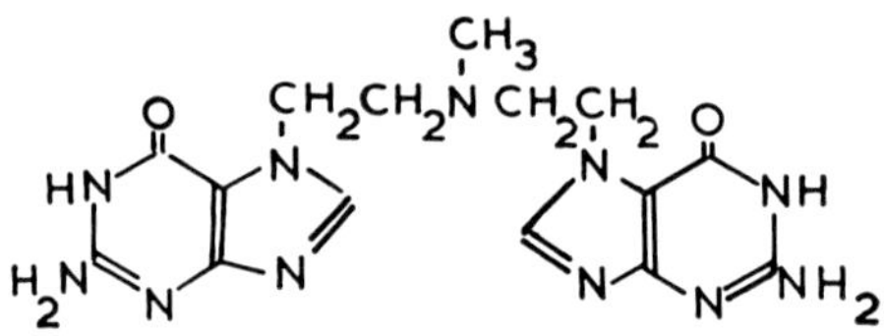

(II)

FIG. 1. 7-Alkylguanine (I) and di–(guanin-7-yl) derivative (II) from reaction of nitrogen mustard, di-(2-chloroethyl) methylamine and guanylic acid or nucleic acid.

for mustard gas (di-[β-chloroethyl] sulphide) (Auerbach and Robson, 1946), and studies of their cytotoxic action, suggested that deoxyribonucleic acid (DNA) was likely to be an important site of alkylation. The greater cytotoxic activity of the difunctional agents was ascribed to their ability to cross-link fibrous macromolecules essential for the processes of cell division (Goldacre, Loveless, and Ross, 1949).

More recently, the mode of combination of mustard gas with nucleic acids at low doses *in vitro*, and *in vivo*, has been established (Brookes and Lawley, 1960), and shown to apply to a variety of alkylating agents (Brookes and Lawley, 1961). The most reactive site toward alkylation in nucleic acids is the N-7 atom of guanine moieties shown in Figure 1 (Lawley, 1957a; Lawley and Wallick, 1957), and it has been confirmed that this is the site of alkylation under conditions when only the most reactive site is attacked, i.e., at low degrees of alkylation *in vitro*, and *in vivo* (Brookes and Lawley, 1960).

With regard to the generally accepted differences between the types of alkylating agents, a comparison was made (Table 1) of Myleran (1, 4-dimethanesulphonoxybutane), a weakly reactive difunctional agent, half sulphur mustard (β-chloroethyl-β-hydroxyethyl sulphide), a highly reactive monofunctional agent, and mustard gas, a highly reactive difunctional agent (Brookes and Lawley, 1961). As expected, Myleran was bound to cellular constituents to a much smaller extent than the two mustards, although given at a higher dose. This might be held to explain its general weakness as a tumor-growth inhibitor, but cannot account for its value against chronic myelogenous leukemia (Haddow and Timmis, 1953).

Mustard gas and the corresponding half mustard were found to be bound to cellular constituents to the same extent (Table 1), but the tumor inhibitory effect of the mustard gas was found to be at least 30 times that of the half mustard. With regard to reaction with nucleic acids, the only difference between the two mustards was found to be that the mustard gas yielded in addition to 7-alkylguanine a cross-linked guanine product di-(β-guanin-7-yl)ethyl sulphide.

TABLE 1

In vivo Reaction of Alkylating Agents with Nucleic Acids of the Ehrlich Ascites Tumor in the Mouse

			Extent of reaction, moles per 10^6 NA nucleotides	
	Dose mg./kg.	Tumor inhibition	RNA	DNA
Mustard gas $^{35}S(CH_2CH_2Cl)_2$	2	+	46	42
Half-S-mustard $ClCH_2CH_2{}^{35}S\,CH_2CH_2OH$	4	—	75	70
Myleran-[^{3}H] $CH_3SO_2O(CH_2)_4OSO_2CH_3$	20	—	1	2

If the difference in biological effect of these mustards is to be ascribed to difference in their mode of combination with nucleic acid, then the formation of the di-(guanin-7-yl) derivative must be of importance. The possible disposition of the two linked guanine moieties within the nucleic acid molecule was therefore investigated. Examination of the Crick-Watson model for DNA (Crick and Watson, 1954) showed that two guanine moieties on opposite strands of the DNA twin spiral could be linked by an extended alkyl chain of four or five atoms, provided the sequence of bases along the DNA chain was guanine-cytosine, in one direction only (Figure 2).

This concept receives experimental support from two sources. First the proportion of cross-linking decreases in the order DNA> denatured DNA> ribonucleic acid (RNA), i.e., as the extent of structure of the twin-spiral type decreases (Brookes and Lawley, 1961). Second, the difunctional mustard is more effective in causing decrease in the molecular weight of DNA than the monofunctional

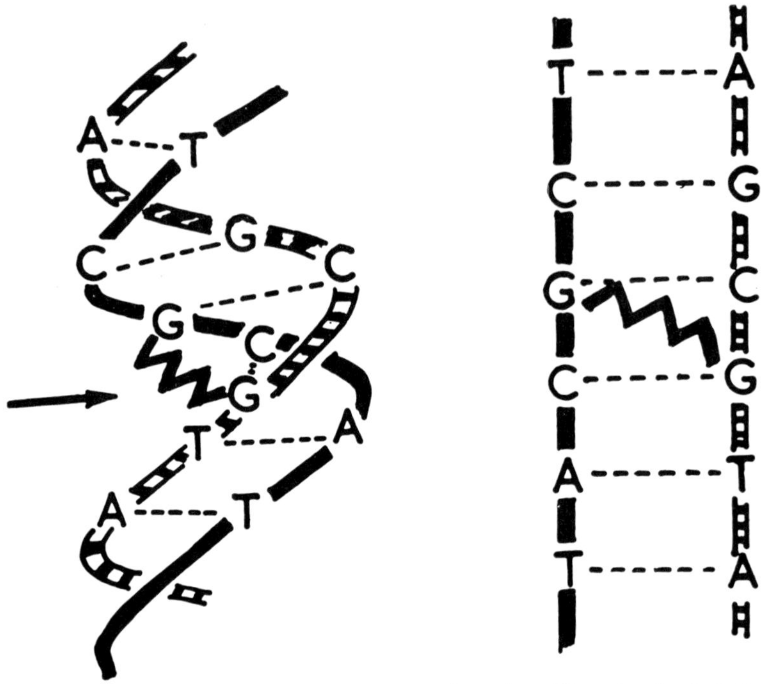

FIG. 2. Diagramatic representation of reaction of a difunctional alkylating agent with DNA. The order of bases along the DNA molecular chain is indicated by their initial letters and the alkyl chain by the zigzag line.

mustard (Lawley *et al.*, 1960).

In order to explain this latter effect, the effect of alkylation on the hydrolysis of DNA must be discussed. It was found that following alkylation of DNA in neutral aqueous solution at 37°C the alkylated guanine products split off (Lawley and Wallick, 1957; Lawley, 1957b; Brookes and Lawley, 1961) and fission of the sugar phosphate chain is thereby potentiated (Brown and Todd, 1954), as shown in Figure 3. Following alkylation of DNA by a monofunctional agent at a low extent of alkylation, breaks in either of the twin strands of the molecule at widely separated points would result which would not be expected to decrease the molecular weight. With the difunctional agent about one quarter of all alkylations would cross-link the strands at nearby points and when both were broken a decrease in molecular weight would result (Figure 4). The rate of splitting off of alkylguanine at neutral pH and 37°C is a much slower process (half life $\sim$ 50 hours) than the initial alkylation (half life $<$ two minutes) and the subsequent fission

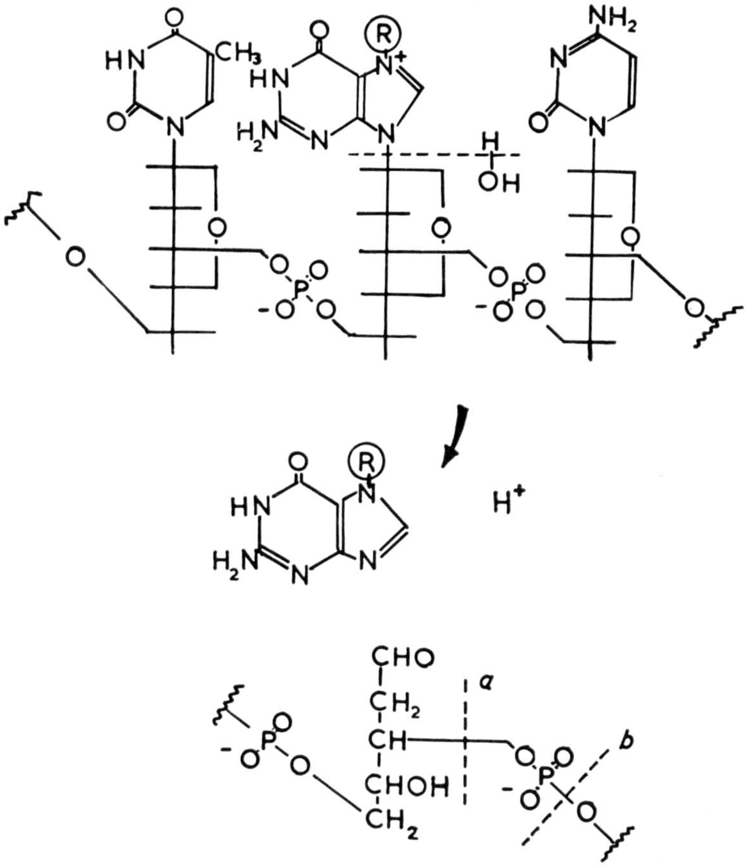

FIG. 3. Hydrolysis of alkylated DNA: the alkyl group is denoted by R, the β-elimination mechanism by a, and the cyclophosphate mechanism by b.

of the twin spiral of DNA much slower again (half life > 50 days).

Returning to the contrast in cytotoxic effects of the mono- and difunctional mustards it is possible to relate this with their mode of reaction with DNA. The Watson-Crick hypothesis (Watson and Crick, 1953) proposes that separation of the twin strands of DNA is essential for cell division. Linkage of these strands by a covalent bond would therefore be expected to inhibit this process.

Mutagenic effects of alkylation can be discussed in terms of the splitting off of 7-alkylguanine products from alkylated DNA (Figure 4). Following deletion of alkylated guanine it is possible that the strand of DNA affected could still serve as a template for

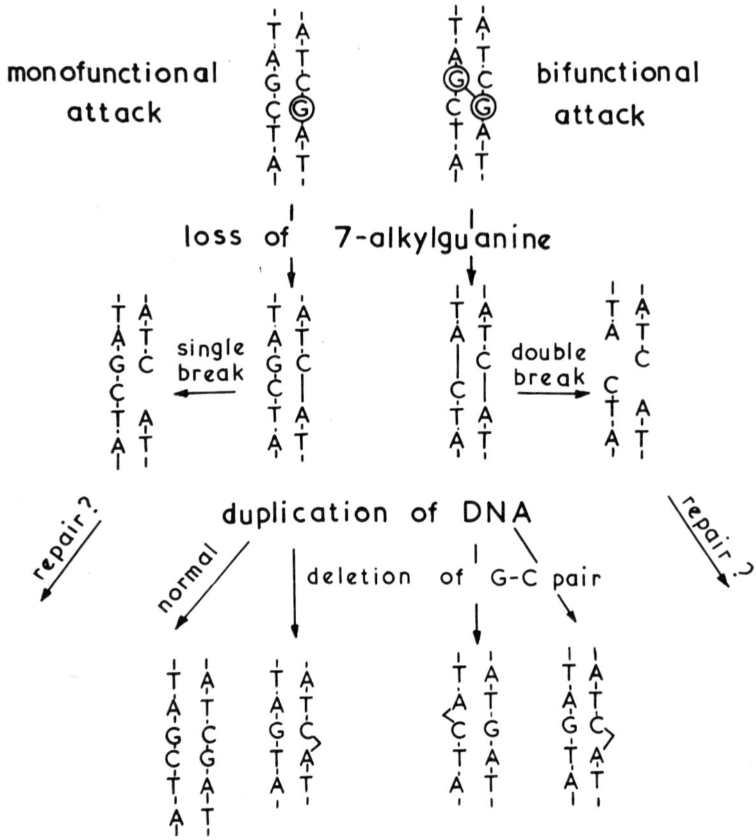

FIG. 4. Effects of the hydrolysis of alkylated DNA on its reduplication according to the Crick-Watson mechanism.

duplication yielding a DNA identical with the original except for loss of a guanine-cytosine pair of bases. This would constitute mutation by loss. Alternatively, if one invokes "repair" mechanisms, insertion of a "wrong" base in place of the deleted guanine could be proposed as a basis for mutation; if the complementary strand resulting from "repair" were guanine instead of cytosine, reversible mutation would result, since a repetition of the deletion and repair processes could lead to restoration of the original base sequence.

Seemingly, "double breaks" following difunctional attack would be more difficult to repair; also, single deletions may correspond to single chromatid mutations. The differences between the mutagenic spectra of mono- and difunctional agents could thus be explained.

I have not considered the initial effects of alkylation in detail although one could assume from steric considerations that this process would affect the binding of DNA and protein. However, no adequate detailed model of this binding is yet available, nor is its biological role understood. It has been proposed that differences between various types of alkylating agents could be connected with the steric relationships of the "prosthetic group" of the agent and the nucleoprotein complex (Fahmy and Fahmy, 1960).

We also at present lack a generally accepted model for the process of carcinogenesis. It was suggested many years ago (cf. review by Strong, 1949) that a relationship existed between mutagenesis and carcinogenesis. The latter, however, is a longer and more complex process. The suggested mechanism by which alkylating agents yield mutation by deletion of guanine-cytosine base pairs from DNA could be envisaged as part of a carcinogenic process since the latter has been suggested to involve deletion of enzymes controlling cell division (cf. Haddow, 1958). Alternatively, one could postulate that fission of the DNA molecule could release a nucleoprotein particle with viruslike properties capable of transforming neighboring cells, thus linking the mutation and virus theories of carcinogenesis (cf. Loveless, as cited by Haddow, 1953). It should be noted here that the proposed mechanism of fission of DNA would be more likely to occur with difunctional agents and would be a slow chemical process.

To conclude, an attempt to compare other types of mutagenic and carcinogenic agents will be made. Ionizing radiation has been shown (Hems, 1960) to yield chemical effects on DNA similar to those subsequent to alkylation, i.e., deletion of bases and fission of the DNA molecular chain. Particular resemblance to difunctional agents would follow from the fact that ionizing radiation yields groups of chemical events within a small volume rather than widely scattered single events. Differences between these agents are that the radiation can destroy the sugar moiety of nucleic acids, and thus break the molecular chain directly, whereas with alkylating agents the break is a secondary process; also evidence for cross-linking of the DNA strands by irradiation with X-rays is lacking; further, the specificity of alkylating agents for attack on one base, guanine, is not found with ionizing radiation since all bases can be destroyed. It is of particular interest, however, that guanosine can be attacked in a specific way by ionizing radiation with fission of the imidazole ring (Hems, 1958).

It is to be expected, therefore, that these differences in effects on DNA superimposed on a general resemblance should be reflected in differences in biological effects, although the term "radiomimetic" applied to alkylating agents still holds true in the broad sense. For example, the mutational spectrum of X-rays differs from that of alkylating agents (Fahmy and Fahmy, 1956). X-rays give more chromosome breaks than difunctional alkylating agents, reflecting their ability to break the DNA molecule directly; their target of attack is larger, giving fewer small deletions; and the distribution of loci of mutation along the chromosome differs, possibly reflecting the variety of bases attacked by X-rays, whereas the chemical agents are restricted to guanine, and are possibly different in their susceptibility to steric interference by protein.

Turning to another important group of carcinogens, those of the aromatic type, hydrocarbons and amines, no similarity with regard to reaction with DNA is evident. In fact, effects of these chemical agents on DNA have not been found although some have been shown to be mutagens (Scherr, Fishman, and Weaver, 1954). It has, however, been shown that reactive molecular species of the type of orthoquinones and orthoquinone imines can result *in vivo* which can bind to proteins (Heidelberger, 1959; Nagasawa and Gutmann, 1959). Two views can be taken in attempting to explain the carcinogenic action of these chemical substances: first, that direct effects are exerted on DNA which have so far not been detected, possibly due to their small extent in comparison to binding of the agents to protein; second, that the binding to protein is able to interfere with mechanisms of cell division possibly by processes related to immunological mechanisms (cf. Green, 1954). This might involve the DNA-protein relationship about which little is known at present. Carcinogenic activity of metals might also involve interference with DNA-protein binding which has been suggested to include metallic linkages (Kirby, 1957).

To summarize, therefore, it may be suggested that the principal biological effects of alkylating agents result from alkylation of DNA since the differences in biological effects between mono- and difunctional agents are reflected in their reactions with DNA, as are their radiomimetic properties. However, it is difficult at present to see how direct action on DNA could provide a mechanism for carcinogenic and mutagenic activity of aromatic hydrocarbons and amines.

ACKNOWLEDGMENTS

This investigation has been supported by grants to the Chester Beatty Research Institute (Institute of Cancer Research: Royal Cancer Hospital) from the Medical Research Council, the British Empire Cancer Campaign, the Jane Coffin Childs Memorial Fund for Medical Research, the Anna Fuller Fund and the National Cancer Institute of the National Institutes of Health, United States Public Health Service.

REFERENCES

Auerbach, C., and J. M. Robson. 1946. Chemical Production of Mutations. *Nature, London*, 157:302.

Brookes, P., and P. D. Lawley. 1960. The Reaction of Mustard Gas and Nucleic Acids *in vitro* and *in vivo*. *Biochemical Journal*, 77:478–484.

———. 1961. The Action of Mono- and Di-functional Alkylating Agents on Nucleic Acids. *Biochemical Journal*, 80:496–503.

Brown, D. M., and A. R. Todd. 1954. "Chemical Bonds in Nucleic Acids," *The Nucleic Acids*, E. Chargaff and J. N. Davidson, Eds., Vol. 1, pp. 409–444. New York, New York: Academic Press, Inc.

Crick, F. H. C., and J. D. Watson. 1954. The Complementary Structure of Deoxyribonucleic Acid. *Proceedings of the Royal Society, Series A*, 223:80–96.

Fahmy, O. G., and M. J. Fahmy. 1956. Differential Genetic Response to the Alkylating Mutagens and X-Radiation. *Journal of Genetics*, 54:146–164.

———. 1960. Mutagenicity in the Sperm of *Drosophila* and the Structure of the "Nitrogen Mustard" Molecule. *Heredity*, 15:115–128.

———. 1961. The Nature of the Mutations Induced by the Mesyloxy Esters in Relation to Molecular Cross-Linkage. *Genetics*, 46:446–458.

Goldacre, R. J., A. Loveless, and W. C. J. Ross. 1949. Mode of Production of Chromosome Abnormalities by the Nitrogen Mustards: The Possible Role of Cross-Linking. *Nature, London*, 163:667.

Green, H. N. 1954. An Immunological Concept of Cancer: A Preliminary Report. *British Medical Journal*, December: 1374–1380.

Haddow, A. 1953. "Mechanisms of Carcinogenesis," *The Physiopathology of Cancer*, F. Homburger and W. H. Fishman, Eds., p. 504. London: Cassell and Co.

———. 1958. Chemical Carcinogens and Their Modes of Action. *British Medical Bulletin*, 14:79–92.

Haddow, A., G. A. R. Kon, and W. C. J. Ross. 1948. Effects upon Tumours of Various Haloalkylarylamines. *Nature, London*, 162:824–825.

Haddow, A., and G. M. Timmis. 1953. Myleran in Chronic Myelogenous Leukemia. *Lancet*, 264:207.

Heidelberger, C. 1959. "The Relation of Protein Binding to Hydrocarbon Carcinogenesis," *Foundation Symposium, Mechanisms of Carcinogenesis*, G. E. W. Wolstenholme and C. M. O'Conner, Eds., pp. 179–192. London: J. and A. Churchill, Ltd.

Hems, G. 1958. Effect of Ionizing Radiation on Aqueous Solutions of Guanylic Acid and Guanosine. *Nature, London,* 181:1721–1722.

———. 1960. Chemical Effects of Ionizing Radiation on Deoxyribonucleic Acid in Dilute Aqueous Solution. *Nature, London,* 186:710–712.

Kirby, K. S. 1957. A New Method for Isolation of Deoxyribonucleic Acids: Evidence on the Nature of Bonds Between Deoxyribonucleic Acid and Protein. *Biochemical Journal,* 66:495–504.

Lawley, P. D. 1957a. Relative Reactivities of Deoxyribonucleotides and of the Bases of Deoxyribonucleic Acid Towards Alkylating Agents. *Biochimica et biophysica acta,* 26:450–451.

———: 1957b. Hydrolysis of Methylated Deoxyguanylic Acid at pH 7 to Yield 7-Methylguanine. *Proceedings of the Chemical Society,* p. 290.

Lawley, P. D., P. Brookes, J. A. V. Butler, D. J. R. Laurence, and K. V. Shooter. 1960. The Action of Alkylating Agents on Nucleic Acids. *Annual Report of the British Empire Cancer Campaign,* 38:10.

Lawley, P. D., and C. A. Wallick. 1957. The Action of Alkylating Agents on Deoxyribonucleic Acid and Guanylic Acid. *Chemistry and Industry,* May 18:633.

Loveless, A., and W. C. J. Ross. 1950. Chromosome Alteration and Tumour Inhibition by Nitrogen Mustards: The Hypothesis of Cross-Linking Alkylation. *Nature, London,* 166:1113–1114.

Nagasawa, H. T., and H. R. Gutmann. 1959. The Oxidation of Orthoaminophenols by Cytochrome C and Cytochrome Oxidase. I. Enzymatic Oxidations and Binding of Oxidation Products to Bovine Serum Albumin. *Journal of Biological Chemistry,* 234:1593–1599.

Scherr, G. H., M. Fishman, and R. H. Weaver. 1954. Mutagenicity of Some Carcinogenic Compounds for *Escherichia coli. Genetics,* 39:141–149.

Strong, L. C. 1949. Induction of Mutations by a Carcinogen. *British Journal of Cancer,* 3:97–108.

Watson, J. D., and F. H. C. Crick. 1953. Genetical Implications of the Structure of Deoxyribonucleic Acid. *Nature, London,* 171:964–967.

Physicochemical Studies on the Deoxyribonucleic Acids of Mouse Tissues

SAUL KIT, PH.D.

Section of Nucleoprotein Metabolism, The University of Texas M. D. Anderson Hospital and Tumor Institute, Houston, Texas

Although there is evidence that the deoxyribonucleic acid (DNA) from animal tissues consists of a heterogeneous collection of molecular types, information as to the nature and extent of the heterogeneity is limited and there is some disagreement as to whether significant differences in heterogeneity have been demonstrated between adult tissues of the same animal, or between normal and diseased tissues (Bendich, Pahl, and Beiser, 1956; Bendich *et al.*, 1959; Kit, 1960a,g). The hypothesis that DNA differences exist, at least between normal and tumor tissues, is an appealing one and is not unreasonable in view of the fact that chromosomal aberrations are frequently encountered in cancer cells. However, this does not lessen the need to scrutinize critically experiments purporting to demonstrate such differences.

Three approaches to the study of DNA heterogeneity have been employed in the author's laboratory: (1) chromatography of DNA preparations on substituted cellulose anion exchangers (Kit, 1960c,d,f), (2) determination of the ultraviolet absorption spectrum of DNA during thermal denaturation (Kit, 1960g), and (3) equilibrium centrifugation of DNA in cesium chloride (CsCl) density gradients (Kit, 1961). Anion exchangers discriminate between DNA species on the basis of molecular size (Bendich, Pahl, and Beiser, 1956; Rosenkranz and Bendich, 1959), while ultraviolet absorption versus temperature curves provide information as to the range of heterogeneity of composition (Doty, Marmur, and Sueoka, 1959; Kit, 1960g). The DNA bands obtained after density gradient centrifugation depend upon both the heterogeneity of composition and the distribution of molecular sizes (Rolfe and Meselson, 1959; Doty, Marmur, and Sueoka, 1959).

The results of chromatographic studies of DNA have previously been reported (Kit, 1960c,d,f). The DNA chromatographic elution profiles of five normal mouse tissues, lymphomas, carcinomas, and melanomas were all similar.

Data on the banding of DNA and the effect of temperature on the ultraviolet absorption spectra will be presented. The results of the present experiments confirm and extend previous observations.

In the course of these investigations, two additional observations of interest came to light. First, DNA preparations from all mouse tissues manifested a characteristic difference from the DNA of other animal species when centrifuged in CsCl density gradients. Second, the DNA from tissue culture cells which had been grown in the presence of bromodeoxyuridine exhibited unusual optical density-thermal denaturation curves. DNA in which bromouracil had partially replaced thymine showed a significantly higher melting temperature (T_m) than did normal DNA.

TABLE 1

Properties of the DNA of Normal Mouse Tissues and Tumors

Tissue	T_m*	2σ*	Per cent Hyper-chromicity	$E^{1\%}_{1cm.}$	$[\eta]^{26}_{dl/g}$	S†
Lung	87.9°	5.4°	45.1	193	49.5	24.1
Brain	87.7°	5.4°	44.0	207	65.0	24.5
Liver	87.8°	5.7°	39.2	207	56.0	25.7
Spleen	87.8°	5.5°	45.0	185	53.5	23.8
Kidney	87.7°	5.7°	44.2	191	53.8	23.3
6C3HED (diploid lymphoma)	87.8°	5.5°	45.2	181	52.3	23.9
6C3HED-DBA to C3H (tetraploid lymphoma)	87.7°	5.5°	45.1	186	58.4	25.4
Ehrlich (hypotetraploid carcinoma)	87.9°	5.4°	42.1	186	62.1	24.9
Lettré-Ehrlich (hyperdiploid carcinoma)	87.8°	5.5°	43.1	195	57.6	24.3
S91A (tetraploid amelanotic melanoma)	87.7°	5.4°	43.8	196	53.0	23.5

* Degrees centigrade.
† Sedimentation coefficients of DNA at 0.005 per cent concentration and 20° C and corrected to the solvent viscosity of water.

THERMAL DENATURATION CURVES OF MOUSE DNA PREPARATIONS

High molecular weight DNA was prepared by modifications of the method of Kirby (Kirby, 1957; Kit, 1960c). From 0.3 to 3.0 Gm. wet weight of tissues were extracted twice with *p*-aminosalicylate-phenol and subsequently further deproteinized with a phenol-saline mixture and with chloroform-octanol. The DNA preparations from all sources were similar with respect to average nucleotide compositions (Kit, 1960d), extinction coefficients ($E^{1\%}_{1cm.}$), intrinsic viscosities $[\eta]^{26}$, and velocity sedimentation coefficients (Table 1) (Kit, 1960g).

The effect of temperature on the ultraviolet absorption of mouse DNA preparations is shown in Figure 1. The ultraviolet absorption increases sharply between 80°C and 95°C due to the "melting" of the hydrogen bonds of the DNA double helix. The midpoint of the thermally induced absorbance increase may be defined as the T_m of the DNA and is a function of the guanine and cytosine (G + C) content of the molecules. The T_m for all mouse DNA preparations investigated were the same within the limits of experimental error (Figure 1; Table 1). This represents a confirmation that the mean molar nucleotide compositions are the same (Kit, 1960d,g).

Doty, Marmur, and Sueoka (1959) have shown that a linear relationship exists between the nucleotide composition of DNA and

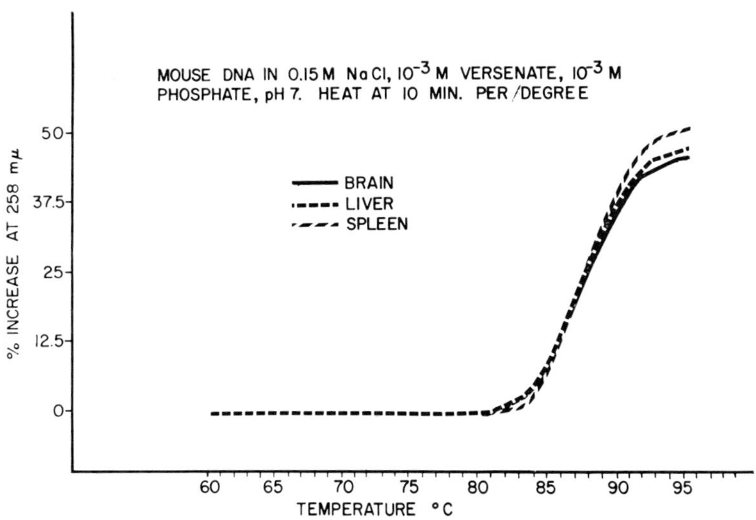

FIG. 1. Per cent increase of optical density with temperature of mouse spleen, liver, and brain DNA. DNA concentration: 0.002 per cent.

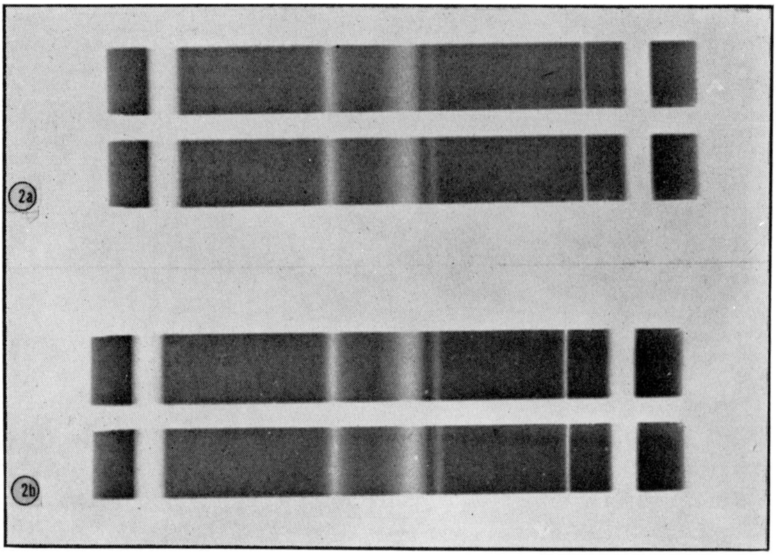

FIG. 2. Resolution of *Streptomyces viridochromogenes* DNA and mouse DNA by density gradient centrifugation. The photograph was taken after centrifugation for 24 hours at 25°C at 44,770 rpm. The *Streptomyces* band ($\rho^{25°} = 1.729$ gcm^{-3}) appears at the left. Two bands with mean densities of 1.701 and 1.690 gcm^{-3} are obtained with mouse DNA. The initial densities of the CsCl solutions were: a) mouse brain, 1.7208 gcm^{-3}; b) mouse lung, 1.7165 gcm^{-3}.

the melting temperature. The slope of the curve, as measured in this laboratory was 2.2 mole per cent (G + C) per degree increase in T_m (Kit, 1960g).

The temperature range (Δ T) over which the absorbance increase (hyperchromicity) takes place is also significant. The temperature range is very narrow for a solution consisting of only one molecular type of DNA. In the case of the adenine-thymine polymer, the middle two thirds of the absorbance rise, that is, 17 to 83 per cent of the observed hyperchromicity, takes place over a temperature range of 3.0°C (Doty, Marmur, and Sueoka, 1959). This value may be taken as an estimate of the natural transition for DNA. When a DNA preparation consists of numerous molecular species differing in nucleotide composition, the melting curve is the composite of the melting curves for each molecular type. Hence, the temperature range of the transition from the double helix to denatured DNA is broadened. An estimate of the compositional distribution can be obtained as follows. By approximating the distributions as Gaussian, twice the standard deviation ($2\,\sigma$) of the distribution about the

TABLE 2

Gradient Centrifugation of Mouse DNA in CsCl

Tissue	$\rho^{25°}$	$\sigma\rho$	$\rho^{25°}$ (minor band)
LM	1.701	0.0043	1.690
Liver	1.701	0.0042	1.690
Brain	1.701	0.0042	1.690
Kidney	1.701	0.0042	1.690
Spleen	1.701	0.0046	1.690
Lung	1.701	0.0044	1.690
6C3HED-DBA to C3H	1.701	0.0042	1.690
Lettré-Ehrlich	1.701	0.0042	1.689
Ehrlich	1.701	0.0042	1.689

All values expressed as gcm.$^{-3}$
2μg. of DNA dissolved in CsCl (density, 1.70–1.72 gcm^{-3}) were centrifuged for 24 hours at 44,770 rpm at 25° C in the Spinco Model E ultracentrifuge. The density of the mouse DNA band was calculated from a *Streptomyces viridochromogenes* DNA marker having a density of 1.729 gcm.$^{-3}$

mean can be derived from the temperature difference, Δ T, between 17 and 83 per cent of the absorbance rise. This result is corrected for the natural transition width by subtracting the corresponding quantity for the adenine-thymine DNA transition (that is, 3.0) and then transformed into the mole per cent guanine plus cytosine scale by multiplying by 2.2. The 2 σ values for all mouse DNA preparations ranged from 5.4 to 5.7°C (Table 1). Hence, the heterogeneity of composition for the middle two thirds of the transition (2σ) is about $(5.5 - 3.0) \times 2.2 = 5.5$ mole per cent (G + C). Heterogeneity of composition, as estimated in this way, was the same for all normal and neoplastic mouse DNA preparations.

Equilibrium Centrifugation of Mouse DNA in CsCl Density Gradients

Photographs illustrating the banding of mouse brain and lung DNA after density gradient centrifugation in CsCl are shown in Figure 2. Two bands with effective buoyant densities of about 1.701 and 1.690 gcm.$^{-3}$ were found. The mouse DNA bands were well separated from the reference *Streptomyces viridochromogenes* band ($\rho^{25°} = 1.729$) shown on the left. Rolfe and Meselson (1959) and Doty, Marmur, and Sueoka (1959) have shown that the mean buoyant densities of DNA bands increase in a linear fashion with the mean molar (G + C) content of the DNA. As shown in Table 2, the mean buoyant densities of DNA from normal and neoplastic mouse tissues are the same. Hence, the similarity in average nucleotide composition is confirmed by a third method.

Since the density of DNA depends on its composition, it follows that a compositional heterogeneity among the various DNA molecules of a given sample will be reflected in a broadening of the band. Molecules of uniform density are distributed in the band region as a result of thermal agitation. Meselson, Stahl, and Vinograd (1957) have demonstrated that the square of the standard deviation, σ^2, (that is, the variance) is inversely proportional to the molecular weight. However, if a distribution of density is superimposed upon the molecules, there will be a further broadening of the band. The σ_ρ values for mouse DNA preparations are shown in Table 2. The values for all tissues are approximately 0.0044 gcm.$^{-3}$, showing that the resultant of the combined heterogeneity of composition and molecular size is the same. The σ_ρ values for mouse DNA are somewhat greater than those obtained for *Serratia marcescens* DNA ($\sigma_\rho = 0.0033$ gcm.$^{-3}$) and *Streptomyces viridochromogenes* DNA ($\sigma_\rho = 0.0031$ gcm.$^{-3}$).

The heterogeneity of composition of mouse brain DNA may be estimated as follows. The square of the total DNA band variance (σ_T^2) is equal to the sum of the squares of the variance (σ^2_{DN}) due to density heterogeneity and the variance (σ^2_{BN}) caused by Brownian motion of molecules which is molecular weight dependent (Doty, Marmur, and Sueoka, 1959; Sueoka, 1959):

$$\sigma_T^2 = \sigma^2_{DN} + \sigma^2_{BN}$$

A reasonable estimate of the number average molecular weight of the cesium salt of mouse brain DNA is 6,000,000 (Kit, 1960g; Sueoka, 1959). Hence, the square of the variance (σ^2_{BN}) caused by Brownian motion of the molecules is, under the conditions of our experiments, approximately 0.000447 cm.^{2} (Meselson, Stahl, and Vinograd, 1957). The observed value for σ_T^2 equals 0.001122 cm.^{2}. Therefore, $\sigma^2_{DN} = 0.000675$ cm.^{2}. The square root of this value is about 0.025 cm. (σ_{DN}). In this case, the distance from the center of the rotor to the mean of the band is 6.432 cm. It can be calculated that the variance due to density heterogeneity ($\sigma_{(DN)}$) is 0.00299 gcm^{-3}. The variance on a mole fraction (G + C) scale is about 10 times this value (Rolfe and Meselson, 1959), or 0.0299 gcm.$^{-3}$ and twice this variance ($2\sigma_{GC}$) is 0.0598. The latter figure is of the same order of magnitude as was calculated from the optical density temperature curves [0.0528 moles (G + C)]. Similarly, an estimate of compositional heterogeneity may be made for the other mouse DNA preparations. In each case, heterogeneity of composition as estimated from the density gradient experiments shows good agreement with that estimated from the optical density temperature curves.

Properties of Rat Kidney and Rat Brain DNA

The chromatographic elution profiles of rat kidney and rat brain DNA have previously been described (Kit, 1960f). The physical properties of these DNA preparations are shown in Table 3. The sedimentation coefficients, extinction coefficients, T_m and $2\ \sigma$ values, and the effective buoyant densities and standard deviations of the density gradient bands of rat brain DNA are all similar to those of rat kidney DNA.

On the basis of the experiments which have been presented, it seems unlikely that gross differences exist between the DNA of normal tissues of the same animal or between the DNA of normal tissues and tumors. The methods so far employed do not discriminate between DNA molecules differing in chain length by a few nucleotides, or between molecules differing slightly in composition or in the sequence of nucleotides. Hence, differences of the latter kind cannot be ruled out but must await the development of improved methods and further studies of the properties of DNA (Shapiro and Chargaff, 1960). There is another possibility, that is, that only a small part of the population of DNA molecules from a given source are distinctive. An apparent example of this is described in the next section.

Specific Differences Between Mouse DNA and the DNA of Other Animal Species

Photographs of the rat brain and rat kidney DNA bands after density gradient centrifugation are shown in Figure 3. These photographs may be compared with those from mouse DNA (Figure 2). In contrast to mouse DNA, only one band is found with rat kidney or rat brain DNA and this band corresponds to the principal mouse DNA band ($\rho^{25°} = 1.701$ gcm^{-3}). Likewise, only one band ($\rho^{25°} = 1.700$ gcm^{-3}) is observed for the DNA derived from a human tissue culture cell line (Lass liver), or the DNA of the golden hamster liver ($\rho^{25°} = 1.700$ gcm^{-3}).

Two interpretations which suggest themselves may account for the differences between the DNA of rat, human, or hamster origin and mouse DNA: (1) the DNA from the mouse tissues includes a

TABLE 3

Properties of Rat Kidney and Rat Brain DNA

	Rat kidney	Rat brain
T_m (in °C)	88.7°	88.7°
2σ (in °C)	6.1°	6.0°
Hyperchromicity	41.5%	42.0%
$\rho^{25°}$ gcm^{-3}	1.701	1.701
σ_ρ gcm^{-3}	0.0044	0.0046
$S_{20,w}$	26.0 S	27.5 S
$E^{1\%}_{1cm.}$	198	216

component which has a relatively high ratio of adenine plus thymine to guanine plus cytosine $\left(\frac{A+T}{G+C}\right)$. The estimated $\frac{A+T}{G+C}$ ratio for the "lighter" mouse DNA component would be approximately 1.9, a value corresponding to the average ratio of $\frac{G+C}{A+U}$ of 80 per cent or more of the total mouse RNA (Kit ,1960b,e); and

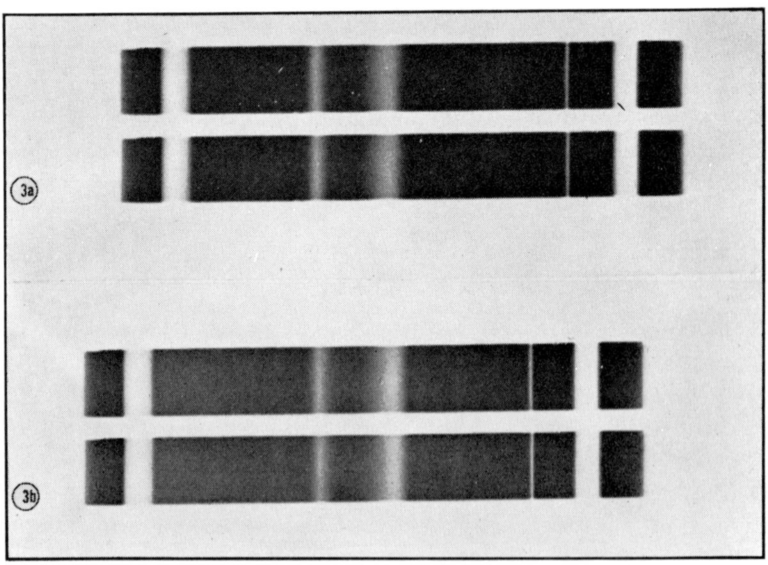

FIG. 3. Resolution of *Streptomyces viridochromogenes* and rat DNA by density gradient centrifugation. The photograph was taken after centrifugation for 24 hours at 25°C at 44,770 rpm. The effective buoyant density of the *Streptomyces* band is 1.729 gcm^{-3}; that of the rat DNA, 1.701 gcm^{-3}. The initial densities of the CsCl solutions were: a) rat brain, 1.729 gcm^{-3}; b) rat kidney, 1.7186 gcm^{-3}.

(2) the mouse DNA may contain a component which is tightly bound to protein. As the density of protein is about 1.3 gcm^{-3}, the buoyant density of this mouse DNA-protein complex would be displaced from the main DNA band toward lighter densities. The confirmation of either of these possibilities awaits the isolaticn of the "lighter" mouse DNA band.

A third possibility, namely, that the "lighter" band is due to the interaction of ribonuclease with DNA, is contraindicted. Although ribonuclease is normally employed in the DNA preparative procedure to eliminate contamination of RNA, the 1.690 gcm^{-3} density mouse DNA band is present even when ribonuclease is not used and the rat, human, or hamster DNA preparations do not manifest the band despite the fact that ribonuclease is used in the latter preparations.

Properties of DNA Containing Bromodeoxyuridine

Bromodeoxyuridine (BUDR), an analog of thymidine, does not affect the respiration, glycolysis, protein synthesis, or ribonucleic acid (RNA) synthesis of cells, but inhibits competitively the incorporation of thymidine into DNA (Kit, Beck, Graham, and Gross, 1958) and is itself incorporated in place of thymidine into bacterial, bacteriophage, or animal cell DNA (Dunn and Smith, 1957; Djordjevic and Szybalski, 1960; Eidinoff, Cheong, and Rich, 1959; Kozinski and Szybalski, 1959; Wacker, Trebst, Jacherts, and Weygand, 1954; Zamenhof and Griboff, 1954; Zamenhof, Rich, and de Giovanni, 1958). Cells containing bromouracil in their DNA are more susceptible to growth inhibition by radiation than normal cells (Djordjevic and Szybalski, 1960). Bromodeoxyuridine is an established mutagenic agent (Litman and Pardee, 1959). Presumably, it induces errors in DNA replication as a result of which adenine-thymine base pairs are replaced by guanine-cytosine base pairs in the DNA (Freese, 1959).

Strain LM mouse cells and strain B14FAF28 Chinese hamster cells have been cultivated in a medium containing from 5 to 25 μg. of BUDR (Kit and Hsu, 1961). Hsu and Somers (1961) have shown that chromosome breakage is enhanced after the Chinese hamster cells have been grown for 12 hours in 25 μg./ml. of BUDR and a great majority of the breaks are found at one spot, the secondary constriction. Chromosome breakage is abundant in LM cells after four to five days of treatment but after 12 weeks of growth in BUDR, the breakage frequency is definitely abated. Hsu

TABLE 4

Physical Properties of DNA from Tissue Culture Cells Grown in the Presence of 10 µg./ml. Bromodeoxyuridine (BUDR)

Cell type	$S_{20,w}$	$[\eta]^{26°}$	$E^{1\%}_{1cm.}$
LM	28.4S	60 dl/g	206
LM (BUDR)	26.2S	55 dl/g	207

and Somers (1961) have suggested that the enhancement of chromosome breaks at specific regions may be the result of, or at least closely related to the BUDR incorporation, and that certain chromosome loci contain DNA molecules with a relatively high adenine-thymine ratio.

In confirmation of the experiment of Djordjevic and Szybalski (1960) we have observed that tissue culture cells which have been growing for five days in a BUDR medium contain no normal density DNA molecules but only molecules whose effective buoyant densities correspond to hybrid "unifilarly" and heavy "bifilarly" substituted DNA. After 13 weeks or more of growth in BUDR medium, all the DNA is "heavy" as reflected by density gradient centrifugation experiments, even though the chromosome breakage frequency is abated and the cells manifest normal growth rates (Kit and Hsu, 1961).

The sedimentation coefficients, intrinsic viscosities, and extinction coefficients of DNA containing BUDR are similar to those of normal DNA (Table 4). The T_m values are, however, abnormal (Table 5). As early as 22 hours after growth in BUDR medium, the T_m value is slightly elevated and subsequently the T_m values increase further to about 90° to 91°C.

Three possibilities may be suggested to explain the enhanced T_m values: (1) The substitution of the bromine atom for the methyl group in thymine alters the electron densities in the bromouracil rings so as to strengthen the hydrogen bonding to the purine base of the complementary DNA chain. (2) A distortion of nucleotide sequence along the DNA chains is induced by growing the cells in the presence of BUDR (Shapiro and Chargaff, 1960) and, possibly, some adenine-thymine hydrogen bonded pairs are replaced by guanine-cytosine (Freese, 1959). (3) Those molecular types of the DNA mixture of molecules in which the adenine-thymine ratio is high are deleted from the cells, or preferentially altered in composition.

TABLE 5

Properties of DNA from LM Cells Grown in the Presence of Bromodeoxyuridine (BUDR) (10 μg./ml.)

Cells	Time in BUDR	T_m	2σ	% Hyper-chromicity
LM (normal)	0	88.0°	5.8°	41.3
LM (BUDR)	22 hours	88.7°	6.0°	40.0
LM (BUDR)	46 hours	90.0°	5.5°	42.1
LM (BUDR)	5 days	90.1°	5.8°	42.6
LM (BUDR)	91 days	89.8°	5.7°	44.7
LM (BUDR)	158 days	91.3°	5.5°	41.1
LM (BUDR)*	161 days	91.4°	6.1°	42.1
LM (BUDR)	70 days, then 12 days in normal growth medium	88.6°	5.4°	42.3
LM (BUDR)*	168 days, then 17 days in normal growth medium	88.5°	5.7°	39.4

* 25 μg./ml.

To test these possibilities, cells which had been grown in BUDR medium for 23 weeks were transferred for 17 days to normal growth medium (Table 5). After density gradient centrifugation, both the "lighter" mouse DNA band ($\rho^{25°} = 1.690$ gcm^{-3}) and the principal band $\rho^{25°} = 1.701$ gcm^{-3}) were still present. Hence, one may exclude the hypothesis that molecules rich in adenine and thymine are preferentially deleted. Also, the T_m value was reduced to 88.5°C, slightly higher than the normal value (Table 5). This demonstrates: (1) that the change in T_m values was not hereditary, or (2) that in the absence of BUDR, persisting cellular types having unaltered DNA could outgrow the population of cells having DNA molecules with enhanced T_m values. Although the hypothesis that there is a permanent distortion of nucleotide sequence and guanine-cytosine substitution for adenine-thymine cannot be completely excluded, the fact that the T_m values are enhanced as soon as 46 hours (two generations) of growth in BUDR medium also argues against this hypothesis. It appears, therefore, that the first possibility mentioned above is more plausible, that is, that substitution of the bromine atom for the methyl group of thymine alters the electron distribution in the bromouracil ring so as to strengthen the hydrogen bonding to the purine base of the complementary DNA chain. Consistent with this hypothesis are the recent experiments of Baldwin, Inman, and Wake (1961) which show that in solutions of low ionic strength, the T_m value of the enzymatically synthesized adenine-bromouracil polymer is approximately 10° higher than that of the adenine-thymine polymer.

ACKNOWLEDGMENTS

These experiments were aided in part by grants from The American Cancer Society (P35B), The Leukemia Society, Inc., and The National Cancer Institute (4064C2 and 4238C2).

David Cullop, Jo Anita Jefferies, and Andrew Cox provided expert assistance. *Serratia marcescens* and *Streptomyces viridochromogenes* DNA were obtained through the kindness of Drs. Julius Marmur and Carl Schildkraut. The author would like to express his thanks to Dr. T. C. Hsu for cultures of strain LM cells and LM cells grown in the presence of BUDR.

REFERENCES

Baldwin, R. L., Inman, R. B., and Wake, R. G. 1961. Hybrid Molecules Containing Strands of dAT and dABrU, Formed Both by Enzymatic and Physico-Chemical Means. *Federation Proceedings*, 20:354.

Bendich, A., G. P. diMayorca, H. S. Rosenkranz, M. Bianchessi, and E. E. Polli. 1959. Chromatographic Studies on Human Deoxyribonucleic Acid (DNA). *Haematologia Latina Estratto, Supplement* 2:33–38.

Bendich, A., H. B. Pahl, and S. M. Beiser. 1956. "Chromatographic Fractionation of Deoxyribonucleic Acids with Special Emphasis on the Transforming Factor of Pneumococcus," *Genetic Mechanisms: Structure and Function* (Cold Spring Harbor Symposia on Quantitative Biology, Vol. 21), pp. 31–48. Cold Spring Harbor, New York: Long Island Biological Association.

Djordjevic, B., and W. Szybalski. 1960. Genetics of Human Cell Lines. III. Incorporation of 5-Bromo- and 5-Iododeoxyuridine into the Deoxyribonucleic Acid of Human Cells and Its Effects on Radiation Sensitivity. *Journal of Experimental Medicine*, 112:509–531.

Doty, P., J. Marmur, and N. Sueoka. 1959. "The Heterogeneity in Properties and Functioning of Deoxyribonucleic Acids," *Structure and Function of Genetic Elements* (Brookhaven Symposia in Biology, No. 12), pp. 1–16. Upton, New York: Brookhaven National Laboratory.

Dunn, D. B., and J. D. Smith. 1957. Effects of 5-Halogenated Uracils on the Growth of *Escherichia coli* and Their Incorporation into Deoxyribonucleic Acids. *Biochemical Journal*, 67:494–506.

Eidinoff, M. L., L. Cheong, and M. A. Rich. 1959. Incorporation of Unnatural Pyrimidine Bases into Deoxyribonucleic Acid of Mammalian Cells. *Science*, 129:1550–1551.

Freese, E. 1959. "On the Molecular Explanation of Spontaneous and Induced Mutations," *Structure and Function of Genetic Elements* (Brookhaven Symposia in Biology, No. 12), pp. 63–75. Upton, New York: Brookhaven National Laboratories.

Hakala, M. T. 1959. Mode of Action of 5-Bromodeoxyuridine on Mammalian Cells in Culture. *Journal of Biological Chemistry*, 234:3072–3076.

Hsu, T. C., and C. E. Somers. 1961. Effect of 5-Bromodeoxyuridine on

Mammalian Chromosomes. *Proceedings of the National Academy of Sciences of the U.S.A.*, 47:396–403.

Kirby, K. S. 1957. A New Method for the Isolation of Deoxyribonucleic Acids. Evidence on the Nature of Bonds Between Deoxyribonucleic Acid and Protein. *Biochemical Journal*, 66:495–504.

Kit, S. 1960a. "The Nucleic Acids of Normal Tissues and Tumors," *Amino Acids, Proteins, and Cancer Biochemistry*, John T. Edsall, Ed., pp. 147–174. New York, New York: Academic Press, Inc.

———. 1960b. "Studies on the Structure, Composition, and Metabolism of Tumor RNA," *Cell Physiology of Neoplasia* (The University of Texas M. D. Anderson Hospital and Tumor Institute, 14th Annual Symposium on Fundamental Cancer Research), pp. 337–373. Austin, Texas: The University of Texas Press.

———. 1960c. Fractionation of Deoxyribonucleic Acid Preparations on Substituted Cellulose Anion Exchangers. *Archives of Biochemistry and Biophysics*, 87:318–329.

———. 1960d. Investigations of the DNA Content, Base Composition, and Chromatography on Ecteola-Cellulose of Normal and Tumor DNA Preparations. *Archives of Biochemistry and Biophysics*, 87:330–336.

———. 1960e. Base Composition of the Ribonucleic Acids of Normal Tissues, Tumors, and Tissue Subfractions. *Archives of Biochemistry and Biophysics*, 88:1–8.

———. 1960f. Chromatographic Profiles of Deoxyribonucleic Acid Preparations from Rat and Mouse Tissues. *Journal of Biological Chemistry*, 235:1756–1760.

———. 1960g. Compositional Heterogeneity of Normal and Malignant Tissue Deoxyribonucleic Acids (DNA). *Biochemistry and Biophysics Research Communications*, 3:361–367.

———. 1961. Density Gradient Centrifugation of DNA from Normal Mouse Tissues and Tumors. *Federation Proceedings*, 20:354.

Kit, S., C. Beck, O. L. Graham, and A. Gross. 1958. Effect of 5-Bromodeoxyuridine on Deoxyribonucleic Acid-Thymine Synthesis and Cell Metabolism of Lymphatic Tissue and Tumors. *Cancer Research*, 18:598–602.

Kit, S., and Hsu, T. C. 1961. Relative Stability to Thermal Denaturation of Deoxyribonucleic Acid (DNA) Preparations Containing Bromodeoxyridine. *Biochemical and Biophysical Research Communications*, 5:120–124.

Kozinski, A. W., and W. Szybalski. 1959. Dispersive Transfer of Parental DNA Molecules to the Progeny of Phage $\phi\chi$-174. *Virology*, 9:260–274.

Litman, R. M., and A. B. Pardee. 1959. Mutations of Bacteriophage T_2 Induced by Bromouracil in the Presence of Chloramphenicol. *Virology*, 8:125–127.

Meselson, M., F. W. Stahl, and J. Vinograd. 1957. Equilibrium Sedimentation of Macromolecules in Density Gradients. *Proceedings of the National Academy of Sciences of the U.S.A.*, 43:581–588.

Rolfe, R., and M. Meselson. 1959. The Relative Homogeneity of Microbial DNA. *Proceedings of the National Academy of Sciences of the U.S.A.*, 45:1039–1043.

Rosenkranz, H. S., and A. Bendich. 1959. Sedimentation Studies of Fractions of Deoxyribonucleic Acid. *Journal of the American Chemical Society*, 81: 902–904.

Shapiro, H. S., and E. Chargaff. 1960. Severe Distortion by 5-Bromouracil of the Sequence Characteristics of a Bacterial Deoxyribonucleic Acid. *Nature, London*, 188:62–63.

Sueoka, N. 1959. A Statistical Analysis of Deoxyribonucleic Acid Distribution in Density Gradient Centrifugation. *Proceedings of the National Academy of Sciences of the U.S.A.*, 45:1480–1490.

Wacker, A., A. Trebst, D. Jacherts, and F. Weygand. 1954. Über den Einbau von 5-bromuracil-[2-^{14}C] in die Desoxyribonucleinsäure verschiedener Bakterien. *Zeitschrift für Naturforschung*, 9b:616–617.

Zamenhof, S., and G. Griboff. 1954. Incorporation of Halogenated Pyrimidines into the Deoxyribonucleic Acids of *Bacterium coli* and its Bacteriophages. *Nature, London*, 174:306–308.

Zamenhof, S., K. Rich, and R. de Giovanni. 1958. Further Studies on the Introduction of Pyrimidines into Deoxyribonucleic Acids of *Escherichia coli*. *Journal of Biological Chemistry*, 232:651–657.

Properties and Applications of Halogenated Deoxyribonucleic Acids

WACLAW SZYBALSKI, D.Sc.

McArdle Memorial Laboratory, University of Wisconsin Medical School, Madison, Wisconsin

Deoxyribonucleic acid (DNA), the "master biopolymer" believed to govern directly or indirectly all of the cell's activities, is composed of only four basic components: two purine and two pyrimidine deoxynucleotides. It is not known exactly how much deviation in the chemical structure of these building blocks is compatible with normal biological functioning of the DNA molecule. Isotopic substitution is without apparent effect on DNA function, other than the inactivation caused by the decay of radioactive isotopes. However, only a very few chemical alterations are known to be tolerated. The present study deals with one particular type of chemical modification of the DNA polymer: substitution at position "5" of thymine by one of the three halogens, chlorine, bromine, or iodine. The similarity between the van der Waals radius of the methyl group and those of the halogens, as quoted by Pauling (1945) and as represented in Figure 1, permits essentially perfect functioning of the DNA molecule even after almost total halogenation. 5-Chloro-, 5-bromo-, and 5-iodouracil (CU, BU, and IU), originally shown by Hitchings, Falco, and Sherwood (1945) to be partial thymine substitutes (CU, BU) in folic acid-deficient bacilli, were first tentatively (Weygand, Wacker, and Dellweg, 1952) and later definitely shown to be incorporated into the DNA of bacteria (Zamenhof and Griboff, 1954; Wacker, Trebst, Jacherts, and

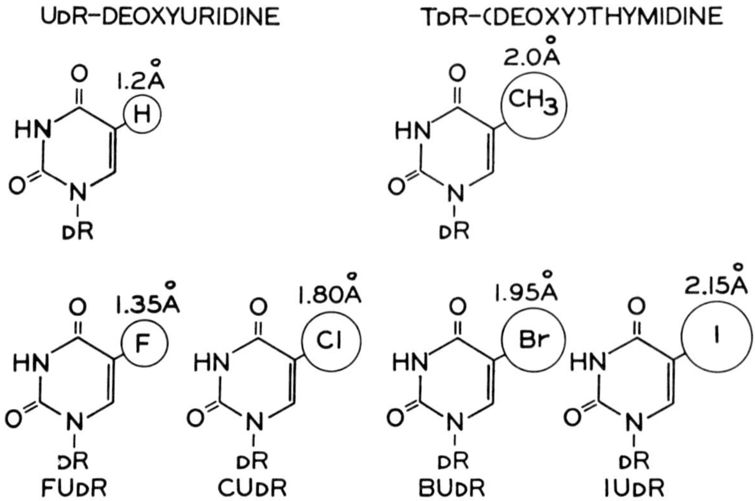

FIG. 1. Chemical structure of deoxyuridine, thymidine, and their analogs. Circles represent the van der Waals radii of the atoms or groups occupying position 5.

Weygand, 1954; Dunn and Smith, 1957), bacteriophages (Litman and Pardee, 1956), and even human and other mammalian cells (Kit, see pages 133 to 146, this volume; Hakala, 1959; Cheong, Rich, and Eidinoff, 1960; Szybalski and Djordjevic, 1959; Littlefield and Gould, 1960; Prusoff, 1960). 5-Halodeoxycytidines were found also to be incorporated into cell DNA, but only in the form of 5-halodeoxyuridines, apparently after their deamination (Frisch, Gregory, and Visser, 1960). Other pertinent references are quoted in the above papers and in the recent review by Handschumacher and Welch (1960).

The methods for effecting the incorporation of halogenated thymidine analogs into DNA, the properties of the modified DNA's and of the cells producing them, and various applications of this technique for chemical labeling of DNA will be briefly discussed.

INCORPORATION OF 5-HALODEOXYURIDINES INTO DNA

Most organisms have the capacity for *de novo* synthesis of nucleic acid constituents. The pathways of pyrimidine nucleotide synthesis and interconversion are represented in Figure 2. Although an exogenous supply of thymine or thymidine is normally not required, the utilization of thymidine for DNA synthesis through the action of thymidine kinase is usually possible. Utilization of the free base,

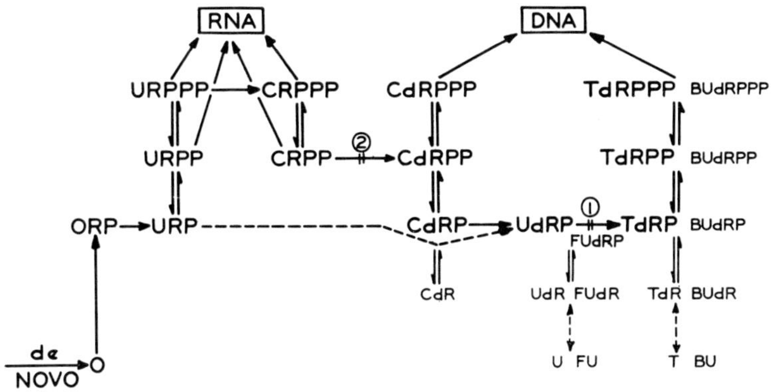

FIG. 2. Simplified map of the synthetic pathways for pyrimidine nucleotides and deoxynucleotides. Heavy lines: *de novo* synthetic pathways; thin lines: preformed pathways; (1): block in thymidylic acid synthesis; (2): feedback inhibition of the cytidine diphosphate to deoxycytidine diphosphate conversion.

thymine, requires an additional enzyme, thymidine phosphorylase, which is apparently lacking in most mammalian cells but present in several bacterial strains. Halogenated thymidine analogs can enter the DNA precursor pool after conversion to nucleotides by thymidine kinase and other kinases along the thymidylic acid pathway. Although some bacteria can also utilize 5-halouracils, 5-halodeoxyuridines are incorporated much more efficiently.

The actual extent of thymine replacement in the DNA depends on the composition of the precursor pool, particularly on the molar ratio of 5-halodeoxyuridylic acids entering through the preformed pathway to *de novo* synthesized thymidylic acids. It follows that selective inhibition of *de novo* synthesis of thymidylic acid (Figure 2, Block 1) should result in more extensive DNA labeling with preformed thymidine analogs. The block in thymidylate synthesis can be of genetic origin (mutation to thymine dependence) or can be produced by metabolic antagonists as follows: (1) specific inhibition of thymidylate synthetase, employing 5-fluorodeoxyuridine (FUdR) (Harbers, Chaudhuri, and Heidelberger, 1959; Cohen *et al.*, 1958), which is converted through phosphorylation to 5-fluorodeoxyuridylic acid, the active inhibitor; or (2) interference with single carbon transfer mechanisms by either (a) inhibiting the synthesis of folic acid through the use of sulfanilamides, or (b) binding folic acid reductase with folic acid analogs, most commonly aminopterin or amethopterin. Method 1, employed by Lorkiewicz and Szybalski (1960), is more efficient and specific than method 2, in which imposed additional requirements for preformed purines and certain amino acids must be satisfied. In the case of bacteria, where aminopterin is not very active and sulfanilamides rather toxic, as well as with mammalian cells, method 1 was found to give higher halodeoxyuridine incorporation with lower toxicity than method 2, especially after two further refinements of the technique were introduced. The first was the addition of deoxycytidine to the medium, the rationale for which was the demonstration by Reichard, Canellakis, and Canellakis (1960), and by Morris and Fisher (1960), that thymidylic triphosphates (or their haloanalogs) inhibit the conversion of cytidylate diphosphate to deoxycytidylate diphosphate (cf. Figure 2, Block 2), virtually depriving the cells of the deoxycytidylate precursors of DNA. The second improvement was the supplementation of the medium with uracil and uridine, which interfere with the catabolism of FUdR and its conversion into 5-fluorouridylates, inhibitors of ribotide metabolism and ribonucleic acid (RNA) function. Employing these supplements, it was possible to maintain the growth of human cells for an indefinite period, even though their DNA was continually chlorinated or brominated to the extent of over 50 per cent thymine replacement. In the case of bacteria (*Bacillus subtilis*), the concentrations of FUdR and 5-halodeoxyuridines required for over 80 per cent thymidine replacement were found to be 50 to 100 times higher than those employed for human cells; but in the course of over two cell generations on deoxycytidine-, uracil- and uridine-supplemented media, quite homogeneous, biologically active (transforming), unifilarly and bifilarly labeled DNA was produced (cf. Figure 7).

Functionality of Halogenated DNA

The incorporation of 5-halodeoxyuridines into growing cells is associated with a variable degree of toxicity. Although one is tempted to equate these two phenomena, closer analysis reveals that it is possible to modify conditions in such a manner (cf. the earlier section) that the toxic effects of the analogs are completely or almost completely eliminated, while their incorporation into DNA is unimpaired. One human cell line, D98/AG, was carried for over a year in the presence of 5-bromodeoxyuridine (BUdR) and FUdR in concentrations sufficient to maintain over 50 per cent replacement of the DNA thymidine by BUdR. Since incorporation was rather homogeneous throughout the DNA, as revealed by analytical ultracentrifugation in the CsCl gradient, and since human cells producing it were fully viable (Djordjevic and Szybalski, 1960), it could be concluded that heavily BUdR-labeled DNA is fully functional.

Another line of evidence for the functionality of the halogenated thymidine analogs derives from their ability to support the growth of human cells under conditions of thymidine dependence (in FUdR-containing medium). In this respect 5-chlorodeoxyuridine (CUdR) and BUdR are both efficient thymidine substitutes, particularly CUdR, while 5-iododeoxyuridine (IUdR) permits only limited growth of FUdR-inhibited cells. On the basis of its van der Waals radius (Figure 1), BUdR should theoretically be the best of the three thymidine substitutes; the radius of chlorine is substantially smaller than that of the methyl group. The approximate equality of CUdR and BUdR indicates that (1) the van der Waals radii for the methyl group in the 5-position of thymine and for the halogens should be re-evaluated, or (2) the partial specific volumes are more closely correlated with biological functionality than the van der Waals radii (Szybalski, 1960b), or (3) still other factors must be considered.

Other organisms, including phages, bacteria, and even tissues of higher animals, e.g. mice, can be labeled with CUdR or BUdR without gross impairment of viability.

A unique test for the functionality of purified DNA from *B. subtilis* cells is the assay of its genetic transforming activity. Heavily bifilarly BUdR- or IUdR-labeled DNA (close to 100 per cent halogenation) was found to have a specific transforming activity indistinguishable from that of unifilarly halogenated DNA or from normal DNA (Szybalski, *et al.*, 1960; Opara-Kubinska and Szybalski, unpublished data). Even IUdR-labeled DNA isolated from very fragile or "dead" cells still transformed with undiminished specific activity, attesting to the full biological functionality of heavily halogenated DNA.

Intrinsic Properties of Halogenated DNA and Properties Conferred on Cells

Although halogenation of DNA does not impair its biological functionality and, in general, is compatible with continued cell multiplication, the physicochemical properties of the molecule are obviously altered, as are certain cellular characteristics. The major

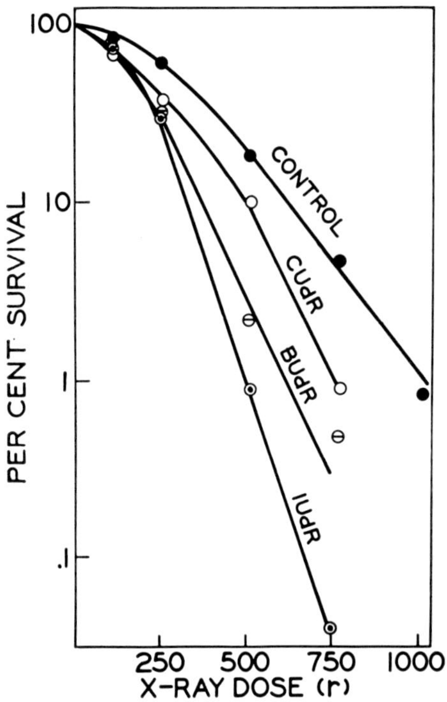

(3a)

FIG. 3. Comparative X-ray (3a) and ultraviolet light (3b) survival of D98/AG cells grown for four days prior to irradiation in the absence (control) or in the presence of 0.004 μg. FUdR/ml. and 2 × 10^{-6} M CUdR, BUdR, or IUdR. (Redrawn from Erikson and Szybalski, 1961).

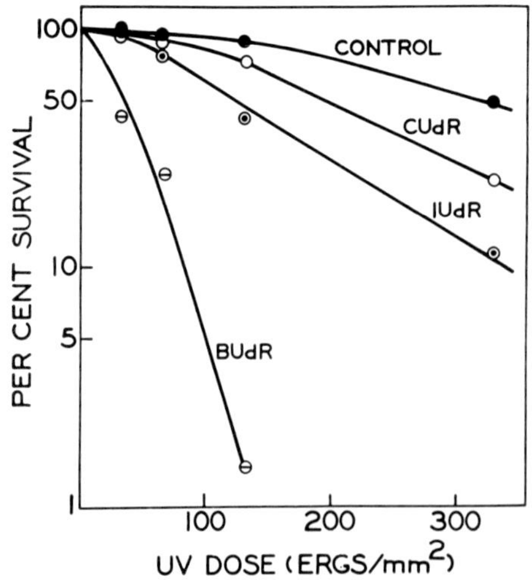

(3b)

biological effects observed on the cellular level are retarded growth rate, enhanced genetic instability, and increased radiation sensitivity. Parallel studies on isolated DNA indicate that, in addition to increased density, halogenation imparts to the molecule a greater lability to various types of chemical and hydrodynamic stresses in its longitudinal structure.

Mutagenic Effects

It has been observed with phages and bacteria that incorporation of BU or IU is accompanied by highly mutagenic effects at certain loci (Litman and Pardee, 1956; Benzer and Freese, 1958; Zamenhof, 1959; Rudner and Balbinder, 1960; Luzzati, 1957). It has been postulated that incorporation of pyrimidine analogs, e.g. BU, results, upon subsequent DNA replication, in more frequent pairing mistakes with consequent "transition", i.e., replacement of an adenine-thymine pair by guanine-cytosine. The reciprocal "transition" would also be possible when BU was mistakenly substituted for cytosine during replication. Thus, mutants produced by BU should also revert at an increased frequency under its influence or in the presence of another analog with similar action, a theoretical notion confirmed experimentally (Freese, 1959). This whole area covering mutagenic effects of base analogs is presently receiving wide attention and is extensively discussed elsewhere (Freese, 1959; Rudner, 1960).

Radiosensitizing Effect

In all organisms so far studied, the incorporation of 5-haloanalogs of thymidine into DNA results in sensitization to various types of radiation. This phenomenon was observed with the most primitive type of DNA-containing organism, BUdR-labeled phage $\phi\chi$-174 (Kozinski and Szybalski, 1959), phages T2 and T4 (Litman and Pardee, 1960; Stahl *et al.*, 1961), bacteria (Zamenhof, 1959; Greer, 1960; Lorkiewicz and Szybalski, 1960), and even with human cells grown *in vitro* (Djordjevic and Szybalski, 1960). Although most of these observations pertained to ultraviolet light effects, sensitization was also observed to X-rays (Djordjevic and Szybalski, 1960; Kaplan and Tomlin, 1960; Erikson and Szybalski, 1961), to visible light (Stahl *et al.*, 1961; Greer, 1960), and to the decay of internally incorporated radioactive phosphorus (P^{32}) (Ragni and Szybalski, in press). In the case of X-rays, the radiosensitizing capacity of the analog increases with the atomic number of the halogen (Figure

3a). Thus, of the three halodeoxyuridines in equimolar concentrations, IUdR is the most potent and CUdR the weakest X-ray sensitizer for human cell lines (Erikson and Szybalski, 1961). With ultraviolet light, however, BUdR represents an exception to the rule. In this case, radiosensitization by CUdR and IUdR closely parallels that observed for X-rays (two- to fivefold in terms of the final slope of the survival curve), while incorporation of BUdR results in a more drastic increase in sensitivity to ultraviolet light (ten- to twentyfold) as compared with X-rays (Figure 3b). The mechanism of this radiosensitizing effect of halogenation has received considerable attention in the author's laboratory.

Mechanism of Radiosensitizing Effect

This problem was approached from one angle by radiobiological studies on normal and halogenated cells, viruses, and biologically active (transforming) DNA, and from another angle by physicochemical characterization of isolated DNA.

Radiobiological Studies on Transforming Principle. Whether the radiosensitizing effect of halogenation for the intact cell reflects an increase in the intrinsic sensitivity of the DNA itself was conveniently tested with extracted transforming principle. As can be seen in Figure 4, BUdR-labeled transforming DNA, isolated from *B. subtilis* cells and purified by CsCl gradient centrifugation, exhibits an increase in its sensitivity to ultraviolet light comparable to that of the intact cells from which it was extracted (Opara-Kubinska, Lorkiewicz, and Szybalski, 1961). This experiment shows not only that halodeoxyuridine incorporation radiosensitizes the cell through a direct effect on its DNA, but also provides the first conclusive evidence that DNA is the most radiosensitive cell component, and thus is the principal target of lethal radiation effects (Szybalski and Opara-Kubinska, 1961; Szybalski and Lorkiewicz, in press). Should survival be dependent upon some more sensitive component, it would be difficult to understand why DNA, probably the only site of halodeoxyuridine incorporation, should exhibit in the purified state the same degree of radiosensitization as the intact cells producing it, when labeled with any of the three analogs under a variety of conditions. These results would seem to exclude various other mechanisms postulated to explain lethal radiation effects (Alper, 1960), including the so-called "enzyme release hypothesis" (Bacq and Alexander, 1960). However, the present

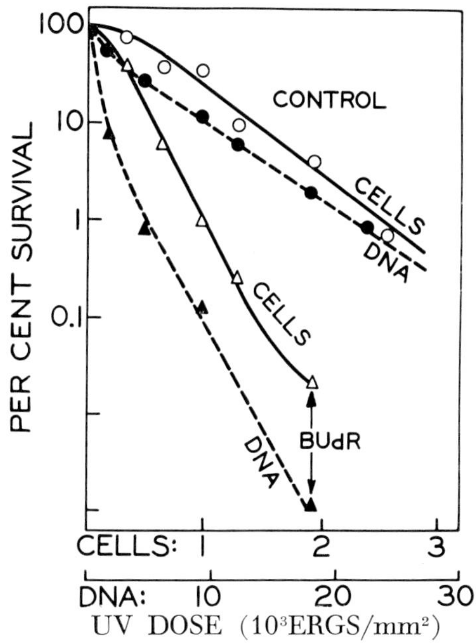

FIG. 4. Ultraviolet light survival (colony-forming ability) of *B. subtilis* cells (solid lines) grown for 3.5 hours in the presence (BUdR) or in the absence (control) of BUdR (200 μg./ml.) and FUdR (4 μg./ml.); and ultraviolet light inactivation of transforming DNA (broken lines) isolated from the above BUdR-free (control) and BUdR-labeled (BUdR) cells. (Redrawn from Opara-Kubinska, Lorkiewicz, and Szybalski, 1961).

data do not pinpoint which of the vital DNA functions is most vulnerable to radiation, although various other studies have indicated that the DNA-mediated synthesis of new enzymes (Bollum, Anderegg, McElya, and Potter, 1960) or other proteins, especially those involved in cell replication, may be primarily affected. However, the replicating capacity of the DNA molecule itself does not appear to be very sensitive to lethal radiation doses, as inferred from the observation that the "priming" capacity of DNA in the *in vitro* synthetic system is rather resistant to scission of the molecule or to other types of radiation damage (Bollum, 1960), and has actually been shown to increase as a result of heavy irradiation (Okada, 1960), although these observations were questioned by Stacey (1961).

Other Radiobiological Studies. These included determination of (1) the differential sensitizing effect of halogenation toward the direct and indirect components of radiation, (2) the relationship between the degree or mode of labeling and radiosensitivity, and (3) the response to various types of radiation.

The increase in radiosensitivity produced by halogenation was essentially the same, whether or not the "indirect" radiation component was eliminated. This was true both for the 10 per cent

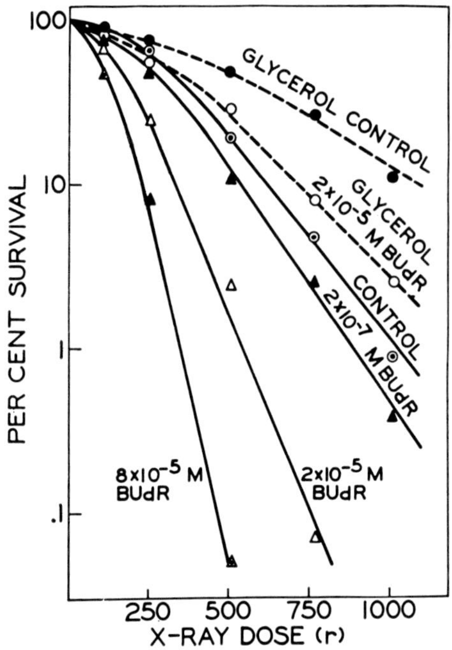

FIG. 5. X-ray survival of D98/AG cells grown at various BUdR concentrations and irradiated in glycerol-free (solid lines) or 10 per cent glycerol-supplemented (broken lines) medium. (Redrawn from Erikson and Szybalski, 1961).

glycerol-protected BUdR-labeled human cells (Figure 5) and for 4 per cent 2-aminoethylisothiouronium bromide hydrobromide (AET) protected transforming DNA, exposed to various doses of X-rays. These data suggest that halogenation affects intrinsic DNA radiosensitivity regardless of the type of radiation effects.

Since the DNA molecule is composed of two complementary strands, two quantitative aspects of halogen labeling must be considered: first, unifilar versus bifilar labeling of the molecule, and second, the actual per cent replacement of thymine by the 5-halouracil. The studies of Djordjevic and Szybalski (1960) indicated that both DNA strands must be halogen labeled to obtain substantial radiosensitization, while substitution in one strand only affects mainly the extrapolation value rather than the slope of the survival curve. The observations of Erikson and Szybalski (1961) on the relationship between the degree of bifilar labeling and the slope of the X-ray survival curve are summarized in Figure 5, and indicate that radiosensitization occurs over a very wide range of analog concentration.

The effect of halogenation on cell death due to the decay of nucleic acid-incorporated P^{32} was evaluated by Ragni and Szybalski (in press). The results were well correlated with the X-ray data, CUdR being the weakest and IUdR the most effective sensitizing agent. Since halogenation cannot alter the rate of P^{32} decay, it must affect the lability of the proximate region of the sister strand irradiated by the P^{32} or exposed to the shock of the recoil. This experiment, together with the results of comparing the effects of BUdR incorporated either into the same strand as P^{32} or into the opposite strand, have led to further elucidation of the mode of inactivation of the double-stranded DNA molecule by P^{32} decay (Ragni and Szybalski, in press).

Physicochemical Studies. Since the molecular mechanism of the radiosensitizing effect of halogenation could not be inferred from the biological studies, it was investigated by physical and chemical means. Several properties of normal and labeled molecules were compared with the following results: (1) The molecular weight of carefully prepared, CsCl gradient purified DNA, as determined by sedimentation in the ultracentrifuge, is not significantly affected by extensive BUdR labeling (Szybalski, 1960b). (2) The halogen-labeled molecule is more sensitive to hydrodynamic shearing forces (Szybalski, unpublished data). (3) The intrinsic viscosity of BUdR-labeled DNA is lower than that of normal DNA exhibiting the same sedimentation constant (Szybalski, 1960b). This observation, however, might have reflected the higher sensitivity of the halogenated DNA to shear. (4) The melting temperature (T_m) of halogenated DNA is slightly increased, more so with the IUdR than with the BUdR label, especially when this value is depressed by the low ionic strength of the "melting" medium or by addition of water-miscible solvents (Lorkiewicz and Szybalski, 1960; Szybalski, 1960b). The differences in T_m observed between normal and BUdR-labeled DNA from natural sources, which were of the order of 2° to 4°C (in 50 per cent methanol, 0.5 mM NaCl), seem to be accentuated in the case of the $d\overline{ABU}$ copolymer (Baldwin, personal communication). The T_m of the $d\overline{ABU}$ (deoxyadenylate-deoxybromouridylate) copolymer at very low ionic strengths is approximately 9°C higher than that of the copolymer of deoxyadenylate and deoxythymidylate (dAT copolymer). At higher ionic strengths the differences in T_m decrease. (5) Halogenated DNA is more sensitive to heat degradation of its longitudinal structure, as inferred from the extensive drop in the molecular weight of high-temperature-separated strands of BUdR-labeled DNA. When a hybrid DNA, which originally banded at a density of 1.738 g × $cm.^{-3}$, was heated for 30 minutes at 100°C in 7 M CsCl solution, in analogy with the experiments of Meselson and Stahl (1958), only one prominent band of density (1.718) and shape corresponding to denatured BUdR-free DNA was observed upon subsequent centrifugation in the CsCl gradient. A second band corresponding to the denatured BUdR-labeled strand was quite broad and barely visible, indicating that the latter was degraded during heating (Szybalski, 1960b). BUdR-labeled bacteria have also been reported to be more sensitive to heat (Greer, 1960). (6) Irradiation results in extensive dehalogenation, as measured chromatographically or by the decrease in buoyant density of halodeoxyuridine-labeled DNA (Wacker, Mennigmann, and Szybalski, in press).

Conclusions Drawn From the Radiobiological and Physicochemical Studies. The present data indicate that DNA is the most radiosensitive cell component, and that damage to this biopolymer is responsible for the lethal effects of radiation. Halogenation of DNA renders it more sensitive to inactivation by radiation, and this in turn results in an enhanced radiosensitivity of the carrier cell. The questions which remain to be answered are: (1) what structural alterations in the halogen-labeled DNA molecule are responsible for its higher radiation lability; and (2) which DNA function is chiefly affected by the coupled effects of halogenation and radiation. Neither of these questions can be answered independently, since separate DNA functions might have individual molecular bases and thus have different susceptibilities to radiation damage. Moreover, radiation can initiate a multitude of chemical alterations; therefore, the answers to questions 1 and 2 can have only statistical significance and can indicate only which type of damage is prevalently responsible for cell death and most easily augmented by halogenation of the DNA molecule.

The most plausible explanation for the increased sensitivity of the halogenated DNA molecule to radiation and to hydrodynamic shear is the postulated instability of the phosphate ester bonds between the 5-bromodeoxyuridylic acid moiety and the adjoining nucleotide on the same DNA strand. The basis for this instability could reside in repulsion between the negatively charged halogen atom and the proximate phosphate group within the large groove of the DNA double helix, as represented in Figure 6. This repulsion would result in considerable strain in the phosphate ester bond, rendering it prone to breakage even at reduced levels of radiation, shear, or thermal stress. By the same token, radiation-caused de-

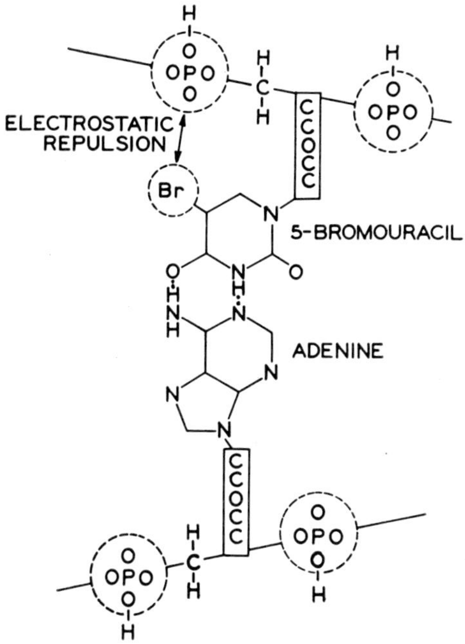

FIG. 6. Steric relationship between halogens and the phosphate groups in the DNA molecule, represented by the adenine-5-bromouracil deoxynucleotide pair.

halogenation (Wacker, Mennigmann, and Szybalski, in press) would also be augmented by repulsion between the bromine and phosphate groups.

While the phosphate-ester bonds are primarily responsible for the longitudinal strength of the DNA structure, the hydrogen bonds between the corresponding purine and pyrimidine moieties hold the two DNA strands together. The latter bonds do not seem to be adversely affected by halogenation; in fact, they appear to be strengthened, as indicated by an increase in the T_m (Szybalski, 1960b).

It is known that irradiation depresses the T_m of DNA (Butler, 1959). When the influence of halogenation on this effect was studied, it was found that the T_m is more severely depressed by irradiation in the case of halogen-labeled (especially with IUdR) than in the case of normal DNA. If one assumes that the decrease in the T_m results from single-strand breaks and localized unraveling in the irradiated DNA double helix (Peacocke and Preston, 1960) and consequent easier melting-out of the hydrogen bonding between the shortened polynucleotides, the augmenting effect of halogenation is consistent with the explanation depicted in Figure 6 and suggested in this section. It is necessary, however, to keep in mind that the breakage of hydrogen bonds in the proximity of the phosphate bond breaks might be more potential than real (Butler, 1959). The pronounced radiosensitizing effect of the BUdR label on phage $\phi\chi$-174 (Kozinski and Szybalski, 1959), which contains only single-stranded DNA, provides another line of evidence that the hydrogen bonds between the DNA strands probably do not play any role in the phenomenon of radiosensitization.

The radiation stability of other bonds might also be affected by halogenation, e.g., the sugar-to-base bond, the halogen-to-uracil bond, the pyrimidine ring structure, and the hydrophobic or other interactions between the stacked base pairs. There is no doubt that the rupture of the halogen-uracil bond is one of the major radiation effects, including the action of visible light (Wacker, Mennigmann, and Szybalski, in press), but very little is known about the influence of halogenation on the radiosensitivity of other bonds.

The radiation sensitivity of two major groups of DNA functions could be affected by halogenation: (1) the genetic or synthetic functions, and (2) the proneness of damaged DNA to enzymatic or other type of repair. It would thus be interesting to ascertain whether halogenation increases the radiation sensitivity of DNA directly, or by decreasing its capacity for repair. The experiments with bacteria (Greer, 1960; Lorkiewicz and Szybalski, 1960) and phages (Stahl *et al.*, 1961) indicate that ultraviolet light-inactivated BUdR-labeled organisms are less susceptible to repair and photoreactivation. Since the molecular mechanism of photoreactivation (and "dark" reactivation) most probably involves the dissociation of thymine dimers produced by ultraviolet light (Beukers and Berends, 1960; Wacker, Dellweg, and Lodeman, 1961), the absence of BU-dimer formation (Wacker, Mennigmann and Szybalski, in press) forms a logical basis for explanation of the absence of reactivation phenomena.

Applications of Halogenated DNA

The ease with which halogen atoms can be introduced into the DNA component of living cells opens several interesting possibilities, from the theoretical, experimental and practical (medical) points of view. It permits chemical labeling of DNA, isolation of the modified molecule on the basis of its higher density, detection and recognition of the halogenated DNA by virtue of its higher radiosensitivity, controlled mutagenesis, radiosensitization of replicating tissue, and introduction (and detection) of gamma-ray-emitting atoms into replicating cells, among other applications.

Density Labeling

Since the molecular weights of Cl, Br, and I are considerably higher (35.5, 80, and 130) than that of the CH_3 group (15), halogen-containing DNA molecules are much heavier and denser than normal DNA. This property permits their separation by centrifugation in the CsCl gradient, e.g., the DNA of *B. subtilis*, which bands in CsCl solution at the buoyant density of 1.703 g $\times$ cm.$^{-3}$, should theoretically band at 1.740 g $\times$ cm.$^{-3}$ if all the CH_3 groups on one strand were replaced by bromine atoms and at 1.776 g $\times$ cm.$^{-3}$ for complete bifilar labeling, calculated for DNA as the cesium salt. Figure 7 is an actual photograph of the bands produced by normal (Figure 7a) and close to 100 per cent unifilarly and bifilarly BUdR-labeled, fully functional (transforming) DNA molecules (Figure 7b) extracted from *B. subtilis* cells. Figure 7b corresponds to approximately two rounds of DNA replication and confirms the semiconservative mode of DNA replication in *B.*

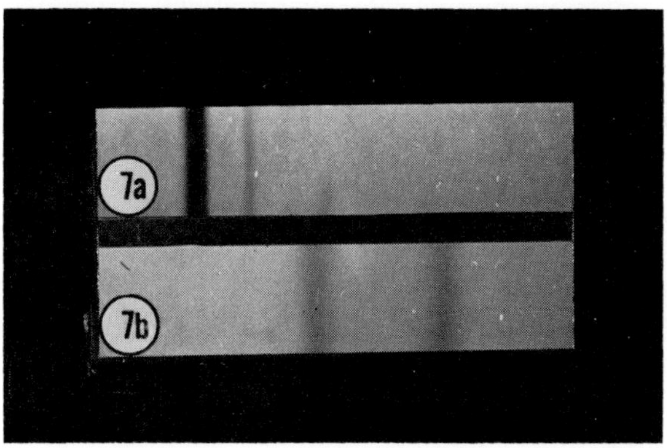

FIG. 7. CsCl gradient equilibrium sedimentation of DNA extracted from *B. subtilis* cells grown for four hours in BUdR-free (Figure 7a) or BUdR + FUdR supplemented medium (Opara-Kubinska, Lorkiewicz, and Szybalski, 1961) (Figure 7b) and centrifuged for 15 hours at 47,660 rpm. The bands from left to right correspond to normal DNA (1.702 g $\times$ cm.$^{-3}$), an artificial density marker (1.726 g $\times$ cm.$^{-3}$) (a disk of ether-washed Saran Wrap plastic, Dow-Corning Co., Szybalski, unpublished data), unifilarly BUdR-labeled DNA (1.744 g $\times$ cm.$^{-3}$), and bifilarly BUdR-labeled DNA (1.781 g $\times$ cm.$^{-3}$).

subtilis cells, in analogy with the results first obtained with the N^{15} label in *Escherichia coli* by Meselson and Stahl (1958). The labeling of DNA by BUdR appears rather homogeneous as measured by the width of the bands. This type of experiment permitted demonstration of the semiconservative mode of DNA replication in human cells (Djordjevic and Szybalski, 1960), fragmentary semiconservative DNA transfer in bacteriophage T4 (Kozinski, 1961), and dispersive transfer in bacteriophage $\phi\chi$-174 (Kozinski and Szybalski, 1959), as well as determination of the molecular fate of transforming principle after its entry into the receptor bacterial cell (Lorkiewicz, Opara-Kubinska, and Szybalski, 1961), among others. The data on the replication of dAT copolymer in an enzymatic system containing BUdR triphosphate, or in the reciprocal system containing dA$\overline{\text{BU}}$ primer and thymidine triphosphate, are also consistent with the semiconservative mode of replication of these DNA-like polymers (Baldwin, Inman, and Wake, 1961; Baldwin, personal communication).

The halogen label should also provide a means of answering the question as to whether biologically active DNA can be synthesized by polymerase in the *in vitro* system. Using "bifilarly" BUdR-labeled transforming DNA (the heaviest band in Figure 7) and the thymidine, cytidine, guanosine, and adenosine triphosphates, it should be possible to separate quantitatively from the "heavy" primer by preparative CsCl centrifugation (Szybalski, 1960) any newly synthesized "light" DNA, and measure its transforming activity, even though the latter were extremely low or extensively degraded by the action of nucleases. Although it might not be meaningful to speak about rounds of DNA replication in non-synchronized, polymerase-mediated, *in vitro* DNA synthesis, the period should be long enough to permit the synthesis of BUdR-free molecules, since the transforming activity of the hybrid molecules, if any, could reflect only the functionality of the "heavy" strand derived from the "heavy" primer.

Low-temperature strand separation ("melting") of normal and bifilarly BUdR-labeled transforming DNA can be employed for the formation of artificial DNA hybrids (Doty, Marmur, Eigner, and Schildkraut, 1960), which can in turn be quantitatively isolated and assayed for possible artificial linkage between markers derived from both parental DNA's.

Potential Medical Application of the Halogenation Process

As discussed earlier (Szybalski, 1961; Djordjevic and Szybalski, 1960), halogenated thymidine analogs have two potential major applications in the field of oncology: (1) selective radiosensitization of replicating tissues, including tumors, and (2) selective introduction of gamma-emitting radioisotopes into tumors for the purpose of localizing malignant lesions by standard scanning procedures.

Since the radiosensitivity of practically all organisms tested becomes enhanced by DNA halogenation, there is little doubt that growing tumors so treated will exhibit the same property. On the basis of the results presented in Figure 3a, IUdR should be the most effective X-ray sensitizing agent, although the lower toxicity of BUdR or CUdR might make their use preferable. It has been shown by Berry and Andrews (1961) that both these analogs strongly radiosensitize intraperitoneally grown mouse leukemia cells without affecting the transplantability of nonirradiated tumor cells. The most important phase of work leading to the practical application of this principle would be the development of methods and routes of administration of the halogenated analogs, paralleled by analytical determination of the extent of halogenation, subjects which have been more extensively discussed elsewhere (Szybalski, 1961). Obviously, direct radiosensitization of DNA by halogenation might be supplemented by the radiosensitizing action of other pyrimidine and purine analogs, the effects of which would be additive and even perhaps synergistic, since their action must involve different mechanisms, probably interference with DNA repair or RNA-mediated synthetic functions of DNA. It was demonstrated earlier that certain purine and pyrimidine analogs, including 8-azaguanine, 8-azahypoxanthine, 6-thioguanine, and 5-fluorouracil, at subinhibitory concentrations, also have a definite capacity to sensitize toward both X-rays and ultraviolet light (Szybalski and Djordjevic, 1959; unpublished data).

A more detailed discussion of the rationale and the possible methods for radiosensitization and diagnostic localization of tumors has been presented elsewhere by Szybalski (1961) and Djordjevic and Szybalski (1960).

Methods for Quantitative Determination of Halodeoxyuridine Incorporation into Tumor Tissue

Analytical centrifugation in the CsCl gradient seems to be the method of choice for the quantitative determination of halodeoxyuridine incorporation. It requires only an extremely small amount of tumor tissue (2 to 8 μg. DNA), and a very simple preparative

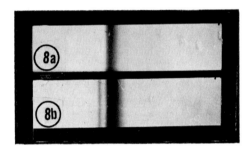

FIG. 8. CsCl gradient equilibrium sedimentation of DNA extracted from human cell line D98/AG (Figure 8a) (Djordjevic and Szybalski, 1960), and from mouse cell line L (Figure 8b), and centrifuged for 15 hours at 44,770 rpm at 25°C. The separate band, sedimenting very sharply at the density approximately 0.010 g $\times$ cm.$^{-3}$ lower than the bulk of the mouse DNA (Figure 8b), was present in all mouse tissue studied (liver, mammary glands, spleen, thymus, embryonic tissue) derived from a variety of mouse strains or from established mouse tissue culture lines (Szybalski, unpublished data).

procedure (lysis with 1 per cent sodium lauryl sulphate solution, alcohol precipitation, and transfer into CsCl solution adjusted to the density 1.710 g $\times$ cm.$^{-3}$). With the analytical rotor F (Spinco Division, Palo Alto, California), adjustable masks in front of the light source and the camera lens, and proper wedge windows, four samples (and even more, when using six-place rotor G or double-sector cells with special half-wedge windows) can be centrifuged simultaneously for 12 to 15 hours and photographed separately with ultraviolet optics (Szybalski, unpublished data). Since human and rat DNA produces only a single band (Figure 8a) the amount and the type of analog labeling is relatively easy to determine from the shift in the position of the bands (Figure 7). In the case of mouse

DNA (Figure 8b), which is heterogeneous and bands at two densities, the interpretation of the sedimentation patterns produced by halogenated DNA is more difficult. Other quantitative methods of halogen detection, including the use of radioactive isotopes, neutron-activation analysis and other microchemical methods, could determine only the over-all degree of halogenation without indicating the mode or heterogeneity of the DNA labeling.

Other Implications of DNA Halogenation

The enhanced radiosensitivity of halogenated DNA molecules permits them to be traced within the intact organism. Thus, Kozinski and Szybalski (1959) used this property to follow the fate of replicating phage ϕx-174. An analogous approach could be utilized for determining whether DNA is responsible for a particular cell function; e.g., it might be possible to ascertain whether the F factor governing bacterial sexuality is DNA or RNA in nature, combining "suicidal" P^{32} labeling with radiosensitization by IUdR or BUdR labeling. Many other experiments along this line are feasible. The property of radiosensitization and desensitization by BUdR was also applied to assess the functionality of DNA produced during inhibition of protein synthesis by puromycin, chloramphenicol or *p*-fluorophenylalanine (Djordjevic and Szybalski, 1960). The mutagenicity of BUdR was applied for the same purpose by Litman and Pardee (1959), Brenner and Smith (1959), and Glass and Novick (1959). Applications of the 5-halodeoxyuridines in mutagenicity studies will not be discussed further here, since the subject was mentioned in earlier sections.

In closing, it should perhaps be mentioned that the perfect functionality of the heavily 5-halodeoxyuridine-labeled DNA has important implications from the point of view of the coding mechanism. It could be inferred that the genetic message is the same whether written with the thymine-adenine "letters" or with BU-adenine "letters". Conversely, one might imagine that only the guanine-cytosine "letters" spell out the genetic message of the code, while the dAT copolymer plays the role of fabric and interspacing (commas). Thus, again the message would be essentially the same whether written out on dAT "fabric", or on "inferior" $d\overline{ABU}$ "paper". That the dAT copolymer may have arisen early in evolution might be inferred from the ease with which it is formed spontaneously in the *in vitro* enzymatic system (Schachman *et al.*, 1960) and by its natural appearance in some organisms (*Cancer borealis*) in amounts up to 30 per cent of the total DNA (Sueoka, 1961, and personal communication). Evolution then would have only introduced the meaningful code into the "meaningless" dAT copolymer ("meaningless" because of its perfectly regular d-ATATATA. . . structure) and thereby have created life in all its forms. If this supposition is correct, the incorporation of guanine or cytosine analogs into DNA should result in much more drastic changes in DNA function than those produced by halogenated thymidine analogs. Whether any of these speculations turn out to be factual will be revealed by further experimentation.

Summary

The molecular configurations of several synthetic pyrimidine deoxyribosides, including CUdR, BUdR, and IUdR, are similar enough to that of the natural deoxynucleoside, thymidine, to permit these analogs to serve as substrates for several enzymes, including kinases and polymerase, and to substitute for thymidine as a component of DNA. CUdR and BUdR behave as the best thymidine substitutes, as judged by their ability to support the growth of thymidine-requiring cells. High concentrations of these analogs, as well as of thymidine, are toxic to the cell, inhibiting the conversion of cytidine nucleotides to deoxynucleotides, a block which can be counteracted by deoxycytidine.

Uni- or bifilarly analog-labeled DNA functions almost perfectly within the cell, permitting it to grow indefinitely under conditions of massive thymidine replacement, and also to serve as fully active transforming principle. Halogenated DNA, however, is chemically less stable, probably as a result of strong electrostatic repulsion between electronegative bromine and phosphorus atoms located on the same DNA strand. This lower stability is manifested by higher sensitivity of the DNA to P^{32} decay, X-rays, ultraviolet light, shear, and heat. Selective halodeoxyuridine incorporation into DNA-synthesizing neoplastic cells and the resultant highly augmented X-ray sensitivity could serve as a practical method for selective radiosensitization of tumors. Several other experimental applications of 5-halodeoxyuridine labeling are outlined.

ACKNOWLEDGMENTS

This study was supported by Grants CY 5415 and CY-3492 from the United States Public Health Service.

I am indebted to Mrs. Zofia Opara-Kubinska, Dr. Giorgio Ragni, and Mr. R. L. Erikson for permitting me to quote our unpublished results.

REFERENCES

Alper, T. 1960. Cellular Radiobiology. *Annual Review of Nuclear Science*, 10:489–530.

Bacq, Z. M., and P. Alexander. 1960. *Fundamentals of Radiobiology*. New York, New York; Oxford, England: Pergamon Press, 555 pp.

Baldwin, R. L. Personal Communication.

Baldwin, R. L., R. B. Inman, and R. G. Wake. 1961. Hybrid Molecules, Containing Strands of dAT and dABrU, Formed Both by Enzymatic and Physico-Chemical Means. (Abstract) *Federation Proceedings*, 20:354.

Bendich, A., H. B. Pahl, and G. B. Brown. 1957. "Chromatographic Fractionation of *E. coli* DNA Containing 5-Bromouracil-2-C^{14}," *The Chemical Basis of Heredity*, W. D. McElroy and B. Glass, Eds., pp. 378–389. Baltimore, Maryland: The Johns Hopkins Press.

Benzer, S., and E. Freese. 1958. Induction of Specific Mutations with 5-Bromouracil. *Proceedings of the National Academy of Sciences of the U.S.A.*, 44:112–119.

Berry, R. J., and J. R. Andrews. 1961. Modification of Radiation Effect Upon the Reproductive Capacity of Tumor Cells *in vivo* with Pharmacologic Agents. (Abstract) *Radiation Research*, 14:452.

Beukers, R., and W. Berends. 1960. Isolation and Identification of the Irradiation Product of Thymine. *Biochimica et biophysica acta*, 41:550–551.

Bollum, F. J. 1960. "General Discussion Following Session 3," *The Cell Nucleus*, J. S. Mitchell, Ed., p. 163. New York, New York: Academic Press, Inc.

Bollum, F. J., J. W. Anderegg, A. B. McElya, and V. R. Potter. 1960. Nucleic Acid Metabolism in Regenerating Rat Liver. VII. Effect of X-Radiation on Enzymes of DNA Synthesis. *Cancer Research*, 20:138–143.

Brenner, S., and J. D. Smith. 1959. Induction of Mutations in the Deoxyribonucleic Acid of Phage T2 Synthesized in the Presence of Chloramphenicol. *Virology*, 8:124–125.

Butler, J. A. V. 1959. Changes Induced in Nucleic Acids by Ionizing Radiations and Chemicals. *Radiation Research*, Supplement 1:403–416.

Cheong, L., M. A. Rich, and M. L. Eidinoff. 1960. Introduction of the 5-Halogenated Uracil Moiety into Deoxyribonucleic Acid of Mammalian Cells in Culture. *Journal of Biological Chemistry*, 235:1441–1447.

Cohen, S. S., J. G. Flaks, H. D. Barner, M. R. Loeb, and J. Lichtenstein. 1958. The Mode of Action of 5-Fluorouracil and Its Derivatives. *Proceedings of the National Academy of Sciences of the U.S.A.*, 44:1004–1012.

Djordjevic, B., and W. Szybalski. 1960. Genetics of Human Cell Lines. III. Incorporation of 5-Bromo-, and 5-Iododeoxyuridine into the Deoxyribonucleic Acid of Human Cells and Its Effect on Radiation Sensitivity. *Journal of Experimental Medicine*, 112:509–531.

Doty, P., J. Marmur, J. Eigner, and C. Schildkraut. 1960. Strand Separation and Specific Recombination in Deoxyribonucleic Acids: Physical Chemical Studies. *Proceedings of the National Academy of Sciences of the U.S.A.*, 46: 461–476.

Dunn, D. B., and J. D. Smith. 1957. Effects of 5-Halogenated Uracils on the Growth of *Escherichia coli* and Their Incorporation into Deoxyribonucleic Acids. *Biochemical Journal*, 67:494–506.

Erikson, R. L., and W. Szybalski. 1961. Molecular Radiobiology of Human Cell Lines. I. Comparative Sensitivity to X-Rays and Ultraviolet Light of Cells Containing Halogen-Substituted DNA. *Biochemical and Biophysical Research Communications*, 4:258–261.

Freese, E. 1959. The Specific Mutagenic Effect of Base Analogues on Phage T4. *Journal of Molecular Biology*, 1:87–105.

Frisch, D. M., J. Gregory, and D. W. Visser. 1960. Effects of 5-Bromodeoxycytidine in *Escherichia coli* and Bacteriophage. *Journal of Bacteriology*, 79: 666–673.

Glass, E. A., and A. Novick. 1959. Induction of Mutation in Chloramphenicol Inhibited Bacteria. *Journal of Bacteriology*, 77:10–16.

Greer, S. 1960. Studies on Ultraviolet Irradiation of *Escherichia coli* Containing 5-Bromouracil in Its DNA. *Journal of General Microbiology*, 22:618–634.

Hakala, M. T. 1959. Mode of Action of 5-Bromodeoxyuridine on Mammalian Cells in Culture. *Journal of Biological Chemistry*, 234:3072–3076.

Handschumacher, R. F., and A. D. Welch. 1960. "Agents Which Influence Nucleic Acid Metabolism," *The Nucleic Acids*, E. Chargaff and J. N. Davidson, Eds., Vol. 3, pp. 453–526. New York, New York: Academic Press, Inc.

Harbers, E., N. K. Chaudhuri, and C. Heidelberger. 1959. Studies on Fluorinated Pyrimidines. VIII. Further Biochemical and Metabolic Investigations. *Journal of Biological Chemistry*, 234:1255–1262.

Hitchings, G. H., E. A. Falco, and M. B. Sherwood. 1945. The Effects of Pyrimidines on the Growth of *Lactobacillus casei*. *Science*, 102:251–252.

Kaplan, H. S., and P. A. Tomlin. 1960. Enhancement of X-Ray Sensitivity of *E. coli* by 5-Bromouracil. (Abstract) *Radiation Research*, 12:447–448.

Kozinski, A. W. 1961. Fragmentary Transfer of P^{32}-Labeled Parental DNA to Progeny Phage. *Virology*, 13:124–134.

Kozinski, A. W., and W. Szybalski. 1959. Dispersive Transfer of the Parental DNA Molecule to the Progeny of Phage ØX-174. *Virology*, 9:260–274.

Litman, R. M., and A. B. Pardee. 1956. Production of Bacteriophage Mutants by a Disturbance of Deoxyribonucleic Acid Metabolism. *Nature, London,* 178:529–531.

———. 1959. Mutations of Bacteriophage T2 Induced by Bromouracil in the Presence of Chloramphenicol. *Virology,* 8:125–127.

———. 1960. The Induction of Mutants of Bacteriophage T2 by 5-Bromouracil. III. Nutritional and Structural Evidence Regarding Mutagenic Action. *Biochimica et biophysica acta,* 42:117–130.

Littlefield, J. W., and E. A. Gould. 1960. The Toxic Effect of 5-Bromodeoxyuridine on Cultured Epithelial Cells. *Journal of Biological Chemistry,* 235: 1129–1133.

Lorkiewicz, Z., Z. Opara-Kubinska, and W. Szybalski. 1961. Molecular Fate of Transforming DNA. (Abstract) *Federation Proceedings,* 20:360.

Lorkiewicz, Z., and W. Szybalski. 1960. Genetic Effects of Halogenated Thymidine Analogs Incorporated During Thymidylate Synthetase Inhibition. *Biochemical and Biophysical Research Communications,* 2:413–418.

Luzzati, D. 1957. Sur le repércussions génétiques de la substitution de la thymine par le 5-iodouracyle dans l'acide désoxyribonucléique de *E. coli* 15T–. *Comptes rendus hebdomadaires des seances de l'Academie des sciences,* 245:1466–1468.

Meselson, M., and F. W. Stahl. 1958. The Replication of DNA in *Escherichia coli. Proceedings of the National Academy of Sciences of the U.S.A.,* 44:671–682.

Morris, N. R., and G. A. Fischer. 1960. Studies Concerning Inhibition of the Synthesis of Deoxycytidine by Phosphorylated Derivatives of Thymidine. *Biochimica et biophysica acta,* 42:183–184.

Okada, S. 1960. Incorporation of Tritium-Labelled Thymidine and Tritium-Labelled Deoxycytidilic Acid into Deoxyribonucleic Acid After Irradition of the Deoxyribonucleic Acid Primer with X-Rays. *Nature, London,* 185:193–194.

Opara-Kubinska, Z., Z. Lorkiewicz, and W. Szybalski. 1961. Genetic Transformation Studies. II. Radiation Sensitivity of Halogen Labeled DNA. *Biochemical and Biophysical Research Communications,* 4:288–291.

Opara-Kubinska, Z., and W. Szybalski. Unpublished data.

Pauling, L. 1945. *The Nature of the Chemical Bond,* p. 189. Ithaca, New York: Cornell University Press.

Peacocke, A. R., and B. N. Preston. 1960. The Action of X-Rays on Sodium Deoxyribonucleate in Solution. III. Denaturation. *Proceedings of the Royal Society series B,* 153:103–110.

Prusoff, W. H. 1960. Incorporation of Iododeoxyuridine into the Deoxyribonucleic Acid of Mouse Ehrlich-Ascites-Tumor Cells *in vivo. Biochimica et biophysica acta,* 39:327–331.

Ragni, G., and W. Szybalski. (in press). Molecular Radiobiology of Human Cell Lines. II. Effects of Thymidine Replacement by Halogenated Analogues on Cell Inactivation by Decay of Incorporated Radiophosphorus. *Journal of Molecular Biology*.

Reichard, P., Z. N. Canellakis, and E. S. Canellakis. 1960. Regulatory Mechanisms in the Synthesis of Deoxyribonucleic Acid *in vitro*. *Biochimica et biophysica acta*, 41:558–559.

Rudner, R. 1960. Mutation as an Error in Base Pairing. *Biochemical and Biophysical Research Communications*, 3:275–280.

Rudner, R., and E. Balbinder. 1960. Reversions Induced by Base Analogues in *Salmonella typhimurium*. *Nature, London*, 186:180.

Schachman, H. K., J. Adler, C. M. Radding, I. R. Lehman, and A. Kornberg. 1960. Enzymatic Synthesis of Deoxyribonucleic Acid. VII. Synthesis of a Polymer of Deoxyadenylate and Deoxythymidylate. *Journal of Biological Chemistry*, 235:3242–3249.

Stahl, F. W., J. M. Crasemann, L. Okun, E. Fox, and C. Laird. 1961. Radiation Sensitivity of Bacteriophage Containing 5-Bromodeoxyuridine. *Virology*, 13:98–104.

Stacey, K. A. 1961. The Inhibition of DNA Synthesis by Calf-Thymus Polymerase by X-Irradiation of the Primer DNA. *Biochemical and Biophysical Research Communications*, 5:486–490.

Sueoka, N. 1961. Variation and Heterogeneity of Base Composition of Deoxyribonucleic Acids: A Compilation of Old and New Data. *Journal of Molecular Biology*, 3:31–40.

———. Personal Communication.

Szybalski, W. 1960a. Sampling of Virus Particles and Macromolecules Sedimented in an Equilibrium Density Gradient. *Experientia*, 16:164.

———. 1960b. "Ultraviolet Sensitivity and Other Biological and Physicochemical Properties of Halogenated DNA," *Progress in Photobiology*. (Proceedings of the Third International Congress on Photobiology), The Finsen Memorial Congress, B. C. Christensen and B. Buchmann, Eds., pp. 542–545. Copenhagen, Denmark: Elsevier Publishing Co.

———. 1961. "The Radiosensitizing Effects of the Halogenated Thymidine Analogs," *Research in Radiotherapy. Approaches to Chemical Sensitization*, R. F. Kallman, Ed., pp. 162–180. Washington, D.C.: National Academy of Sciences, National Research Council.

———. Unpublished data.

Szybalski, W., and B. Djordjevic. 1959. Radiation Sensitivity of Chemically Modified Human Cells. (Abstract) *Genetics*, 44:540–541.

Szybalski, W., and Z. Lorkiewicz. (in press). "On the Nature of the Principal Target of Lethal and Mutagenic Radiation Effects." *Erwin-Baur-Gedächtnisvorlesungen. Abhandlungen der Deutschen Akademie der Wissenschaften zu Berlin*, Berlin.

Szybalski, W., and Z. Opara-Kubinska. 1961. DNA as Principal Determinant of Cell Radiosensitivity. (Abstract) *Radiation Research*, 14:508–509.

Szybalski, W., Z. Opara-Kubinska, Z. Lorkiewicz, E. Ephrati-Elizur, and S. Zamenhof. 1960. Transforming Activity of Deoxyribonucleic Acid Labelled with 5-Bromouracil. *Nature, London*, 188:743–745.

Wacker, A. Personal Communication.

Wacker, A., H. Dellweg, and E. Lodeman. 1961. Strahlenchemische Veränderung der Nucleinsäure. *Angewandte Chemie*, 73:64–65.

Wacker, A., H. D. Mennigmann, and W. Szybalski. (in press). Mechanism of Photochemical Inactivation of Halogenated DNA. *Federation Proceedings 1962.*

Wacker, A., A. Trebst, D. Jacherts, and F. Weygand. 1954. Über den Einbau von 5-Bromouracil-(2-^{14}C) in die Desoxyribonucleinsäure verschiedener Bakterien. *Zeitschrift für Naturforschung*, 9b:616–617.

Weygand, F. A. Wacker, and H. Dellweg. 1952. Stoffwechseluntersuchungen bei Mikroorganismen mit Hilfe Radioactiver Isotope. II. Kompetitive und nichtkompetitive Enthemmung von 5–^{82}Br–Uracil. *Zeitschrift für Naturforschung*, 7b:18–25.

Zamenhof, S. 1959. Further Studies on the Unstable and "Unnatural" Desoxyribonucleic Acid. *Annals of the New York Academy of Sciences*, 81: 784–787.

Zamenhof, S., and G. Griboff. 1954. Incorporation of Halogenated Pyrimidines into the Deoxyribonucleic Acids of *Bacterium coli* and its Bacteriophages. *Nature, London*, 174:306–307.

Mutagenesis and the Functioning of Genetic Material in Phage

IRWIN TESSMAN, PH.D.

Department of Biological Sciences,
Purdue University,
Lafayette, Indiana

The double-stranded Watson-Crick structure of deoxyribonucleic acid (DNA) provokes theories concerning the role of the individual strands in the transmission of genetic information to progeny and in the physiologic expression of the genetic information. If the two strands of the DNA duplex are truly complementary, any information contained in one strand would necessarily be contained in the other. But, at the same time, each strand would be chemically distinct from its complement. This distinctiveness means that the genetic information is stored in two different chemical forms within each DNA duplex. Macroscopically, these two chemical forms appear the same, but, in detail, they are different. Although I will refer to the two chemical forms as the two individual strands of a DNA duplex, no implication that the DNA functions in a single-stranded state is intended. The questions I will discuss concern only the location of genetic information, and not the complete mechanism of its transmission or expression.

Since the genetic information is embodied in two distinct chemical strands, the following questions arise:

1. Can each strand transmit the genetic information to progeny?
2. Can each strand function in expressing the genetic information that controls the physiological behavior of the organism?

The problems may be illustrated by the specific case illustrated in Figure 1, in which a normal duplex has had one of the strands altered, producing a singular region containing a pair of noncomplementary bases. The letters A, B, C, and D represent the four bases, with A normally pairing with B, and C normally pairing with D. In the region indicated by brackets A pairs abnormally with C. Each strand of this duplex corresponds to a different normal duplex; i.e., each strand contains the information for two distinct genotypes and phenotypes. The questions stated above can be rephrased:

1. In replication, what genotypes will the progeny contain? Will two types of progeny result, corresponding to each of the two strands, or will one type result, corresponding to only one of the strands, or will there be other possibilities?

2. In physiological function, what phenotypes will be expressed? Will two phenotypes result, corresponding to each of the two

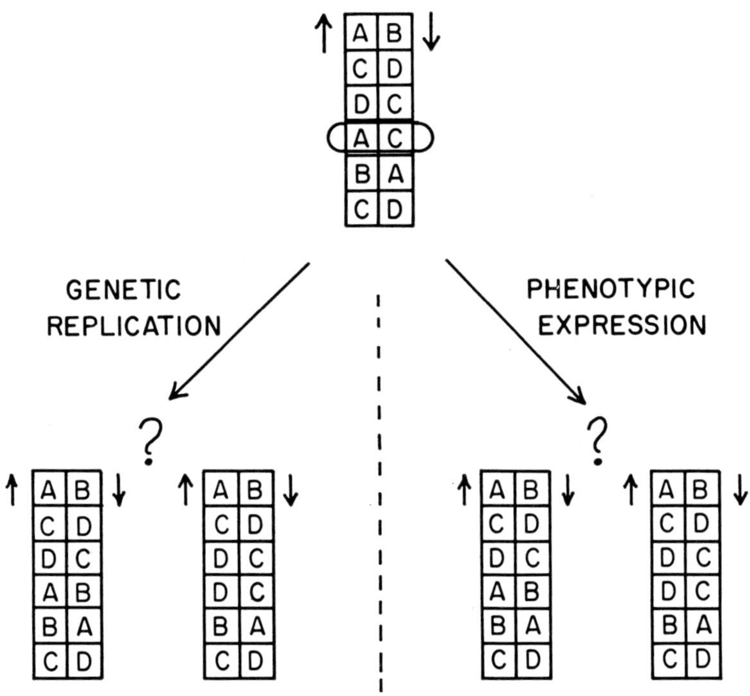

FIG. 1. Schematic representation of the informational content of a DNA duplex having noncomplementary base pairing.

strands, or will one phenotype result, corresponding to only one of the strands, or will there be other possibilities?

I will not attempt a detailed picture of the nebulous realm of "other possibilities."

These questions have been approached by altering the DNA *in vitro* by nitrous acid treatment to approach the condition illustrated in Figure 1. Following the suggestion of Schuster and Schramm (1958), it was found that the deamination of ribonucleic acid (RNA) and DNA with nitrous acid leads to the production of mutants (Mundry and Gierer, 1958; Litman and Ephrussi-Taylor, 1959). Although it has not been rigorously proven, it is expected that such nitrous acid treatment would produce singular regions in DNA in which a base pair would not consist of complementary bases. The situation would differ from that shown in Figure 1, in that one member of the noncomplementary pair would be an abnormal base, not normally occurring in DNA, but nevertheless similar in hydrogen-bonding properties to a normal base. We could now hope to answer the two main questions by asking how the chemically-produced heterozygotic duplex would transmit and express its information.

Mutant progeny of nitrous acid-treated phages T2 and T4 have been found to arise usually in mixed clones containing both mutant and wild-type phage (Vielmetter and Wieder, 1959; Tessman, 1959). Figure 2a illustrates this interpretively. The interpretation is that the nitrous acid alters the information in one of the strands, leading to mutant progeny; but, because the other strand is intact and also capable of transmitting information to progeny, wild-type phage is also found in the same clone. Therefore, such experiments are consistent with the theory that each strand is capable of transmitting the genetic information to progeny, the altered strand leading to mutant progeny.

The alternative explanation that only one strand can transmit the genetic information is not completely excluded. It is conceivable that the deamination of the base leads to an unstable condition in which the strand transmits wild-type information at one time and mutant information at a subsequent duplication. Two facts argue against this:

1. In mixed clones, the two types occur in roughly equal amounts (Tessman, 1959). An unstable situation might be more favorable to one type than to the other.

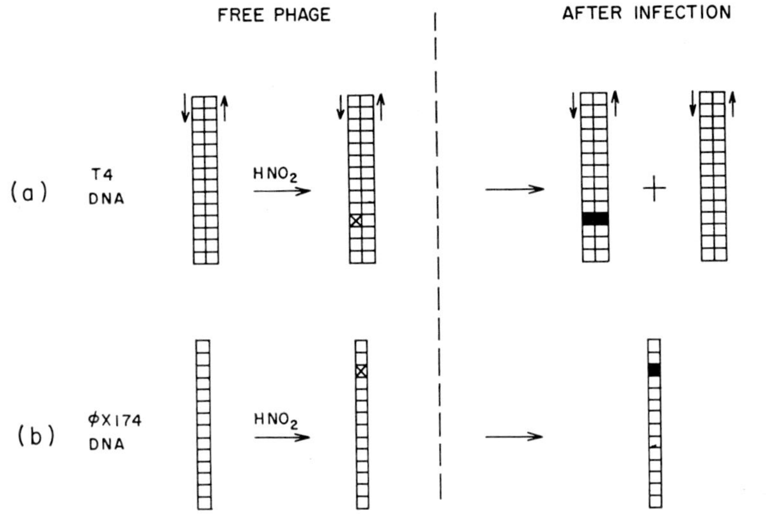

FIG. 2. Schematic representation of the *in vitro* nitrous acid induction of T4 mutants in mixed clones and φX174 mutants in pure clones.

2. More convincing is a control experiment (Figure 2b) with a phage (φX174) containing a single strand of DNA (Tessman, 1959). In this case the mutant clones are pure, arguing against, but not completely excluding, the possibility of an unstable condition in T2 or T4. The production of T4 heterozygotes using 5-bromodeoxyuridine (5-BUDR) (Pratt and Stent, 1959) adds to the evidence that each strand can transmit genetic information to progeny.

The problem of the expression of the genetic information is more difficult to approach. In this case, we examined the consequences of assuming that only one strand can express the information physiologically. We call this hypothetical strand the active (A) strand and the complementary strand the inactive (I) strand. The I strand is considered passive and its information content has no effect on the ability of the A strand to express its information. Therefore, damaging or altering the I strand alone should have no physiological effect, while damaging or altering the A strand alone should destroy some physiological function of the DNA.

The function studied is that controlled by the *r*II region of phage T4. The physiological expression of the *r*II$^+$ function is easily detected by the ability of the phage to grow in *Escherichia coli* K12(λ) (designated simply as K), where the *r*II$^+$ function is needed (Benzer, 1955). The *r*II$^+$ function is not needed for growth in *E. coli* strain B (designated simply as B). A study of the relative production of *r*II mutants in both B and K provides a test of a possibly disparate role for the two strands of the DNA duplex in physiological expression.

Figure 3a illustrates a case in which the nitrous acid reacts with a base in the A strand, and Figure 3b illustrates a case in which the nitrous acid reacts with a base in the I strand. Only those cases are considered in which subsequent growth in B leads to an *r*II mutant (generally occurring in mixed clones as already described). The actual distinction between the two cases occurs when the growth is in K. When the A strand is altered (Figure 3a), growth cannot occur and no mutant is produced. When the I strand is altered (Figure 3b), growth is possible because the unaltered A strand can express the $r\text{II}^+$ function and mutant phage can then be produced from the altered I strand. (A necessary condition for production of phage progeny in K appears to be that the $r\text{II}^+$ information be contained in the infecting phage particles [Epstein, 1958; Krieg, 1959]; thus, an A strand produced from an I strand would not be effective.)

From Figure 3 it is seen that, if the two strands react with equal frequency with nitrous acid, as would be expected *a priori*, the proportion of *r*II mutants obtained by subsequent growth in B should be approximately double the proportion obtained in K. Preliminary experiments (Tessman, unpublished data) have shown this to be the case, in complete agreement with the hypothesis that there is an active and an inactive strand.

But, is the active strand unique? Or can the designation be equally well applied to either strand, provided only that, in any particular infection, one of the strands is active and the other inactive? If the active strand is unique, not only should the frequency of *r*II mutants obtained from B exceed the frequency obtained from K, but the mutants obtained from B should cover a larger number of genetic sites than the mutants obtained from K. For example, if a genetic site were represented by an adenine-thymine pair in the DNA and if the adenine were in the active strand, then a mutant at that site should only be obtained by growing in strain B, since no way is known for nitrous acid to alter the I strand at that site. If the active strand is not unique, the same genetic sites could be represented among the *r*II mutants obtained in B and in K.

Experimentally, the same number of genetic sites seem to be found using either host. Thus, it would seem that both strands can express the information physiologically, as if the cell were capable of reading the message in either of its two chemical forms. And to

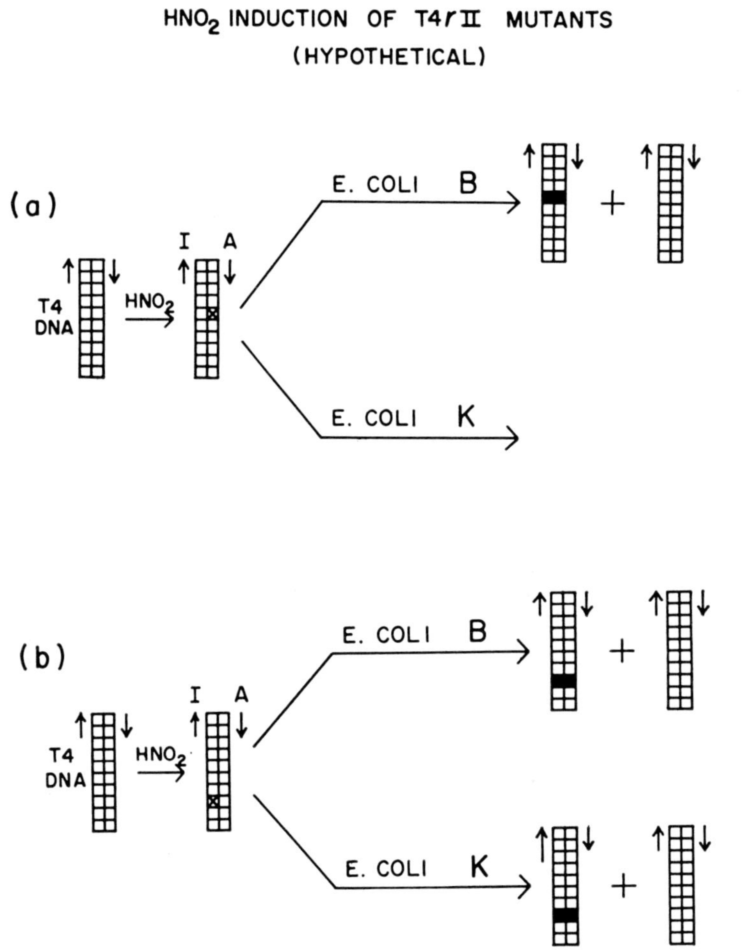

FIG. 3. Schematic representation of the *in vitro* nitrous acid induction of T4 mutants with subsequent growth in *E. coli* B and *E. coli* K. The hypothesis is that the DNA consists of a functionally active (A) strand and a functionally inactive (I) strand.

explain the higher frequency of *r*II mutants obtained in B compared with those obtained in K, it would be necessary to assume that the message can be read from only one of the two strands in any particular infection, the individual strand not being unique. Therefore, in 50 per cent of the cases one strand would be read, and in the other 50 per cent of the cases the other strand would be read. Such a theory would be consistent with the observed frequency and spectra of *r*II mutants.

However, I wish to propose an alternative possibility that involves a considerable departure from current theory. It is that in phage T4 the ultimate site of the mutation may not be the same as the original site of the chemical reaction. It would then be possible to maintain that the active and the inactive strands are unique and it would no longer be necessary to explain the identical genetic spectra in the B and K experiments. The prediction concerning the number of sites affected by the nitrous acid concerns only the initial site of the chemical reaction. Different initial sites may be translated to give the same ultimate mutational site. Furthermore, although it is certainly not the only explanation, it would also explain why 95 per cent of the nitrous acid-induced mutants occur at approximately only 30 genetic sites, whereas chemical evidence combined with mutational studies predicts that there should be approximately 370 sites (Vielmetter and Schuster, 1960). In other words, the phenomenon of "hot spots" (Benzer and Freese, 1958) would be explained. Since mutants of diverse origin fall into "hot spots" (Benzer, 1961) the implication would be that in most mutagenic situations an alteration is translated in some form from an initial to an ultimate site, the ultimate sites possibly being fewer in number than the initial sites. This proposal is being tested.

We know that approximately 10 per cent of the nitrous acid-induced mutants show ultimate mutational sites that are not all the same as the initial sites of chemical reaction. It is because this fraction of mutants are deletions (Tessman, unpublished data). However, it is not yet clear whether this represents an exceptional situation or the commonly occurring one.

For purposes of illustration the discussion has been in terms of the individual strands of the DNA duplex. However, in the absence of conclusive evidence that we are dealing with two-stranded DNA molecules, a cautious approach would be to refer to DNA subunits without a complete commitment about the relation of the subunits to the DNA strands.

It can be concluded that in T4 phage the DNA has at least two subunits, each of which can transmit the information to progeny. Only one of the subunits is active at any time in expressing the information phenotypically, but whether the active subunit is unique or whether either subunit can function has not been settled. If the subunit is unique and constitutes one of the strands of the duplex, the mutagenic action of nitrous acid must be different from that previously imagined. The induction of deletions by nitrous acid indicates that, under some circumstances, at least, the mutational process cannot be simply described in terms of the hydrogen-bonding properties of certain deaminated bases.

ACKNOWLEDGMENT

I am particularly indebted to Mrs. Carol Phares for assistance with the unpublished experiments cited in this paper.

ABBREVIATIONS

Abbreviations used in this paper are as follows: DNA, deoxyribonucleic acid; RNA, ribonucleic acid; 5-BUDR, 5-bromodeoxyuridine.

REFERENCES

Benzer, S. 1955. Fine Structure of a Genetic Region in Bacteriophage. *Proceedings of the National Academy of Sciences of the U.S.A.*, 41:344–354.

———. 1961. On the Topography of the Genetic Fine Structure. *Proceedings of the National Academy of Sciences of the U.S.A.*, 47:403–416.

Benzer, S., and E. Freese. 1958. Induction of Specific Mutations With 5-Bromouracil. *Proceedings of the National Academy of Sciences of the U.S.A.*, 44:112–119.

Epstein, R. H. 1958. A Study of Multiplicity-Reactivation in the Bacteriophage T4. *Virology*, 6:382–404.

Krieg, D. R. 1959. A Study of Gene Action in Ultraviolet-Irradiated Bacteriophage T4. *Virology*, 8:80–98.

Litman, R. M., and H. Ephrussi-Taylor. 1959. Inactivation et Mutation des Facteurs Génétiques de l'Acide Désoxyribonucléique du Pneumocoque par l'Ultraviolet et par l'Acide Nitreux. *Comptes rendus hebdomadaires des séances de l'Académie des sciences*, 249:838–840.

Mundry, K. W., and A. Gierer. 1958. Die Erzeugung von Mutationen des Tabakmosaikvirus durch chemische Behandlung seiner Nucleinsäure *in vitro*. *Zeitschrift für Vererbungslehre*, 89:614–630.

Pratt, D., and G. S. Stent. 1959. Mutational Heterozygotes in Bacteriophages. *Proceedings of the National Academy of Sciences of the U.S.A.*, 45:1507–1515.

Schuster, H., and G. Schramm. 1958. Bestimmung der biologisch wirksamen Einheit in der Ribosenucleinsäure des Tabakmosaikvirus auf chemischem Wege. *Zeitschrift für Naturforschung*, 13b:697–704.

Tessman, I. 1959. Mutagenesis in Phages ϕX174 and T4 and Properties of the Genetic Material. *Virology*, 9:375–385.

———. Unpublished data.

Vielmetter, W., and C. M. Wieder. 1959. Mutagene und inaktivierende Wirkung salpetriger Säure auf freie Partikel des Phagen T2. *Zeitschrift für Naturforschung*, 14b:312–317.

Vielmetter, W., and H. Schuster. 1960. Die Basenspezifität bei der Induktion von Mutationen durch salpetrige Säure im Phagen T2. *Zeitschrift für Naturforschung*, 15b:304–311.

Polymerization-Depolymerization of Tobacco Mosaic Virus Protein

MAX A. LAUFFER, B.S., M.S., PH.D.

Professor of Biophysics, and Dean, Division of the Natural Sciences, University of Pittsburgh[1], *Pittsburgh, Pennsylvania*

HISTORICAL INTRODUCTION

Stanley (1935) precipitated tobacco mosaic virus (TMV) in the form of rodlike paracrystals. In succeeding years, Bawden and Pirie (1937), Stanley (1938) and Loring (1939) showed that tobacco mosaic virus was a ribonucleoprotein containing about 5 per cent nucleic acid. Within a few years after its crystallization, tobacco mosaic virus was decomposed by various means into small protein fragments and ribonucleic acid. Included in these methods are treatment with urea (Stanley and Lauffer, 1939), with dilute alkali, pyridine and other organic chemicals (Pfankuch, 1940; Bawden and Pirie, 1940; Knight and Lauffer, 1942), with heat (Bawden and Pirie, 1937; Lauffer and Price, 1940) and with high pressures (Lauffer and Dow, 1941). Sedimentation coefficients as low as 1.6 or 1.7 $\overline{S}$ were obtained for the urea-treated material, indicative of molecular weights of the order of 15,000, and particles of comparable size were found when heat-denatured virus was dissolved in 6 M urea or 0.1 M sodium hydroxide (Lauffer and Stanley, 1943). Amino acid analyses, interpreted on the assumption that the protein

---

[1] Publication No. 90 of the Department of Biophysics.

subunits of tobacco mosaic virus are uniform in composition and that the least abundant amino acid occurs to the extent of one residue per subunit, also indicated molecular weights of the order of 18,000 for protein subunit. Complete amino acid analyses of tobacco mosaic virus and several of its strains were reported by Knight (1947), but the crucial analysis of cysteine, the least abundant amino acid, was first reported by Ross (1940).

The tendency of tobacco mosaic virus to aggregate was commented on by Bawden and Pirie as early as 1937. Loring, Lauffer, and Stanley (1938) showed that double refraction of flow increased when tobacco mosaic virus was subjected to three or four repeated cycles of high-speed centrifugation, thereby indicating the formation of longer particles. The nature of this aggregation was clarified when Lauffer (1938) interpreted quantitatively ultracentrifugation results obtained by Wyckoff (1937), which showed the existence of components with sedimentation coefficients of 174 $\overline{S}$ and 200 $\overline{S}$ in some preparations of tobacco mosaic virus, but only a single component with the lower sedimentation rate in the most carefully prepared virus samples, in terms of aggregation of the basic virus particle into particles of the same thickness but double the length. That low molecular weight, nucleic acid-free protein subunits are also capable of aggregation was pointed out by Knight and Lauffer (1942). Schramm (1943) showed that nucleic acid-free, rodlike particles, somewhat resembling tobacco mosaic virus but lacking biological activity, were obtained when the protein subunits, isolated by mild alkaline treatment of the virus, were allowed to aggregate. Franklin (1955) studied the X-ray diffraction patterns of such nucleic acid-free rods and showed that the structure was similar to that of the intact virus, except for the absence of nucleic acid. Therefore, the protein subunits are arranged in a giant helix around a hollow core.

Schramm (1943) succeeded in obtaining nucleoprotein rods by permitting fragments to aggregate. Later (1947) he showed that protein and nucleic acid could be reconstituted into nucleoprotein preparations which, in two out of 15 cases, showed significant increase of biological activity over the dissociated material. Fraenkel-Conrat and Williams (1955) and Lippincott and Commoner (1956) demonstrated, beyond question, that tobacco mosaic virus reconstituted by copolymerization of protein subunits and ribonucleic acid (RNA) possessed appreciable biological activity. This result was at first interpreted as a reactivation of formerly inactivated material, thereby evoking a great deal of general speculation about the synthesis of life. In 1956, however, two lines of evidence converged to establish that the nucleic acid is the bearer of infectiousness. Gierer and Schramm (1956) and Fraenkel-Conrat (1956) showed that isolated tobacco mosaic virus-ribonucleic acid preparations are infectious. Lauffer, Trkula, and Buzzell (1956) showed that X-ray inactivation of tobacco mosaic virus is correlated with breaking the ribonucleic acid chain and concluded that the intactness of the ribonucleic acid, but not of the protein, was essential for infection.

The ill-fated speculation concerning the synthesis of life, precipitated by the "reactivation" conclusion, has tended to obscure the true significance of the reconstitution of tobacco mosaic virus from its protein and nucleic acid subunits. The tobacco mosaic virus particle is a remarkable structure. Based on evidence published in fragments beginning in 1938 and presented in critical detail in 1944, the author (Lauffer, 1944) showed that the tobacco mosaic virus particle is a rod about 20 times as long as thick, with a molecular weight of about 40 million. Numerous subsequent studies have substantiated and refined this conclusion. The presently accepted values for the dimensions of the tobacco mosaic virus particle are length, 300 mμ, over-all diameter, 180 mμ,, and molecular weight, 40 million. Details of the fine structure of tobacco mosaic virus have also been worked out. The virus particle is considered to be composed of a giant helix of more than 2,000 protein subunits intermeshed with a helix of the same pitch representing a single RNA particle of molecular weight two million, as represented diagramatically in Figure 1. The principal evidence from which this structure was deduced comes from X-ray diffraction studies of Watson (1954) and of Franklin and Holmes (1958) and electron microscopy studies of Schramm and associates (1955) and Hart (1955).

The remarkable thing about the reconstitution of tobacco mosaic virus from its protein subunits and nucleic acid is the demonstration that this beautifully intricate biological structure will, under proper conditions, form spontaneously. The secret, therefore, to the formation of this and perhaps other biological structures lies in the synthesis of subunits with the proper physical and chemical characteristics. Much effort in our laboratory has been devoted to an elucidation of the mechanism of this biologically important reaction. As a first step, my colleagues, students, and I have turned our attention to the polymerization of protein subunits in the absence

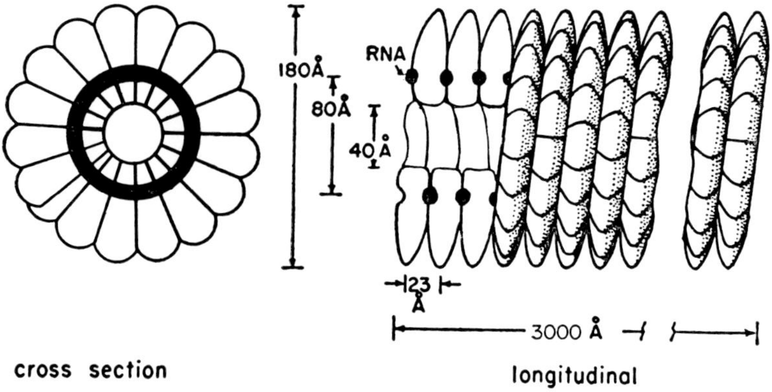

FIG. 1. Structure of tobacco mosaic virus. Modified from Stanley (1956).

of nucleic acid. This choice was made because this polymerization is basically simpler than copolymerization with the nucleic acid.

Knight and Lauffer (1942) pointed out that aggregation of alkaline degradation products of tobacco mosaic virus was accelerated by a rise in temperature. Harrington and Schachman (1956), in the course of an investigation of the kinetics of degradation of tobacco mosaic virus in alkaline solutions, showed that, at 0°C, protein with a sedimentation coefficient of about 4 $\overline{S}$ was obtained at pH 9.8 but that when the reaction was carried out at 25°C nucleic acid-free protein particles with a much higher sedimentation coefficient were obtained. They established that some of these larger particles were produced by polymerizing the 4$\overline{S}$ component. Lauffer, Ansevin, Cartwright, and Brinton (1958) discovered that the protein prepared by degrading tobacco mosaic virus at pH 10.3 and purified by means of electrophoresis and high-speed centrifugation, when placed in 0.1 ionic strength phosphate buffer at pH 6.5, polymerized at room temperature and depolymerized in the cold.

Effect of Temperature on Polymerization-Depolymerization

Four lines of evidence establish the reversibility of the polymerization of protein subunits in phosphate buffer at pH 6.5 and 0.1 ionic strength.

(1) Opital densities were measured with the Beckman spectrophotometer at wave length 320 mμ. on solutions at various temperatures. The results are shown in Table 1. The same solution was used at all temperatures and the sequence of measurements was that indicated in the table from top to bottom.

TABLE 1

Optical Density of Tobacco Mosaic Virus Protein at Various Temperatures at pH 6.5

Temperature 0° C	Optical Densities
23	0.409
30	0.430
11	0.063
5	0.059
10	0.054
27	0.420

(Lauffer, Ansevin, Cartwright and Brinton, 1958.)

(2) Viscosity measurements were made on a solution of tobacco mosaic virus protein in pH 6.5 phosphate buffer of 0.1 ionic strength at 2°C and at 25°C. The results are shown in Table 2. The temperature was changed rapidly in the sequence shown in the table from top to bottom. The symbol η is the viscosity of the solution and η_0 is the viscosity of the buffer solvent, both measured at the same temperature. The errors indicated in the table are standard errors.

Both of these lines of evidence show clearly that large anisometric particles exist at the higher temperatures and smaller more symmetrical particles at the lower temperatures.

(3) Further evidence was obtained with the ultracentrifuge. Sedimentation analyses were carried out in a Spinco ultracentrifuge at three temperatures. At 4.8°C all of the material had a sedimentation coefficient of approximately 4 $\overline{S}$. At 12°C components with sedimentation coefficients of 4 $\overline{S}$ and 22 $\overline{S}$ were observed and at 30°C components with sedimentation coefficients of 40 $\overline{S}$ and 220 $\overline{S}$ were found. A summary of the sedimentation results is found in Table 3. The sedimentation coefficients were corrected to water at 20°C and the concentrations were estimated from the areas associated with each schlieren pattern. These results also show that high molecular

TABLE 2

Viscosity of a Tobacco Mosaic Virus Solution at pH 6.5 as a Function of Temperature

Temperature 0° C	$(\eta/\eta_0)-1$
2° C	0.035±0.0005
25° C	0.099±0.0004
2° C	0.037±0.0003

(Lauffer, Ansevin, Cartwright and Brinton, 1958.)

TABLE 3

Sedimentation of Tobacco Mosaic Virus Protein in 0.1 Ionic Strength Phosphate Buffer at pH 6.5 as a Function of Temperature

Temperature 0° C	S_w^{20}	Concentration (mg./ml.)
30	40	0.7
	220	0.7
12.0	4.5	1.3
	22	0.5
4.8	3.8	1.7

(Lauffer, Ansevin, Cartwright and Brinton, 1958.)

weight components predominate at higher temperatures and low molecular weight components predominate at lower temperatures.

(4) The electron microscope has also provided evidence of reversibility of the polymerization. A tobacco mosaic virus protein preparation in 0.1 ionic strength phosphate buffer at pH 6.5, with

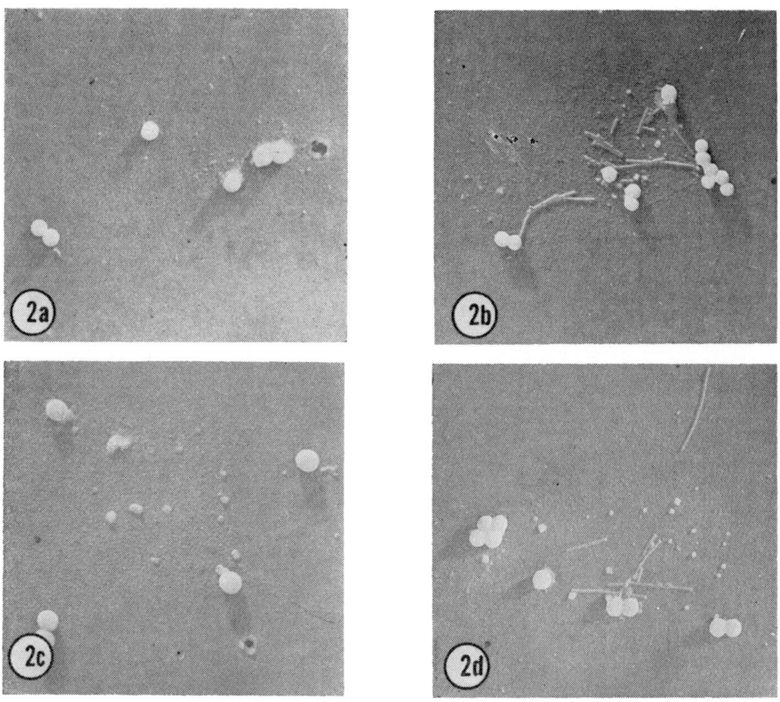

FIG. 2. Electron micrographs of the same tobacco mosaic virus protein solution (with polystyrene latex indicator particles) sprayed on grids and dried at different temperatures in the sequence indicated a, 4°C; b, 30°C; c, 4°C; d, 25°C. Magnification—ca. 2,000.

a small amount of polystyrene latex as indicator particles, was alternately sampled in the cold and at room or higher temperatures. Samples were sprayed onto electron microscope grids and dried at the sampling temperature. The results are shown in Figure 2. In Figure 2a the sampling and the drying were carried out at 4°C. The temperature was then raised to 30°C and a sample was taken, sprayed and dried (Figure 2b). The temperature of the same solution was then lowered to 4°C and 2c was obtained in the same manner as 2a. Finally, the temperature was raised to 25°C and 2d was obtained in the same manner as was 2b. This process can be carried through an unlimited number of cycles. The polymerization and the depolymerization are extremely rapid reactions.

Reversal of polymerization with temperature is not observed in 0.1 M phosphate buffers at pH 5.0 or at pH 7.7. Optical density measurements similar to those carried out at pH 6.5 demonstrate this conclusion. The results are shown in Tables 4 and 5. At pH 5.0 the protein exists in the polymerized state at all temperatures studied between 8.0°C and 29.5°C. At pH 7.7, the protein exists in

TABLE 4

Optical Density for Solution of Tobacco Mosaic Virus Protein at Various Temperatures and at pH 5.0

Temperatures 0° C	Optical Density
23.8	0.326
8.0	0.325
29.5	0.326

(Lauffer, Ansevin, Cartwright and Brinton, 1958.)

TABLE 5

Optical Density for Solution of Tobacco Mosaic Virus Protein at Various Temperatures and at pH 7.7

Temperatures 0° C	Optical Density
5.0	0.016
14.5	0.016
20.2	0.018
25.6	0.019
7.0	0.018
25.5	0.020
29.0	0.026
7.0	0.027

(Lauffer, Ansevin, Cartwright and Brinton, 1958.)

the unpolymerized state at all temperatures between 5.0°C and 29.0°C. Recent results, however, establish that reversible endothermic aggregation is also obtained in 0.1 ionic strength Michaelis buffer at pH 2.84 (Ansevin and Lauffer, in preparation).

Chemical Nature of Reversible Polymerization of Tobacco Mosaic Virus Protein

Depolymerization by lowering the temperature of an aggregated tobacco mosaic virus protein preparation was found to be accompanied by a decrease in pH when the reaction was carried out in an unbuffered medium (Ansevin and Lauffer, 1959a). Measurements of pH were made with a pH meter on an unbuffered solution containing 0.5 per cent nucleic acid-free protein. At the higher temperatures, the protein is in the polymerized state and at the lower temperatures it is in the dissociated state. Control measurements were made on tobacco mosaic virus nucleoprotein under identical conditions. In this case, there is a steady increase in pH reading as the temperature is lowered. These results, presented in Figure 3, can be interpreted to mean that polymerization of protein subunits is accompanied by either binding of hydrogen ions or dissociation of hydroxyl ions. Since the protein is on the alkaline side of its isoelectric point, the total net negative charge is less in the polymerized than in the depolymerized state.

Electrophoretic mobility determinations were made on tobacco mosaic virus protein in 0.05 ionic strength phosphate buffer at pH 6.5 in the depolymerized state at 2°C and in the polymerized state at 24°C (Ansevin and Lauffer, 1959a). The measured mobilities were then corrected for viscosity of the medium by multiplying by the ratio of the viscosity of water at the temperature of the measurement to that of water at 20°C. The results are shown in Table 6. It can be seen that, in spite of the higher total net negative charge, there is a much lower negative mobility of the depolymerized material than of the polymerized material. Lower negative electrophoretic mobilities for depolymerized protein in contrast with polymerized protein were also observed by Kleczkowski (1959), who used ultraviolet irradiation to cause polymerization, and by Kramer and Wittmann (1958), who demonstrated a sharp hiatus at pH 6 in the pH-mobility graph. The explanation for the lower mobility of depolymerized protein in spite of higher net charge is that electrophoretic mobility depends on surface density of charge. Even though the negative charge is increased when polymerized protein

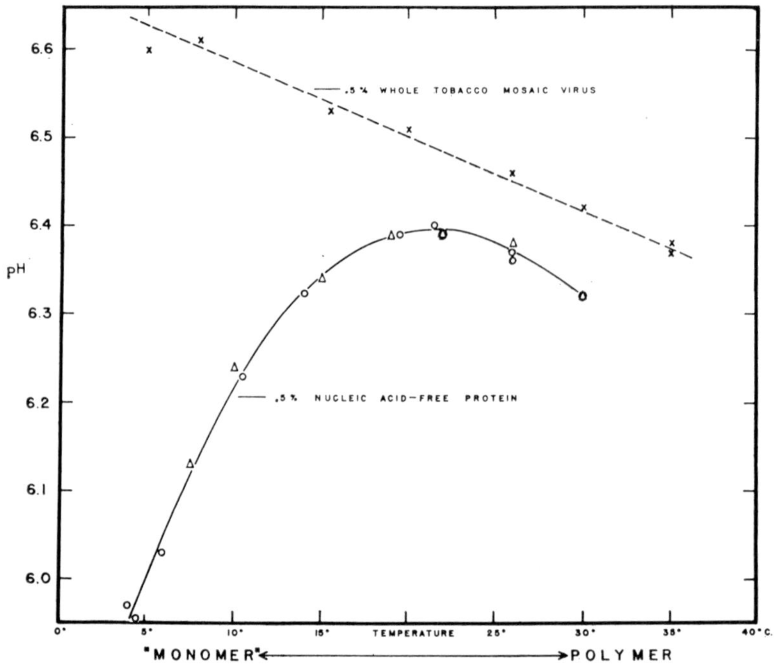

FIG. 3. pH as a function of polymerization of unbuffered tobacco mosaic virus protein. Data of Ansevin and Lauffer, 1959a.

depolymerizes, the total surface increases even more and, therefore, the surface density of charge decreases.

Kinetic studies (Ansevin and Lauffer, in preparation) show that as pH is lowered from a value somewhat above neutrality, the rate of polymerization of protein fragments increases. This is consistent with the finding that there is a pH increase associated with polymerization in nearly neutral, unbuffered solutions. There is,

TABLE 6

Electrophoretic Mobility of Tobacco Mosaic Virus Protein at 2° C and at 24° C Corrected for Viscosity of Water at 20° C

	Mobility cm.²/volt sec. $\times 10^5 \times \eta_w^T/\eta_w^{20}$	% in boundary
2° dissociated	— 7.5	100
24° associated	—21.5	82
	—18.5	9
	— 9.0	9

however, a maximum in the rate of polymerization at approximately pH 3.7. This result is also consistent with the known behavior of tobacco mosaic virus because the protein subunits can be isolated by both mild alkaline and mild acidic digestion.

The disintegrating action of urea on tobacco mosaic virus nucleoprotein was referred to previously (Lauffer and Stanley, 1943). Kinetic studies (Lauffer, 1943) demonstrated an unusual dependence of the specific reaction velocity (K) on the absolute temperature. As is illustrated in Figure 4, the reaction had a minimum rate at room temperature and higher rates at both lower and higher temperatures. This result was interpreted to mean that loss of turbidity was accomplished by two parallel reactions, one of which dominates below and the other above room temperature. Further kinetic studies showed that at 0°C reaction rate varied with the eighth power and at 45°C with the sixth power of urea concentration.

Recent experiments (Smith and Lauffer, in preparation) on the

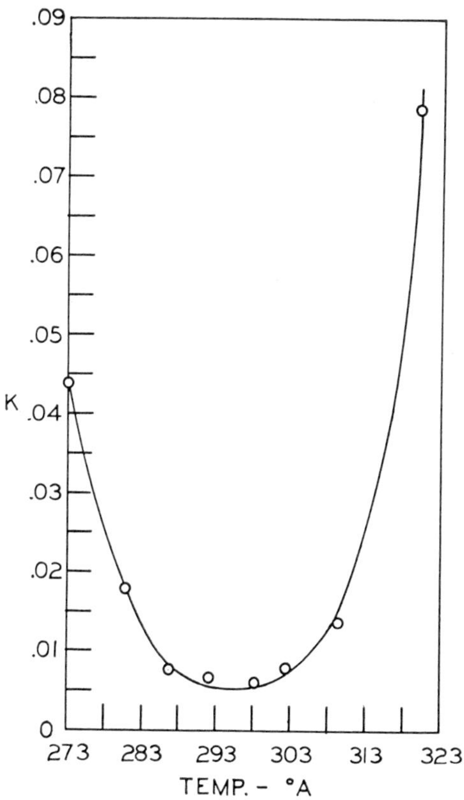

FIG. 4. Rate constants for denaturation of TMV in 6 M urea plotted against absolute temperature (From Lauffer, 1943).

effect of urea on the reversible polymerization of TMV protein supplement and illuminate this earlier finding. When 1.8 M urea was added to polymerized TMV protein at pH 6.6 in 0.1 ionic strength potassium phosphate buffer at 23°C, almost instantaneous loss of turbidity followed by gradual irreversible increase in turbidity was observed. If the temperature was lowered immediately after clearing took place and if the urea was then removed by dialysis at 2°C, the TMV protein retained its ability to polymerize reversibly when temperature was subsequently raised. This shows that there are two effects of urea, one of which results in the dissociation of the polymerized TMV protein into smaller units and the other of which involves irreversible changes in solubility or denaturation. Further studies at pH 6.5 in 0.1 ionic strength phosphate buffer show that the temperature range over which polymerized protein dissociates is about 2°C higher in the presence of 0.2 M urea than in its absence. This latter observation confirms the conclusion that one of the effects of urea is to promote or favor dissociation of polymer into smaller units.

This dissociating action of urea on TMV protein is a reaction which is favored by lowering the temperature. It is, in this respect, comparable to one of the rate-determining reactions leading to the disintegration of tobacco mosaic virus in concentrated urea solutions, the one whose rate increases when temperature is lowered (Figure 4).

Smith and Lauffer (1961) also studied the effect of tetra-n-butyl ammonium ion on the polymerization-depolymerization of TMV protein. This ion is, according to Frank and Wen (1957), a structure maker in water. Well-buffered solutions of tobacco mosaic virus protein at pH 6.5 and at a constant ionic strength of 0.1 were prepared with different amounts of tetra-n-butyl ammonium bromide. Ionic strength was kept constant by using compensating amounts of potassium bromide. When 0.05 M tetra-n-butyl ammonium ion was added to polymerized tobacco mosaic virus protein at room temperature, a very rapid depolymerization occurred, followed by a slower irreversible decrease in solubility or denaturation. If the reaction mixture was cooled immediately after the depolymerization, as indicated by a drop in optical scattering, and if it was then dialyzed to remove the tetra-n-butyl ammonium ion, apparently unaltered protein subunits, still capable of polymerization at room temperature, were isolated. This shows that the first step in the action of tetra-n-butyl ammonium ion is dissociation of the polymer into subunits and that the denaturation is a secondary reaction which can be avoided in the manner indicated. When 0.03 M tetra-n-butyl ammonium ion is added to polymerized tobacco mosaic virus protein at room temperature and then the temperature is lowered slowly, the temperature range over which depolymerization, indicated by a drop in optical scattering, occurs is significantly higher than for the protein in the absence of tetra-n-butyl ammonium ions. When 0.02 M tetra-n-butyl ammonium ion is added to unpolymerized tobacco mosaic virus protein in the cold and then the temperature raised to room temperature, the rate of polymerization is slower than for tobacco mosaic virus protein subunits in the absence of the ion. All of these results show that the tetra-n-butyl ammonium ion favors dissociation and inhibits polymerization. This ion is similar to urea in its gross effect on TMV protein; it promotes deploymerization and it also causes denaturation.

The Role of Water in Depolymerization of Tobacco Mosaic Virus Protein

As was described previously, tobacco mosaic virus protein subunits in 0.1 ionic strength phosphate buffer at pH 6.5 polymerize spontaneously at room temperature and depolymerize in the cold (Lauffer, Ansevin, Cartwright, and Brinton, 1958). Polymerization, therefore, involves an increase in enthalpy. Since polymerization at room temperature is a spontaneous reaction it must be accompanied by a decrease in free energy. In view of the endothermic nature of this reaction, there must, therefore, be an increase in entropy. An uncomplicated process involving the collection of small subunits distributed at random into a single ordered structure, such as the tobacco mosaic virus protein rod with its helical arrangement of subunits, would involve a decrease in entropy. It is, therefore, necessary to postulate that the total reaction of the polymerization process must involve the release of something which is bound to the subunits in addition to the joining together of the subunits in the polymerized rod. This something could be any constituent of the solution, an ion, a trace constituent, water, etc. For many reasons, however, water is the prime suspect. It is the most obviously abundant constituent of the environment. Furthermore, intact tobacco mosaic virus nucleoprotein has a rather low degree of hydration, something of the order of 0.25 Gm. H_2O/Gm. nucleoprotein (Schachman and Lauffer, 1949). It is probable, therefore, that polymerized tobacco mosaic virus protein also has a relatively

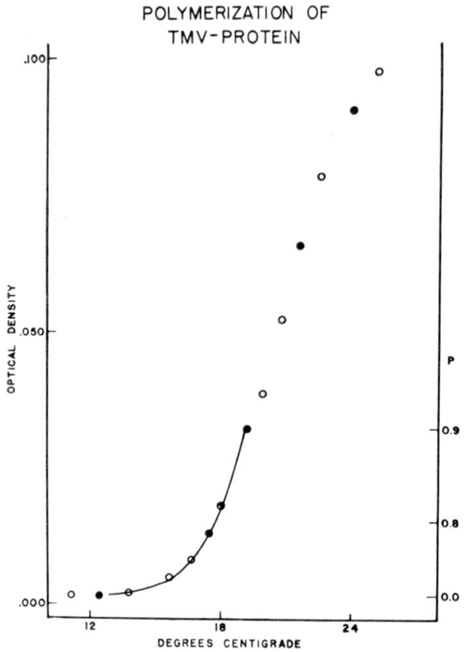

FIG. 5. Reversible polymerization of tobacco mosaic virus protein dissolved in 0.1 ionic strength phosphate buffer at pH 6.5. ○ corresponds to rising temperatures and ● to falling temperatures. Curve calculated for equilibrium reaction. Left ordinate is O. D. and right ordinate is fraction of linkages formed. (Data of Smith and Lauffer, 1961).

low degree of hydration. It is easily conceivable that the virus protein subunits, with their much greater surface area/unit of weight, bind more water/unit weight than the polymerized material.

An estimate of the amount of water involved in the formation of a single link when TMV protein polymerizes can be obtained by studying the energetics of the reaction. As is shown in Figure 5, when temperature is changed slowly, almost the same turbidities are obtained upon increase as upon decrease (Smith and Lauffer, 1961). This result is a necessary condition for calculation of equilibrium constants for polymerization.

The simplest assumption one can make is that this reaction is a condensation polymerization. The prime requisite for this mechanism is that the reactivity of a free end is independent of the length of chain attached to the other end of the same monomeric unit. The existence of apparently stable intermediates in the polymerization of TMV protein[1] warns that this view is oversimplified;

[1] Buzzell (1959; 1962) has isolated stable intermediates in the urea disintegration of tobacco mosaic virus. To explain this observation, she advanced the thesis that TMV protein subunits are not homogeneous with respect to acid amide content. If such postulated inhomogeneity accounts for the formation of stable intermediates during degradation of the virus, it would also account for stable intermediates in the polymerization of TMV protein subunits. It should be observed, however, that the theory applied in the present study is assumed to be valid only for rods very much shorter than the intermediates discussed by Buzzell.

nevertheless, the deductions made through its use might still be instructive. Flory (1936) has shown, from statistical consideration, that, in condensation polymerization, the weight average molecular weight of the polymer, $\overline{Mw}$, should be given by the equation, $\overline{Mw} = Mo \frac{1+p}{1-p}$, where Mo is the molecular weight of monomer and p is the fraction of the ends of the monomeric units joined to form linkages. Since, in a dilute solution of small molecules, the turbidity, τ, is given by the equation, $\tau = Hc\,\overline{Mw}$, where H is the scattering factor and c is concentration (Oster, 1948), one can write, $\tau = Hc\,Mo \frac{1+p}{1-p} = \tau_0 \frac{1+p}{1-p}$, where τ_0 is the turbidity when p is 0. An equilibrium constant, K, can be defined for condensation polymerization by the equation, $K = p/c\,(1-p)^2$, where c is the initial molarity of monomer. From the thermodynamic relationships, $-RT \ln K = \Delta F_0 = \Delta H_0 - T\,\Delta S_0$, where R is the gas constant, T the absolute temperature and ΔF_0, ΔH_0 and ΔS_0 are, respectively, the standard free energy, enthalpy and entropy changes, and the above equation, one can derive:

$$\ln \frac{(1-p)^2}{P}\; p = \frac{\Delta H_0}{R}\frac{1}{T} - \frac{\Delta S_0}{R} - \ln c$$

The curve in Figure 5 was obtained by converting p as a function of T to O.D. proportional to τ as a function of T for parameters of 190 k cal./mole for ΔH_0, 682 entropy units (e.u.) for ΔS_0, 8×10^{-6} molar for c and 0.004 cm.$^{-1}$ for τ_0. It should be observed that the data fit the curve reasonably well for p values between 0 and 0.9 Since the theory of condensation polymerization predicts infinite turbidity for $p = 1$, it is unrealistic to expect the curve to fit the data for values of p much higher than 0.9.

Frank and Evans (1945) suggested that water might be organized in the form of "icebergs" in the region of hydrophobic groups. Another possibility is that water is condensed around dipolar ions. If such water has the same entropy of "melting" as ordinary ice, 5.3 e.u., the + 680 e.u. change associated with forming a mole of linkages in TMV protein could be achieved by releasing 130 moles of bound water.

If the view is accepted that water is bound by the smaller units when TMV protein polymer dissociates, then one can rationalize the effects of urea and tetra-n-butyl ammonium ion by postulating that they are bound in competition with the water. Mechanisms by which these substances are bound are not necessarily the same. The only essential postulate is that, in both cases, the binding must be of such a nature that, at any given temperature in the range studied, the free energy decrease accompanying dissociation of these reagents from the subunits and the polymerization of the subunits must be less than for the case involving water.

Preliminary experiments (Stevens and Lauffer, in preparation) indicated that the water, assumed to be released when TMV protein subunits polymerize, can be weighed directly by an application of Archimedes' principle. A cellophane bag containing about 100 mg. of TMV protein dissolved in about 3 ml. of buffered glycerol solution of a density of approximately 1.06 was suspended on a delicate coiled quartz fiber in a buffered glycerol solution of exactly the same density (Figure 6). The temperature was carefully controlled at 4°C. The experimental set-up was such that the external glycerol solution could be replaced with another glycerol solution of about the same density but different pH.

In principle, the extension of the fiber should be proportional to the difference between the weight of the bag, the protein contained in it, and any water bound by the protein not free to dissolve glycerol and the weight of the glycerol solution displaced. Since the cellophane bag is permeable to glycerol solution, complete equilibrium should be achieved and the amount of glycerol solution inside the bag should be immaterial because it is completely canceled by buoyancy.

Polymerization was brought about in these experiments by changing the pH of the external buffer and, after equilibrium, of the protein solution inside the bag from approximately seven to approximately five. This procedure introduces complications of its own. One is associated with the Donnan effect because the apparatus should be sensitive to changes in buoyant weight accompanying redistribution of ions when the net charge on the protein is altered. A further major complication was disclosed by preliminary experiments which showed that there is a weight change when the protein subunits polymerize even when the reaction is carried out in dilute buffer solution in the absence of added glycerol. If water is being released when the protein polymerizes, this must mean that there is an accompanying change in partial specific volume. A detailed analysis of the theory showed that if control experiments are done on a material which changes charge to the same extent as the TMV protein inside the bag, then the Donnan effect and certain other

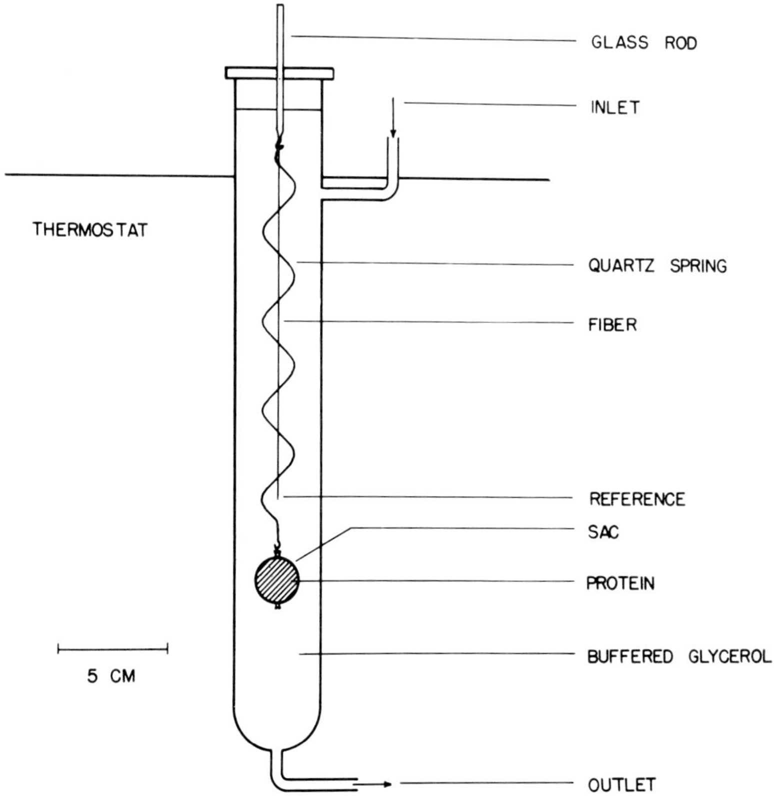

FIG. 6. Diagram of apparatus for determining the effective weight change accompanying polymerization of TMV protein. (Stevens and Lauffer, in preparation).

conceivable effects accompanying charge change can be compensated for experimentally. Further, if measurements on both control and TMV protein are carried out in media of at least two different densities, for example, buffer at a density of 1.0 and buffered glycerol at a density of 1.06, both the change in partial specific volume and the amount of water released can be determined. In our experiments, tobacco mosaic virus, which does not polymerize appreciably when the pH is changed from about seven to about five, was chosen as an appropriate control. The detailed theory can be summarized by the equation:

$$\left(\frac{\Delta W_a}{w_a} - \frac{\Delta W_b}{r w_b}\right) = -\rho\left(\Delta V_a - \frac{\Delta V_b}{r}\right) + \left(d - \rho\right)\left(\Delta h_a - \frac{\Delta h_b}{r}\right)$$

In this equation, the subscript a refers to TMV protein and b to the control (TMV); Δ W means the effective weight of the bag and contents suspended in the medium at pH 7 minus that at pH 5; w means the weight of material inside the bag; r is the ratio of the net charge change/gram for the control to that for TMV protein; ρ means the bulk density of the liquid outside the bag; Δ V means the partial specific volume at approximately pH 7 minus that at approximately pH 5; d means the bulk density of water and Δ h means the difference between the hydration at pH 7 and at pH 5.

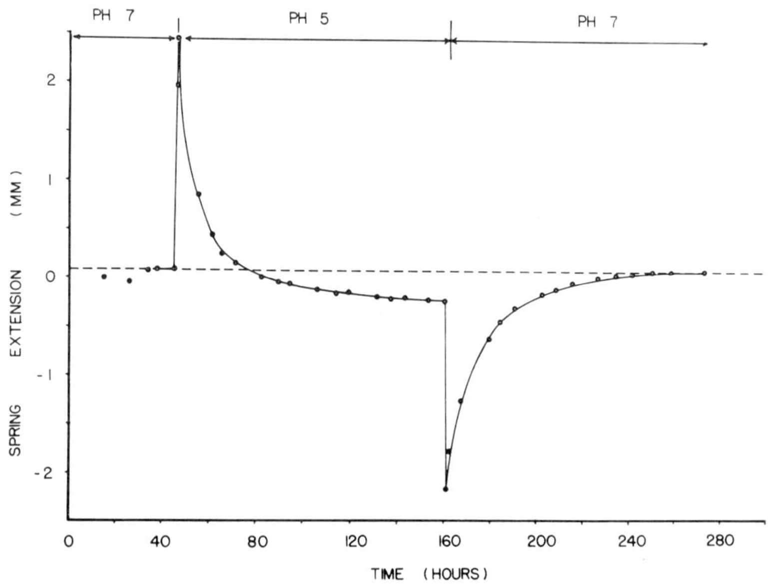

FIG. 7. Representative measurement of change in effective weight of protein inside analysis bag accompanying change in pH. (Stevens and Lauffer, in preparation).

When an experiment is actually carried out, results such as those illustrated in Figure 7 are obtained. It can be seen that the quartz spring extension comes to an equilibrium value at pH 7 and then when pH 5 buffer is substituted outside the bag there is an immediate change in extension followed by a gradual approach to an equilibrium value characteristic of pH 5. When pH 7 buffer is returned to the system, the ultimate equilibrium spring extension is the same as the original value at pH 7. The difference between the equilibrium values at pH 7 and at pH 5 can be converted into the change in effective weight accompanying change in pH. The results of preliminary experiments are shown in Table 7. From these results one can calculate:

$$\left(\Delta V_a - \frac{\Delta V_b}{r}\right) = -.0029 \text{ ml./Gm.} = -150 \text{ ml./mole}$$

$$\left(\Delta h_a - \frac{\Delta h_b}{r}\right) = +.043 \text{ ml./Gm.} = +130 \text{ moles/mole}$$

The first term in parentheses has as an approximate meaning—the change in partial specific volume accompanying depolymerization; and the second term in parentheses has as an approximate meaning—the change in bound water accompanying depolymerization. In both cases, ml./Gm. was converted to ml./mole by multiplying by the molecular weight of the polymerizing material under the actual conditions of the experiment.

TABLE 7

ΔW/*100 mg.*

	TMV protein (a)	TMV control (b)
Buffer ($\rho = 1$)	+0.48 mg.	+0.19 mg.
Buffered glycerol ($\rho = 1.06$)	+0.18 mg.	+0.12 mg.

Abbreviation: TMV, tobacco mosaic virus.

It can be seen that these measurements indicate that 130 moles of water are bound/mole of unpolymerized TMV protein on dissociation or released on polymerization. This quantity agrees with that indicated by the thermodynamic considerations.

The results indicate further that, associated with depolymerization, there is a decrease in partial specific volume of 150 ml./mole. It is possible that this comes about by exposing, when linkages are broken, dipolar ions which bind water by electrostriction. Edsall (1943) has estimated that the electrostriction accompanying the formation of dipolar ions averages 13.3 ml./mole. Thus, the electrostriction observed in this case would correspond to exposing 11 dipolar ions each time a link between two TMV subunits is broken or concealing those dipolar ions each time such a linkage is formed.

The Size of the Tobacco Mosaic Virus Protein Subunits

As was pointed out previously, X-ray diffraction data on tobacco mosaic virus have been interpreted in terms of protein repeat units with a molecular weight of approximately 18,000 arranged in a helix (Franklin and Holmes, 1958). Further, amino acid analyses and end group titrations yield a similar value (Knight, 1954). Neither of these studies, however, answers the question of whether the ultimate molecular weight is 18,000 or some integral multiple of it. Comparable low molecular weights have been reported for denatured protein of tobacco mosaic virus (Lauffer and Stanley, 1943; Anderer, 1959). Nevertheless, the protein degradation products obtained from mild alkaline digestion or mild acidic digestion of tobacco mosaic virus normally have sedimentation coefficients of about 4 $\overline{S}$ and molecular weights of about 10^5 (Schramm and Zillig, 1955). Ansevin and Lauffer (1959b) have presented evidence that at extremely low concentrations these 10^5 molecular weight units dissociate into smaller particles with physicochemical parameters consistent with a molecular weight of 18,000 and that these small particles are still native in the sense that they can be repolymerized into nucleic acid-free, rodlike helices and that they can be reconstituted with nucleic acid into nucleoprotein rods.

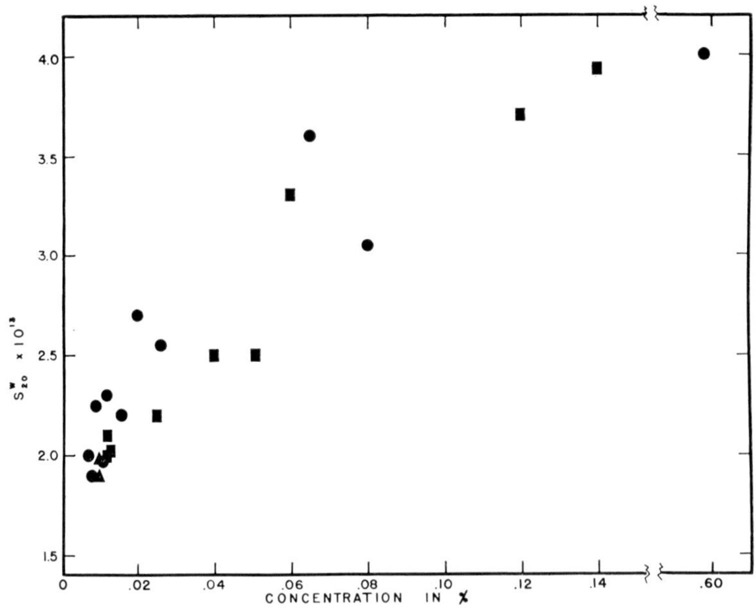

FIG. 8. Sedimentation coefficients of tobacco mosaic virus protein at different concentrations.
■ 0.1 mμ. phosphate buffer, pH 6.5
▲ 0.05 mμ. phosphate buffer, pH 7.0
● 0.10 mμ. borate buffer, pH 9.0
(Ansevin and Lauffer, 1959b).

Sedimentation measurements were made in the synthetic boundary cell of a Spinco untracentrifuge at temperatures between 0°C and 6°C. The protein was prepared by treatment of tobacco mosaic virus at pH 10.3. It was later diluted to concentrations as low as 0.01 per cent with 0.05 ionic strength phosphate buffer at pH 7, with 0.1 ionic strength phosphate buffer at pH 6.5 or with 0.1 ionic strength borate buffer at pH 9. The centrifuge speed was 59,780 rpm. Boundary migration was followed by means of schlieren optics. Sedimentation coefficients, corrected to water at 20°C are shown as a function of protein concentration in Figure 8. It can be seen that when the protein is diluted to values as low as 0.01 per cent the sedimentation coefficient decreases from the usual value of about 4 $\overline{S}$ to a minimum value of 1.9 $\overline{S}$. If X-ray diffraction data have been interpreted correctly, the ultimate particle of tobacco mosaic virus protein must be a truncated wedge with a length of 70 Å, a thickness of 23 Å and a maximum width of 34.8 Å. A highly schematized drawing is shown in Figure 9. If one employs the reasoning introduced by Lauffer and Szent-Györgyi (1955), one postulates that the coefficient of friction of the tobacco mosaic virus protein subunit depicted in Figure 9 lies between those of the two elongated ellipsoids of revolution, also shown in the figure, both with major semiaxes of 35 Å and one with a minor semiaxis of 11.5 Å and the other with a minor semiaxis of 17.4 Å. The coefficient of friction, f, for translational motion of randomly oriented ellipsoids of revolution is given by the equation:

$$f = \frac{6\pi\eta b \sqrt{1 - a^2/b^2}}{\ln\left(\frac{1 + \sqrt{1 - a^2/b^2}}{a/b}\right)}$$

where b is the major semiaxis, a is the minor semiaxis and η is the coefficient of viscosity. The coefficients of friction calculated to correspond to water at 20°C for the larger and for the smaller ellipsoids are 4.52×10^{-8} and 3.49×10^{-8} cgs. units, respectively. The formula,

$$s = \frac{M\,(1 - V\rho)}{Nf},$$

where M is the molecular weight, N is Avogadro's number, V is the partial specific volume, ρ is the density of the medium and s is the sedimentation coefficient corrected to water at 20°C, can be used to calculate the molecular weights. By substituting values of 0.74

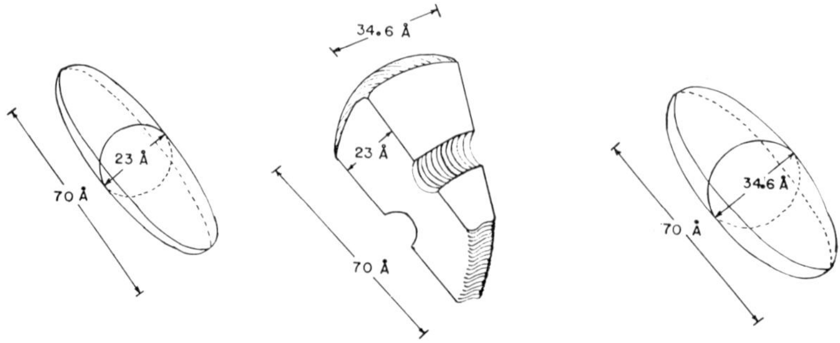

FIG. 9. Model for the tobacco mosaic virus protein subunit.

ml./Gm. for V (Schramm and Zillig, 1955), 1.9×10^{-13} cgs. units for *s* and the above mentioned values for f, one obtains molecular weights of 15,000 and 20,000, respectively, to correspond to the higher and the lower friction coefficients. Inasmuch as these values bracket 18,000, it can be concluded that the sedimentation coefficient of 1.9 $\overline{S}$ is concordant with the protein repeat unit suggested by X–ray diffraction studies (Ansevin and Lauffer, 1959b).

Attempts have been made to measure the coefficient of diffusion of the protein subunits at extremely high dilutions using the method of diffusion into agar gels. Diffusion studies carried out in phosphate buffer at pH 6.5 were not successful. However, one diffusion experiment carried out in carbonate buffer at pH 10.2 could be interpreted in terms of a diffusion coefficient of 10×10^{-7} cgs. units after correction to water at 20°C (Schantz and Lauffer, in preparation). This value, combined with the sedimentation coefficient, 1.9 $\overline{S}$, yields a molecular weight of 17,400. It seems, therefore, that at extreme dilution a protein particle is obtained which corresponds, in general, to the 18,000 molecular weight repeat unit indicated as the smallest possible unit by chemical and X-ray diffraction considerations.

This highly diluted material can be reconcentrated. The most successful method used thus far involves dialysis against a 30 per cent aqueous solution of polyvinylpyrrolidone. Tenfold reconcentrations and recoveries of better than 50 per cent were obtained for material initially diluted in 0.05 ionic strength phosphate buffer at pH 7. When the reconcentrated protein was adjusted to pH 6.5, it polymerized into rods at 25°C as described by Lauffer, Ansevin, Cartwright, and Brinton (1958) for the usual protein subunits. Figure 10 is an electron micrograph of rodlike particles obtained upon the polymerization of protein which had been dissociated to

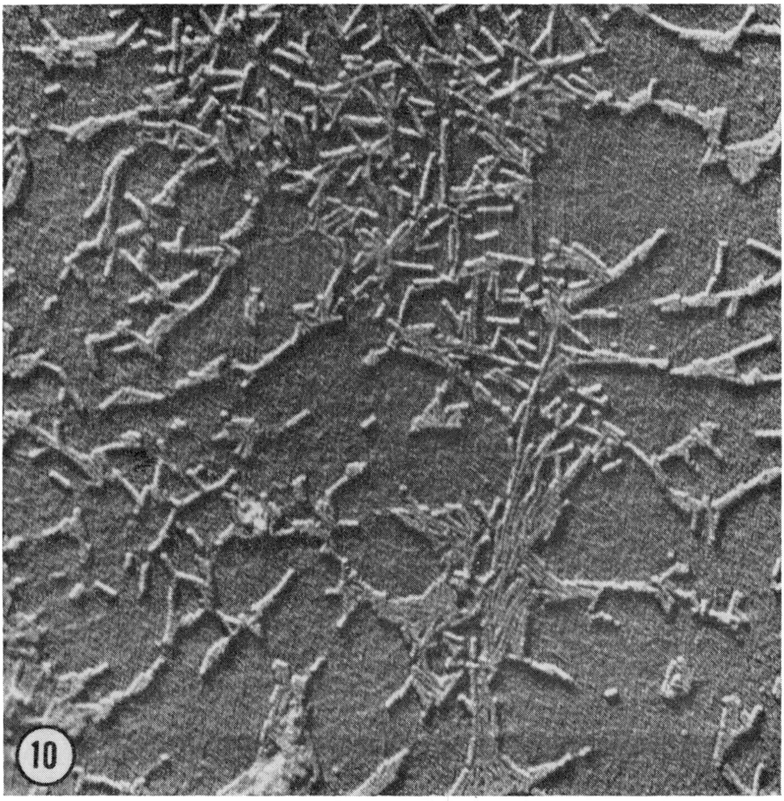

FIG. 10. Polymerized TMV protein rods obtained from protein previously dissociated to the $\overline{S}$ 1.9 state by dilution to 0.01 per cent and later reconcentrated.

the 1.9 $\overline{S}$ state. This reconcentrated material can also be reconstituted with tobacco mosaic virus nucleic acid into rodlike nucleoprotein particles. It seems, therefore, that the protein on dissociation remains native at least to the extent that it is still capable of polymerizing both with and without the nucleic acid (Ansevin and Lauffer, 1959b). This work then constitutes direct experimental evidence for the existence of a native subunit of tobacco mosaic virus protein with a molecular weight of approximately 18,000 postulated for the interpretation of X-ray diffraction patterns.

Summary and Conclusions

Tobacco mosaic virus protein polymerizes reversibly by an endothermic process. To provide a mechanism for this observation, it is postulated that TMV protein subunits are more highly hydrated than polymer. Equilibrium constants were evaluated for polymerization, and from the variation with temperature the enthalpy and entropy of polymerization were calculated to be plus 190 kcal./mole and plus 680 e.u. If the entropy change associated with the release of water from the subunits is the same as for melting ice at the same temperature, this entropy increase suggests that several hundred molecules of water are released each time a linkage is formed between subunits. Urea and tetra-n-butyl ammonium ion both shift the equilibrium in the direction of dissociation. They both cause denaturation also, but the two reactions are separate. The dissociating effect of these two reagents can be explained on the assumption that they are bound to the subunits in competition with water.

Another factor which affects polymerization is pH. Both high and low pH values favor depolymerization, while pH values near the isoelectric point find the protein in the polymerized state at all ordinary temperatures. When the protein dissociates in unbuffered media in the neighborhood of pH 6.5, there is a sharp drop in pH, indicating that hydrogen ions are released. The extent of depolymerization also depends on concentration. At pH 6.5, the predominant particle obtained upon depolymerization has a molecular weight of about 10^5 when the reaction is carried out at protein concentrations of the order of 0.1 per cent. When the concentration is reduced to 0.01 per cent the protein dissociates to the ultimate monomeric unit with a molecular weight of approximately 18,000.

These observations can be accounted for by the assumption that so-called entropy bonds, that is, the entropy decrease associated with combining of water or reagents like urea or tetra-n-butyl ammonium ion with subunits, contribute to the stability of the polymerized form. Opposing this is electrostatic repulsion between subunits, repulsion at a minimum near the isoelectric point and at high values at pH values far removed from the isoelectric point. Also opposing is the entropy factor associated with release of small protein units from the helical structure of the polymerized rods. A further contribution to nonstability at pH values above the isoelectric point is the dissociation of hydrogen ions which accompany dissociation of the protein. It must be remembered that all of this applies to the TMV protein alone. In the virus, there is obviously additional bonding between protein and RNA, because the virus itself is much more stable that the protein polymer.

Studies on the polymerization of tobacco mosaic virus protein point up the possibility that water may play an extremely important role in the formation of the tobacco mosaic virus protein rod from its constituent subunits. The potentiality exists that this phenomenon is general, and that water is uniquely responsible for many aspects of structure formation in living systems.

REFERENCES

Anderer, F. A. 1959. Das Molekulargewicht der Peptideinheit im Protein des Tabakmosaikvirus. *Zeitschrift für Naturforschung*, 14b:24–28.

Ansevin, A. T., and M. A. Lauffer. 1959a. The Disaggregation and Repolymerization of Purified Protein from Tobacco Mosaic Virus. (Abstract) *Program and Abstracts*, The Biophysical Society, 1959 Meeting, February 25, 26, 27, Pittsburgh, Pennsylvania.

———. 1959b. Native Tobacco Mosaic Virus Protein of Molecular Weight 18,000. *Nature, London*, 183:1601–1602.

Ansevin, A. T., and M. A. Lauffer. Polymerization and Depolymerization of Tobacco Mosaic Virus Protein. (In preparation).

Bawden, F. C., and N. W. Pirie. 1937. The Isolation and Some Properties of Liquid Crystalline Substances from Solanaceous Plants Infected with Three Strains of Tobacco Mosaic Virus. *Proceedings of the Royal Society of London, Series B*, 123:274–324.

———. 1940. The Effects of Alkali and Some Simple Organic Substances on Three Plant Viruses. *Biochemical Journal*, 34:1278–1292.

Buzzell, A. 1959. Action of Urea on Tobacco Mosaic Virus. *Journal of the American Chemical Society*, 82:1636–1641.

———. (in press). Action of Urea on Tobacco Mosaic Virus. II. The Bonds between Protein Subunits. *Biophysical Journal.*

Edsall, J. T. 1943. *Apparent Molar Volume, Heat Capacity, Compressibility and Surface Tension of Dipolar Ions in Solution, in Proteins, Amino Acids and Peptides*, E. J. Cohn and J. T. Edsall, Eds., pp. 155–176. New York, New York: Reinhold Publishing Corporation.

Flory, P. J. 1936. Molecular Size Distribution in Linear Condensation Polymers. *Journal of the American Chemical Society*, 58:1877–1885.

Fraenkel-Conrat, H. 1956. The Role of the Nucleic Acid in the Reconstitution of Active Tobacco Mosaic Virus. *Journal of the American Chemical Society*, 78:882–883.

Fraenkel-Conrat, H., and R. C. Williams. 1955. Reconstitution of Active Tobacco Mosaic Virus from Its Inactive Protein and Nucleic Acid Components. *Proceedings of the National Academy of Sciences of the U.S.A.*, 41:690–698.

Frank, H. S., and M. W. Evans. 1945. Free Volume and Entropy in Condensed Systems. III. Entropy in Binary Liquid Mixtures; Partial Molal Entropy in Dilute Solutions; Structure and Thermodynamics in Aqueous Electrolytes. *Journal of Chemical Physics*, 13:507–532.

Frank, H. S., and W. Y. Wen. 1957. Structural Aspects of Ion-Solvent Interaction in Aqueous Solution: A Suggested Picture of Water Structure. *Faraday Society Discussions*, 24:133–140.

Franklin, R. E. 1955. Structural Resemblance Between Schramm's Repolymerized A-Protein and Tobacco Mosaic Virus. *Biochimica et biophysica acta,* 18:313–314.

Franklin, R. E., and K. C. Holmes. 1958. Tobacco Mosaic Virus: Application of the Method of Isomorphous Replacement to the Determination of the Helical Parameters and Radial Density Distribution. *Acta Crystallographica,* 11:213–220.

Gierer, A., and G. Schramm. 1956. Infectivity of Ribonucleic Acid from Tobacco Mosaic Virus. *Nature, London,* 177:702–703.

Harrington, W. F., and H. K. Schachman. 1956. Studies on the Alkaline Degradation of Tobacco Mosaic Virus. I. Ultracentrifugal Analysis. *Archives of Biochemistry and Biophysics,* 65:278–295.

Hart, R. G. 1955. Electron-Microscopic Evidence for the Localization of Ribonucleic Acid in the Particles of Tobacco Mosaic Virus. *Proceedings of the National Academy of Sciences of the U.S.A.,* 41:261–264.

Kleczkowski, A. 1959. Aggregation of the Protein of Tobacco Mosaic Virus With and Without Combination with Nucleic Acid. *Virology,* 7:385–393.

Knight, C. A. 1947. The Nature of Some of the Chemical Differences Among Strains of Tobacco Mosaic Virus. *Journal of Biological Chemistry,* 171:297–308.

———. 1954. The Chemical Constitution of Viruses. *Advances in Virus Research,* 2:153–182.

Knight, C. A., and M. A. Lauffer. 1942. A Comparison of the Alkaline Cleavage Products of Two Strains of Tobacco Mosaic Virus. *Journal of Biological Chemistry,* 144:411–417.

Kramer, E., and H. G. Wittmann. 1958. Elektrophoretische Untersuchungen der A-Proteine dreier Tabakmosaikvirus Stämme. *Zeitschrift für Naturforschung,* 13b:30–33.

Lauffer, M. A. 1938. The Viscosity of Tobacco Mosaic Virus Protein Solutions. *Journal of Biological Chemistry,* 126:443–453.

———. 1943. Denaturation of Tobacco Mosaic Virus by Urea. II. Kinetic Aspects. *Journal of the American Chemical Society,* 65:1793–1802.

———. 1944. The Size and Shape of Tobacco Mosaic Virus Particles. *Journal of the American Chemical Society,* 66:1188–1194.

Lauffer, M. A., A. T. Ansevin, T. E. Cartwright, and C. C. Brinton, Jr. 1958. Polymerization-Depolymerization of Tobacco Mosaic Virus Protein. *Nature, London,* 181:1338–1339.

Lauffer, M. A., and R. B. Dow. 1941. The Denaturation of Tobacco Mosaic Virus at High Pressures. *Journal of Biological Chemistry,* 140:509–518.

Lauffer, M. A., and W. C. Price. 1940. Thermal Denaturation of Tobacco Mosaic Virus. *Journal of Biological Chemistry,* 133:1–15.

Lauffer, M. A., and W. M. Stanley. 1943. Denaturation of Tobacco Mosaic Virus by Urea. I. Biochemical Aspects. *Archives of Biochemistry,* 2:413–424.

Lauffer, M. A., and A. G. Szent-Györgyi. 1955. Comments on the Structure of Myosin. *Archives of Biochemistry and Biophysics,* 56:542–548.

Lauffer, M. A., D. Trkula, and A. Buzzell. 1956. Mechanism of Inactivation of Tobacco Mosaic Virus by X-Rays. *Nature, London,* 177:890.

Lippincott, J. A., and B. Commoner. 1956. Reactivation of Tobacco Mosaic

Virus Infectivity in Mixtures of Virus Protein and Nucleic Acid. *Biochimica et biophysica acta*, 19:198–199.

Loring, H. S. 1939. Properties and Hydrolytic Products of Nucleic Acid from Tobacco Mosaic Virus. *Journal of Biological Chemistry*, 130:251–258.

Loring, H. S., M. A. Lauffer, and W. M. Stanley. 1938. Aggregation of Purified Tobacco Mosaic Virus. *Nature, London*, 142:841–842.

Oster, G. 1948. The Scattering of Light and Its Application to Chemistry. *Chemical Reviews*, 43:319–365.

Pfankuch, E. 1940. Über die Spaltung von Virusproteinen der Tabakmosaik-Gruppe. *Biochimische Zeitschrift*, 306:125–129.

Ross, A. F. 1940. The Sulfur Distribution in Tobacco Mosaic Virus Protein. *Journal of Biological Chemistry*, 136:119–129.

Schachman, H. K., and M. A. Lauffer. 1949. The Hydration, Size and Shape of Tobacco Mosaic Virus. *Journal of the American Chemical Society*, 71:536–541.

Schantz, E. J., and M. A. Lauffer. Diffusion Measurements in Agar Gel. (In preparation).

Schramm, G. 1943. Über die Spaltung des Tabakmosaikvirus in niedermolekulare Proteine und die Rückbildung hochmolekularen Proteins aus den Spaltstucken. *Die Naturwissenschaften*, 31:94–96.

———. 1947. Über die Spaltung des Tabakmosaikvirus und die Wiedervereinigung der Spaltstucke zu höhermolekularen Proteinen. *Zeitschrift für Naturforschung*, 2b:249–257.

Schramm, G., and W. Zillig. 1955. Über die Struktur des Tabakmosaikvirus. IV. Mitt.: Die Reaggregation des nucleinsäure-freien Proteins. *Zeitschrift für Naturforschung*, 10b:493–499.

Schramm, G., G. Schumacher, and W. Zillig. 1955. An Infectious Nucleoprotein from Tobacco Mosaic Virus. *Nature, London*, 175:549–550.

Smith, C. E., and M. A. Lauffer. 1961. Evidence for Participation of Water in Polymerization-Depolymerization of TMV Protein. (Abstract SB 2) Fifth Annual Biophysical Society Meeting, February 16–18, St. Louis, Missouri.

———. Factors Affecting the Polymerization-Depolymerization of TMV Protein. (In preparation).

Stanley, W. M. 1935. Isolation of a Crystalline Protein Possessing the Properties of Tobacco Mosaic Virus. *Science*, 81:644–645.

———. 1938. "Biochemistry and Biophysics of Viruses," *Handbuch der Virusforschung*, R. Doerr and C. Hallauer, Eds., 1:447–546. Vienna, Austria: Julius Springer.

———. 1956. Virus Composition and Structure—25 Years Ago and Now. *Federation Proceedings*, 15:812–818.

Stanley, W. M., and M. A. Lauffer. 1939. Disintegration of Tobacco Mosaic Virus in Urea Solutions. *Science*, 89:345–347.

Stanley, W. M., and H. S. Loring. 1938. "Properties of Virus Proteins," *Protein Chemistry* (Cold Spring Harbor Symposia on Quantitative Biology, Vol. 6), pp. 341–360. Cold Spring Harbor, New York: Long Island Biological Association.

Stevens, C. L., and M. A. Lauffer. Direct Weighing of Water Released Upon

Polymerization of TMV Protein. (In preparation).

Watson, J. D. 1954. The Structure of Tobacco Mosaic Virus. I. X-Ray Evidence of a Helical Arrangement of Subunits Around the Longitudinal Axis. *Biochimica et biophysica acta*, 13:10–19.

Wyckoff, R. W. G. 1937. Molecular Sedimentation Constants of Tobacco Mosaic Virus Proteins Extracted from Plants at Intervals After Inoculation. *Journal of Biological Chemistry*, 121:219–224.

Nuclear Proteins of Neoplastic Tissues

HARRIS BUSCH, M.D., PH.D., PAUL BYVOET, M.D., PH.D., AND JOSEPH R. DAVIS,* M.D., PH.D.

Departments of Biochemistry and Pharmacology,
Baylor University College of Medicine,
Houston, Texas

Our interest in nuclear proteins has arisen from two types of observations made in our laboratory. In the first of these, shown in Figure 1, the effect of the aminouracil mustard, prepared by Lyttle and Petering (1959), was determined with regard to labeling of nuclear proteins of the Walker tumor (Busch, Amer, and Nyhan, 1959). An early effect of the mustard is suppression of labeling of the acid-insoluble nuclear proteins. In the period from 12 to 24 hours, there was marked suppression of labeling of the histones or the acid-soluble nuclear proteins. A particularly important point was that there was no suppression, at any period up to 24 hours, of amino acid incorporation into the proteins of the cytoplasmic sap, the mitochondrial proteins or microsomal proteins. This investigation suggested that antitumor agents were exerting a more specific effect on biosynthesis of nuclear proteins than was hitherto shown to occur.

The second type of experiment which aroused our interest in nuclear proteins is that indicated in Figure 2, which is a chromatogram of the acid-soluble nuclear proteins of the Jensen sarcoma following the administration of L-lysine-U-C^{14} to rats bearing this

---

* Postdoctoral Fellow of the American Cancer Society.

tumor (Davis and Busch, 1960). There are five protein peaks, and in this case, two radioactive peaks. Radioactive peak 2 and peak 3 are so named because of their relationship to the patterns for other tissues. Radioactive peak 2 is a peak which thus far has been found only in neoplastic tissues, including the Walker tumor, the Flexner-Jobling carcinosarcoma, the Ehrlich ascites tumor, a human malignant melanoma, the Morris hepatoma, and sarcoma 180. (Figure 2).

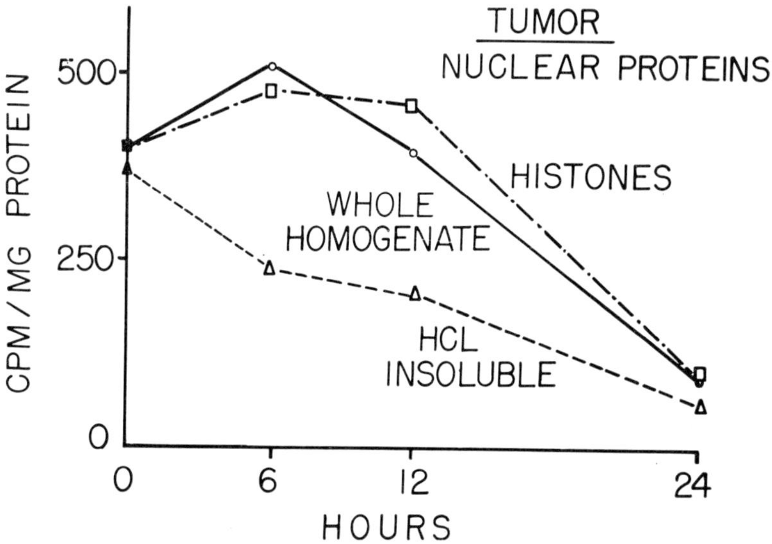

FIG. 1. Kinetics of the effects on amino acid incorporation into the nuclear proteins of the tumor by the aminouracil mustard. One hour prior to the designated time, 7.5 μc. of L-arginine-U-C^{14} were injected intraperitoneally.

INTRANUCLEAR DISTRIBUTION OF PROTEIN

Chromosomes

With these two findings in mind, let us explore the biological and chemical approaches to the types of nuclear proteins.

In Figure 3 is a schematic impression of the binding of protein and deoxyribonucleic acid (DNA) in the chromosomes (Zubay and Doty, 1959). The concept presented is that along the surface of DNA there are proteins which are of small molecular weight placed in such a way that they cover certain of the surface layers of the DNA. The type of nuclear protein, linked to the chromosomes, which has been labeled "histone," is linked very tightly to the nucleic acid. The pictures made by Horn and Ward (1957) show that

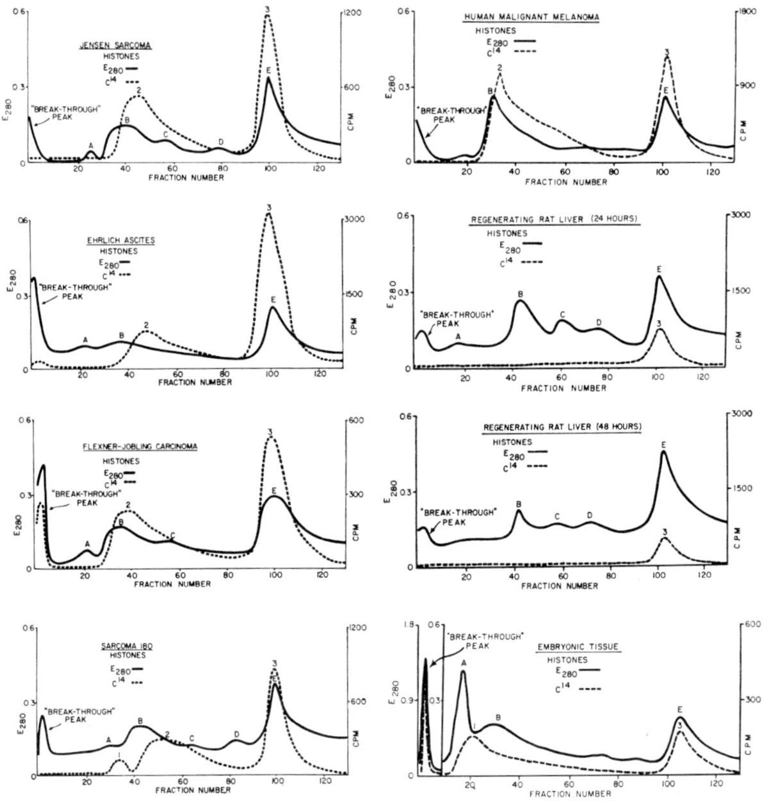

FIG. 2. Chromatographic patterns of both radioactivity and protein concentration for acid-soluble nuclear proteins of the Jensen sarcoma, Ehrlich ascites tumor, Flexner-Jobling carcinoma, sarcoma 180, a human malignant melanoma, 24-hour regenerating rat liver, 48-hour regenerating rat liver and rat embryonic tissue.

wherever there is a band of DNA along the chromosome there is also a protein band which rapidly takes the stain with Fast Green. This unique combination of protein and DNA accounts for only one type of chromosomal protein.

In addition to the histones, there is much chromosomal protein in the heterochromatin, along with some ribonucleic acid (RNA). In all probability, there are some specific proteins linked with the RNA. The chromatin would then appear to contain at least three types of nuclear protein: DNA-bound, RNA-bound, and the protein of the "heterochromatin."

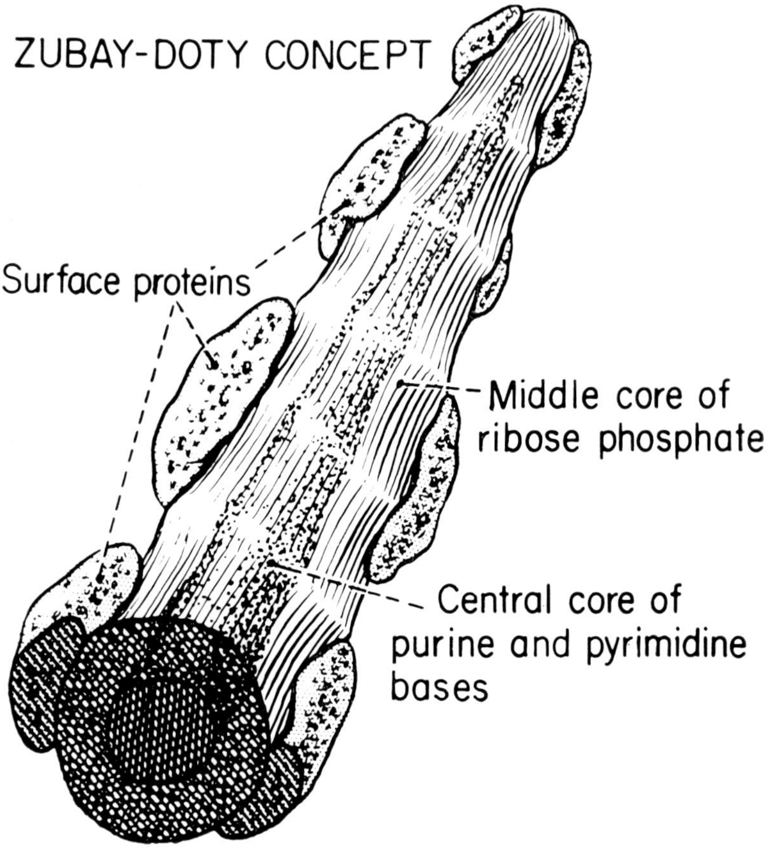

FIG. 3. Schematic illustration of the relationship of histones to DNA in the chromosomal fiber.

Nuclear particles

The nucleolus is a unique organelle which is apparently important in RNA biosynthesis. Following the report of Albertini (1959), the nucleolus would appear to have a surface layer of protein, rich in sulfhydryl groups. There is probably another kind of protein within the nucleolus, as illustrated by electron microscopy studies showing substructures of nucleoli, i.e., nucleolini and nucleolar sap. Thus, at least two more types of nuclear protein are probably present in the nucleolus. In addition to these nuclear proteins, there are also proteins of the nuclear ribosomes, structures whose existence has been suggested by Allfrey, Mirsky, and Osawa (1955–

1957), and later by Osawa, Takata, and Hotta (1958). These ribonucleoproteins may contain at least two different types of particles, i.e., those remaining in the nucleus and those transferred out with "messenger RNA."

The Nuclear Sap

The nuclear sap is rather different from the cytoplasmic sap in a number of important respects. One of the positive differences is the state of these two different protoplasmic entities. The nuclear sap is a gelatinous, semisolid material, perhaps made so, in part, by the chromatin which is present. Its constitution is different from that of the semiliquid state of the cytoplasmic sap, and probably the proteins present are different from those already mentioned. In addition, the nucleus probably contains enzymes for important synthetic reactions (Allfrey, Mirsky, and Osawa, 1955, 1957; Rees and Rowland, 1961). In summary, the nucleus would appear to contain four groups of proteins in its components: chromosomal proteins, nucleolar proteins, proteins of the ribosomes, and the proteins of the nuclear sap.

Cytoplasmic Proteins Resembling Nuclear Proteins

A number of recent studies have provided evidence of the presence in cytoplasmic ribonucleoproteins of proteins resembling the nuclear proteins in a relatively higher content of the basic amino acids than is usually found. In many animal proteins, the ratio of acidic amino acids to basic amino acids is approximately 1.5. Such proteins include plasma proteins, muscle proteins, and proteins of a number of tissues. However, in the acid-soluble nuclear proteins, the concentration of the acidic amino acids is decreased, and this ratio is inverted (Busch and Davis, 1958). A similar result was obtained by Butler, Cohn, and Simson (1960) in recent studies on fractions obtained from microsomal proteins. As indicated in Table 1, in the whole microsomal protein, the acidic amino acids comprised 21.6 per cent of the total amino acid while the basic amino acids, lysine, arginine, and histidine, comprised 18.7 per cent of the total amino acids. In fractions obtained by treatment of the microsomes with Lubrol or perfluorooctanoate, the acidic amino acids accounted for approximately 19 per cent of the total amino acids, while the basic amino acids accounted for 18 per cent of the total amino acids. In the acid-extracted proteins of the perfluorooctanoate pellet, the concentrations of the basic amino acids were increased to 27.8 per cent of the total amino acids, as compared with the 18.9 per cent of the total amino acids found in the acidic amino acids.

TABLE 1

*Amino Acid Composition of Ribonucleoproteins of Microsomes**

	Crampton and Peterman (1959)	Butler, Cohn and Simson (1960)		
Amino acid	Microsomes	Microsomes	Lubrol	Perfluoro-octanoate
Alanine	8.2	7.5	8.1	8.0
Arginine	7.0	7.2	6.7	7.9
Aspartic acid	8.1	9.5	9.1	7.9
Glutamic acid	8.7	12.1	10.7	10.7
Glycine	7.5	7.1	7.5	8.1
Histidine	6.7	2.5	2.6	2.5
Isoleucine	5.0	. .	. .	. .
Leucine	8.8	. .	. .	. .
Lysine	9.0	6.7	8.0	8.2
Methionine	2.1	0.5	0.4	. .
Phenylalanine	3.7	5.4	5.1	5.3
Proline	4.9	5.9	5.6	5.0
Serine	5.0	6.2	6.6	5.6
Threonine	5.0	5.4	5.4	5.2
Tyrosine	3.1	1.4	2.2	2.2
Valine	7.2	8.0	. .	8.4

* Values are per cent of total moles of amino acids recovered in the particular amino acid. Some of the data are recalculated from the original papers.

Crampton and Peterman (1959) also reported a similar result in their studies on the ribonucleoproteins of the liver, which were obtained by ultracentrifugation in salt solutions. The concentrations of the amino acids in their proteins were not strikingly different from those obtained by Butler, Cohn, and Simson (1960), with the exception of histidine, which was present in a higher percentage in their ribonucleoproteins, and the acidic amino acids which were present in a slightly lower concentration (Table 1). The similarity of these proteins to histones and their possible role in contributing to specificity of the templates have been discussed by these authors.

Chemical Fractionation of Nuclear Proteins

Figure 4 illustrates the types of chemical fractionation of the nuclear proteins (Busch and Davis, 1958). Isolated nuclei have been subjected to a wide variety of procedures for extraction of the chromosomal proteins or histones. Such extractions have been carried

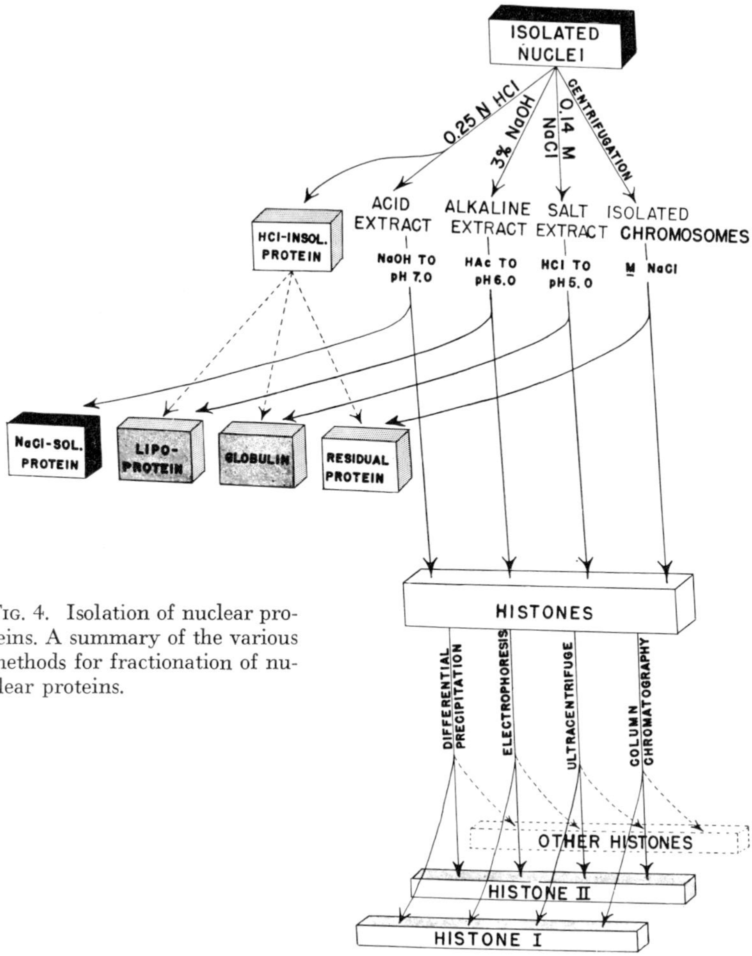

FIG. 4. Isolation of nuclear proteins. A summary of the various methods for fractionation of nuclear proteins.

out with many aqueous solutions: salt solutions, alkali, acids and even with water. The fractions which contain the histones are then subjected to a number of additional procedures for extraction of the histones. In the residue after acid extraction, there are proteins which have been variously termed "lipoproteins," "globulins," "residual proteins" and "NaCl soluble proteins." These are all fractions obtainable from the broad group of "acid-insoluble" nuclear proteins. It is rather disappointing that greater identification of the nuclear proteins has not been achieved despite the efforts in recent years by a number of groups. Nuclear proteins had not been isolated in highly purified form until recently and, even yet, no crystalline nuclear protein has been obtained.

Incorporation of Amino Acids Into Nuclear Proteins

In vitro and *in vivo*

The data which aroused our interest in the nuclear proteins are illustrated in the following figures. Figure 5 illustrates the distribution of radioactive amino acids such as lysine, alanine, or aspartic acid in proteins of liver slices after one hour of incubation

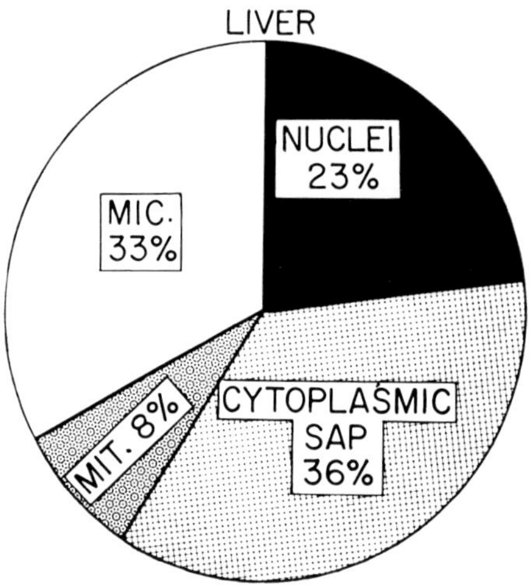

Fig. 5. Total protein incorporation from L-aspartate-U-C^{14} in slices of liver. The data are expressed as percentage of the total isotope incorporated into protein of the tissue slice. MIC. = microsomes; MIT. = mitochondria.

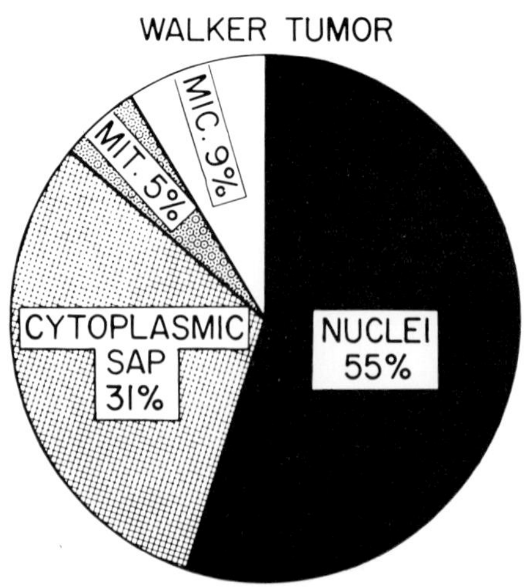

Fig. 6. Total protein incorporation from L-aspartate-U-C^{14} in slices of Walker 256 carcinosarcoma. MIC. = microsomes; MIT. = mitochondria.

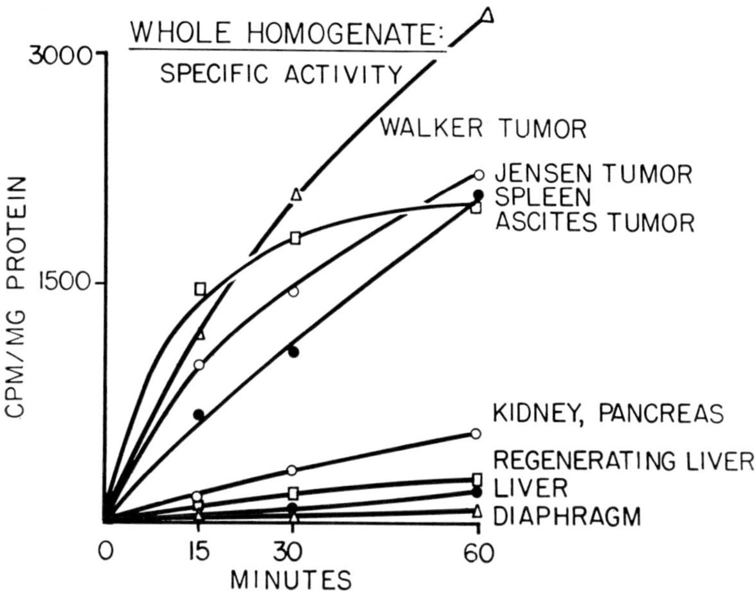

FIG. 7. Kinetics of labeling of the proteins of the whole homogenate of the tissues following *in vitro* incubation with L-arginine-U-C^{14}.

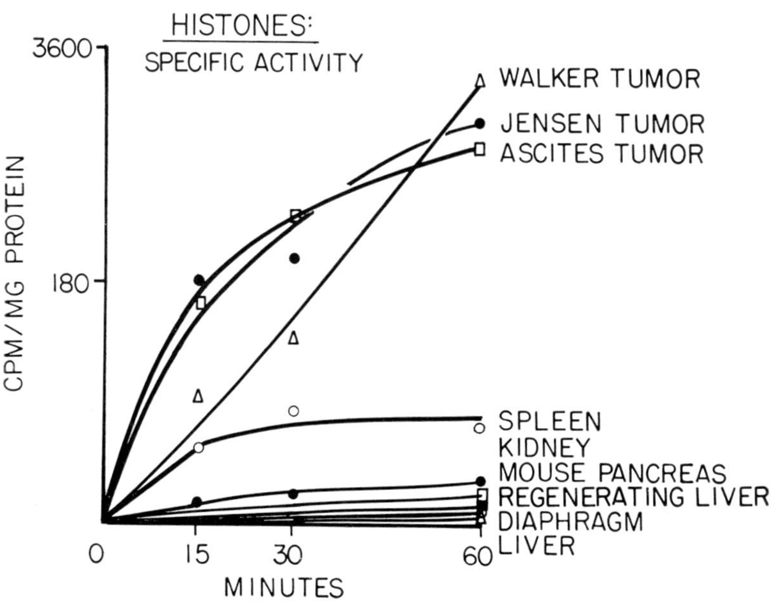

FIG. 8. Kinetics of labeling of the histones of the tissues following *in vitro* incubation with L-arginine-U-C^{14}.

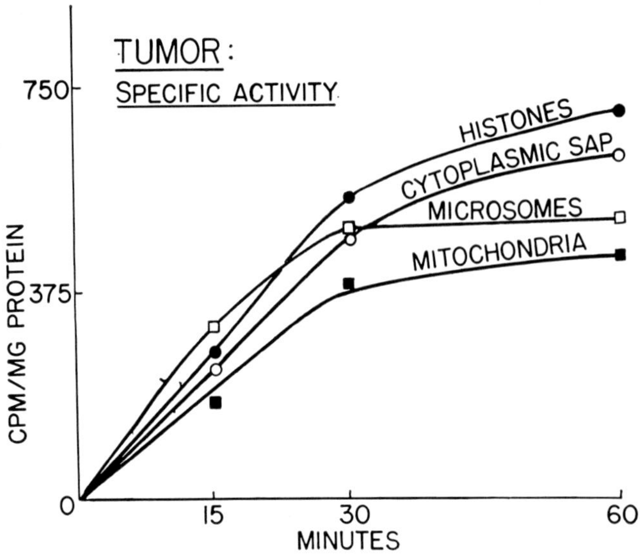

FIG. 9. Time course of specific activities of proteins of various cellular fractions of the Walker 256 carcinosarcoma after *in vivo* injection of L-lysine-U-C^{14} into a tumor-bearing rat.

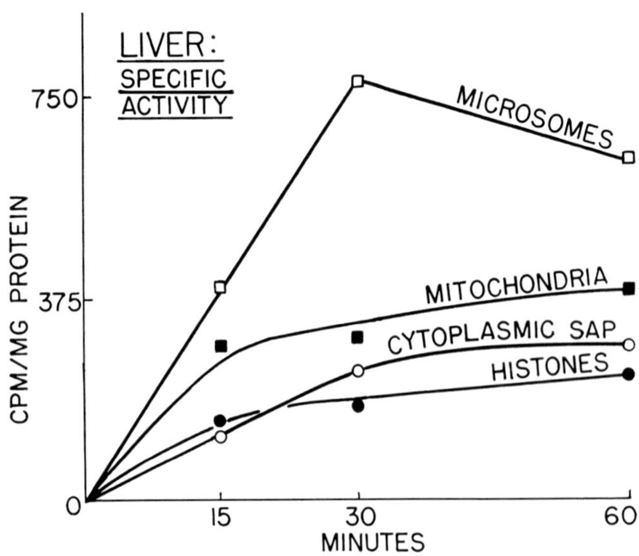

FIG. 10. Time course of specific activities of proteins of various cellular fractions of liver after *in vivo* injections of L-lysine-U-C^{14} into a tumor-bearing rat.

with the tracer (Davis and Busch, 1958). Approximately one third of the total radioactivity is incorporated into the proteins of the microsomes and another third is incorporated into the proteins of the cytoplasmic sap. A relatively small percentage of the radioactivity entered the mitochondrial proteins and approximately 23 per cent entered the nuclear proteins of liver slices. A rather different result is shown for the Walker tumor (Figure 6). In this case, approximately 55 per cent of the total radioactivity entered the nuclear proteins and only 9 per cent entered the microsomal proteins. In further studies on slice systems *in vitro* (Figure 7), it was shown that some tumors and the spleen incorporated radioactivity into the total cellular proteins at approximately equal rates (Starbuck and Busch, 1960). Somewhat lower rates of incorporation of isotopes into proteins of the slices were found for other tissues. However, virtually a qualitative difference was found in the labeling of the histones of the tumors as compared with the other tissues studied (Figure 8).

This very large difference in the labeling of the intracellular proteins of the tumors *in vitro* led to experiments on the fate of

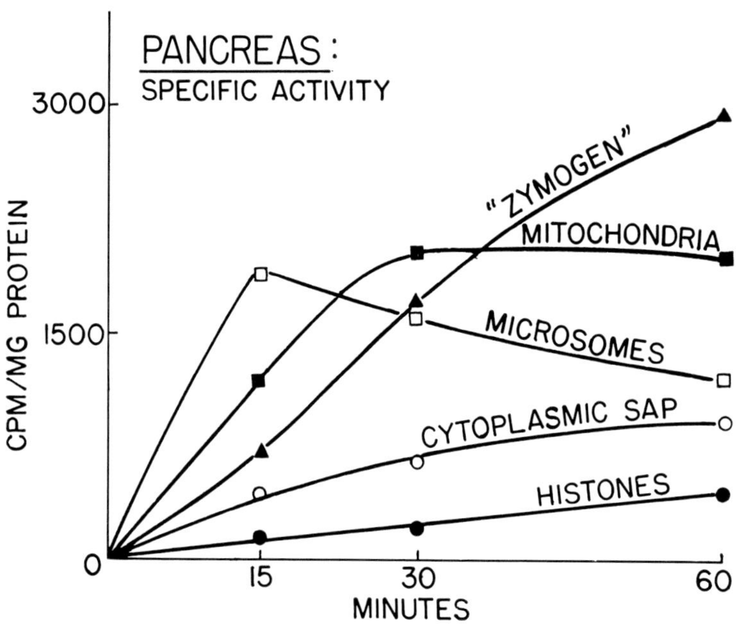

FIG. 11. Time course of specific activities of proteins of various cellular fractions of pancreas after *in vivo* injection of L-lysine-U-C^{14} into a tumor-bearing rat.

radioactive lysine *in vivo* (Busch, Davis, and Anderson, 1958). Figure 9 indicates that the increase in the specific activity of the histones of the Walker tumor was greater than that of the other proteins at a very short time after the radioactivity was injected into the tumor-bearing rat. In the liver (Figure 10), the labeling of microsomal proteins exceeded that of proteins of the mitochondria and of the nuclear fractions. In the pancreas (Figure 11), an even more marked labeling of cytoplasmic proteins was evident. The zymogen granules became enormously labeled compared to the nuclear proteins. These results led us to the concept illustrated in Figure 12, which shows that in most tissues the amino acids are used for production of proteins essential to homeostasis but that in the tumors nuclear protein synthesis was a predominant pathway (Busch *et al.*, 1959). This conclusion was arrived at after studies with 17 different radioactive amino acids.

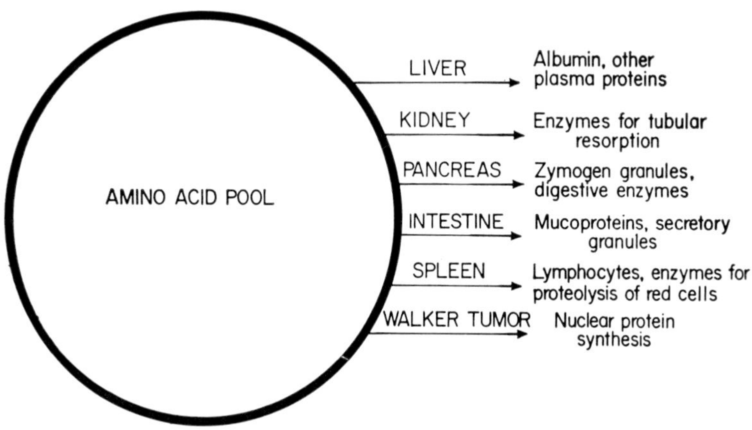

FIG. 12. Summary of the specific roles of various tissues in utilization of amino acids.

RADIOACTIVE PEAK 2, WITH L-LYSINE-U-C^{14} AS THE AMINO ACID PRECURSOR (RP2-L)

Chromatography was employed to determine whether the proteins being labeled were the same in the tumors and other tissues (Davis and Busch, 1959). Figure 13 presents the chromatogram of the Walker 256 carcinosarcoma and shows the presence of RP2-L, a peak emerging between fraction numbers 35 and 55 in this tumor and highly radioactive. A variety of nongrowing nontumorous

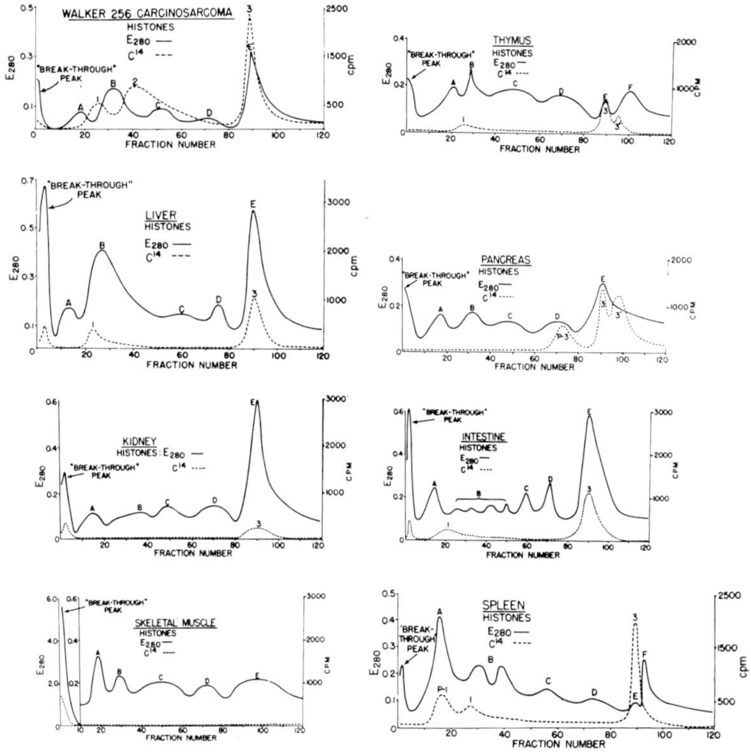

Fig. 13. Chromatographic patterns of both radioactivity and protein concentration for acid-soluble nuclear proteins of the Walker 256 carcinosarcoma, liver, kidney, skeletal muscle, thymus, pancreas, small intestine, and spleen.

tissues were also studied and did not contain RP2-L (Figure 13). Figure 2 shows that peak 2 was found also in the Flexner-Jobling carcinoma, a human malignant melanoma, the sarcoma 180, and the Ehrlich ascites tumor. However, growing, nontumorous tissues, such as the regenerating rat liver, did not contain RP2-L, nor did embryonic tissue (Figure 2). It should be emphasized that in all of these cases the radioactive amino acid injected was lysine uniformly or randomly labeled. With the aid of chromatographic methods and the employment of radioactivity, specific patterns were obtained for most of the nontumor tissues studied.

Biochemistry of RP2-L

In an effort to learn more about RP2-L of the Walker tumor, extracts of large quantities of tumors were rechromatographed in

TABLE 2

Molecular Data on Cationic Nuclear Proteins

	Liver	Walker 256 Carcinosarcoma	
	Peak B	Peak B	RP2-L
Sedimentation constant ($S_{20,w}$)	1.34	1.26	1.79
Diffusion constant* ($D_{20,w}$)	6.80	6.72	4.58
Physical molecular weight	17,100	16,400	34,200
Chemical molecular weight	17,500	17,600	33,900

* Apparent diffusion constant calculated from the boundary spreading observed in the ultracentrifuge by the maximal ordinate-area method.

large amounts on the carboxymethyl cellulose columns. Table 2 indicates the data regarding RP2-L as compared with peak B, the neighboring and contaminating protein. In the purified product, 51 per cent of the N-terminal amino acids were alanine and 9 per cent were valine. The ultracentrifugation pattern is shown in Figure 14. The sedimentation constant and diffusion constant for RP2-L were 1.79 and 4.6 approximately. A minimal molecular weight calculated from chemical data is 8,170 and the physical molecular weight is about 34,000, so that the molecular weight based on analysis of amino acids would be about 33,000. The total number of amino acid residues found was 300, as compared to 160 in peak B, the neighboring and contaminating protein. Estimates of purity were based upon the fact that peak B protein was the most likely contaminant. In view of the lower molecular weight of peak

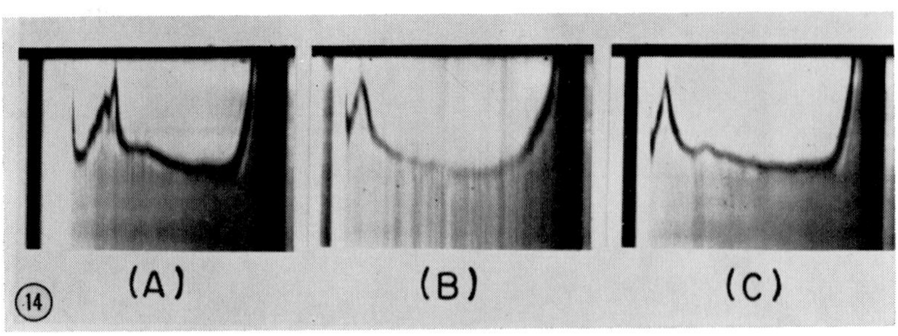

FIG. 14. Sedimentation patterns of cationic nuclear proteins of the Walker 256 carcinosarcoma. Speed 52,640 rpm, 26°C, 0.25 N HCl, after 60 minutes.
(A): Crude RP2-L. (B): Protein Peak B. (C): Purified RP2-L.

B, the purity of RP2-L was calculated to be approximately 96 per cent by weight, assuming that peak B was the only contaminant.

Origin of RP2-L

A critical question was which of these possible structural types of nuclear proteins was RP2-L (i.e., chromosomal, nucleolar, ribosomal or in the nuclear sap). An effort has been made in recent studies to determine whether the protein was DNA bound. Water extracts were made from nuclei of tumors which were prelabeled with radioactive lysine, as was indicated previously. The water extract was then treated with NaCl to make a final concentration of 0.15 M. Both the precipitate and the supernatant solution were treated with 0.25 N HCl and chromatographed as indicated

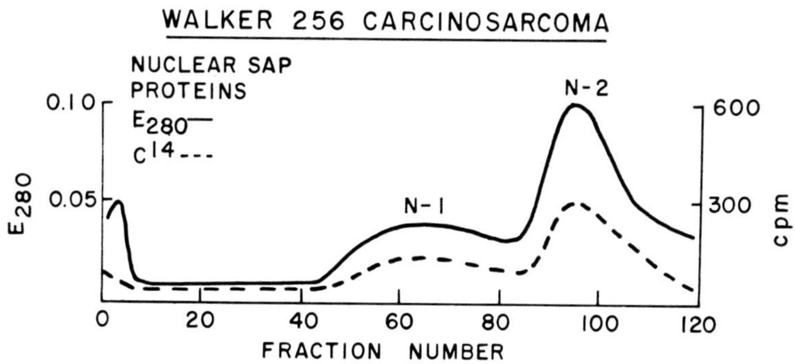

FIG. 15. Chromatographic patterns of both radioactivity and protein concentration for nuclear sap proteins of the Walker 256 carcinosarcoma.

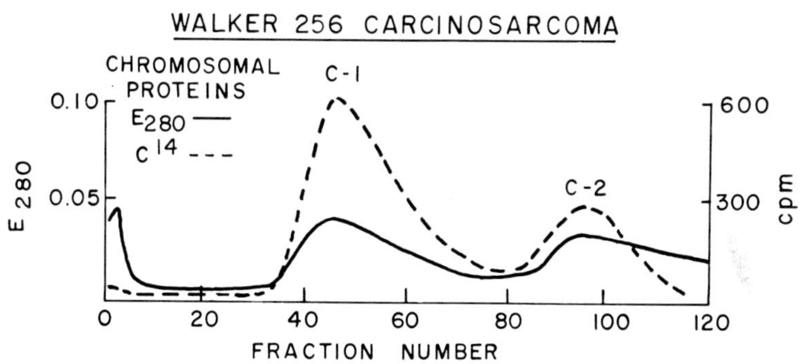

FIG. 16. Chromatographic patterns of both radioactivity and protein concentration for chromosomal proteins of the Walker 256 carcinosarcoma.

previously (Davis and Busch, 1959). The supernatant solution would contain the proteins of the nuclear sap and other nonchromosomal proteins as well as the chromosomal proteins soluble in dilute salt solutions. Conversely, the precipitate contains deoxyribonucleoprotein, as was determined by direct measurement of the DNA of the fractions. The data indicate that the supernatant solution primarily contains the protein of peak E and the radioactivity of those proteins (Figure 15). However, the precipitate or the deoxyribonucleoprotein complex (Figure 16) contained the protein of RP2-L as indicated by three parameters: (1) position of elution, (2) the total amount of isotope in the peak was approximately 35 per cent of that in the acid-extracted nuclear proteins of the Walker tumor, and (3) the very high specific activity of these proteins. In each of these cases, the results were in agreement with the data obtained in the initial chromatograms shown earlier.

Functional Role of These Proteins

Origin

Some attempt needs to be made to correlate these nuclear proteins with a functional role in the nucleus and the site of their biosynthesis. It is possible that these proteins are biosynthesized directly on the DNA. Another possibility which exists is that these proteins are biosynthesized in the nucleoli or on the nuclear ribosomes and are then linked with the DNA. At the moment, no satisfactory resolution of this problem is available.

Function

Another question, of course, is what could such proteins do. What function might abnormal nuclear proteins have? One possible function is illustrated in Figure 17, which proposes that such proteins might serve as accelerators for the neoplastic process by functioning as activators for the DNA formation of cancer RNA in a kind of cyclical process inside tumor cells (Busch, 1961). In conclusion, a significant difference has been demonstrated between the nuclei of neoplastic tissues and other tissues with these studies. It is hoped that these studies may be of value in providing a basis for understanding the genetic change in the DNA of tumor cells, and perhaps providing a basis for chemotherapy of neoplastic disease.

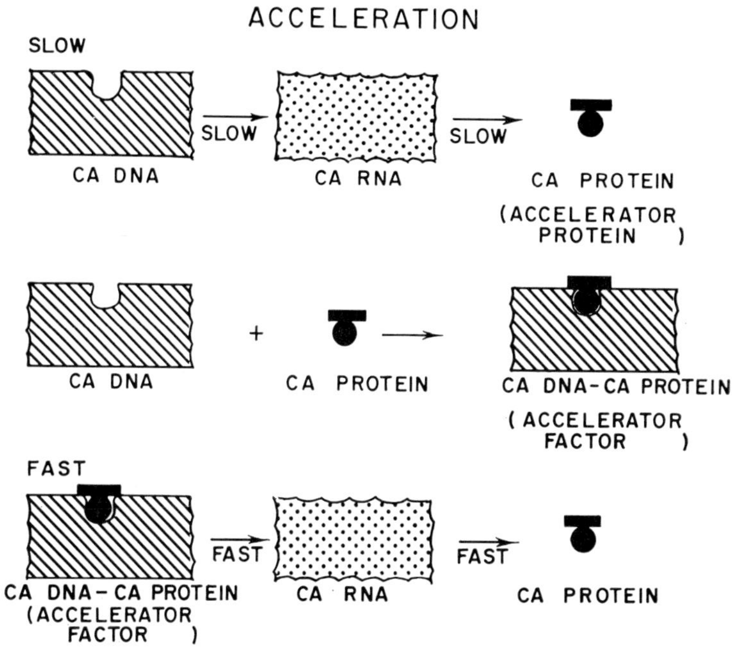

FIG. 17. Stage of acceleration in carcinogenesis. Initial slow reactions leading to the formation of cancer RNA and the accelerator protein. The accelerator protein functions as a cofactor for the rapid formation of cancer RNA which in turn forms more of the accelerator protein.

ACKNOWLEDGMENTS

The original studies reported were supported in part by grants from the United States Public Health Service, the American Cancer Society, the Jane Coffin Childs Fund, and the Anna Fuller Fund.

REFERENCES

Albertini, Louis. 1959. Étude Cytophotométriques des Protéines—SH Nucleoaires de la Racine de Jacinthe; Répartition Précise de ces Composés au Sein du Nucleole. *Comptes rendus hebdomadaires des séances de l'Académie des sciences,* 248:3476–3478.

Allfrey, V. G., A. E. Mirsky, and S. Osawa. 1955. Protein Synthesis in Isolated Cell Nuclei. *Nature, London,* 176:1042–1049.

———. 1957. Protein Synthesis in Isolated Cell Nuclei. *Journal of General Physiology,* 40:451–490.

Busch, H. 1961. Biochemistry of Carcinogenesis: A Theory. *Texas Reports on Biology and Medicine,* 19:1–15.

Busch, H., S. M. Amer, and W. L. Nyhan. 1959. Inhibition of Uptake of L-Arginine-U-C^{14} into Nuclear Proteins by 5-Bis(2-Chloroethyl)Aminouracil. *Journal of Pharmacology and Experimental Therapeutics*, 127:195–199.

Busch, H., and J. R. Davis. 1958. Nuclear Proteins of Tumors and Other Tissues: A Review. *Cancer Research*, 18:1241–1256.

Busch, H., J. R. Davis, and D. C. Anderson. 1958. Labeling of Histones and Other Nuclear Proteins With L-Lysine-U-C^{14} in Tissues of Tumor-Bearing Rats. *Cancer Research*, 18:916–926.

Busch, H., J. R. Davis, G. R. Honig, D. C. Anderson, P. V. Nair, and W. L. Nyhan. 1959. The Uptake of a Variety of Amino Acids into Nuclear Proteins and Other Tissues. *Cancer Research*, 19:1030–1039.

Butler, J. A. V., P. Cohn, and P. Simson. 1960. The Presence of Basic Proteins in Microsomes. *Biochimica et biophysica acta*, 38:386–388.

Crampton, C. F., and M. L. Peterman. 1959. The Amino Acid Composition of Proteins Isolated From the Ribonucleoprotein Particles of Rat Liver. *Journal of Biological Chemistry*, 234:2642–2644.

Davis, J. R., and H. Busch. 1958. Rate-Limiting Factors in the Uptake of Radioactive Amino Acids into Proteins of Tumor Slices. *Cancer Research*, 18:718–724.

———. 1959. Chromatographic Analysis of Radioactive Cationic Nuclear Proteins of Tissues of Tumor-Bearing Rats. *Cancer Research*, 19:1157–1166.

———. 1960. Chromatographic Analysis of Cationic Nuclear Proteins of a Number of Neoplastic Tissues. *Cancer Research*, 20:1208–1213.

Horn, E. C., and C. L. Ward. 1957. The Localization of Basic Proteins in the Nuclei of Larval *Drosophila* Salivary Glands. *Proceedings of the National Academy of Sciences of the U.S.A.*, 43:776–779.

Lyttle, D. A., and H. G. Petering. 1959. 5-Bis(2-Chloroethyl)Aminouracil, a New Antitumor Agent. *Journal of the National Cancer Institute*, 23:153–162.

Osawa, S., K. Takata, and Y. Hotta. 1958. Nuclear and Cytoplasmic RNA of Calf Thymus. *Biochimica et biophysica acta*, 28:271–277.

Rees, K. R., and G. F. Rowland. 1961. The Metabolism of Isolated Rat-Liver Nuclei. *Biochemical Journal*, 78:89–94.

Starbuck, W. C., and H. Busch. 1960. Kinetics of Incorporation of L-Arginine-U-C^{14} into Nuclear Proteins of Tumors and Other Tissues *in vitro*. *Cancer Research*, 20:891–896.

Zubay, G., and P. Doty. 1959. The Isolation and Properties of Deoxyribonucleoprotein Particles Containing Single Nucleic Acid Molecules. *Journal of Molecular Biology*, 1:1–20.

PROTEIN CONFORMATION AND SEQUENCE

The Conformation of Globular Proteins in Solution and Its Relation to the Study of Enzyme Action

CHARLES TANFORD, PH.D.

Department of Biochemistry,
Duke University Medical Center,
Durham, North Carolina

PRINCIPLES GOVERNING THE CONFORMATION OF PROTEINS IN AQUEOUS SOLUTION

The "conformation" of a protein molecule is a term which describes those aspects of the structure which are not completely determined by primary chemical bonds. It includes the manner in which polypeptide chains are arranged in space, the disposition of side chains, and the association of polypeptide chains with each other where such association is not due to primary chemical bonds.

In the absence of special attractive forces, any polymer molecule will be in a randomly coiled conformation: the precise arrangement of chain elements undergoes continuous change, and will at a given instant be different for each molecule in a solution. The average conformation is spread over a large volume of space, as illustrated by the schematic representation U of Figure 1. Random coils have a high entropy, and, where other considerations are not important, would thus have a lower free energy than any organized structure.

Native protein molecules are usually not randomly coiled. We find, instead, that they possess rigid compact structures, and that they frequently consist of two or more polypeptide chains joined in a specific way (but not generally by primary bonds). In many

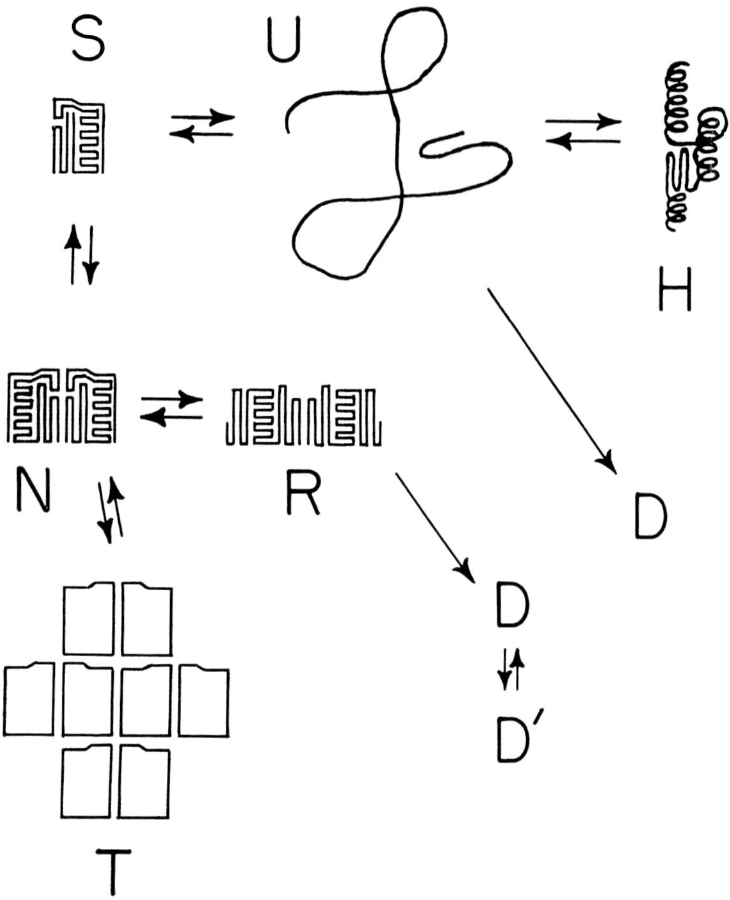

FIG. 1. Schematic representation of the known conformations of β-lactoglobulin in solution. Each of the boxlike parts of conformation T represents a single chain folded as in conformations S and N. The two disulphide cross-links per chain, which presumably remain unaltered in all the reversible transitions, have not been shown, as their locations are not known.

examples this compact conformation has been established to be the equilibrium conformation, so that special forces must exist which lead to a positive, rather than a negative, free energy change for the reaction:

$$\text{Compact Structure} \leftrightarrows \text{Random Coil}$$

The forces which are most likely to be involved are:

1. Intramolecular hydrogen bonds. The carbonyl and imino

groups of the polypeptide chain backbone and some side chain groups are capable of entering into the formation of intramolecular hydrogen bonds (N — H · · · O or O — H · · · O). Because of the greater abundance of backbone groups it is generally believed that the optimum use of hydrogen-bonding capacity is achieved in most cases if the major part of the backbone is in the form of an α-helix (Pauling, Corey, and Branson, 1951).

2. Electrostatic Forces. About one fourth of the side chains of a protein molecule bear single units of charge. These charged groups will be stable if they are in intimate contact with water or other polar solvents or if they are associated as pairs of opposing charge. Single charges in a nonpolar medium will be highly unstable (Tanford and Kirkwood, 1957).

3. Solvent Structure. Liquid water has a preferred three-dimensional structure, the origin of which lies in the strong hydrogen bonds between water molecules. Ionic or polar groups may usually be absorbed into this structure quite readily, but absorption of nonpolar groups results in formation of a more than normally ordered water structure about the holes, which the nonpolar groups create in the normal structure. The result is a decrease in entropy and an increase in free energy (Kauzmann, 1959). Similar considerations may apply to liquids other than water, but the effects are usually likely to be smaller in terms of calories of free energy.

If we ask which of these forces is most likely to be primarily responsible for giving the compact structure of native globular proteins *in aqueous solutions* a lower free energy than a randomly coiled structure, we are forced to conclude that only the third force, the force of solvent structure, can be given serious consideration. In a randomly coiled structure, all nonpolar groups are immersed in the solvent. If the compact structure is formed in such a way as to remove nonpolar groups from contact with the solvent, a decrease in free energy will result which may amount to 2,000 or 3,000 cal. for each nonpolar group. The nonpolar groups in the compact structure will, in effect, be bonded to each other and their cohesion is, in fact, most commonly called hydrophobic bonding (Kauzmann, 1959).

By contrast, little gain in free energy can result from formation of intramolecular hydrogen bonds or from the action of electrostatic forces. The hydrogen bond-forming groups of the protein molecule are fully hydrogen bonded to water molecules in the randomly coiled conformation and the gain in free energy which might result from formation of somewhat stronger hydrogen bonds in a compact structure cannot be large. Similarly, the ionic sites are in their preferred, fully solvated state in the randomly coiled conformation and it is difficult to see how creation of a compact structure can result in an interaction pattern of appreciably lower free energy.

The conclusion we have just reached does not imply that hydrogen bonds and electrostatic forces are unimportant in the compact structure of globular proteins. It must be recognized that the polar, nonpolar, and ionic groups of protein molecules are linked in specific arrangements, so that the removal of nonpolar groups from contact with solvent is likely to be accompanied by the removal of some of the polar and ionic groups. If these groups are left isolated in a nonpolar environment, then a *positive* contribution to the free energy results, which may more than cancel the decrease in free energy of the vicinal solvent. Therefore, hydrophobic bonding will lead to a stable compact structure only if ionic groups are situated at the surface of the particle, in contact with solvent, or if they form ion pairs in the interior. Similarly, most of the groups capable of hydrogen bonding must be hydrogen bonded in the compact conformation. However, the optimum use of intramolecular hydrogen bonding capacity (formation of α-helices) is not required. For example, regions of β-structure with lateral hydrogen bonds between carbonyl and imino groups (Pauling and Corey, 1951) are entirely feasible. For a polypeptide chain in a vacuum or in a nonpolar solvent, the β-structure would be ustable because a large number of unsatisfied hydrogen bonding groups would remain on the surface; in aqueous solution these groups would be hydrogen bonded to the solvent. Another possibility is hydrogen bonding of polar side chains, not only with one another, but also with backbone carbonyl and imino groups.

Existence of Several Different Conformations

One of the consequences of the foregoing theory of protein structure is that there may exist several different conformations of a protein molecule which differ relatively little in free energy, and therefore in stability. Moreover, slight changes in environment (e.g., in pH) may alter the value of ΔF (free energy change) for a conformational change, so that different conformations may have lowest free energy under different environmental conditions.

This fact need not be of practical significance if sizable potential energy barriers impede the transition from one conformation to another. In that event, the protein molecule would remain frozen in whatever conformation was adopted at the site of protein synthesis. Drastic conditions would be required to alter the conformation, and under such conditions the transition would tend to be directly to a randomly coiled structure. To return to the original conformation would, in all likelihood, be difficult or even impossible. For practical purposes, we would have only two attainable states of the protein molecule: a single native conformation and an irreversible denatured state.

Experimental studies of recent years indicate, however, that this is not the typical situation. Drastic conditions (such as high temperature) do indeed lead to irreversible denaturation, but for no protein has it been unequivocally demonstrated that irreversible unfolding occurs in the absence of changes in primary bonds (such as disulfide bridges). It has, however, been unequivocally established that ribonuclease, serum albumin, β-lactoglobulin, and other proteins may be unfolded reversibly at a rapid rate. This implies that the transition between different possible conformations, including even the randomly coiled structure, is generally easy, so that dynamic equilibrium between all possible conformations is maintained. Under these conditions, changes in conformation will be expected to occur whenever thermodynamic considerations dictate.

The Conformations of β-lactoglobulin

A striking example of a protein which may exist in several stable conformations is provided by recent studies of β-lactoglobulin. Eight different structures of this protein have been identified. Six of them are simply different conformations without differences in covalent structure, and transition between them is rapid and reversible. The other two structures may be reversibly converted into one another, but are separated from the other six structures by an irreversible step. It is highly probable that this step involves a change in covalent bonding.

Schematic diagrams of the eight conformations are shown in Figure 1. Their characteristics may be described as follows:

1. Native conformation (N). The native molecule consists of two polypeptide chains, which are probably identical. The molecule is a typical, compact, globular protein with low intrinsic viscosity and frictional coefficient. The optical rotatory properties indicate that the principal folding of the polypeptide backbone is not that of an α-helix (Tanford, De, and Taggart, 1960). Titration

studies show that one carboxyl group of each polypeptide chain is buried in the interior of the molecule (Nozaki, Bunville, and Tanford, 1959). Conformation N is the stable conformation in aqueous solutions at 25° C and ionic strength 0.15, from about pH 7.5 to about pH 3.

2. Single chain (S). The native molecule dissociates readily into single chains without other perceptible change; i.e., the single chains appear to be compact and globular with the same kind of folding as in conformation N. Conformation S is stable at low pH, more so if the ionic strength is low (Townend, Weinberger, and Timasheff, 1960). This conformation is also produced when small amounts of organic substances, such as dioxane, are added to aqueous β-lactoglobulin (Tanford and De, 1961).

3. Tetramer (T). At low temperature, near pH 4.65, a tetramer of N is formed. It is again compact and globular and again seems to have essentially the same folding of the polypeptide chains as conformation N (Townend, Winterbottom, and Timasheff, 1960; Townend and Timasheff, 1960). A dimer of N must be an intermediate in the formation of conformation T, but it does not have sufficient stability to be present at any time in detectable quantity (except in the genetic variant β-lactoglobulin B. The present discussion applies to β-lactoglobulin A or to a mixture of the two genetic forms).

4. Refolded Conformation (R). Near pH 7.5 conformation N is transformed reversibly into conformation R (Tanford, Bunville, and Nozaki, 1959; Tanford and Taggart, 1961). The molecule still consists of two chains, and it is only slightly less compact than in conformation N. The specific rotation is about double that of N, but rotatory dispersion again indicates the absence of helical regions (Tanford, De, and Taggart, 1960). The carboxyl groups which were buried in the interior in conformation N are exposed in conformation R.

5. Helical Conformation (H). β-Lactoglobulin is soluble in aqueous dioxane, ethanol, propanol, dimethyl formamide, chloroethanol, *N*-methyl propionamide, and presumably many other organic substances, up to about a 75 per cent content of the organic substance. These conditions convert most of the molecules to a new conformation; it consists of single chains which are rigid but not globular. The intrinsic viscosity is 12 cc./Gm., indicative of a rodlike shape with a ratio of length to width of about 10:1. Optical rotatory dispersion in this conformation indicates that the conformation has a high

content of α-helical structure (Tanford, De, and Taggart, 1960).

It is of interest that a predominantly helical conformation is formed only when the protein is placed in an environment largely devoid of water. Under these conditions the structure of the solvent is drastically altered, and it will more readily admit nonpolar side chains. Moreover, the hydrogen bonding ability of the solvent is reduced. Thus, intramolecular hydrogen bond formation is favored.

6. Unfolded Conformation (U). β-Lactoglobulin is reversibly unfolded by the addition of urea or formamide at pH 3 (Tanford and De, 1961). A similar form also occurs as an intermediate between conformations S and H during the addition of organic reagents such as dioxane. The unfolded form consists of single chains. One cannot be sure that it is a completely random coil, as small regions with specific structure could remain. However, hydrodynamic, optical rotatory, and spectroscopic data are all consistent with a structure which is random except for the restrictions imposed by the presence of disulfide bonds.

7. Irreversible Denaturation. The six conformations enumerated above may all be reversibly converted into one another. Above pH 9.5, however, conformation R is slowly converted to an unfolded conformation which cannot be reconverted to the native form (Bunville, 1959). Refolding to a new conformation which is fairly compact does occur when the pH is reduced, but the new conformation is not the same as any of those described above. The reaction of β-lactoglobulin with urea at pH 7.8 leads to a conformational change which is also irreversible (Kauzmann and Simpson, 1953). It is possible that the conformation produced in this way is the same as that produced at high pH in the absence of urea. The fact that the irreversible change occurs in alkaline solution suggests that the irreversibility results from a disulfide exchange reaction,

$$\text{–S–S–} + \text{–S}^- \rightarrow \text{–S}^- + \text{–S–S–}.$$

Thermodynamics of Conformational Change

A quantitative study of the reversible equilibrium between two conformations can be used to determine the changes in free energy, enthalpy, and entropy, which accompany the change in conformation. The free energy of reaction has been evaluated in this way for all of the reversible reactions of β-lactoglobulin. The values of ΔH and ΔS have been obtained for the reactions $N \rightarrow R$, $4N \rightarrow T$, $S \rightarrow U$, and $U \rightarrow H$.

The thermodynamic parameters determined in this way apply,

of course, to the experimental conditions under which the change from one conformation to another occurs; e.g., the data for the reaction, N → S, are obtained in aqueous solution at pH 3.5 and below. For this reaction, as well as for the other two reversible reactions which are observed in purely aqueous solutions, it is, however, possible to extrapolate all the observed data to the isoelectric point of the protein, so that a measure of the stability of conformation N may be obtained.

TABLE 1

Free Energy Changes for Configurational Changes of β-Lactoglobulin at pH 5.2, 0.1 Ionic Strength, 25° C

Reaction	Free energy change (ΔF^0) cal./mole*	Free energy change (ΔF^1) cal./mole**
N → R	3,500	3,500
N → 2S	11,300	6,400
4N → T	— 9,900	4,600

* Standard state is 1 mole/L.
** Standard state is 1 Gm./100 cc.

The free energy differences obtained in this way have been tabulated in Table 1. The listed values of free energy changes (ΔF^0) refer to the usual standard conditions, in which both reactants and products are present at a concentration of 1 mole/L. As these conditions are so far removed from any possible experimental conditions, we have also calculated free energy changes (ΔF^1) which refer to standard conditions in which both reactants and products are at a concentration of 1 Gm./100 cc. These values give a more realistic picture of the stability of the native conformation, and show quite clearly that the margin of stability is small.

It is noteworthy that the stability of conformation N would be even lower under physiological conditions. At pH 7 and 38°C in an aqueous medium we would expect that about 10 per cent of the molecules will be in conformation R. The presence of sugar and other substances in milk would have an additional effect. They could produce some dissociation to single chains.

Table 1 contains no data on the free energy required to convert conformation N to the unfolded or helical conformation. These reactions have been studied in mixed solvents only and the dependence of the equilibrium constants on the concentration of the organic component is too large to permit a meaningful extrapolation to a purely aqueous medium.

The Site of Enzyme Action

The protein, β-lactoglobulin, has no biological activity, so that we have no possibility of using it to study the connection between structure and enzyme activity (or other biological action). There is, however, good reason for believing that detailed study of proteins with enzymatic activity will often lead to similar conclusions about the molecular conformation. In fact, dissociation-association equilibriums have already been discovered in a number of enzymes.

The possible existence of multiple conformations is a factor which must be kept in mind in studies pertaining to the mechanism of enzyme action and to the elucidation of the structure of the active sites of enzyme proteins. For example, the pH-dependence of enzymatic catalysis is commonly interpreted in terms of the ionization of acidic groups, which are supposedly part of the active site and which must be in a particular ionization state for activity. Such an explanation is, of course, reasonable and may often be correct. It may, however, sometimes be incorrect, since a pH-dependent conformation change, such as the $N \rightleftarrows R$ or the $4N \rightleftarrows T$ transition of β-lactoglobulin, with one conformation active and the other inactive, would lead to comparable experimental enzyme kinetics. Moreover, the pH at which such a transition occurs cannot be taken as indication of the normal pK and thereby as identification of a titratable group associated with the transition. The $N \rightleftarrows R$ transition of β-lactoglobulin has an apparent pK of 7.74, but the titratable group with which it is associated is a carboxyl group (Tanford and Taggart, 1961).

A second aspect of configurational multiplicity concerns structural studies of enzymes and the attempt to construct models on which the active site may be located. There is a possibility that binding of substrate or cofactors may sometimes alter the conformation of the enzyme molecule, so that the component parts of the active site may be widely separated in the enzyme molecule when it is in the free state.

These possibilities are, of course, not being suggested here for the first time. However, the studies of β-lactoglobulin show how real they are, and suggest that studies of enzyme conformation should routinely accompany studies of enzyme kinetics.

ACKNOWLEDGMENTS

The investigations described in this paper have been supported by research grants from the National Science Foundation and from the

Institute of Arthritis and Metabolic Diseases, the National Institutes of Health, United States Public Health Service.

REFERENCES

Bunville, L. G. 1959. *The pH Dependence of the Configuration of β-Lactoglobulin.* Ph.D. Dissertation. State University of Iowa, Iowa City, Iowa.

Kauzmann, W. 1959. Some Factors in the Interpretation of Protein Denaturation. *Advances in Protein Chemistry*, 14:1–63.

Kauzmann, W., and R. B. Simpson. 1953. The Kinetics of Protein Denaturation. III. The Optical Rotations of Serum Albumin, β-Lactoglobulin and Pepsin in Urea Solutions. *Journal of the American Chemical Society*, 75:5154–5157.

Nozaki, Y., L. G. Bunville, and C. Tanford. 1959. Hydrogen Ion Titration Curves of β-Lactoglobulin. *Journal of the American Chemical Society*, 81: 5523–5529.

Pauling, L., and R. B. Corey. 1951. Configurations of Polypeptide Chains with Favored Orientations around Single Bonds. Two New Pleated Sheets. *Proceedings of the National Academy of Sciences of the U.S.A.*, 37:729–740.

Pauling, L., R. B. Corey, and H. R. Branson. 1951. The Structure of Proteins: The Hydrogen-Bonded Helical Configurations of the Polypeptide Chain. *Proceedings of the National Academy of Sciences of the U.S.A.*, 37:205–211.

Tanford, C., L. G. Bunville, and Y. Nozaki. 1959. The Reversible Transformation of β-Lactoglobulin at pH 7.5. *Journal of the American Chemical Society*, 81:4032–4036.

Tanford, C., and P. K. De. 1961. The Unfolding of β-Lactoglobulin at pH 3 by Urea, Formamide and Other Organic Substances. *Journal of Biological Chemistry*, 236:1711–1715.

Tanford, C., P. K. De, and V. G. Taggart. 1960. The Role of the α-Helix in the Structure of Proteins. Optical Rotary Dispersion of β-Lactoglobulin. *Journal of the American Chemical Society*, 82:6028-6034.

Tanford, C., and J. G. Kirkwood. 1957. Theory of Protein Titration Curves. I. General Equations for Impenetrable Spheres. *Journal of the American Chemical Society*, 79:5333–5339.

Tanford, C., and V. G. Taggart. 1961. Ionization-Linked Changes in Protein Conformation. II. The N → R Transition in β-Lactoglobulin. *Journal of the American Chemical Society*, 83:1634–1638.

Townend, R., and S. N. Timasheff. 1960. Molecular Interactions in β-Lactoglobulin. III. Light Scattering Investigation of the Association between pH 3.7 and 5.2. *Journal of the American Chemical Society*, 82:3168–3174.

Townend, R., L. Weinberger, and S. N. Timasheff. 1960. Molecular Interactions in β-Lactoglobulin. IV. The Dissociation of β-Lactoglobulin below pH 3.5. *Journal of the American Chemical Society*, 82:3175–3179.

Townend, R., R. J. Winterbottom, and S. N. Timasheff. 1960. Molecular Interactions in β-Lactoglobulin. II. Ultracentrifugal and Electrophoretic Studies of the Association of β-Lactoglobulin Below Its Isoelectric Point. *Journal of the American Chemical Society*, 82:3161–3168.

Optical Rotatory Dispersion and Structure of Nonhelical Globular Proteins

BRUNO JIRGENSONS, DR. CHEM.

Department of Biochemistry,
The University of Texas M. D. Anderson Hospital and Tumor Institute,
Houston, Texas

The structure of proteins is studied by different methods. While the amino acid sequence is determined by chemical methods, the manner of folding of the polypeptide chain, i.e., conformation, is studied chiefly by physical methods. The optical rotatory dispersion method is now established as one of the most efficient that yields information on protein conformation in solutions (Schellman and Schellman, 1956, 1958; Yang and Doty, 1957; Jirgensons, 1956; Jirgensons and Straumanis, 1957; Jirgensons, 1958a,b,c; 1959a,b,c; 1960a, b). Listings of the pertinent literature can be found in recent reviews (Schellman and Schellman, 1961; Jirgensons, 1961a).

The present paper deals only with the aqueous solutions of globular proteins, such as the proteins of blood serum, and most of the discussion will be focused on the proteins having exceptional interest in the biochemistry of neoplastic growth. Serum gamma globulins, myeloma globulins, and the urinary Bence-Jones proteins have in this paper a preferential treatment. New results will be reported, and the discussion will be based on these and former findings.

As reported before (Jirgensons, 1958b), all globular proteins, with respect to their optical rotatory behavior, can be classified into three classes: Class I, those proteins possessing high values of 245 to 290 mμ. for the dispersion constants (λ_c); Class II, those having low dispersion constants of 220 to 245 mμ.; Class III, globular proteins which have, when in the native state, abnormally low λ_c below 220 mμ. Representative examples of these classes are shown in Table 1, and complete listings of the 47 globular proteins studied

TABLE 1

Classification of Globular Proteins on the Basis of Rotatory Dispersion Data

Class I λ_c = 245–290 mμ.	Class II λ_c = 220–245 mμ.	Class III λ_c = below 220 mμ.
Albumin, egg white	Amylase, α	Bence-Jones proteins
Albumin, serum	Casein, α	Casein, β
Aldolase	Chymotrypsin	Gamma globulin, serum
Amylase, β	Chymotrypsinogen	Gamma globulin, milk
Amylase, taka	Deoxyribonuclease	Luteinizing hormone
Carboxypeptidase	Elastase	Macroglobulins
Dehydrogenase, alcohol	Lactoglobulin, β	Myeloma globulins
Dehydrogenase, lactic acid	Ovomucoid	Pepsin
Ficin	Papain	Rennin
Insulin	Ribonuclease	Trypsin inhibitor, soybean
Lysozyme	Thyroglobulin	
Prolactin	Trypsin	
Somatotropin	Trypsinogen	

thus far can be found in a recent review (Jirgensons, 1961a). Although this classification is somewhat arbitrary, there are strong indications that the proteins of each class are related with respect to their macromolecular conformation. Thus the Class I proteins possessing high dispersion constants of 245 to 290 mμ. seem to be largely α-helical, i.e., large portions of the polypeptide chains in the macromolecules of these proteins seem to have the α-helical conformation. The proteins of Class III, on the contrary, seem to be nonhelical, and those of Class II probably have little of α-helical segments in their polypeptide chains. The gamma globulins, Bence-Jones proteins, myeloma globulins, and macroglobulins all belong to Class III, and thus seem to be nonhelical. The intriguing question is: what is the conformation of these proteins? There is no doubt that these proteins cannot be treated as disordered random-chain macromolecules. For example, the gamma globulins as antibodies must have a definite unique conformation. The presently available experimental data do not permit formation of a definite concept of what these conformations may be, yet we are beginning to understand the forces involved in folding the chains in these macromolecules.

Experimental Results of Further Studies on the Proteins of Class III

Methods of Study

The optical rotatory power was determined with an O. C. Rudolph & Sons model 80 photoelectric spectropolarimeter. Most of the determinations were made at room temperature of 23° to 25°C. Some series of measurements were performed at higher temperatures. In these series, the jacketed tube was warmed by means of a Brinkmann-Haake constant temperature circulator. The tubes were 10.0 cm. long, and equipped with fused silica windows. (In a few measurements, a 1.0 cm. short cell also was employed.) The performance of the instrument was checked with a quartz control plate certified by the National Bureau of Standards. Two light sources were used: a Hanovia SH type mercury burner, and a Westinghouse SAH-250 lamp, and the rotatory power was determined at the wave lengths of 578, 546.1, 435.8, 404.7, 390.6, 366.3, 365.0, 334.1, and 313.1 mμ. The width of the slit never exceeded 0.5 mm. The dispersion constant was calculated by the method of Yang and Doty (1957), and the experimental errors were evaluated by the usual statistical methods.

The proteins and their methods of isolation and purification are briefly described in each case in the following sections. The solutions used for polarimetry were practically free of colored impurities, and they were liberated from coarse particles by filtration through a layer of Cellite filter on sintered glass. The concentration of the proteins was determined either by gravimetric method or by micro-Kjeldahl nitrogen analyses, or by both methods. The proteins were characterized by determining the sedimentation constants in the Beckman-Spinco analytical ultracentrifuge at 56,100 rpm, and by free boundary or paper electrophoresis. The free boundary electrophoresis was performed in a Perkin-Elmer model 38A instrument, and the paper electrophoresis with Bender and Hobein's Elphor instrument.

Optical Rotatory Properties of Serum Gamma Globulins from Various Species

Materials

The gamma globulins from human blood sera or plasmas were isolated according to the method of Cohn *et al.* (1950), and the Fraction II proteins were purified and subfractionated on the DEAE (diethylaminoethyl) cellulose columns after Sober, Gutter, Wyckoff, and Peterson (1956). Bovine, horse, pig, dog, and rabbit gamma globulins were obtained from Pentex Inc., Kankakee, Illinois. These globulins, according to the specifications, have been isolated by a similar method (Oncley *et al.*, 1949), and they were purified and subfractionated in our laboratory in the same way as the human globulins. Some of the samples which were not subfractionated were purified by extensive dialysis of their solutions. The ion exchange fractionation of the globulins was accomplished always in the same way, i.e., a 2 × 60 cm. jacketed column was packed with 25 Gm. of pure washed DEAE cellulose, and a solution of 500 mg. of globulin was washed down with 0.005 M sodium phosphate buffer of pH 8.0. The effluent was collected in 5 ml. aliquots by an automatic fraction collector, and after collecting 85 tubes, the salt concentration was increased by introducing in a mixing chamber of 500 ml. volume 0.3 M sodium phosphate of pH 8.0. The column was cooled to +5°C by circulating cold water around it. This method of fractionation, independent of the source of the gamma globulin, always yielded two major subfractions. Subfraction I was eluted with the diluted buffer and appeared in tubes numbered 30 to 60, whereas Subfraction II could be eluted only with more concentrated buffer and appeared in tubes numbered 130 to 160 (or a similar range). An example of the elution diagram is shown in Figure 1. In addition, several minor peaks were observed in the elution diagram, but paper electrophoresis tests revealed these as impurities possessing in the sodium barbiturate buffer (pH 8.3) higher mobility rates than the gamma globulins. The eluted major subfractions of the gamma globulins were dialyzed at +4°C, and lyophilized. For polarimetry, the globulins were dissolved either in 0.20 M sodium bromide or 0.1 M phosphate buffer.

Comparison of the Subfractions I and II. Sedimentation experiments in the analytical ultracentrifuge revealed that the subfractions were homogeneous with respect to sedimentation, and that the sedimentation constant of Subfraction I was the same as that of Subfraction II. For example, the sedimentation constant of a 0.8 per cent porcine gamma globulin Subfraction I at a mean temperature of 23.5°C was found to be 6.6 S (± 0.2), whereas that of the Subfraction II under similar conditions was 6.4 S. The electrophoretic mobilities of the Subfractions I and II, however, were found to be different. This Subfraction I of the porcine globulin, in 0.1 M sodium barbiturate buffer of pH 8.3, had a low mobility of − 1.23

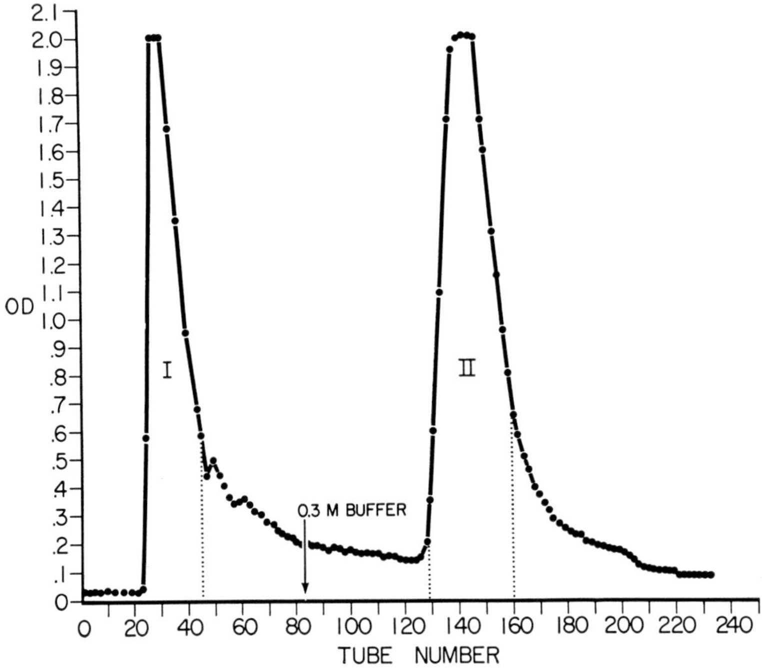

FIG. 1. Chromatographic subfractionation of porcine gamma globulin on DEAE cellulose. Subfraction I is eluted with 0.005 M sodium phosphate buffer of pH 8.0. Subfraction II is eluted with more concentrated buffer of the same pH. On the abscissa is plotted the tube number and on the ordinate the optical density obtained with the Folin-Lowry reagent.

$\times 10^{-5}$ cm.^{2}/sec. volt, whereas the Subfraction II had a mobility of − 2.48 units. Similarly, the mobility of Subfraction I of bovine gamma globulin was found to be − 1.77 units, whereas that of Subfraction II was − 2.69 units. Hence it is possible that the subfractions eluted with the diluted buffer (Subfraction I) differ from the more tightly bound macromolecular species (Subfraction II) only in charge density, e.g., that Subfraction I has more amidated carboxyl groups per macromolecule than Subfraction II. The similarity in macromolecular conformation of the subfractions was ascertained by rotatory dispersion measurements.

Optical Rotatory Properties of the Globulins

Dependence of the Specific Rotation on pH. The dependence of the specific rotation of human gamma globulin on pH of the solutions has been studied earlier (Jirgensons, 1954, 1957). It was found that within the pH limits of 4 to 10, there was no detectable change in the rotatory power, but a strong negative shift was observed in more strongly acid or alkaline solutions. Since the intrinsic viscosity of the solutions increased in the same manner as the levorotation, it was concluded that the observed negative shift is caused by conformational changes associated with expansion of the macromolecules. The earlier measurements were made with sodium light, and it seemed worthwhile to remeasure the rotatory power with the more efficient ultraviolet light, as well as to compare the globulins of the various species. The globulins were dissolved in 0.25 M sodium bromide, and the pH was varied by adding sodium hydroxide or hydrochloric acid. The rotatory power was determined with ultraviolet light of 365 mμ. wave length. It was found that the various gamma globulins and their subfractions at pH 4 to 10 had the $[\alpha]_{365}$ of −175 to −185°. The differences may be due to slight compositional and structural differences, as well as to impurities and experimental errors, but they are not caused by the change of acidity. If one and the same preparation is used, the lavorotation between pH 4 to 10 is constant as shown in Figure 2. In all instances the levorotation increased when the pH was below 4, and when the alkalinity was raised above pH 10.5. Also the DEAE cellulose treated specimens had somewhat higher levorotation values than untreated samples.

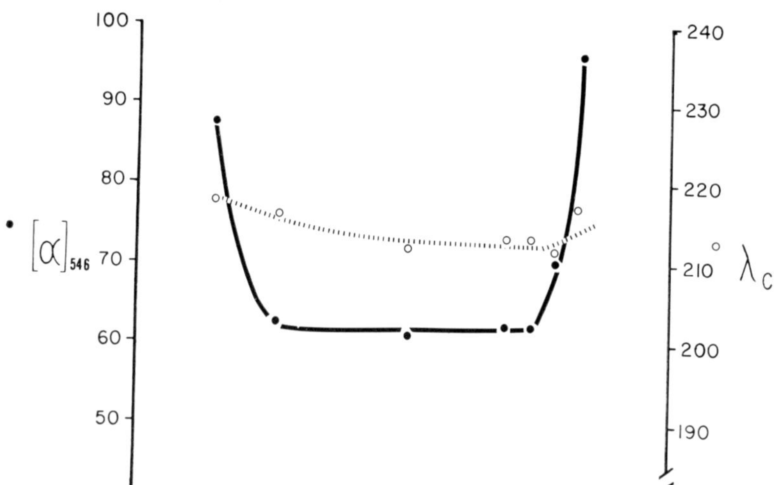

FIG. 2. Dependence of the specific rotation and the dispersion constant of canine gamma globulin on pH of the solutions. The specific rotation is represented by discs, the dispersion constant by open circles.

Dependence of the Specific Rotation on the Wave Length of the Light. Dependence of the specific rotation on the wave length was studied on the unfractionated (Cohn's Fractions II) as well as on the subfractionated globulins. Representative graphs illustrating this dependence are shown in Figure 3. It is obvious that the rotatory dispersion of the rabbit serum gamma globulin Subfraction I is essentially the same as the dispersion of the porcine gamma globulin Subfraction II. The rotatory dispersion constants of the various globulins and their subfractions are compiled in Table 2. According to these data, the dispersion constants (λ_c) in all cases are very low, and they are the same within the limits of experimental error. Moreover, the constants are not affected by pH variations, in pH limits of 3 to 11. The effect of ionic strength on the dispersion constant also is insignificant. There are, however, slight differences in the rotatory power: the bovine globulins seem to have smaller and the porcine globulins greater levorotation values than the other globulins. In Table 3 are compiled results on the optical rotatory dispersion of denatured gamma globulins, and two examples of denatured globulins are shown also in Figure 3. Dispersion constant

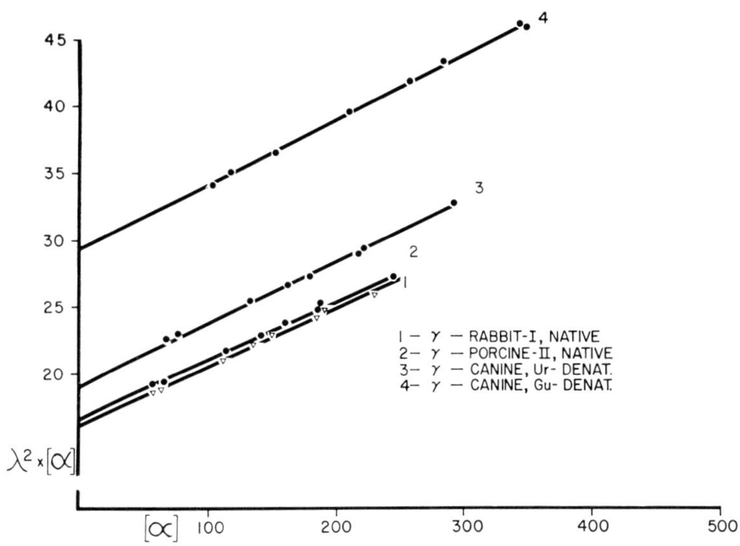

FIG. 3. The optical rotatory dispersion of native and denatured gamma globulins in the form of Yang-Doty plots. On the abscissa is plotted the specific rotation and on the ordinate the product of the squared wave length and specific rotation. The wave length is given in microns, the rotation in degrees. All values on the graph are negative.

TABLE 2

Optical Rotation Data of Native Serum Gamma Globulins from Several Species Concentration of the Protein 0.70 to 1.97 Per Cent. Ionic Strength (Sodium Bromide) 0.20. Acidity, pH 6.7 to 9.3

Gamma Globulin	$-[\alpha]^{24}_{546}$, degrees	K*	λ_c, mμ.
Bovine, Subfraction I	55.9	14.4	210 ±8
Bovine, Subfraction II	57.6	14.6	215 ±5
Equine, Subfraction I	60.0	15.2	214 ±3
Equine, Subfraction II	62.7	16.0	210 ±5
Human, Subfraction I	62.5	15.8	212 ±3
Human, Subfraction II	60.4	15.4	213 ±2
Porcine, Subfraction I	70.3	18.2	205 ±8
Porcine, Subfraction II	65.0	16.7	210 ±4
Rabbit, Subfraction I	63.1	16.4	203 ±6
Rabbit, Subfraction II	56.9	14.6	211 ±6

* The constants K and λ_c were calculated from the straight line relationship between the product $\lambda^2 \times [\alpha]$ and $[\alpha]$, i.e. the rearranged Drude rule

$$\lambda^2 \times [\alpha] = \lambda_c^2 \times [\alpha] + K,$$

where λ is the wave length, K the rotatory constant, and λ_c the dispersion constant. If λ is given in mμ, the K-values in the Tables should be multiplied by 10^{-6}.

(λ_c) is represented by the slope of the lines, and it is obvious that it has not changed (or has slightly increased) upon the disorganization of these macromolecules. The levorotation of these serum gamma globulins, however, increases considerably, i.e., it is shifted toward the negative direction upon the expansion and disorganization. The fact is noteworthy that 4.6 M urea had a much lesser disorganizing effect on these macromolecules than 2.0 M guanidine thiocyanate. The guanidine thiocyante containing solution precipitated on dilution with water, whereas the urea containing solution remained clear when so diluted. The differences in the specific rotation also are conspicuous.

Alkali has a very complex effect on the gamma globulins. A strong negative shift of the specific rotation occurs, and the dispersion constant is slightly enhanced. Sedimentation runs in the ultracentrifuge showed that at pH 11.2 to 11.6 the macromolecules aggregate, while both aggregation and dissociation occur when the pH is raised to 11.8 and higher. At pH of 11.0 to 11.5, the specific rotation changes slowly with time. For example, at pH 11.3 the specific rotation of canine gamma globulin, as measured with the wave length of 365 mμ. was $-216°$ when the measurement was

TABLE 3

Dispersion Constants and Specific Rotation Values of Denatured Gamma Globulins

Globulin	Denaturing agent	$-[\alpha]^{24}_{546}$, degrees	K	λ_c, mμ.
Gamma globulin, canine	4.6 M urea	76.2	19.3	213 ±3
Gamma globulin, canine	2.0 M guanidine-HCNS	117.2	29.5	219 ±2
Gamma globulin, rabbit	2.0 M guanidine-HCNS	111.1	27.5	224 ±5
Gamma globulin, rabbit	3.2 M guanidine-HCNS	118.6	30.0	216 ±3
Gamma globulin, equine	4.6 M urea	72.8	18.4	213 ±2
Gamma globulin, equine	6.0 M urea	96.1	23.4	214 ±1
Gamma globulin, equine	2.0 M guanidine-HCNS	126.9	31.7	220 ±1

made immediately after adding alkali. This value rose in 30 minutes to − 221°, and in four hours the specific rotation attained an even higher value of − 226°. After two more hours a slight drop could be observed, and after two days the specific rotation had dropped to − 209°. At the same time, the pH had diminished gradually from 11.3 to 10.6. At a starting pH of 10.5 to 11.1 and room temperature, the changes of the specific rotation were very slow, whereas at pH 11.6 to 11.9, the equilibrium was reached in 30 to 60 minutes. Slight changes of the rotatory power with time were observed also with the solutions of the globulins which contained 3 to 6 M urea, whereas the denaturation with 2 M guanidine thiocyanate was practically instantaneous and independent of temperature. The results quoted are the final values, when no further significant change of the rotatory power with time could be observed.

Optical Rotatory Dispersion of Myeloma Globulins

Materials

Myeloma globulins. Five specimens of myeloma globulins were used in the experiments described in this section. One of the specimens, P, was described in a previous paper (Jirgensons, 1960a). All specimens were isolated from the sera of patients with established diagnosis of multiple myeloma. In all instances the globulins were found in high concentrations, and in all cases they appeared in Fraction II upon fractionating the sera after the method of Cohn *et al.* (1950). The specimen EV was subfractionated on DEAE cellulose in the same manner as the gamma globulins described above, and two major subfractions were obtained. Electrophoretic mobility determinations in sodium barbiturate buffer of pH 8.3 showed that they were between − 2.9 and − 4.1 mobility units. The major component represented 80 to 90 per cent of the total, the rest being more rapidly or more slowly moving components. Sedimentation tests showed that the specimens CU and SH, as well as the subfractions of the specimen EV, were homogeneous, and that the sedimentation constants had the values of 6 to 7 S (uncorrected). Specimen P, in addition to this major component, contained two faster sedimenting components in small amounts, whereas sample KA contained about 10 per cent of a slow impurity. A corrected $s^0_{20,w}$ value of a 1 per cent solution of Subfraction I of specimen EV was found to be 6.6 S, and specimen SH yielded a $s^0_{20,w}$ value of 6.8 S (± 0.1). From the latter value and the intrinsic viscosity of the solution (0.060), the molecular weight of the myeloma globulin SH was calculated to be 163,000 (± 5,000) (see Scheraga and Mandelkern, 1953; Schachman, 1957). For the polarimetric measurements, the myeloma globulins, like the formerly described gamma globulins, were dissolved in 0.20 M or 0.25 M sodium bromide.

Optical Rotatory Dispersion of the Globulins

Native myeloma globulins. The results obtained with the native myeloma globulins are compiled in Table 4. It is obvious that the

TABLE 4

Dispersion Constants and Rotatory Power of Myeloma Globulins in the Native State

Specimen	pH of solution	$-[\alpha]^{24}_{546}$, degrees	K	λ_c, mμ.
EV, Subfraction I	9.6	63.5	16.1	213 ±4
KA	8.2	61.0	15.4	220 ±3
SH	5.9	55.0	14.0	212 ±2
SH	10.7	58.4	14.8	216 ±5
CU	6.3	54.2	13.6	218 ±3
CU	10.5	59.7	15.2	215 ±5

rotatory properties of these globulins are essentially the same as those of the normal gamma globulins. The results reported here agree well with earlier published data obtained by studying several other individual specimens of myeloma globulins (Jirgensons, 1960a).

Denatured myeloma globulins. The effect of disorganization of native macromolecules on the rotatory properties is demonstrated by the data shown in Table 5. Denaturation with either alkali or guanidine thiocyanate produces a strong negative shift, while the λ_c either does not change or increases slightly. Thus the effects are the same as those described earlier with the normal gamma globulins. Especially interesting are the results using the detergent sodium dioctylsulphosuccinate (Aerosol OT) as denaturing agent. It is noteworthy that the detergent is able to disorganize the macromolecules of these globulins at extremely low concentrations of the detergent. While it is necessary to have approximately 4 to 5 M urea or 1.0 to 1.5 M guanidine thiocyanate for achieving a measurable disorganization, the surface active OT acts at a concentration of 0.1 to 0.2 per cent or 0.002 to 0.004 mole/L. solution. Noteworthy are two other facts: the positive effect of temperature, and the unexpected increase of the dispersions constant above ordinary limiting

TABLE 5

Dispersion Constants and Rotatory Power of Denatured Myeloma Globulins

Specimen	Denaturing agent	$-[\alpha]^{24}_{546}$, degrees	K	λ_c, mμ.
EV, Subfraction I, 0.50%	OT, 0.25%, 24° C	73.0	18.4	216 ±3
Do	Do, 37° C, 2 hours	77.1	19.1	221 ±4
Do	Do, 50° C, 2 hours	79.4	19.3	233 ±4
EV, Subfraction II, 0.77%	OT, 0.25%, 50° C, 2 hours	80.4	19.6	230 ±2
KA, 1.24%	OT, 0.34%, 50° C, 2 hours	77.3	19.2	226 ±1
P, 1.0%	Guanidine-HCNS, 2 M, 50° C, 2 hours	113.6	28.4	219 ±4
P, 1.4%	OT, 0.50%, 24° C	76.0	19.3	217 ±5
Do	Do, 50° C, 2 hours	83.0	20.4	235 ±4
SH, 0.86%	Alkali, pH = 11.8, 24° C	96.3	24.3	218 ±3
SH, 1.5%	OT, 0.5%, 25° C	67.7	17.0	219 ±2
Do	Do, 37° C, 2 hours	70.9	17.6	221 ±2
Do	Do, 50° C, 2 hours	75.3	18.4	231 ±2

value of 212 to 230 mμ. Thus the disorganizing effects of OT differ strongly from the effects produced by the alkali or the guanidine salt. A similar increase of the dispersion constant under the influence of surface active agents was observed recently in this laboratory with normal gamma globulins, and with several other proteins of Class III.

Examination in the ultracentrifuge showed that denaturation with the detergent has produced only relatively small changes in molecular size. In the case of specimen SH (see last item in Table 5), only one symmetrical peak appeared in the sedimentation picture, and the corrected sedimentation constant was 5.1 S. In the instance EV, Subfraction II, the picture was similar, and the sedimentation constant was 5.0 S. Thus the macromolecules seem to be only expanded, and no significant dissociation or aggregation could be observed.

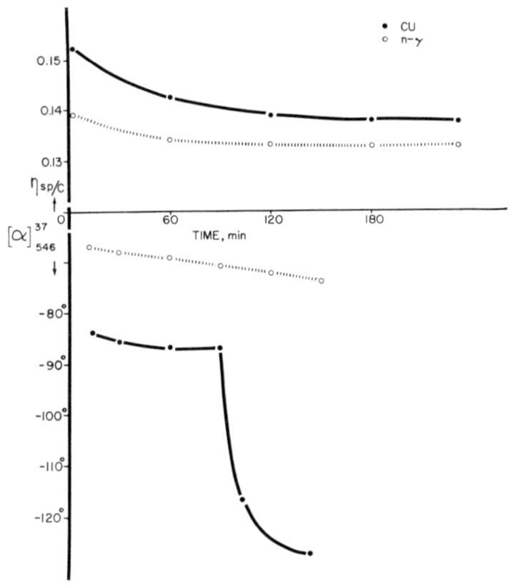

FIG. 4. The change of specific rotation and reduced specific viscosity with time for the myeloma globulin CU and normal human gamma globulin. The solid curves represent CU, the broken curves the normal gamma globulin. pH at the start was 11.4, and at the end it was 10.2. The temperature was 37.0°C.

The effect of alkali on the myeloma globulins was studied to a considerable extent, and some of the results have been reported in another paper (Jirgensons, 1961a). Attempts were made to find some differences between the normal and myeloma globulins with respect to the alkali stability. It was found that normal human gamma globulins were more stable to alkali than myeloma globulins, but exceptions were also found. While individual normal human gamma globulins were similar in their stability to alkali, the myeloma globulins exhibited striking individuality. Observations on an alkaline solution (pH 11.4 at the start, and 10.2 at the end of the experiment) of the myeloma globulin CU at 37°C showed that the specific rotation in the first 90 minutes was nearly constant and then suddenly increased, while a normal globulin under the same conditions showed a slight uniform rise of the rotatory power (see Figure 4). Similarly performed experiments with the specimens SH, P, and KA, however, showed that the break in the rotatory power versus time curve observed with specimen CU is not a general phenomenon. Specimen CU appeared also sensitive to detergent OT in that not only the conformation but also the molecular size was affected. In contrast, the molecular size of specimens EV and SH was not affected by warming with OT at 50°C.

Further Studies on Bence-Jones Proteins

Materials

Two individual specimens (HE and PI) of Bence-Jones proteins were isolated from the urine of two patients suffering from multiple myeloma. The urine was filtered, and the pH was adjusted with acetic acid to 5.1. The protein was precipitated with a saturated solution of ammonium sulphate at about 65 per cent saturation. The precipitate was removed from the liquid, dissolved in water, and dialyzed against distilled water. The aqueous solution of the protein was lyophilized, and the proteins were further purified by the same method of ion exchange chromatography as the gamma globulins and myeloma globulins. Elution from the column was started with a 0.005 M sodium phosphate buffer of pH 8.0, and the ionic strength was increased gradually with phosphate buffers of pH 7.0; the final concentration of the buffer was 0.5 M. In case HE, only one major component appeared in the effluent; in case PI, the major peak was relatively broad and possibly could be separated in several components. All of the colored impurities were removed in the ion exchange treatment. The solutions were liberated from electrolytes by dialysis, and water was removed by lyophilization. The resulting Bence-Jones proteins were readily soluble in water, the solutions flocculated at 50° to 55°C, and the precipitate almost fully redissolved on boiling.

Both HE and PI appeared to be homogeneous in paper electrophoresis tests, and the electrophoretic mobility was in the range of beta globulins. The aqueous solution of HE appeared homogeneous in sedimentation runs, and the corrected sedimentation constant $s^o_{20,w}$ was found to be 2.4 S. From this value and the intrinsic viscosity, which was 0.0338, a molecular weight of 25,700 was computed for this protein. Complete amino acid analysis of this sample also was performed, and the composition was found similar to that of other Bence-Jones protein specimens (e.g., Jirgensons, Ikenaka, and Gorguraki, 1959).

Optical Rotatory Dispersion of Native and Denatured Bence-Jones Proteins

The dependence of the specific rotation on the wave length of light is illustrated in the form of Yang-Doty plots (Yang and Doty, 1957) in Figure 5 and the constants are compiled in Table 6. In accord with previously published results (Jirgensons, 1959b), it was found that the dispersion constants (λ_c) of both specimens are below 220 mμ., and that these values increase upon the disorganization of the native macromolecules. While, by the use of guanidine

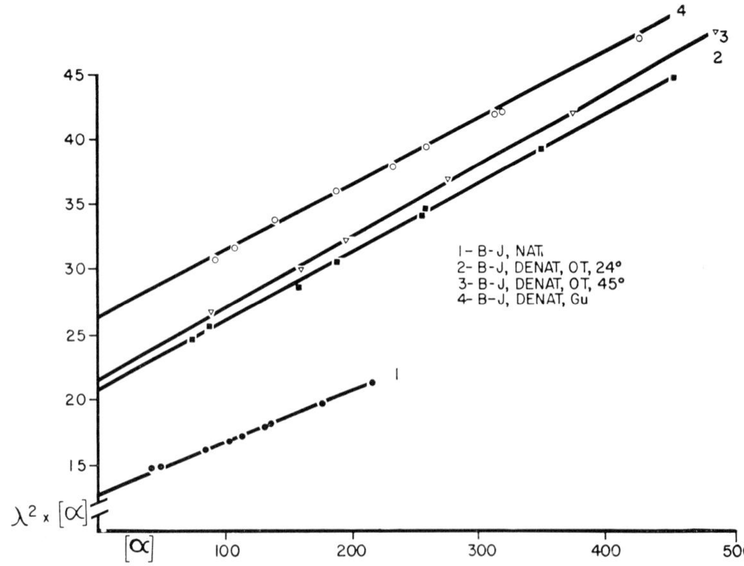

FIG. 5. The Yang-Doty plots of rotatory dispersion for native and denatured Bence-Jones protein.

TABLE 6

Dispersion Constants and Rotatory Power of Native and Denatured Bence-Jones Proteins. pH of the Solutions 7.0 to 7.4. Protein Concentration 1.6 to 2.2 Per Cent

Specimen	Solvent, treatment	$-[\alpha]^{24}_{546}$, degrees	K	λ_c, mμ.
HE, native	Water	49.2	12.9	196 ±2
PI, native	Water	45.4	11.5	207 ±4
HE, denatured	Guanidine-HCNS, 2 M 50° C	105.9	26.6	220 ±2
HE, denatured	OT, 0.36%, 24° C	80.7	20.0	227 ±1
Do	Do, 50° C, 1 hour	89.2	21.6	233 ±3
Do	Do, 50° C, 1 hour, cooled to 24° C	85.5	21.0	227 ±3
PI, denatured	OT, 0.25%, 22° C	67.8	17.0	214 ±2
Do	Do, 1 hour at 50° C, cooled to 24° C	73.0	18.1	224 ±2
Do	Do, 1 hour at 70° C, cooled to 24° C	75.2	18.5	228 ±4

thiocyanate as a denaturing agent, the λ_c was raised to only 220 mμ., the detergent OT was able to enhance this value to approximately 230 mμ. The effects produced by guanidine salt and detergent on the Bence-Jones proteins are generally the same as described above

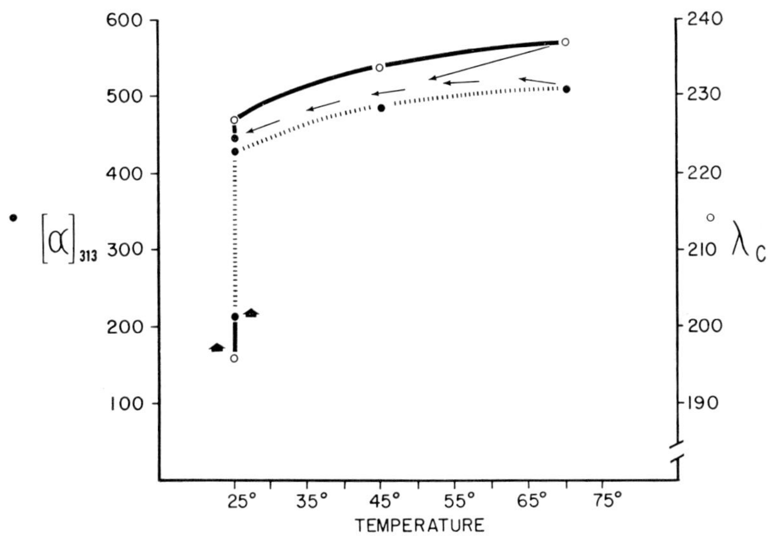

Fig. 6. Dependence of the specific rotation values (discs) and rotatory dispersion constants (open circles) of Bence-Jones protein on temperature in the presence of the surface active OT. Long arrows indicate the changes on cooling. Protein concentration 0.56 per cent, OT 0.36 per cent.

in the discussion of myeloma globulins. Heating the solutions that contained the detergent always facilitated disorganization of the macromolecules (Figure 6), and led to an increase of λ_c, whereas the temperature increase had only a slight effect on the denaturation with guanidine thiocyanate. The guanidine salt, however, always produced a greater negative shift of the rotatory power than the detergent.

Discussion

The most straightforward evidence about the geometry of polypeptide chains in macromolecules of proteins is furnished by X-ray structural analysis, and an excellent recent review on this matter was published by Crick and Kendrew (1957). The now popular α-helix (Pauling and Corey, 1950) did not appear as a product of ingenious imagination but as a result of painstaking X-ray diffraction measurements and structural analysis on crystals of amino acids and simple peptides. The presence of this conformation was first established, or made strongly probable, in several fibrous proteins such as myosin and certain keratins, again on the basis of X-ray diffraction data. The presence of α-helical conformation in globular proteins was not directly ascertained by these X-ray studies until very recently, when these spirals were shown to be present in crystals of myoglobin (Kendrew *et al.*, 1960). The optical rotation method appeared as an aid in these studies of chain geometry somewhat later, and the semiempirical conclusions regarding soluble proteins were made on the basis of studies on synthetic polyaminoacids (e.g., Doty, Bradbury, and Holtzer, 1956; Yang and Doty, 1957; Blout, 1960). Theoretical studies lead to the conclusion that hydrogen bonded α-helical conformation must be present in proteins which have a weakly negative or positive specific rotation and a high dispersion constant λ_c. Another fact that should indicate the presence of α-helical structures in the macromolecules of dissolved proteins is deviation of the rotatory dispersion function from the one term Drude rule, and it was somewhat surprising to find that aqueous protein solutions always followed the one term Drude rule, if the rotatory power was measured between the wave length limits 350 to 700 mμ. (Schellman and Schellman, 1956, 1958; Yang and Doty, 1957; Jirgensons and Straumanis, 1957; Jirgensons, 1958a,b,c 1959 a,b,c). According to Yang and Doty (1957), the experimental results could be brought in accord with the requirements of theory if one should assume that part of the macromolecule of the protein is α-helical and another represents a random chain. Any kind of denaturation then would mean a disorganization of the hydrogen bonded α-helices into random coils, viz., "melting" of these helices. This concept, which excluded any ordered conformations other than α-helices, however, was limited in its validity by the strange behavior of the Class III proteins (Jirgensons, 1958a,b,c; 1960a,b). The gamma globulins, Bence-Jones proteins, pepsin, and a number of others did not fit in the simple helix-random chain framework, since the λ_c values of the native proteins were very low and increased somewhat on disorganization of the unique native conformation. The experimental results of this paper furnish additional evidence indicating the possibility of specific chain conformations which are neither α-helices nor any nonspecific random arrangements in space.

What are these other ordered spatial arrangements of the polypeptide chains in such macromolecules as those of gamma globulin, myeloma globulin, or Bence-Jones protein? The absence of α-helices at once raises the question of the forces responsible for the compact folding of the chains. In the helical proteins, the regular twists are stablized by hydrogen bonds between the CO and NH groups of the peptide bonds within the same chain. This is the so-called secondary structure of the protein. Since in globular proteins the chains are folded, one has to consider also the way of folding or the tertiary structure. What makes the chains fold? Why do the helical chains of myosin remain straight, and why are they so compactly folded in serum albumin and globulins? One obvious reason, in the instance of albumin, is the presence of many disulfide bridges that link parts of the single chain of albumin; but there must be other forces, since there are globular proteins which do not have any disulfide bonds. Interchain hydrogen bonds, electrostatic interactions between polar groups, and other covalent bonds besides the disulfide bridges have been suggested and partially ascertained. However, more important than all these factors seems to be the hydrophobic nature of the amino acid side chains which tend to escape water (Kauzmann, 1954, 1959; Tanford, 1958; Tanford, De, and Taggart, 1960). It is possible that the twisting and folding of the polypeptide chain in a globular protein is due chiefly to the tendency of the hydrophobic groups and segments to escape water, whereby these hydrophobic parts are turned inside the coil and the polar groups remain in contact with water. According to this concept, the folding is enforced by the same factors that make detergent molecules, when placed into water, associate into micelles. It seems likely that the hydrophobic force is not the only factor which causes folding; it seems that the causes are always more than one, and that their importance differs from protein to protein (Tanford, 1958). In Class I proteins, such as the albumins, lysozyme, and prolactin, the hydrophobic forces may be less important than in Class II, and especially in Class III. According to a recent study by Tanford, De, and Taggart (1960), β-lactoglobulin, a protein of Class II, is nonhelical in aqueous solutions, but the chains become helically twisted under the influence of organic solvents such as alcohol. These authors conclude that the α-helical conformation in the proteins of Class II is insignificant. According to Schellman and Schellman (1961), the rotatory dispersion anomalies of the Class III may be due to the presence of interchain hydrogen bonds producing the so-called β-conformation, known to be present in silk as well as in some denatured proteins (Imahori, 1960). There is, however, no positive proof that the β-conformation might be present in the macromolecules of native serum gamma globulin or other proteins of Class III.

Results of this paper support the contention that in the proteins described here the folding of polypeptide chains is caused chiefly by hydrophobic forces rather than hydrogen bonds. The major argument in favor of such a decision is the effectiveness of the surface active agents in unfolding and disorganizing these macromolecules. As demonstrated in Tables 5 and 6, myeloma globulins or Bence-Jones proteins can be denatured with 0.25 to 0.5 per cent sodium dioctylsulphosuccinate (OT). When recalculated in molar concentration, this is a surprisingly low concentration of 0.0056 to 0.0112 moles/L.; and even lower concentrations of 0.001 moles/L. were found active, although to a lesser extent. Such ordinary denaturing agents as urea or guanidine salts are needed in thousand-fold higher concentrations. This effectiveness of the surface active agents has been demonstrated only with some of the proteins of Class III. In comparison, serum albumin (Jirgensons, 1959a) or taka-amylase (Isemura and Takagi, 1959) have been found much more resistant to the disorganizing effect of detergents than the globulins described in this paper. This is probably due to the fact that the folding of chains in albumin and taka-amylase is caused chiefly by hydrogen bonding, electrostatic attraction, and disulfide bonding, whereas in myeloma globulins, gamma globulins, and Bence-Jones proteins the folding is due chiefly to hydrophobic forces. Additional support to this contention was furnished in another study in which it was shown that disorganizing activity of surface active agents depends on the size of the hydrophobic portion of the detergent molecule (Jirgensons, 1961b). The mechanism of disorganization of the globulins by the detergents can be explained as a wedging of the hydrophobic tails of the detergent molecules into the folds of the polypeptide chain. The macromolecules of the protein usually are only partially unfolded, as has been ascertained by sedimentation and viscosity measurements. Electrophoretic mobility determinations proved that the detergent is bound to the protein in such a manner that the negatively charged heads remain on the surface since the mobility was strongly increased. Similar ideas for the mechanism of the denaturation of thyroglobulin by sodium dodecylsulphate have been expressed recently by other authors (Edelhoch and Lippoldt, 1960).

It is noteworthy that denaturation by means of guanidine thiocyanate resulted in a larger negative shift of specific rotation than denaturation with the detergent. The dispersion constant, on the contrary, was changed by the detergent more than by the guanidine salt. This indicates that the mechanisms are different in each case. The abnormal rise of λ_c to 230 mμ., observed on warming with the detergent, may be regarded as an indication of a limited α-helix formation of the partially disorganized chains. Such interpretation has been given for other protein systems, e.g., aqueous solutions of β-lactoglobulin to which were added various organic solvents (Tanford, De, and Taggart, 1960). Thus, the globular proteins, which are nonhelical in the native state, can be transformed after disorganizing the native compact conformation into partially helical form, which in this case is an unnatural conformation.

Summary

The optical rotatory dispersion of serum gamma globulins, myeloma globulins, and Bence-Jones proteins was studied by means of photoelectric spectropolarimetry. The rotatory dispersion constants λ_c of these proteins, when in the native state, were found to be in the low range of 196 to 220 mμ. Only slight differences could be found between the rotatory properties of serum gamma globulins from various mammal species, as well as between normal gamma globulins and myeloma globulins. Denaturation of these proteins by various agents resulted in a negative shift of the specific rotation and in a slight increase of the dispersion constants. Denaturation of myeloma globulins and Bence-Jones proteins with the surface active sodium dioctylsulphosuccinate (OT) at 50°C raised the λ_c to 230 mμ. It was concluded that the folding of the polypeptide chains in the described proteins is caused chiefly by the hydrophobic forces, viz., tendency of the hydrophobic side chains of the protein to escape water.

ACKNOWLEDGMENTS

This study was supported in part by Grant NCI-1785 from the National Cancer Institute, National Institutes of Health, United States Public Health Service; by Grant G-051 from the Robert A. Welch Foundation, Houston; and by Institutional Grants from The American Cancer Society.

ABBREVIATIONS

Abbreviations used in this paper are: [α], specific rotation, degrees; DEAE, diethylaminoethyl; K, rotatory constant; λ, wave length of the light; λc, dispersion constant; OT, sodium dioctylsulphosuccinate; S, sedimentation constant in Svedberg units; s_{20}, sedimentation constant at 20°C; $s^{o}_{20,w}$ corrected sedimentation constant.

REFERENCES

Blout, E. R. 1960. "Polypeptides and Proteins," *Optical Rotatory Dispersion*, C. Djerassi, Ed., pp. 238–273. New York, New York: McGraw-Hill Book Co., Inc.

Cohn, E. J., F. R. N. Gurd, D. M. Surgenor, B. A. Barnes, R. K. Brown, G. Derouaux, J. M. Gillespie, F. W. Kahnt, W. F. Lever, C. H. Liu, D. Mittelman, R. F. Mouton, K. Schmid, and E. Uroma. 1950. A System for Separation of the Components of Human Blood: Quantitative Procedures for the Separation of the Protein Components of Human Plasma. *Journal of the American Chemical Society*, 72:465–474.

Crick, F. H. C., and J. C. Kendrew. 1957. X-Ray Analysis and Protein Structure. *Advances in Protein Chemistry*, 12:133–214.

Doty, P., J. H. Bradbury, and A. M. Holtzer. 1956. Polypeptides. IV. The Molecular Weight, Configuration, and Association of Poly-γ-benzyl-L-glutamate in Various Solvents. *Journal of the American Chemical Society*, 78:947–954.

Edelhoch, H., and R. E. Lippoldt. 1960. The Properties of Thyroglobulin. II. The Effects of Sodium Dodecyl Sulfate. *Journal of Biological Chemistry*, 235:1335–1340.

Imahori, K. 1960. Rotatory Behavior of Protein Denaturation. *Biochimica et biophysica acta*, 37:336–341.

Isemura, T., and T. Takagi. 1959. Interaction of Taka-Amylase-A with Surface Active Agent. *Journal of Biochemistry*, 46:1637–1644.

Jirgensons, B. 1954. Optical Rotation and Viscosity of Native and Denatured Proteins. III. The Bence-Jones Protein and Human γ-Globulin. *Archives of Biochemistry and Biophysics*, 48:154–166.

———. 1956. Optical Rotation and Viscosity of Native and Denatured Proteins. VII. Human Serum Albumin in Alkaline Solutions. *Die makromolekulare Chemie*, 28/29:48–61.

———. 1957. Optical Rotation and Viscosity of Native and Denatured Proteins. IX. Some Plasma Proteins at Various pH. *Archives of Biochemistry and Biophysics*, 71:148–161.

———. 1958a. Optical Rotation and Viscosity of Native and Denatured Proteins. X. Further Studies on Optical Rotatory Dispersion. *Archives of Biochemistry and Biophysics*, 74:57–69.

———. 1958b. Optical Rotation and Viscosity of Native and Denatured Proteins. XI. Relationships between Rotatory Dispersion, Ionization, and Configuration. *Archives of Biochemistry and Biophysics*, 74:70–83.

———. 1958c. Dependence of Optical Rotatory Dispersion of Globular Proteins on Ionization and Denaturation. *Archives of Biochemistry and Biophysics*, 78:235–244.

———. 1959a. Spectropolarimetric Studies on Stabilization of Serum Albumin with Surface Active Salts. *Texas Reports on Biology and Medicine*, 17:106–113.

———. 1959b. The Optical Rotatory Dispersion of Bence-Jones Proteins. *Archives of Biochemistry and Biophysics*, 85:89–96.

———. 1959c. Optical Rotatory Dispersion of Crystallized Enzyme Proteins. *Archives of Biochemistry and Biophysics*, 85:532–539.

———. 1960a. Optical Rotatory Properties of Some Abnormal Serum Globulins. *Archives of Biochemistry and Biophysics*, 89:48–52.

———. 1960b. Optical Rotatory Dispersion of Some Pituitary Hormones. *Archives of Biochemistry and Biophysics*, 91:123–129.

———. 1961a. Further Studies on Rotatory Dispersion and Structure of Globular Proteins. *Die makromolekulare Chemie*, 44/46:123–137.

———. 1961b. Effect of Detergents on the Conformation of Proteins. I. *Archives of Biochemistry and Biophysics*, 94:59–67.

Jirgensons, B., T. Ikenaka, and V. Gorguraki. 1959. Concerning Chemistry and Testing of Bence-Jones Proteins. *Clinica chimica acta*, 4:876–882.

Jirgensons, B., and L. Straumanis. 1957. Optical Rotation and Viscosity of Native and Denatured Proteins. VIII. Rotatory Dispersion Studies. *Archives of Biochemistry and Biophysics*, 68:319–329.

Kauzmann, W. 1954. "Denaturation of Proteins and Enzymes," *The Mechanism of Enzyme Action*, W. D. McElroy and B. Glass, Eds., pp. 70–120. Baltimore, Maryland: The Johns Hopkins Press.

———. 1959. Some Factors in the Interpretation of Protein Denaturation. *Advances in Protein Chemistry*, 14:1–63.

Kendrew, J. C., R. E. Dickerson, B. E. Strandberg, R. G. Hart, D. R. Davies, D. C. Phillips, and V. C. Shore. 1960. Structure of Myoglobin. A Three-Dimensional Fourier Synthesis at 2Å. Resolution. *Nature, London*, 185:422–427.

Oncley, J. L., M. Melin, D. A. Richert, J. W. Cameron, and P. M. Gross. 1949. The Separation of the Antibodies, Isoagglutinins, Prothrombin, Plasminogen, and β_1-Lipoprotein into Subfractions of Human Plasma. *Journal of the American Chemical Society*, 71:541–550.

Pauling, L., and R. B. Corey. 1950. Two Hydrogen Bonded Spiral Configurations of the Polypeptide Chain. *Journal of the American Chemical Society*, 72:5349.

Schachman, H. K. 1957. "Ultracentrifugation, Diffusion, and Viscometry," *Methods in Enzymology*, S. P. Colowick and N. O. Kaplan, Eds., Vol. 4, pp. 32–103, New York, New York: Academic Press, Inc.

Schellman, C., and J. A. Schellman. 1958. Optical Rotation and Protein Configuration. *Comptes rendus des travaux du Laboratoire Carlsberg, serie chimique*, 30:463–500.

Schellman, J. A., and C. G. Schellman. 1956. The Rotary Dispersion of Amino Acids and Proteins. *Archives of Biochemistry and Biophysics*, 65:58–69.

———. 1961. Use of Rotatory Dispersion in the Determination of Protein Structure. *Journal of Polymer Science*, 49:129–151.

Scheraga, H. A., and L. Mandelkern. 1953. Consideration of the Hydrodynamic Properties of Proteins. *Journal of the American Chemical Society*, 75: 179–184.

Sober, H. A., F. J. Gutter, M. M. Wyckoff, and E. A. Peterson. 1956. Chromatography of Proteins. II. Fractionation of Serum Protein on Anion-Exchange Cellulose. *Journal of the American Chemical Society*, 78:756–763.

Tanford, C. 1958. "The Configuration of Globular Proteins in Aqueous Solution and its Dependence on pH." *Symposium on Protein Structure*, Albert Neuberger, Ed., pp. 35–65. London, England: Methuen & Co.; New York, New York: John Wiley & Sons, Inc.

Tanford, C., P. K. De, and V. G. Taggart. 1960. The Role of the α-Helix in the Structure of Proteins. Optical Rotatory Dispersion of β-Lactoglobulin. *Journal of the American Chemical Society*, 82:6028–6034.

Yang, J. T., and P. Doty. 1957. The Optical Rotatory Dispersion of Polypeptides and Proteins in Relation to Configuration. *Journal of the American Chemical Society*, 79:761–775.

The Substructure of the Myosin Molecule

ALFRED HOLTZER, PH.D., SUSAN LOWEY, PH.D., AND
TODD M. SCHUSTER

Department of Chemistry, Washington University, St. Louis, Missouri; Children's Cancer Research Foundation, Boston, Massachusetts; and Adolphus Busch III Laboratory of Molecular Biology, Washington University, St. Louis, Missouri

The central role played by myosin as a major structural element in muscle, and as a major part of the contractile machinery, makes the precise characterization of the myosin molecule particularly important. In spite of the attention focused upon the problem, however, there is still disagreement about the basic molecular parameters, in particular the molecular weight. In view of the history of this subject (at one time everyone concurred that the molecular weight was 850,000, a value entirely incorrect), it would seem that agreement among various investigators is not necessarily an essential or desirable goal; yet, surely disagreement can never be satisfactory.

Recently, values for the molecular weight have clustered in the region 400,000 to 500,000 (Gergely, Kohler, and Ritschard, 1958; Mommaerts and Aldrich, 1958; Von Hippel, Schachman, Appel, and Morales, 1958; Holtzer and Lowey, 1959; Brahms, 1959). However, since a very recent study of myosin showed an unexpectedly large second virial coefficient and yielded a molecular weight value of 620,000, this entire question was reopened (Kielley and Harrington, 1960).

For a structural protein the myosin molecule falls apart in solution with disturbing ease. The formation of more or less well-defined fragments results when the protein is treated with proteolytic enzymes (Szent-Gyorgyi, 1953), hydroxide ions (Kominz, Carroll, Smith, and Mitchell, 1959), and guanidine hydrochloride (Kielley and Harrington, 1960), among other reagents. The attempted characterization of some of the fragments has also led to controversy (Lowey and Holtzer, 1959a; Laki, 1961).

The best characterized fragments are undoubtedly the meromyosins. Measurement of the molecular weights by the Archibald method gave values of 126,000 for light (L) meromyosin and for heavy (H) meromyosin, 320,000 (Lowey and Holtzer, 1959a). The need for a molecular weight determination by an independent method is obvious. In addition, the molecular sizes of the meromyosins have hitherto not been determined, although viscosity measurements have revealed that both molecules are asymmetric (Szent-Gyorgyi, 1953; Szent-Gyorgyi, Cohen, and Philpott, 1960; Lowey and Cohen, in preparation).

The stoichiometric reconstruction (in imagination) of myosin from the meromyosins obviously could not be placed on a firm basis until the question of the molecular weight of the intact molecule was solved. Furthermore, the geometrical arrangement of the meromyosins in the native myosin molecule could not be determined with confidence until more was known about the molecular extension of the meromyosins.

Since light-scattering studies provide exactly these parameters, we have used this method to redetermine the molecular weight and size of myosin, to check the molecular weights of the meromyosins, and to measure, for the first time, the molecular sizes of the meromyosins. Several circumstances made it possible to increase the reliability of these measurements:

1) The light-scattering photometer was modified so that the light intensity is measured by a null method, increasing somewhat the precision of the experimental angular envelopes and hence producing better definition of the extrapolated values (Townsend, Schuster, and Holtzer, unpublished data).

2) Semiautomatic procedures were developed for pipetting solutions out of the centrifuge tubes and for delivering them into the scattering cell. These procedures produce slow movement of the solutions, minimizing gradients, and reducing the amount of manipulative skill required by the operator (Schuster and Holtzer,

unpublished data). The pipettes used had a minimum bore of 4 mm. to avoid formation of aggregates caused by velocity gradients.

3) Szent-Gyorgyi, Cohen, and Philpott (1960), using fractional precipitation with alcohol, prepared an L-meromyosin (Fraction I) that is ultracentrifugally homogeneous and completely helical. In our experiments, solutions of this material proved far easier to clean for light scattering than the crude L-meromyosin (which we found to be impossible to clean), and, in any case, Fraction I is probably of greater significance for the reconstruction of the parent myosin (Lowey and Cohen, in preparation).

4) Recently, methods have been developed for the preparation of ultracentrifugally homogeneous H-meromyosin (Lowey and Cohen, in preparation). Studies on this preparation are obviously of greater significance than those on earlier preparations which showed a pronounced "slow shoulder" in the ultracentrifuge (Lowey and Holtzer, 1959a).

It will be seen below that the present results indicate, as before, that the molecular weight of myosin is about 500,000 (Holtzer and Lowey, 1959) and that one myosin molecule consists essentially of one L-meromyosin and one H-meromyosin unit arranged end-to-end (Lowey and Holtzer, 1959a; Geiduschek and Holtzer, 1958).

Materials and Methods

Proteins

Myosin

Myosin was prepared as described previously (Holtzer and Lowey, 1959). Instead of 0.6 M KCl, the solvent used was 0.5 M KCl, 0.05 M phosphate buffer, pH 6.7. The phosphate buffer serves not only to control the pH but also to inhibit myosin aggregation (Lowey and Holtzer, 1959b).

Light Meromyosin

Light meromyosin, Fraction I, was prepared as described by Szent-Gyorgyi, Cohen, and Philpott (1960).

Heavy Meromyosin

Heavy meromyosin was prepared by the method of Lowey and Cohen (in preparation).

Physical Measurements

Light Scattering

The Brice-Phoenix light-scattering photometer was modified to make it a null instrument, and a semiautomatic pipetting and delivery system was used (Schuster and Holtzer, unpublished data). These techniques will be described elsewhere. All the other details have been previously reported (Holtzer and Lowey, 1959). Results were plotted as c/R_θ or Kc/R_θ versus $\sin^2(\theta/2)$, where $R_\theta = i_\theta r^2/I_0(1 + \cos^2\theta)$, with i_θ the excess intensity scattered at an angle θ to the incident beam by a unit volume of solution, I_0 the incident intensity of unpolarized light, and r the distance from the scattering volume to the detector; and where c = concentration of protein in Gm./cc.; and $K = 2\pi^2 n_0^2 (dn/dc)^2/N_0\lambda^4$, with n_0 the solvent refractive index, N_0 Avogadro's number, λ the wave length of incident light in vacuum, and dn/dc the refractive increment of the solution.

Refractive Increment

The refractive increments of myosin and the meromyosins were measured using a Phoenix differential refractometer. The values obtained for the refractive increment (*dn/dc*) of myosin do not agree with our previous results or with results of other workers (who do not agree with each other). The difficulty probably lies in the concentration measurement. Therefore, it is advisable to use one's own value, since in forming the ratio Kc/R_θ the concentration error may partially cancel out (Holtzer and Lowey, 1959). The values found in the present study were 0.181 ml./Gm. for myosin, 0.186 ml./Gm. for H-meromyosin, and 0.176 ml./Gm. for L-meromyosin. We are currently examining the problem of the refractive increments of the muscle proteins in detail and the results of these studies will be reported elsewhere.

Concentration

Protein concentrations were determined by volumetric sampling and micro-Kjeldahl analysis. A nitrogen factor of 6.2 was assumed for all three proteins. This is also subject to doubt and is being reevaluated. The molecular weights reported here are directly proportional to the nitrogen factor used; hence, any alteration in the nitrogen factor will require a corresponding change in the molecular weights.

Results

Graphs of some of the light-scattering data, plotted in the conventional way, are shown in Figures 1 and 2. The measured angular

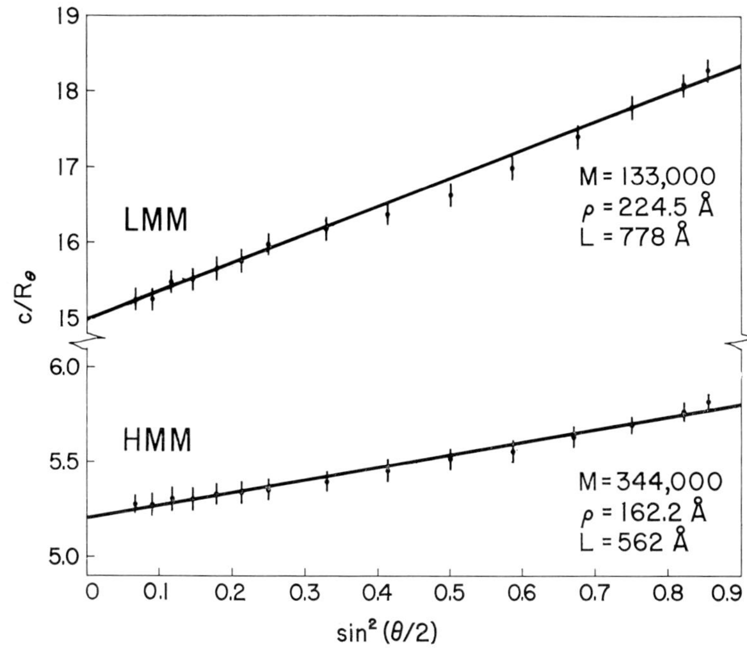

FIG. 1. Light-scattering envelopes of the meromyosins. HMM, heavy meromyosin; LMM, light meromyosin; M, molecular weight; ρ, radius of gyration; L, length.

envelopes for the meromyosins are linear as expected for monodisperse substances in this size range over the span of angles experimentally available. The myosin angular envelope is curved, as observed previously (Holtzer and Lowey, 1959). It was assumed in all cases that the second virial coefficient is zero since no concentration dependence of Kc/R_θ was observed in the rather narrow range of concentrations accessible in scattering studies. In any case, the concentrations used are so low that no reasonable virial coefficient can alter the results appreciably.

The molecular weights, radii of gyration, and molecular lengths obtained are summarized in Table 1. The reproducibility is seen to be quite good for these molecular parameters, with the exception of the results for the radius of gyration of H-meromyosin. In this case the dissymmetry of scattering is so small that the radius cannot be measured as precisely. The molecular weight and radius of gyration of myosin agree with our previous measurements of these quantities (Holtzer and Lowey, 1959), and the meromyosin molecular

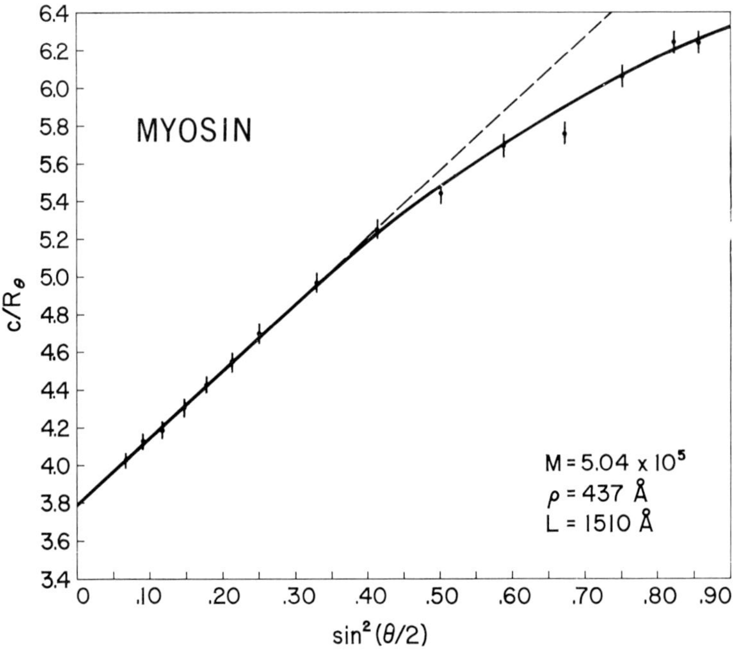

FIG. 2. Light-scattering envelope of myosin. L, length; M, molecular weight; ρ, radius of gyration.

TABLE 1
Light-Scattering Data from Myosin and Meromyosins

Myosin

Concentration (%)	M × 10⁻³	ρ (Å)	L (Å) (rod)
0.0181	504	437	1510
0.0193	499	433	1500
0.0203	532	426	1475
0.0248	523	440	1520
0.0286	541	430	1490
0.0367	526	439	1520
Average	525	434	1503

H-Meromyosin

Concentration (%)	M × 10⁻³	ρ (Å)	L (Å) (rod)	L (Å) (ellipse)
0.0505	347	183	634	820
0.0302	330	176	608	788
0.0522	340	160	554	716
0.0292	322	156	541	699
0.0265	346	178	615	796
0.0348	344	162	562	725
0.0279	350	147	510	658
Average	340	166	575	743

L-Meromyosin

Concentration (%)	M × 10⁻³	ρ (Å)	L (Å) (rod)
0.0263	138	221	766
0.0334	136	226	783
0.0376	132	215	745
0.0424	133	225	780
Average	135	222	769

Abbreviations: L, length; M, molecular weight; ρ, radius of gyration.

weights also agree with previous determinations by the Archibald method (Lowey and Holtzer, 1959a).

Discussion

The Myosin Molecular Weight

Recent determinations of the myosin molecular weight show values between 620,000 and 420,000 (Gergely, Kohler, and Ritschard, 1958; Mommaerts and Aldrich, 1958; Von Hippel, Schachman, Appel, and Morales, 1958; Holtzer and Lowey, 1959; Brahms, 1959; Kielley and Harrington, 1960). Ignoring precedents to the contrary (Kielley and Harrington, 1960), we resist the temptation to average these and thus produce a value in agreement with ours. It is more to the point to examine each value critically to find some reasonable basis for making a choice since it is not only possible, but probable that the average of two incorrect determinations is also incorrect.

Difficulties in obtaining the light-scattering molecular weight of myosin are generally conceded to be caused by three factors: dn/dc, aggregation, and dust.

We have remeasured dn/dc to check this point. While our results do not agree with earlier work, when the values are used in the manner described above, the errors apparently cancel out sufficiently so that the molecular weights agree within experimental error. Since micro-Kjeldahl analysis is a more reliable method for absolute determinations of nitrogen content than the Nessler procedure used previously, it is likely that our current value of dn/dc is the correct one in an absolute sense.

Since we have worked rapidly, in the cold, and in the presence of phosphate, which retards the aggregation (Lowey and Holtzer, 1959b), we do not expect that aggregation to dimers, trimers, etc., is a serious possibility. Low temperature ultracentrifuge runs performed at essentially the same time as the light-scattering studies showed no evidence of the presence of these aggregates.

The presence or absence of macroscopic particles, whether large aggregates formed in handling or extraneous "dust," is less easy to establish objectively, the only recourse being careful visual examination and judgment based on past experience. Solutions of myosin are usually not as clean as solutions of, say, synthetic polymers, but the ones reported here were acceptably clean, and the cleanest ones of them compare favorably with those encountered in studies of synthetic polymers. Because of the possible influence of dust, we consider it highly unlikely that the true molecular weight of myosin is greater than the value reported here. Since solutions found to be cleanest on careful scrutiny in a strong light beam yielded molecular weights close to 500,000, we expect that the true molecular weight may be somewhat closer to 500,000 than to the average of all values, 525,000. It must not be inferred from this that the dust problem in a light-scattering investigation makes it impossible to obtain molecular weights that are too low. Obviously, it is possible, if the solvent and solutions are subjected to different cleaning procedures, to obtain solutions that are cleaner than the solvent. In that event, of course, the calculated molecular weights would be too small. There is no doubt in our minds that in this investigation this was not the case.

The studies reported here thus offer no support for the contention that the molecular weight of myosin is 620,000. In that connection, it should be noted again that these light-scattering studies were performed at such low concentrations (~0.02 per cent) that even if the second virial coefficient were as high as reported by Kielley and Harrington (1960) using the Archibald method, the molecular weights tabulated here would change by only 2 per cent. Furthermore, in a recent study of the myosin molecular weight by the Archibald method (Lowey and Cohen, in preparation), it was found that the second virial coefficient is difficult to characterize accurately for such a high molecular weight material. However, the measurements definitely indicated a value for this parameter considerably less than that found by Kielley and Harrington (1960); in fact, least squares treatment of the data of Lowey and Cohen (in preparation) gave a value of 0.186×10^{-4} mole-cc/Gm.^{2} for the second virial coefficient and showed a myosin molecular weight of 497,000, in agreement with the value reported here.

The experimental data and theoretical predictions available in the literature and used by Kielley and Harrington (1960) in support of their result on the second virial coefficient of myosin also are open to question. Measurement of osmotic pressure in aqueous systems is a difficult feat and it has never been demonstrated that it is experimentally feasible for proteins of such high molecular weight. The study adduced by Kielley and Harrington (Portzehl, 1950), requiring as it did measurements of pressure differences to ± 0.003 cm. of water at the lower concentrations, can hardly be expected to be any more reliable on the question of second virial coefficient than it has been on the question of molecular weight, where it is over 50 per cent in error. The same may be said of determinations of the concentration dependence of the ratio of the diffusion coefficient to the sedimentation coefficient, when those same measurements give a molecular weight of 770,000 (Parrish and Mommaerts, 1954). Finally, the theoretical calculation of excluded volume (Zimm, 1946; Kielley and Harrington, 1960), while it gives a value for the second virial coefficient of the same order as found by Kielley and Harrington, must not be used indiscriminately. The second virial coefficient shown by a given system is a result of a complex set of thermodynamic interactions involving the solvent and the macromolecule, and it is absurd to single out the excluded volume effect as though it were the only one involved. This is particularly true of charged macromolecules in aqueous salt solutions. In the case of collagen, for example, the observed second virial coefficient is only 60 per cent of that expected from the excluded volume (Boedtker and Doty, 1956). In solutions of deoxyribonucleic acid (DNA) the second virial coefficient calculated from the excluded volume is 2 to 3 $\times$ 10^{-4} mole-cc/Gm.^{2}; the observed value is zero (Geiduschek and Holtzer, 1958). In myosin, a decrease in ionic strength from the traditional 0.6 to below 0.4 results in considerable aggregation (Holtzer and Lowey, 1959). The protein-protein interactions responsible for this association could well persist sufficiently at the higher ionic strength to lead to a second virial coefficient substantially below the value computed from the excluded volume alone.

While we can offer no cogent explanation for the results of Kielley and Harrington (1960), we would like to suggest that the different method of preparation adopted by these investigators may be responsible. Almost all of the physical studies on myosin reported in the literature have been on myosin prepared, with minor modifications, by the Szent-Gyorgyi method (Szent-Gyorgyi, 1951). The myosin thus made has been extensively studied and it is apparent that, with proper precautions, material that is homogeneous in the analytical ultracentrifuge results. The method used by Kielley and Harrington (1960), involving ammonium sulphate precipitation, has, to our knowledge, never been shown to be satisfactory in this respect. In view of the theoretical studies of Yphantis (1959) and the observed concentration dependence of the sedimentation coefficients of myosin monomer and dimer (Holtzer and Lowey, 1959; Lowey and Holtzer, 1959b) it is apparent that claims of the efficacy of the Archibald method in detecting such inhomogeneity (Kielley and Harrington, 1960) should be discounted. In this system it is not expected that the apparent molecular weight would show any trend in the course of the time taken by these experiments, even if aggregates were present. Consequently, such heterogeneity could not have been detected in the studies reported by Kielley and Harrington (1960). It is worth noting that myosin has been found to aggregate rather rapidly at high ionic strength (Lowey and Holtzer, 1959b) and exposure to high concentrations of ammonium sulphate would appear to be a highly suspect procedure.

While the authors are in a critical mood, it may not be amiss to discuss another molecular weight value reported for myosin. It has become popular recently to use the value 420,000, which is quoted as the result of agreement (again) among three methods of measurement in three different laboratories (Von Hippel, Schachman, Appel, and Morales, 1958; Mommaerts and Aldrich, 1958; Gergely, Kohler, and Ritschard, 1958). A fourth study, also supporting this value is discussed below. The methods employed in the three studies were, respectively, the Archibald method with schlieren optics, the Archibald method with Rayleigh optics, and light scattering. The value from the first of these studies (Von Hippel, Schachman, Appel, and Morales, 1958) was apparently based on a single determination at a single, rather high (0.5 per cent) concentration of a single sample, assuming a second virial coefficient of zero. The second study (Mommaerts and Aldrich, 1958), based on a method which is still of doubtful validity (Schachman, 1959), was also done largely at high concentrations, and, in fact, a value of 380,000, not 420,000, was obtained. This was corrected to 420,000 because of putative "interaction effects," i.e., a second virial coefficient of 0.25×10^{-4} mole-cc./Gm.^{2} was assumed. The same interaction effects, applied to the first study, would result in a molecular weight of 470,000, not 420,000. In all fairness, it cannot be said, therefore, that these two determinations agree to better than 10 per cent (which is not surprising), and the exact value to be chosen is in doubt. The report of the final study in question (Gergely, Kohler, and Ritschard, 1958) has appeared thus far only in abstract form. No details are yet available concerning dn/dc, concentration measurement, tests of homogeneity, etc. Under the circumstances, the continued uncritical devotion of workers in the field to the value 420,000 may be dismissed as frivolity. The fact is that molecular weight determinations for macromolecular substances are not yet matters of routine; consequently, accurate molecular characterization will never be achieved unless all the experimental and procedural details of relevant studies are published, allowing careful and critical scrutiny of the results by other workers.

The Meromyosin Substructure of Myosin

Molecular Weights

The meromyosin molecular weights shown in Table 1 add up to 475,000. If 5 per cent is added to account for dialyzable fragments produced by the tryptic digestion (Lowey and Cohen, in preparation) we find a molecular weight of close to 500,000 for a molecule made up of one L-meromyosin and one H-meromyosin unit. This agrees closely with the value found for myosin, and provides support for an LH structure. Studies of the weight fraction of the two meromyosins present in myosin show that L-meromyosin is 25 to 30 per cent of the total; nondialyzable material and H-meromyosin, 70 to 75 per cent (Lowey and Holtzer, 1959a; Lowey and Cohen, in preparation). The assumption of an LH structure and our molecular weight data lead to $135/475 = 0.28$ as the expected fraction L-meromyosin present, in agreement with the value found. These percentage composition data should form an important part of any attempts to "reconstruct" the myosin molecule from the meromyosins. The L_2H structure proposed by Kielley and Harrington (1960) and Laki (1961) would require a proportion of L-meromyosin almost double that found experimentally.

Molecular Sizes

It is obvious from the experimental radii of gyration in Table 1 that the one H-meromyosin and one L-meromyosin must be arranged end-to-end if the resulting particle is to have a radius of gyration anywhere near that found for myosin. We must now examine this situation in more detail. First we will treat the problem from a general point of view and then apply the results to our particular case.

General theory. The molecular dimension obtained from light scattering in monodisperse systems, the so-called radius of gyration, ρ, is given by (Geiduschek and Holtzer, 1958):

$$N\rho^2 = \sum_{n=1}^{N} r_{on}^2 \qquad (1)$$

where N is the total number of "scattering centers" in the molecule and r_{on} is the distance from scattering center n to the point o in the molecule, where

$$\sum_{n=1}^{N} r_{on} = O \qquad (2)$$

The N scattering centers are assumed to be equivalent in scattering power; i.e., each would scatter the same amount of light if they were isolated.

Of course, if the distribution of equivalent scattering centers in the molecule corresponds to the mass distribution, i.e., if each equivalent scattering center has the same mass, then the point o in the molecule, defined by equation (2), is also the center of the mass of the molecule. In ordinary cases this is assumed to be true and it is assumed, therefore, that the parameter deduced from the Zimm plot (Zimm, 1948) is the "radius of gyration about the center of gravity." In general, however, the distribution of mass need not coincide with the distribution of equivalent scattering centers. The scattering power of a given region of a molecule depends not only on its mass but on its refractive increment. A massive portion of a molecule, if it had the same refractive index as the solvent, would contribute nothing to the scattering, whereas a lighter region with a high refractive increment would contribute. Thus, in a molecule nonuniform in refractive increment, light scattering would provide the "radius of gyration about the center of scattering power," defined by equation (2), rather than about the center of gravity. We must now inquire explicitly into the proper means of assigning relative numbers of equivalent scattering centers to different regions of a molecule that may differ in mass and refractive index.

The intensity of light scattered at infinite dilution by unit volume of a solution of molecules that are small compared to the wavelength of light (or at zero angle, if the particles are large), may be written in terms of Rayleigh's ratio R_0, as:

$$R_0 = KcM \qquad (3)$$

At infinite dilution the molecules will be scattering incoherently; so, if there are ν molecules/cc., the light intensity scattered/molecule is simply R_o/ν. *Since* $\nu = N_o c/M$, we find for the intensity scattered/molecule:

$$R_o/\nu = \frac{KM^2}{N_o} \qquad (4)$$

We can now divide the molecule into regions of uniform refractive index. Each uniform region, i, would, if it were isolated, scatter an amount of light given by equation (4), i.e., $K_iM_i^2/N_o$. Now we wish to divide each uniform region into N_i equivalent scattering centers and we want to determine the relative number of these to assign to each region. Within a uniform region, the N_i centers are scattering coherently so that if each center, when isolated, were to scatter light of intensity A^2 (amplitude A), the total scattering of this uniform region would be: $(N_iA)^2 = K_iM_i^2/N_o$, and the number of scattering centers to be assigned to this region is:

$$N_i = \frac{M_i}{A}\sqrt{\frac{K_i}{N_o}} \tag{5}$$

Thus, we can think of any two regions (say L and H) of different refractive index and mass as being made up of scattering centers that individually would scatter the same amount of light (A^2), and the relative number of these equivalent centers to be assigned to each region is:

$$\frac{N_{\mathrm{H}}}{N_{\mathrm{L}}} = \frac{M_{\mathrm{H}}\sqrt{K_{\mathrm{H}}}}{M_{\mathrm{L}}\sqrt{K_{\mathrm{L}}}} = \frac{M_{\mathrm{H}}(dn/dc)_{\mathrm{H}}}{M_{\mathrm{L}}(dn/dc)_{\mathrm{L}}} \tag{6}$$

Thus, the "center of scattering power," alluded to above can be seen to be, not the "center of mass," but the "center of the product of mass and refractive increment," and would be obtained from:

$$\sum_i m_i(dn/dc)_i r_{oc} = O \tag{7}$$

where m_i and $(dn/dc)_i$ are, respectively, the mass and refractive increment of the uniform region i, and r_{oc} is the distance from the centroid of i (which is also its center of scattering power) to the center of scattering power of the whole molecule. Equation (7), of course, defines the ordinary centroid for a particle of uniform dn/dc.

Now that we are clear on the exact meaning of the parameter obtained from light scattering, we consider the calculation of the expected light-scattering radius of gyration for a generalized molecule made up of two parts, each of known light-scattering radius of gyration (Figure 3).

The radius of gyration of the whole molecule is given by equation (1) and if we break the sum into two parts, summing over

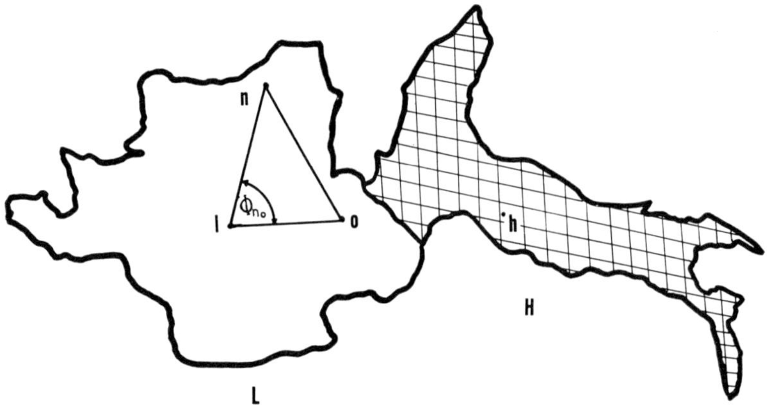

FIG. 3. Generalized molecule consisting of two regions, L and H, differing in mass and refractive increment; other definitions are given in text.*

each of the two regions separately, we have:

$$N\rho^2 = \sum_{n=1}^{N_L} r^2_{on} + \sum_{n=1}^{N_H} r^2_{on} \tag{8}$$

where $N = N_L + N_H$. It should be emphasized that r_{on} is the distance from the point n in the L region or H region to the center of scattering power (obtained from equation 7) of the whole molecule.

Experimentally, we know the radius of gyration of each region:

$$N_L\,\rho^2_L = \sum_{n=1}^{N_L} r^2_{ln}$$

and (9)

$$N_H\,\rho^2_H = \sum_{n=1}^{N_H} r^2_{hn}$$

where l (or h) designates the center of scattering power of the L (or H) region (Figure 3). We must now use the information in equation (9) to perform the summations required in equation (8).

From the law of cosines we have:

$$r^2{}_{no} = r^2{}_{lo} + r^2{}_{ln} - 2\,r_{ln}r_{lo}\cos\phi_{no}$$

so:

$$\sum_{n=1}^{N_L} r^2_{no} = \sum_{n=1}^{N_L} r^2_{lo} + \sum_{n=1}^{N_L} r^2_{ln} - 2\sum_{n=1}^{N_L} r_{ln}r_{lo}\cos\phi_{no}$$

* (Apparently, the author has used this map of a portion of Southern Europe so that the reader will recognize that the molecule under discussion is indeed a generalized molecule and of no specific conformation. Editor)

The first term on the right is simply $N_L r^2_{lo}$; the second is $N_L \rho^2_L$; and the third is zero (Geiduschek and Holtzer, 1959), so that we have:

$$\sum_{n=1}^{N_L} r^2_{no} = N_L r^2_{lo} + N_L \rho^2_L \qquad (10)$$

with an analogous equation for the H region. Thus, equation (8) becomes

$$\rho^2 = (N_L/N)\,\rho^2_L + (N_H/N)\,\rho^2_H + (N_L/N) r^2_{lo} + (N_H/N) r^2_{ho} \qquad (11)$$

which gives the light-scattering radius of the whole molecule in terms of the light-scattering radii of the individual regions, the relative number of scattering centers in each region, and the distance between the center of scattering power of each region and the center of scattering power of the molecule.

Application to Myosin. Since the meromyosins apparently do not undergo any severe structural changes on being split from myosin (Cohen and Szent-Gyorgyi, 1957), the most obvious simple hypothesis is that both the meromyosins are uniform rods and are joined end-to-end in myosin. Using the results obtained for the meromyosins in this investigation (molecular weights and radii for the meromyosins were increased by 5 per cent to correct for loss of fragments in digestion) and using equation (6), we have:

$$(N_L/N) = M_L (dn/dc)_L / M\ (dn/dc)$$

with $M = M_L + M_H$ and (dn/dc) the refractive increment of myosin. Thus, $(N_L/N) = (142{,}000)\ (0.176)/(500{,}000)\ (0.181) = 0.276$ and $(N_H/N) = 0.724$. It is evident from this that the effect of the inhomogeneity in refractive increment is small in this case, the quantity 0.176/0.181 differing little from unity. The lengths of the meromyosins, assuming they are rods, may be calculated from the measured, corrected radii ($\rho_L = 223$ Å; $\rho_H = 174$ Å), and the model of myosin that results is shown in Figure 4a. The relative diameters are not important here since, in any case, they are small compared to the wave length of light used. If the subunits are themselves uniform, the individual centers of scattering power are located in the middle of each rod subunit. The center of scattering power of the

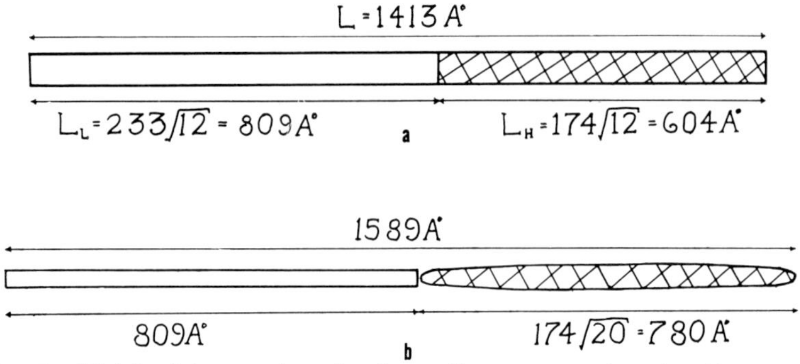

FIG. 4. Models of the myosin molecule: a—Two meromyosin rods colinear and end-to-end; b—L-meromyosin rod and H-meromyosin ellipsoid colinear and end-to-end. L, over-all length of the myosin molecule; L_L, length of the L-meromyosin portion; L_H, length of the H-meromyosin portion.

intact rod is then found from equation (7), which reduces in this case to:

$$M_L(dn/dc)_L r_{lo} = M_H(dn/dc)_H r_{ho} \tag{12}$$

and since $r_{lo} + r_{ho} = (L/2)$, with L the over-all length of the myosin molecule, we obtain:

$$r_{lo} = \frac{M_H(dn/dc)_H L}{2[M_H(dn/dc)_H + M_L(dn/dc)_L]} = \frac{N_H L}{2N} \tag{13}$$

and an analogous equation for r_{ho}. In this case we have, therefore, $r_{lo} = 511$ Å, and $r_{ho} = 195$ Å. The expected radius for myosin may now be calculated from equation (11), and we obtain $\rho = 370$ Å, whereas the measured value for myosin is 434 Å. Thus, the radius for myosin expected from the meromyosin data is 15 per cent lower than that found. Considering the experimental errors of all the quantities used in the calculation, this is not bad agreement. However, since the corrected molecular weights of the meromyosins add up to a value only 5 per cent lower than that measured for myosin, and because of the precision shown in Table 1, we suggest that this discrepancy is not a result of experimental imprecision, but a real property of the system. In seeking a cause for the difficulty there are two obvious possibilities: (1) polydispersity, and (2) the model is wrong. We will consider each in turn.

Polydispersity could account for the results if the heterogeneity is of a type that includes some longer molecules, and if the extent of such heterogeneity is greater in myosin than in the meromyosins. In that event, the radius obtained for myosin would represent a higher average than that obtained for the molecular weight (Geiduschek and Holtzer, 1958) and the radii of the meromyosins would add up to a value not quite that found for the intact molecule. One argument in favor of this is that the model of two meromyosins rods joined end-to-end does not seem to be sufficient to explain the shape of the myosin angular envelope (Schuster and Holtzer, unpublished data). The extra heterogeneity observed may be caused by variations from molecule to molecule, but it may also be caused by variations within the molecule along the lines suggested below.

A preliminary report of work on chromatographic fractionation of myosin (Brahms, 1959) seems to indicate that all myosin molecules may not be alike, although it is hard to tell from this report what relation exists between the fractions described and the preparation of myosin described in our studies. Light-scattering experiments gave a molecular weight for one of the fractions of 430,000 (Brahms, 1959), but in view of the lack of information about (1) the possibility of the presence of the other (heavier) fraction in the unfractionated samples studied hitherto, (2) the concentrations employed in the light scattering, and (3) the concentration method used in evaluating dn/dc (0.209 ml./Gm. was used), etc., we will perhaps be pardoned for not sharing this author's optimistic view that agreement of the light-scattering and Archibald methods has been demonstrated.

In addition to polydispersity, another possible explanation for the data on the radii of gyration exists: the model of two meromyosin rods joined end-to-end may be incorrect. All of the physical studies on purified L-meromyosin clearly indicate that this molecule consists almost entirely of two α-helices packed side-to-side, and probably twisted about one another (Szent-Gyorgyi, Cohen, and Philpott, 1960; Lowey and Cohen, in preparation). In all probability, therefore, the assumption of a rodlike configuration for the L-meromyosin is justified. For the H-meromyosin portion, however, no such definitive statement can be made. Although viscometry indicates that this fragment is asymmetric (Lowey and Cohen, in preparation) there is no cogent reason for preferring a rod shape to, say, a prolate ellipsoid. Furthermore, rotatory dispersion studies suggest that only part of the molecule is in helical form (Cohen and Szent-Gyorgyi, 1957). In fact, if we suppose that the H-meromyosin molecule is not quite a uniform rod but instead has more of its mass distributed closer to its center of gravity—in brief, if it is fatter in the middle—then, as we will see, it is possible to explain the discrepancy between the calculated and measured radii of myosin.

The simplest model for an asymmetric particle that is fat in the middle is a prolate ellipsoid of revolution. For this model, the factor for converting radius of gyration to length is $\sqrt{20}$ (if the ellipsoid is very thin) as opposed to $\sqrt{12}$ for the uniform rod. This difference arises from the obvious physical difference between the two; if a rod and ellipsoid are to have the same radius of gyration, the ellipsoid, being thicker in the middle, must compensate for this by being longer. If the H-meromyosin data are interpreted in this way, the myosin model becomes that of Figure 4b. In this figure the diameters are drawn to scale. The diameter of L-meromyosin was determined from the light-scattering length, from the axial ratio as determined by viscometry, and from the Kirkwood-Riseman (1950) equation for rods. The H-meromyosin diameter was obtained from the same type of data using Simha's (1940) equation for ellipsoids. The myosin radius of gyration calculated for this model using equation (11) is 404 Å. This is only 7 per cent lower than the experimental value and is well within the experimental error. Furthermore, a slight increase in the amount of material placed near the center of gravity would obviously produce even better agreement; the ellipsoid is an arbitrary choice. The entire discrepancy could thus be explained in this way. It is worth noting that the over-all length of the myosin molecule calculated for this model is somewhat greater than for the rod model.

It is interesting to note too that a similar proposal for the structure of H-meromyosin has previously been made, on quite different grounds, by Cohen (in press). At the moment, however, it can only be supported by rather indirect evidence.

The picture of the myosin molecule that best fits our light-scattering data, then, is of a rod 1,590 Å long and of molecular weight 500,000. One rodlike L-meromyosin fragment of molecular weight 140,000 (in the intact molecule) and length 809 Å is joined end-to-end and is colinear with an ellipsoidal H-meromyosin fragment of molecular weight 360,000 and length 780 Å. These data and viscometry results (Lowey and Cohen, in preparation) suggest a diameter of 18 Å for the L-meromyosin fragment and 27 Å for the minor axis of the H-meromyosin fragment.

The Structure of the Thick Filaments of Muscle

Data on the mass and extension of the myosin molecule must

eventually be brought to bear on the recent findings concerning the structure of muscle. It now appears clear that the myosin molecules in muscle are located in a hexagonal array of thick filaments; contraction is postulated to be a result of cross bridging of these thick filaments with another array of (thin) filaments made up of actin molecules (Huxley, 1960).

From a detailed consideration of the studies of the protein content and the spacing of filaments in whole striated muscle, Huxley calculated that each thick filament contains 432 myosin molecules (using the molecular weight we have found here this figure would have to be changed to 370 molecules/filament—a trivial change considering the other errors involved), but from the electron microscope photographs he concluded that the number of cross bridges from any given thick filament to the actin filaments is only about 216 (Huxley, 1960). Two possibilities were enumerated by Huxley to explain this difference: (1) that each observed bridge actually corresponds to two linkages, and (2) that estimates of the myosin content of muscle are too large by a factor of two. The results of our experiments open up still a third possibility, which we must now consider.

If we assume that the thick filaments are all myosin, the weight and density of these filaments are then known. Since the electron micrographs show a filament length of 15,000 Å, and show the shape to be roughly ellipsoidal (Huxley, 1960), we may calculate the minor axis of the thick filament. This calculation yields 165 Å for this parameter, in agreement with the thickness measured in the middle of the filaments, i.e., in the H-zone (Huxley, 1953). While it is dangerous to refer measurements on dried, fixed, stained material to the living tissue, this result lends credence to the view that these filaments are all myosin and that the myosin in them is tightly packed. If it is assumed that the molecular axis is parallel to the fiber axis, the ratio of the filament length to the molecular length (about 10) requires that about 40 myosin molecules appear in a cross section of a single filament. If the arrangement is simply one of close packing, such an array as shown in Figure 5 would represent a molecular picture of a cross section of a thick filament. Completion of four concentric layers of closely packed (but not necessarily in register) rods requires 37 molecules, sufficiently close to the required 40. Using the molecular diameter found in solution studies on myosin (Holtzer and Lowey, 1959), we would expect this filament to have a diameter of about 150 Å in agreement with

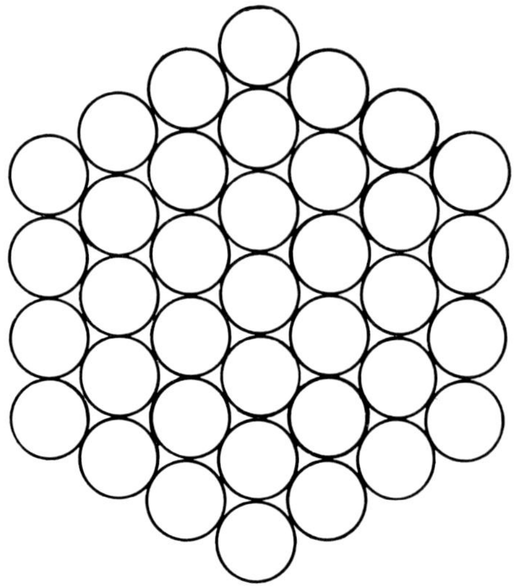

FIG. 5. Putative cross section of a thick filament of straited muscle in the H zone.

both the value calculated above, and that found in the electron microscope experiments.

If we adopt this picture of the filament, the nature of the third possible explanation of the discrepancy between the total number of myosin molecules and the number of observed cross bridges becomes obvious. About half of the myosin molecules are buried inside the filament where cross-bridging to actin is impossible. We thus raise the question whether it might not be that about half of the myosin molecules (perhaps differing in some subtle way from the others) are allowed to participate, with the others, in maintaining the structure of the filaments but not in the interaction directly responsible for contraction.

Obviously, it is only the observation of a difference between the number of cross bridges and the number of molecules that gives rise to these speculations, because it is not difficult to imagine structures, in agreement with the other facts, that could expose part of every myosin molecule at the surface of the filament. For example, even the centrally located molecule in Figure 5 could be made to have one end in the middle of the filament and the other on the periphery by merely tilting the molecule to make an angle of 3° with the fiber axis. An angle as small as this could not be detected by methods currently available.

ACKNOWLEDGMENT

This investigation was supported by Grant RG-5488 from the Division of General Medical Sciences, United States Public Health Service.

REFERENCES

Boedtker, H., and P. Doty. 1956. Native and Denatured States of Soluble Collagen. *Journal of the American Chemical Society*, 78:4267–4280.

Brahms, J. 1959. Chromatography of Myosin. *Journal of the American Chemical Society*, 81:4997.

Cohen, C. (in press). *American Chemical Society Symposium on Microstructure of Proteins, Journal of Polymer Science.*

Cohen, C., and A. G. Szent-Györgyi. 1957. Optical Rotation and Helical Polypeptide Chain Configuration in α-Proteins. *Journal of the American Chemical Society*, 79:248.

Geiduschek, E., and A. Holtzer. 1958. "Application of Light Scattering to Biological Systems," *Advances in Biological and Medical Physics*, C. Tobias and J. Lawrence, Eds., Vol. 6, pp. 431–551. New York, New York: Academic Press, Inc.

Gergely, J., H. Kohler, and W. Ritschard. 1958. Physicochemical and End-group Studies on Proteolytic Fragments of Myosin. (Abstract) *Biophysical Society*, 2:46.

Holtzer, A., and S. Lowey. 1959. The Molecular Weight, Size and Shape of the Myosin Molecule. *Journal of the American Chemical Society*, 81:1370–1377.

Huxley, H. 1953. Electron Microscope Studies of the Organization of the Filaments in Striated Muscle. *Biochimica et biophysica acta*, 12:387–394.

———. 1960. "Muscle Cells," *The Cell*, J. Brachet and A. Mirsky, Eds., Vol. 4, pp. 365–481. New York, New York: Academic Press, Inc.

Kielley, W., and W. Harrington. 1960. A Model for the Myosin Molecule. *Biochimica et biophysica acta*, 41:401–421.

Kirkwood, J. G., and J. Riseman. 1950. Intrinsic Viscosity, Translational and Rotational Diffusion Constants of Rod-Like Macromolecules in Solution. *Journal of Chemical Physics*, 18:512–516.

Kominz, D., W. Carroll, E. Smith, and E. Mitchell. 1959. A Subunit of Myosin. *Archives of Biochemistry and Biophysics*, 79:191–199.

Laki, K. 1961. The L-Meromyosin Content of Myosin. *Archives of Biochemistry and Biophysics*, 92:221–225.

Lowey, S., and C. Cohen. Structure of Myosin. (In preparation).

Lowey, S., and A. Holtzer. 1959a. Homogeneity and Molecular Weights of the Meromyosins and their Relative Proportions in Myosin. *Biochimica et biophysica acta*, 34:470–484.

———. 1959b. Aggregation of Myosin. *Journal of the American Chemical Society*, 81:1378–1383.

Mommaerts, W. F. H. M., and B. Aldrich. 1958. Determination of the Molecular Weight of Myosin. *Biochimica et biophysica acta*, 28:627–636.

Parrish, R. G., and W. F. H. M. Mommaerts. 1954. Studies on Myosin. II. Some Molecular Kinetic Data. *Journal of Biological Chemistry*, 209:901–913.

Portzehl, H. 1950. Masse und Masze von L-Myosin. *Zeitschrift für Naturforschung*, 5b:75–78.

Schachman, H. 1959. *Ultracentrifugation in Biochemistry*. New York, New York: Academic Press, Inc., p. 183.

Schuster, T., and A. Holtzer. Unpublished work.

Simha, R. 1940. Influence of Brownian Movement on Viscosity of Solutions. *Journal of Physical Chemistry*, 44:25–34.

Szent-Györgyi, A. 1951. *Chemistry of Muscular Contraction*. New York, New York: Academic Press, Inc., 162 pp.

Szent-Györgyi, A. G. 1953. Meromyosins, the Subunits of Myosin. *Archives of Biochemistry and Biophysics*, 42:305–320.

Szent-Györgyi, A. G., C. Cohen, and D. Philpott. 1960. Light Meromyosin Fraction I. *Journal of Molecular Biology*, 2:133–142.

Townsend, J., T. Schuster, and A. Holtzer. Unpublished work.

Von Hippel, P. H., H. Schachman, P. Appel, and M. Morales. 1958. On the Molecular Weight of Myosin. *Biochimica et biophysica acta*, 28:504–507.

Yphantis, D. 1959. Ultracentrifugal Molecular Weight Averages During the Approach to Equilibrium. *Journal of Physical Chemistry*, 63:1742–1747.

Zimm, B. 1946. Application of the Methods of Molecular Distribution to Solutions of Large Molecules. *Journal of Chemical Physics*, 14:164–179.

———. 1948. The Scattering of Light and the Radial Distribution Function of High Polymer Solutions. *Journal of Chemical Physics*, 16:1093–1099.

The Structure of Nucleoproteins

GEOFFREY ZUBAY*

The Rockefeller Institute,
New York, New York

A lecture entitled "The Structure of Nucleoproteins" must necessarily be greatly condensed. There are many different types of nucleoproteins, and it would be possible to devote an entire talk to almost any one of them. I hope that something may be gained by making comparisons between a few of the more prominent classes of naturally occurring nucleoprotein complexes. Accordingly, I shall discuss the two main classes of deoxynucleoproteins found in the cell nucleus: nucleohistone and nucleoprotamine. The main ribonucleoprotein found in the cell cytoplasm is referred to as a microsomal particle, or ribosome, depending on whether it has its origin in the endoplasmic reticulum or in free ribonucleoprotein particles. I shall discuss ribosomes from the bacterium *Escherichia coli* and the spherical ribonucleoprotein turnip yellow mosaic virus (TYMV), which might be said superficially to resemble the ribosome in a structural sense. For clarity, the discussion will be divided into four parts, and each of the nucleoproteins will be compared in each part.

The first question to be considered is that of the secondary structure of the nucleic acid itself. In the case of deoxyribonucleic acid (DNA), we know, primarily from the study of X-ray diffraction (Langridge *et al.*, 1960, 1960), that the DNA molecule exists as a double helical structure with pairs of hydrogen bonds formed regularly between opposing bases from the two polynucleotide chains of

* Present address: Biology Department, Brookhaven National Laboratory, Upton, L. I., New York.

the double helix. Hydrogen bonds are only formed between guanine and cytosine and between adenine and thymine. These two hydrogen-bonded base pairs contain the same type of hydrogen bonds, and the distance between the glycosidic bonds in the two base pairs is exactly the same. This means that, regardless of the sequence of base pairs along the double helix axis, the sugar phosphate backbone is regularly disposed. Since the only close contacts between adjacent double helices in a hydrated fiber of DNA are formed between their respective ribose phosphate chains, we can see why, under ideal conditions, the DNA is able to pack in an extremely regular paracrystalline manner as observed by X-ray diffraction.

The likelihood that this uniformly hydrogen-bonded double helical structure is preserved in solution has been shown by various physicochemical studies (Doty, 1956). One of the most convenient and informative assays of the degree and strength of this type of hydrogen-bonded structure is obtained by measuring the optical density as a function of temperature. When the nucleic acid is heated, the hydrogen bonds are broken. This hyperchromicity generally occurs over a narrow range of temperature, as might be expected for the melting of a regularly hydrogen-bonded structure.

In the case of ribonucleic acid (RNA), studies of the secondary structure have not led to such a simple answer. Thus in X-ray diffraction, the patterns obtained are less clear (Rich and Watson, 1954a,b; Rich, 1959a,b; Zubay and Wilkins, 1960; Brown and Zubay, 1960); although they contain the main elements of the double helical diffraction pattern, they do not show the same high degree of regularity. That there is some kind of double helical structure in RNA has also been indicated by solution studies (Doty *et al.*, 1959). In particular, the increase in optical density on heating is observed as in DNA. In contrast to DNA, however, the total increase in optical density is less, about 28 per cent increase in RNA and about 40 per cent increase in DNA; it occurs over a broad range of temperature from about 30° to 80°C. The exact range of temperature depends upon the precise solvent conditions and the particular RNA species being studied, but the results are generally the same. This smaller and more gradual increase in optical density with temperature observed in RNA suggests that the internucleotide hydrogen bonding is less regular than in DNA, and, together with the X-ray diffraction data, leads us to the conclusion that RNA has a double helical structure with less regularity in the base pairing. Different views on the detailed manner in which hydrogen bonds are made in RNA have been expressed (Zubay and Wilkins, 1960; Fresco, Alberts, and Doty, 1960). We (Zubay and Wilkins, 1960) have suggested that in the irregular double helix of RNA, bases between the two polynucleotide chains are randomly matched. We have also emphasized that the most stable hydrogen bonds in RNA will probably be those formed between 6-keto and 6-amino bases. The fact that most naturally occurring RNA's have approximately equal amounts of 6-keto and 6-amino bases (Elson and Chargaff, 1954) may be related to this.

We now ask whether the secondary structure observed in isolated nucleic acid is also found in nucleoproteins. In the case of the two deoxynucleoproteins we are considering, the regularly hydrogen-bonded structure is almost certainly preserved. Thus, the same type of X-ray diffraction pattern indicative of the double helical structure is observed for deoxynucleoproteins as is observed for DNA, although the packing of the double helices next to one another does not have the same degree of crystalline regularity. Also, when dispersed in solution the nucleohistone molecule shows the same sharp increase in optical density on heating as is shown by DNA (Zubay and Doty, 1959). Nucleoprotamine cannot be dispersed, (Zubay and Doty, 1959), and so comparable solution studies on this deoxynucleoprotein have not been made.

In the case of ribonucleoproteins, the situation is less clear, except for tobacco mosaic virus, where it has been firmly established by Franklin, Caspar, and Klug (1959), that the RNA molecule exists as a single extended polynucleotide chain with no internucleotide hydrogen bonding. This case may be exceptional, however, because of the small amount of RNA in that system, and when we consider the most common ribonucleoproteins of the cell, the ribosomes, we find that the X-ray diffraction data and the optical density data point to the double helical structure as it is observed for isolated RNA (Zubay and Wilkins, 1960; Schlessinger, 1960; Hall and Doty, 1959). Also, in the case of spherical ribonucleoprotein viruses, the hyperchromic data argues in favor of some double helical character in the RNA (Zubay and Wilkins, 1960; Schlessinger, 1960).

The present evidence, then, suggests that in the four nucleoprotein systems being considered, the nucleic acid preserves its double helical structure when complexed with protein, whether this is a regular double helix as in the deoxynucleoproteins, or an irregular double helix as in ribosomes. The underlying structural principle involved appears to be one of thermodynamic stability. Thus, the most stable situation for the nucleic acid is that containing the maximum number of hydrogen bonds, and hydrogen bonds are formed most easily and efficiently when two polymeric nucleic acid chains interact in a helical duplex. In the case of nucleohistone and ribosomes, there are good indications from hyperchromic data (Zubay and Wilkins, 1960; Zubay and Doty, 1959) that the nucleic acid hydrogen-bonded configuration is considerably stabilized in the nucleoprotein.

The second aspect of nucleoprotein I should like to consider is the nature of the secondary structure of the protein component. In X-ray diffraction we have found (Wilkins, Zubay, and Wilson, 1959; Zubay and Wilkins, unpublished data) that the nucleic acid and the protein behave partly like a mixture, even though they are known to be bonded to one another as a molecular complex. For instance, in nucleohistone and nucleic acid part of the diffraction pattern seen at high humidity disappears upon dehydration, and one is left with two diffraction rings at 9.7 Å and 4.7 Å. Pure histone gives a diffraction pattern similar to dehydrated nucleohistone. For this reason we believe the dehydrated nucleohistone pattern to be due to the protein component alone. This change in the nucleohistone diffraction pattern upon dehydration is completely reversible. The 9.7 Å and 4.7 Å diffraction rings show no orientation in nucleohistone samples where the DNA component is well oriented. The diffraction pattern of the hisone has been interpreted (Zubay and Wilkins, to be published) as being caused by an α-helix configuration.

A similar situation exists regarding these two strong diffraction rings in both ribosomes and TYMV (Zubay and Wilkins, 1960), although no orientation studies have been made. In contrast to the others, dehydrated nucleoprotamine shows only one strong diffraction ring in the 4.3 Å region in the X-ray pattern (Zubay and Wilkins, unpublished data). A similar strong diffraction ring is observed in isolated preparations of protamine. These studies suggest that the group of four nucleoproteins we are considering may be divided into two classes with respect to the secondary structure of the protein component: nucleohistone, ribosomes and TYMV, which give the two strong diffraction rings at 4.7 Å and 9.7 Å in the dried material, and nucleoprotamine, which gives only one strong diffraction ring in the 4.3 Å region.

Rate of deuteration studies on the same materials have supported this division into two groups (Wilkins, Wilkinson, and Zubay, unpublished data). Here it has been found that a large number of the peptide N-H groups in nucleohistone, ribosomes and TYMV take several weeks to deuterate, whereas the peptide N-H groups in nucleoprotamine deuterate completely in a matter of hours. This evidence is consistent with the X-ray data, and with it suggests that a substantial portion of the protein in the first three nucleoproteins are in the folded or alpha form, while in nucleoprotamine the polypeptide chain exists completely in an extended beta or an unhydrogen-bonded form. In the case of nucleohistone, earlier measurements by optical dispersion suggested that about two thirds of the histone is in the alpha form (Zubay and Doty, 1959).

With the secondary structure of the nucleic acid and protein in mind, we now approach the question of how the protein is arranged about the nucleic acid. Let us first consider the deoxynucleoproteins. One approach to this problem has been to compare the observed X-ray diffraction pattern for the nucleoproteins with that calculated for possible molecular models. Here we take advantage of the fact that the configuration of DNA is accurately known. The surface of the DNA molecule contains two helical grooves. The smaller of these grooves is about 12 Å across, the larger about 18 Å. If the protein combines regularly with the DNA in these grooves, it should change the relative intensity on the different layer lines in the helical part of the diffraction pattern. The most striking difference between the transformation of nucleoprotamine and that of DNA itself is found to be an intensified first layer line in the nucleoprotamine. By exploring various molecular models for nucleoprotamine, Feughelman and his associates (1955) found that a most reasonable way to achieve this type of transform was to place the backbone of the polypeptide chain of protamine as an extended chain in the narrow groove of DNA so as to wind around an individual DNA molecule. The disposition of the protein relative to the DNA in nucleohistone is more complicated (Wilkins, Zubay, and Wilson, 1959; Zubay and Wilkins, unpublished data). First, the diffraction pattern is less clear and the lattice is uncertain, making a quantitative evaluation of the X-ray data impossible. Second, there are additional spacings not present in the diffraction pattern of DNA at all. On the basis of the present X-ray data it is not possible to say with certainty where the protein is situated relative to the DNA. However, some possible molecular models can be ruled out. Thus, a model with two extended polypeptide chains in both grooves would not be possible, for this would lead to a clear intensification of the fourth layer. This layer line is very faint in the diffraction pattern. The transformation of nucleohistone with regard to relative intensities on the different layer lines is not very different from that of DNA itself. Calculations of the molecular transforms show that this is consistent with, but not strong support for, the model proposed by Doty and myself (Zubay and Doty, 1959) for nucleohistone with the polypeptide chain consisting primarily of an interrupted α-helical chain wound around the DNA in the large groove.

In ribosomes, the diffraction data are too vague to allow any judgments to be made about the position of the protein relative to the RNA. In the case of TYMV, Markham demonstrated that the protein occurs as a shell around the nucleic acid (Markham, 1951). This arrangement of a spherical virus with a protein shell and a nucleic acid core is believed to be quite general (Franklin, Caspar, and Klug, 1959; Crick and Watson, 1956; Klug and Finch, 1960), and may be conveniently demonstrated in the electron microscope by use of a complex technique of staining (Huxley and Zubay, 1960). An electron micrograph of TYMV illustrating this technique is presented in Figure 1. Here we see an array of TYMV particles. The centers of the particles have been strongly stained with uranyl acetate, and the entire particles are surrounded by phosphotungstic acid (PTA). Under these conditions, the protein shell of the virus shows up by negative contrast, since it is much less dense than the uranyl acetate-stained nucleic acid core or the PTA outside the virus. When this technique of outlining the protein shell is applied to *E. coli* ribosomes (Huxley and Zubay, 1960b), no evidence for a protein shell is found. We conclude that in *E. coli* ribosomes the existence of a closely packed protein shell is most unlikely.

The final aspect of structure we shall consider is the tertiary structure of the nucleoproteins. X-ray diffraction studies have shown that it is common for nucleoprotamine to consist of well-oriented and nearly close-packed DNA and protein molecules. We know, both from X-ray diffraction (Feughelman *et al.*, 1955) and from solution studies (Zubay and Doty, 1959) that naturally occurring nucleoprotamines will only swell to a very limited extent and show no tendency to disperse in solution. This indicates a rigid cross-linked network in nucleoprotamine which is not easily broken (Zubay and Doty, 1959). It seems reasonable that the protamine provides this cross-linking network by making occasional bridges between two or more DNA molecules.

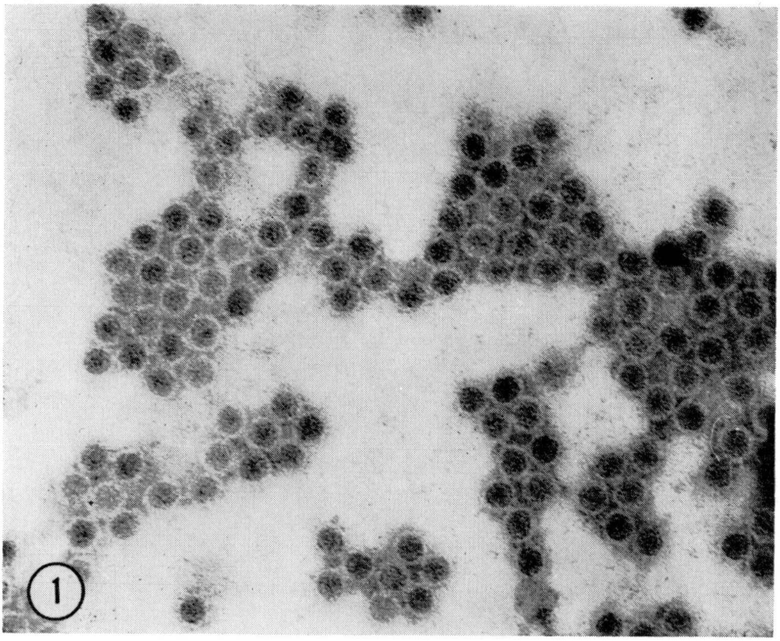

FIG. 1. Electron micrograph of turnip yellow mosaic virus (TYMV) illustrating staining technique for outlining protein shell of virus.

The tertiary structure of nucleohistone is less clearly understood, but also, perhaps, more interesting, because nucleohistone appears to be involved in a considerably greater amount of metabolic activity. A good deal of information about the tertiary structure of nucleohistone comes from X-ray diffraction and electron microscopy. In X-ray diffraction, nucleohistone gives a spacing not present in DNA or histone diffraction patterns with meridional orientation in oriented samples of nucleohistone (Wilkins, Zubay, and Wilson, 1959). We believe this is due to histone bridges formed between DNA molecules. When the degree of hydration is increased, as it would be *in vivo*, we find that the average distance between DNA molecules increases to more than 35 Å, and becomes so irregular beyond this point that we no longer obtain a diffraction spot for the distance between DNA molecules. In spite of this, the spacing suggestive of a bridged structure remains. X-ray diffraction, then, gives us the impression of readily extendible protein bridges existing between DNA molecules.

Unlike nucleoprotamine, it is possible to disperse nucleohistone indefinitely in aqueous medium until one obtains a solution of individual nucleohistone molecules consisting of one DNA molecule and an approximately equal weight of histone (Zubay and Doty, 1959). This testifies to the lability of these histone bridges in nucleohistone. However, nucleohistone molecules possess a pronounced tendency to gel, and if the concentration of nucleohistone is increased above 0.1 per cent in aqueous solution, a gel structure is formed. This gel structure is indicative of substantial interaction between nucleohistone molecules which is very likely to be mediated by the protein bridges observed in X-ray diffraction. A study of artificially stretched nucleohistone in the electron microscope has confirmed the existence of bridges between the DNA molecules (Huxley and Zubay, unpublished data). From a preliminary study of whole thymus tissue in the electron microscope, we can say that the nucleohistone occurs as fibrils about 70 to 110 Å in diameter. This is considerably greater than the diameter of an individual nucleohistone molecule, and similar types of histone bridges might hold these fibrils together. The main advantage of these readily extendible histone bridges from a biochemical point of view would appear to be that they provide the nucleohistone with structural integrity in a flexible network, giving greater access to the DNA in chemical reactions.

Finally, let us consider the tertiary structure of ribonucleoproteins. In TYMV we know very little about the tertiary structure of the nucleic acid core, except for the recent information from Klug and Finch (1960) that it must be arranged inside the TYMV particle with cubic symmetry. For the protein, however, we know much more. Thus, in X-ray diffraction the protein of TYMV shows cubic symmetry as well as strong indications of fivefold axes of symmetry (Klug, Finch, and Franklin, 1957). These results, together with recent results from electron microscopy, have made it possible to demonstrate that the TYMV coat consists of 32 subunits, 20 of one type and 12 of another, arranged very nearly as they would be in a regular geometric figure, the rhombic triacontahedron (Huxley and Zubay, 1960b). A selected group of electron micrographs of the TYMV particles showing different faces of the virus is illustrated in Figure 2. These are compared with appropriate models made from ping-pong balls. In Figure 3 we see a drawing of the faces in the rhombic triacontahedron. The 32 protein subunits would lie on the vertices in this figure, so arranged that no very large cavities exist in the structure, consistent with their serving as a barrier to inhibit the nucleic acid from escaping and to

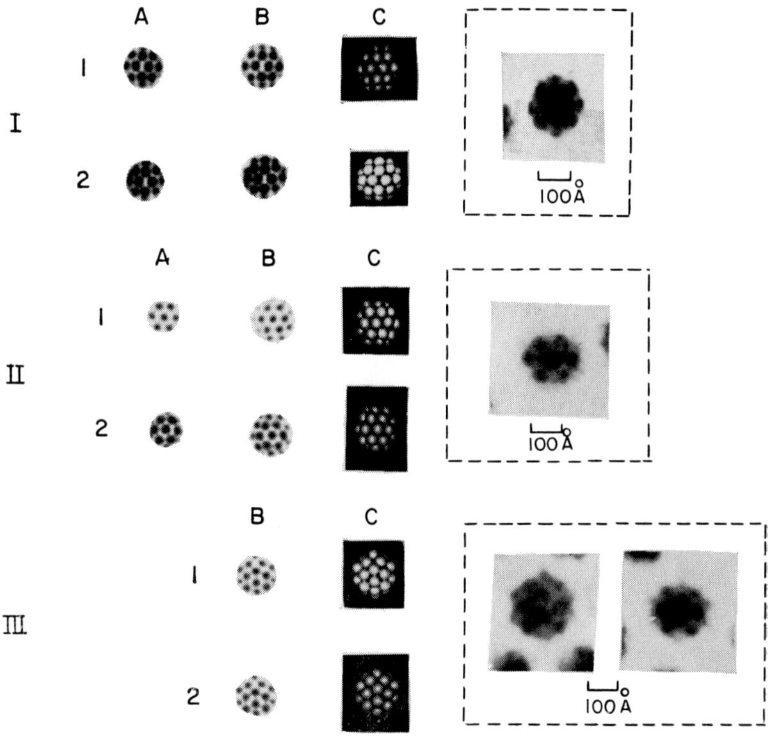

FIG. 2. Different views of the turnip yellow mosaic virus (TYMV) particle in the electron microscope compared with ping-pong ball models.

I. Orientation of TYMV particle is such as to show a diamond- or rhombus-shaped group of four subunits near the center of the particle. In many instances this can be seen to be the central group of subunits in two overlapping sets of [6 + 1] subunits. We consider that this corresponds to a view of the particle looking down a twofold axis. 1, Rhombic triacontahedron. 2, Pentakis dodecahedron.

II. Orientation of TYMV particle is such as to show a hexagonal ring of six subunits about a central subunit [6 + 1] on a face of the particle. We believe this view represents the appearance of the particle seen down a threefold axis. 1, Rhombic triacontahedron. 2, Pentakis dodecahedron.

III. Orientation of TYMV particle is such as to show two "intersecting" sets of [6 + 1] subunits (on the left and right side of the particle) having a common edge, two subunits near the centre of the particle being shared between the two sets. This corresponds, we believe, to a view of the particle looking along a direction in between two threefold axes, and is a particularly favorable one for it shows about half (14 out of 32) of the total number of subunits present.

The ping-pong ball models have been printed in different ways: A, printed through a mask so that only the group of subunits nearest the observer is seen. Contrast reversed.; B, Printed without mask, so that all subunits on the side facing the observer are seen. Contrast reversed; C, Printed with normal contrast.

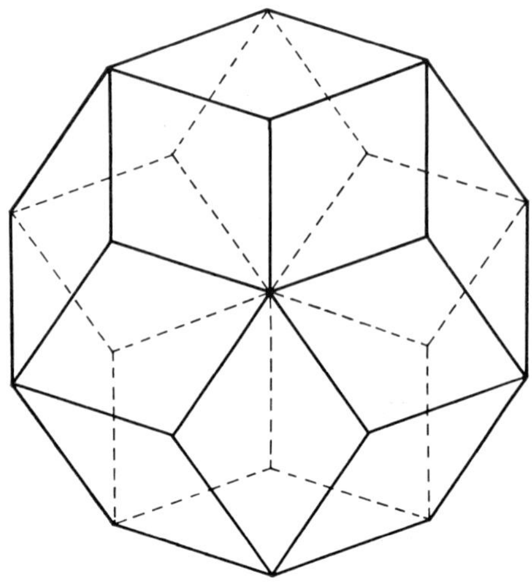

FIG. 3. Rhombic triacontahedron.

prevent destructive enzymes from entering.

The tertiary structure of the *E. coli* ribosomes is different from the viral nucleoprotein, and seems to be suited to their active metabolic role. From X-ray diffraction (Zubay and Wilkins, 1960) and electron microscopy (Huxley and Zubay, 1960a) we can say that the protein is not closely packed, nor does it form a tight shell around the nucleic acid. Rather, the nucleic acid and protein interact to form discrete nucleoprotein subunits containing the same relative amounts of nucleic acid and protein. The existence of nucleoprotein subunits was deduced from sedimentation studies (T'so, Bonner, and Vinograd, 1956; Chao and Schackman, 1956; Tissières and Watson, 1958), in which it was found that there is one subunit with a sedimentation constant of 50 Svedbergs (S), and one with a sedimentation constant of 30 S. These may aggregate to form a single component with a sedimentation constant of 70 S, and two 70 S components in turn dimerize to form a 100 S molecule. A negatively stained electron micrographic profile of a mixture of 70 S and 100 S ribonucleoprotein particles is shown in Figure 4. The field appears to contain primarily two types of particles, dimers and tetrameters with linearly arranged subunits in the latter. From a study of electron micrographs of this type and of the individual subunits, Huxley and I arrived at a model for the 100 S ribonucleoprotein shown in Figure 5. This 100 S particle is about 380 Å in length, and 150 Å in width. It would seem to have approximate

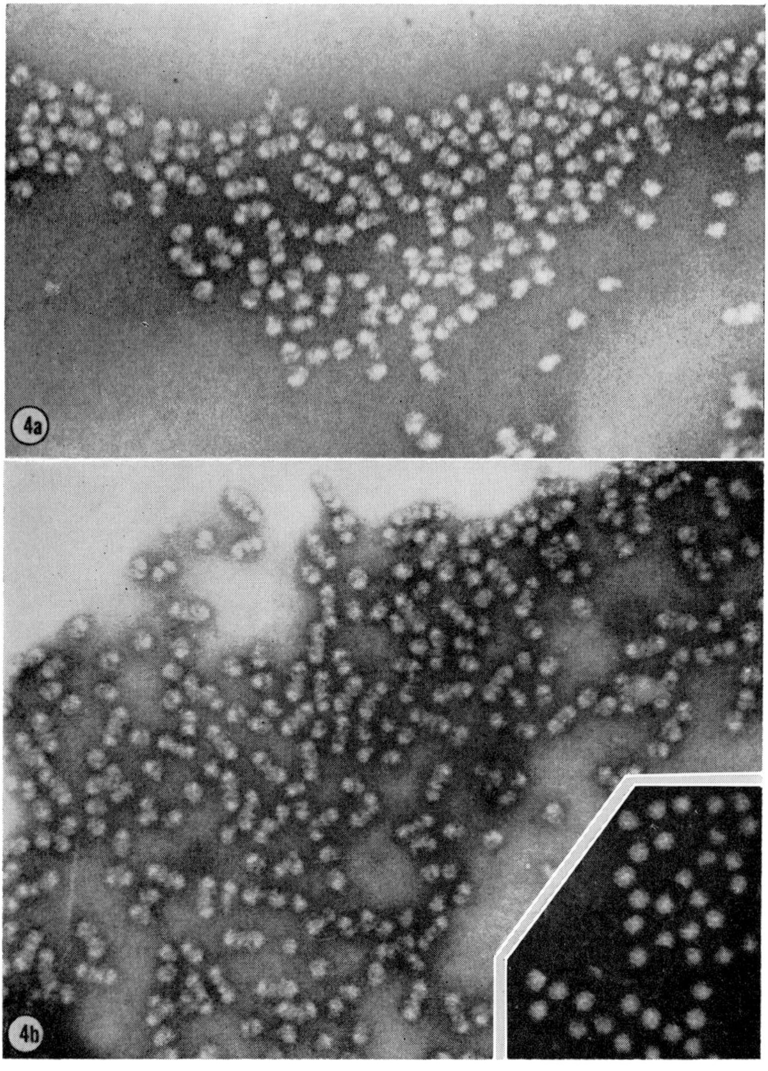

FIG. 4. Electron micrograph of negatively stained 70 to 100 S ribosomes.

cylindrical symmetry. In the region between the 50 S and 30 S subunits there exists a groove-shaped cavity about 25 Å across. The two interconnected 30 S subunits usually show a wedge-shaped cavity on one side. It is not known why this particular construction of the 100 S particle is most suitable for the ribosomes' role in protein synthesis. However, it is virtually a logical necessity for the RNA

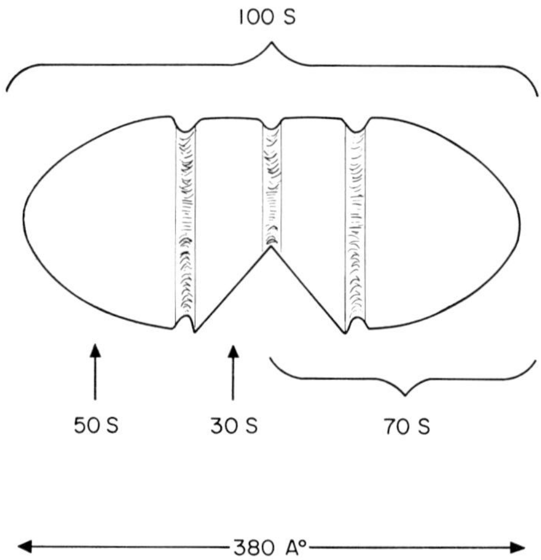

FIG. 5. Diagram of 100 S ribonucleoprotein molecule.

template to be carried by a single covalently linked sequence of nucleotides. In spite of this, *in vivo* and *in vitro* experiments (Lamborg and Zamecnik, 1960; McQuillen, Roberts, and Britten, 1959; Tissières, Schlessinger, and Gros, 1960) suggest that the 30 S and the 50 S subunits must be combined for effective protein synthesis to take place. Since there is no evidence for the breakage of primary valence bonds when these two unequally sized subunits are dissociated, it would seem likely that the RNA template is completely housed in only one of the subunits. If this is the case, we might wonder what the function of the other subunit is. It becomes an obvious speculation that the other subunit helps maintain the growing polypeptide chain in proper register. The fact that the effective ribonucleoprotein particle in protein synthesis is constructed of readily movable components strongly suggests that during some stage of protein synthesis the components move, one relative to the other. The possible types of motion we might consider are translational or rotational. In the case of translational motion, we might visualize the two ribonucleoprotein subunits as coming apart at one phase of protein synthesis, such as the termination of the synthesis of a polypeptide chain. The other type of action would be a rotational motion, where one subunit rotates relative to the other around the axis joining them. This would presumably be a regular stepwise motion, reflecting the stepwise synthesis of the polypeptide chain. I would like to go further and suggest that the guanosine triphosphate (GTP) (Hoagland *et al.*, 1958) known to be required at this final stage of peptide synthesis is used to supply the energy necessary for this regular movement of the two ribonucleoprotein subunits.

In summary, I would like to emphasize the structure-function relationship in our four nucleoproteins. In TYMV the nucleic acid is inaccessible insofar as it is confined to the inside of the virus. Similarly, in nucleoprotamine the nucleic acid is confined, not by being surrounded by protein as in the virus, but by being involved in a tightly cross-linked network with protein consisting of an almost close-packed array of double helices. In both of these nucleoproteins, the nucleic acid might be said to be in a resting state, and the function of the protein must be primarily to protect the nucleic acid and to hold it together in proper order. By contrast, in nucleohistone and ribosomes, these protective and integrating functions of the protein are combined to give a more flexible and open structure in which the nucleic acid is free to play an active biosynthetic role. The results of structural investigations so far represent only a beginning in the understanding of how the protein in nucleoproteins does its job so well.

In concluding, I should like to point out some aspects of nucleoprotein structure related to the subject of this conference—intracellular regulatory mechanisms in neoplastic tissue. Since there is no state in bacteria such as *E. coli* corresponding to neoplastic growth, we might inquire into those types of intracellular regulatory mechanisms which are unique to higher organisms where neoplasia occurs. Regulatory mechanisms involved in cellular differentiation come into this category. Most cells in higher organisms carry a full complement of chromosomal DNA. Despite this, it is clear that in any particular type of cell a great deal of the genetic information is turned off, not temporarily as in the case of inducible enzymes, but permanently. It is entirely plausible that the arrangement of histone plays a fundamental role in this type of regulation. In our studies of the structure of nucleohistone in higher organisms we have found that the histone is deposited rather uniformly about most of the DNA (Zubay and Doty, 1959; Wilkins, Zubay, and Wilson, 1959). In regions where it is present, histone may inhibit the DNA from its major interphase function of producing nuclear RNA. Thus, in any particular cell, only limited segments of the DNA molecule may be free of histone and function in the production of nuclear RNA. In *E. coli*, where there is little or no histone and the bulk of the DNA is not coated with protein (Zubay and Watson, 1959; Wilkins and Zubay, 1959), this type of regulatory mechanism could not exist. Possibly in a cancerous cell the arrangement of the histone becomes disturbed so that the disposition of active or inactive DNA regions is altered. The type of metabolic chaos which could result from a haphazard disruption of the histone reflects that existing in neoplastic tissue.

ACKNOWLEDGMENTS

I should like to thank my colleagues, M. H. F. Wilkins and H. E. H. Huxley, for their advice and technical assistance which made our work possible. I should also like to acknowledge the assistance rendered by G. R. Wilkinson in stimulating discussions on infrared spectroscopy.

REFERENCES

Brown, G. L., and G. Zubay. 1960. Physical Properties of the Soluble RNA of *Escherichia coli*. *Journal of Molecular Biology*, 2:287–296.

Chao, F. C., and H. K. Schachman. 1956. The Isolation and Characterization of a Macromolecular Ribonucleoprotein from Yeast. *Archives of Biochemistry and Biophysics*, 61:220–230.

Crick, F. H. C., and J. D. Watson. 1956. Structure of Small Viruses. *Nature, London*, 177:473–475.

Doty, P. 1956. The Properties of Biological Marcromolecules in Solution. *Proceedings of the National Academy of Sciences of the U.S.A.*, 42:791–800.

Doty, P., H. Boedtker, J. R. Fresco, R. Haselkorn, and M. Litt. 1959. Secondary Structure in Nucleic Acids. *Proceedings of the National Academy of Sciences of the U.S.A.*, 45:482–499.

Elson, D., and E. Chargaff. 1954. Regularities in the Composition of Pentose Nucleic Acids. *Nature, London*, 173:1037–1038.

Feughelman, M., R. Langridge, W. E. Seeds, A. R. Stokes, H. R. Wilson, C. W. Hooper, M. H. F. Wilkins, R. K. Barclay, and L. D. Hamilton. 1955. Molecular Structure of Deoxyribose Nucleic Acid and Nucleoprotein. *Nature, London*, 175:834–838.

Franklin, R. E., D. L. D. Caspar, and A. Klug. 1959. Plant Pathology: Problems and Progress, 1908–1958. *Golden Jubilee Volume of the American Phytopathological Society*, p. 447. Madison, Wisconsin: The University of Wisconsin Press.

Fresco, J. R., B. M. Alberts, and P. Doty. 1960. Some Molecular Details of the Secondary Structure of Ribonucleic Acid. *Nature, London*, 188:98–101.

Hall, B., and P. Doty. 1959. The Preparation and Physical Chemical Properties of Ribonucleic Acid from Microsomal Particles. *Journal of Molecular Biology*, 1:111–126.

Hoagland, M. B., M. L. Stephenson, J. F. Scott, L. I. Hecht, and P. C. Zamecnik. 1958. A Soluble Ribonucleic Acid Intermediate in Protein Synthesis. *Journal of Biological Chemistry*, 231:241–257.

Huxley, H. E., and G. Zubay. 1960a. Electron Microscope Observations on the Structure of Microsomal Particles from *Escherichia coli. Journal of Molecular Biology*, 2:10–18.

———. 1960b. The Structure of the Protein Shell of Turnip Yellow Mosaic Virus. *Journal of Molecular Biology*, 2:189–196.

Huxley, H. E., and G. Zubay. Unpublished data.

Klug, A., and J. T. Finch. 1960. The Symmetries of the Protein and Nucleic Acid in Turnip Yellow Mosaic Virus: X-Ray Diffraction Studies. *Journal of Molecular Biology*, 2:201–215.

Klug, A., J. T. Finch, and R. E. Franklin. 1957. The Structure of Turnip Yellow Mosaic Virus: X-Ray Diffraction tudies. *Biochimica et biophysica acta*, 25:242–252.

Lamborg, M. R., and P. C. Zamecnik. 1960. Amino Acid Incorporation into Protein by Extracts of *Escherichia coli. Biochimica et biophysica acta*, 42:206–211.

Langridge, R., D. A. Marvin, W. E. Seeds, H. R. Wilson, C. W. Hooper, M. H. F. Wilkins, and L. D. Hamilton. 1960. The Molecular Configuration of DNA. II. Molecular Models and Their Fourier Transforms. *Journal of Molecular Biology*, 2:38–64.

Langridge, R., H. R. Wilson, C. W. Hooper, M. H. F. Wilkins, and L. D. Hamilton. 1960. The Molecular Configuration of DNA. I. X-Ray Diffraction Study of Crystalline Form of the Lithium Salt. *Journal of Molecular Biology*, 2:19–37.

Markham, R. 1951. Physiochemical Studies of the Turnip Yellow Mosaic Virus. *Discussions of the Faraday Society*, 11:221–227.

McQuillen, K., R. B. Roberts, and R. J. Britten. 1959. Synthesis of Nascent Protein by Ribosomes in *Escherichia coli. Proceedings of the National Academy of Sciences of the U.S.A.*, 45:1437–1447.

Rich, A. 1959a. "The Bearing of Structural Studies on Relationships Between DNA and RNA." *A Symposium on Molecular Biology*, R. E. Zirkle, Ed., pp. 47–69. Chicago, Illinois: The University of Chicago Press.

———. 1959b. "Physical Studies on Ribonucleic Acid," *Structure and Function of Genetic Elements*, (Brookhaven Symposium in Biology, No. 12), pp. 17–26. Upton, New York: Brookhaven National Laboratory.

Rich, A., and J. D. Watson. 1954a. Some Relations Between RNA and DNA. *Proceedings of the National Academy of Sciences of the U.S.A.*, 40:759–764.

———. 1954b. Physical Studies on Ribonucleic Acid. *Nature, London*, 173:995–996.

Schlessinger, D. 1960. Hypochromicity in Ribosomes from *Escherichia coli. Journal of Molecular Biology*, 2:92–95.

Tissières, A., D. Schlessinger, and F. Gros. 1960. Amino Acid Incorporation into Proteins by *Escherichia coli* Ribosomes. *Proceedings of the National Academy of Sciences of the U.S.A.*, 46:1450–1463.

Tissières, A., and J. D. Watson. 1958. Ribonucleoprotein Particles From *Escherichia coli. Nature, London*, 182:778–780.

T'so, P. O. P., J. Bonner, and J. Vinograd. 1956. Microsomal Nucleoprotein Particles from Pea Seedlings. *The Journal of Biophysical and Biochemical Cytology*, 2:451–465.

Wilkins, M. H. F., G. R. Wilkinson, and G. Zubay. Unpublished data.

Wilkins, M. H. F., and G. Zubay. 1959. The Absence of Histone in the Bacterium *Escherichia coli.* II. X-Ray Diffraction of Nucleoprotein Extract. *The Journal of Biophysical and Biochemical Cytology,* 5:55–58.

Wilkins, M. H. F., G. Zubay, and H. R. Wilson. 1959. X-Ray Diffraction Studies of the Molecular Structure of Nucleohistone and Chromosomes. *Journal of Molecular Biology,* 1:179–185.

Zubay, G., and P. Doty. 1959. The Isolation and Properties of Deoxyriboprotein Particles Containing Single Nucleic Acid Molecules. *Journal of Molecular Biology,* 1:1–20.

Zubay, G., and M. R. Watson. 1959. The Absence of Histone in the Bacterium *Escherichia coli.* I. Preparation and Analysis of Nucleoprotein Extract. *Journal of Biophysical and Biochemical Cytology,* 5:51–54.

Zubay, G., and M. H. F. Wilkins. 1960. X-Ray Diffraction Studies of the Structure of Ribosomes from *Escherichia coli. Journal of Molecular Biology,* 2:105–112.

———. Unpublished data.

The Human Hemoglobins: Chemical Structure and Genetic Significance

V. M. Ingram, D.Sc., Ph.D.

Division of Biochemistry,
Department of Biology,
Massachusetts Institute of Technology,
Cambridge, Massachusetts

In recent years, studies on the chemical structure of the abnormal human hemoglobins have enabled us to illustrate several fundamental concepts of genetics, such as the chemical effect of mutation, allelism, effects of multiple heterozygosity, etc. This success is, in large measure, because of the concerted efforts of a large number of clinical and biochemical laboratories.

The peptide chains of the human hemoglobins are controlled by four distinct genes: called the α, β, γ, and δ genes (Ingram, 1960). They behave as if they were located on different chromosomes and, therefore, independently, with the exception of the β and δ genes, which seem to be linked (Cepellini, 1959), i.e., located near one another on the genetic map. These genes are thought to control the primary structure (Crick, 1958) of the corresponding α-, β-, γ-, and δ-peptide chains and, thereby, also their secondary and tertiary structure. The molecules of the different hemoglobin types are built up from these chains (Schroeder, 1959). The normal adult type is Hb-A = $\alpha_2^A\beta_2^A$, the normal fetal type Hb-F = $\alpha_2^A\gamma_2^F$, and the normal minor (about 2.5 per cent) component Hb-A_2 = $\alpha_2^A\delta_2^{A_2}$. There is considerable evidence that structurally the α chains are common to the three hemoglobin types and that they are under the control of *one and the same* α-chain gene. The present paper summarizes briefly some of the recent studies on the chemical structure of the inherited abnormal human hemoglobins as examples of the effect of gene mutations on the primary structure of a protein (Ingram, 1960). Only those cases will be mentioned in which, at the time of writing February 1961), an amino acid substitution has been assigned to a particular position or to a particular fragment of the molecule of the abnormal hemoglobin.

TABLE 1*

Some Abnormal Human Hemoglobins

α-Chain Variants		*Reference*
Hb–D_{α}	$\alpha_2^{TpIV}\beta_2^A$	(Benzer, Ingram, and Lehmann, 1958)
—$G_{Philadelphia}$	$\alpha_2^{68Lys}\beta_2^A$	(Baglioni and Ingram, 1961)
—$G_{Honolulu}$	$\alpha_2^{30GluNH_2}\beta_2^A$	(Hill, unpublished material)
—I	$\alpha_2^{16Asp}\beta_2^A$	(Murayama and Ingram, 1959)
—"Norfolk"	$\alpha_2^{57Asp}\beta_2^A$	(Baglioni, 1961)
β-Chain Variants		
Hb–S	$\alpha_2^A\beta_2^{6Val}$	(Ingram, 1957, 1959; Hunt and Ingram, 1959)
—C	$\alpha_2^A\beta_2^{6Lys}$	(Hunt and Ingram, 1958, 1959, 1960)
—$G_{San\ José}$	$\alpha_2^A\beta_2^{7Gly}$	(Hill and Schwartz, 1959)
—E	$\alpha_2^A\beta_2^{26Lys}$	(Hunt and Ingram, 1959)
—D_{β}	$\alpha_2^A\beta_2^{TpIII}$	(Benzer, Ingram, and Lehmann, 1958)
—$D_{\beta\ Punjab}$	$\alpha_2^A\beta_2^{125GluNH_2}$	(Bowman and Ingram, in preparation)
—$D_{\gamma} = D_{\beta\ Punjab}$		(Benzer, Ingram, and Lehmann, 1958; Baglioni, in preparation; Bowman and Ingram, 1961)
γ-Chain Variants		
None localised to a particular peptide		
δ-Chain Variants		
None localised to a particular peptide		
Others		
Hb–H	β_4^A	(Jones, Schroeder, Balog, and Vinograd, 1959)
—"Barts"	γ_4^F	(Hunt and Lehmann, 1959)

* The superscripts "TpIV", etc., indicate that the abnormality is known to reside in the fourth tryptic peptide in the α or β chain, numbering from the N-terminus of the chain (Braunitzer *et al.*, 1960a,b). The superscripts "16Asp", etc., denote that, in the particular hemoglobin chain, the 16th amino acid from the N-terminus has been replaced by an aspartic residue. This provisional system of nomenclature was proposed by a group of workers in the field at the Hemoglobin Structure Workshop, Boston, December, 1960 (Gerald and Ingram, 1961).

Some of the results available at present are shown in Table 1. New examples are being added to this list almost every month. It can be seen that mutational alterations are distributed between both α and β chains and are not confined to a particular region of the molecule. In several other hemoglobin variants, it is already known or suspected that the mutation is located on the α or the β chain. There is apparently no correlation between the location or type of amino acid substitution and the degree of malfunctioning of the abnormal molecule. Presumably the explanation of abnormal behavior is to be sought in the altered three-dimensional structure of the molecule, which very likely results from a particular amino acid substitution. In addition, it is becoming apparent that the primary structure of hemoglobin from individuals in a normal population is fairly constant (Ingram, unpublished data), indicating rather close control of very stable genetic material over the synthesizing mechanism.

An interesting example of this is the simultaneous occurrence

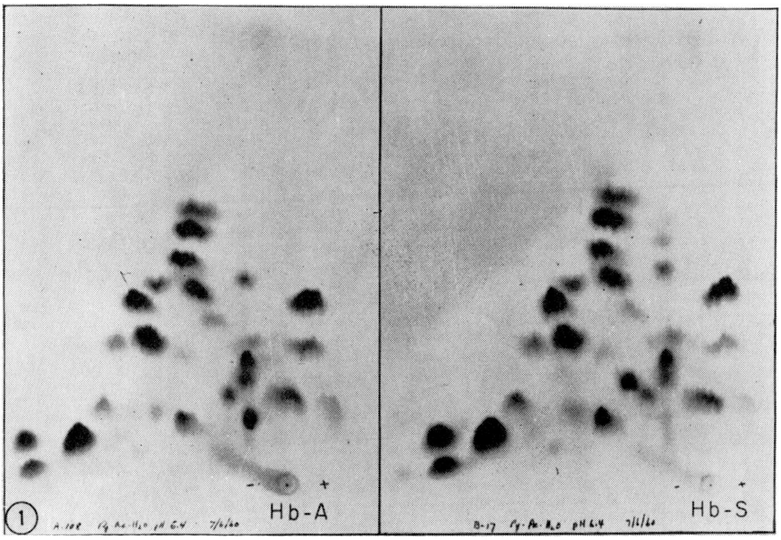

FIG. 1. Fingerprints of tryptic digests of hemoglobin A and S (courtesy of Dr. C. Baglioni). The electrophoresis was performed, as usual, in pyridine acetate buffer at pH 6.4 and chromatography in the vertical direction in pyridine: isoamyl alcohol: water. The tryptic peptide βTpI (originally called "number 4") clearly occupies different positions in the two fingerprints; this peptide carries the amino acid substitution referred to in Table 1. The method of fingerprinting has proved useful in the investigation of the chemical abnormalities in the abnormal hemoglobins.

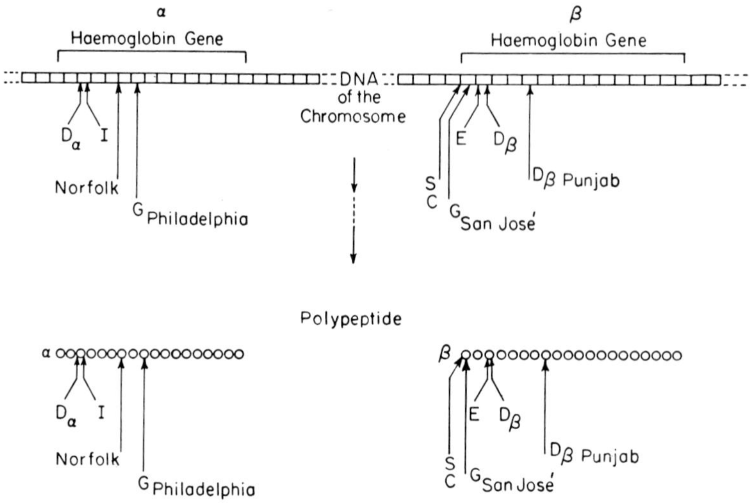

FIG. 2. Scheme of relation between gene and protein. The placing of mutations on the gene is deduced from their occurrence on the peptide chains.

of four distinct adult hemoglobins in one individual (Atwater, Schwartz, and Tocantins, 1960; Baglioni and Ingram, 1961). This person possesses roughly equal proportions of hemoglobin A ($\alpha_2^A\beta_2^A$), hemoglobin $G_{Philadelphia}$ ($\alpha_2^{68Lys}\beta_2^A$), hemoglobin C ($\alpha_2^A\beta_2^{6Lys}$), and hemoglobin "X" ($\alpha_2^{68Lys}\beta_2^{6Lys}$). Clearly, she is a double heterozygote for the G and C abnormalities on the α and the β gene, respectively. This person does not appear to suffer any ill effects from these abnormalities; in addition, it is clear that each gene makes the hemoglobin subunit characteristic of itself and that these subunits then associate in all possible combinations to form the hemoglobins.

It seems likely that the sequences in the γ-peptide chains of Hb-F will show that this chain is in many respects similar in its amino acid sequences to the β chain of Hb-A. This is particularly true of the first 30 amino acids of the chains, starting with the N-terminus. Interestingly enough, not only are there several single amino acid substitutions when comparing the γ chain of Hb-F with the β chain of Hb-A, but there is also an inversion of a sequence of two amino acids (Schroeder *et al.*, 1961). This is the first example of an inversion to be reported in related peptide chains. Whether this arose as the result of genetic inversion is, of course, completely unknown.

β Chain:—.Val.*Asp.Glu*.Val.Gly.Gly.—(positions 20–25)
(Braunitzer *et al.*, 1960a,b)

γ Chain:—.Val.*Glu.Asp*.Thr.Gly.Gly.—(Naughton, unpublished data; Schroeder *et al.*, 1961)

Stretton, (1960, 1961), has shown that the δ-peptide chains of hemoglobin A_2 differ from the closely related β chains in only five amino acid substitutions, though a few more might yet come to light. The substitutions for β chain $\rightarrow$ δ chain are: serine $\rightarrow$ asparagine, threonine $\rightarrow$ serine (2×), glutamic acid $\rightarrow$ alanine and ? $\rightarrow$ lysine. The reason for the presence of this minor hemoglobin component in normal blood has not been clearly explained. Even if it is confirmed that hemoglobin A_2 has a higher affinity for oxygen (Meyering, Israels, Sebens, and Huisman, 1960), it is difficult to see how this can be of use to the organism, since hemoglobin A_2 comprises only 2.5 per cent of all hemoglobins.

From a study of the amino acid composition and of the length of the hemoglobin peptide chains, and more particularly from their three-dimensional structure, their "fingerprints," and from sequence analysis, it has become clear that there is an over-all "family resemblance" in the structures of these chains. In other words, the α-, β-, γ-, and δ-peptide chains appear to be rather closely related. On the basis of such evidence, a scheme has been proposed (Braunitzer *et al.*, 1961b. Ingram, 1961) which pictures the evolution of the four modern hemoglobin genes as having been derived from one ancestral gene by processes involving gene duplication and translocation. Recently, the work of Braunitzer *et al.* (1961a,b), has lent great

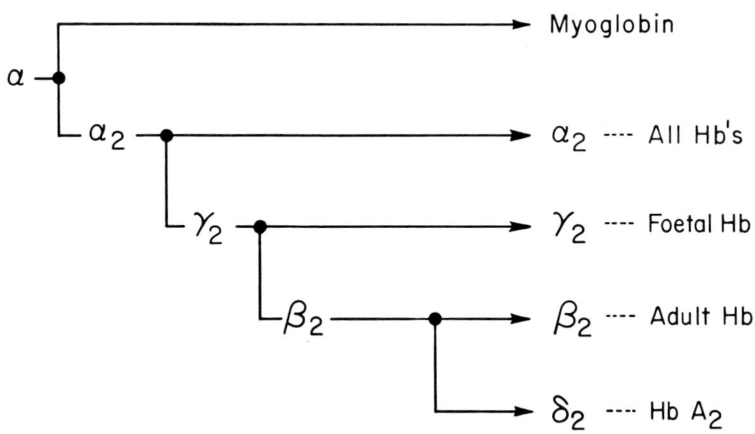

FIG. 3. Scheme for the evolution of the genes controlling the α-, β-, γ-, and δ-peptide chains of hemoglobin. The related muscle protein myoglobin is also included.

support to such a scheme. Their analysis of the human α and β chains shows strong evidence for the evolution of these chains from a common ancestral chain; they show an amazing degree of correspondence in their sequences.

In the evolutionary scheme (Ingram, 1961), the total number of genes increases, which to many people is a likely possibility. Presumably such a scheme covers the evolution of all the rather closely related vertebrate hemoglobins, culminating in the human hemoglobins. The hypothesis seeks to explain the fact that the amino acid sequences of β and δ chains are very closely similar (Stretton and Ingram, 1960; Ingram and Stretton, 1961) and that the sequences of the β and γ chains are more similar than either is to the α-peptide chain. The usual assumption is made that similarity in structure implies relatively recent divergence, and vice versa.

The combination of the recent X-ray work of Perutz *et al.* (1960) with the chemical investigations of Braunitzer *et al.* (1961a,b), Schroeder (1959); Schroeder *et al.* (1961), Konigsberg *et al.* (1961), Naughton (unpublished data), Stretton and Ingram (1960, 1961) and their colleagues is producing a detailed understanding of the structure of the hemoglobin molecule. We can expect that these studies will soon be complete. This will enable us to place the mutational alterations of the abnormal hemoglobins in their correct three-dimensional position in the molecule and to try to understand the reasons for their physiological malfunctioning; in addition, such knowledge will enable us to tackle, with more insight, the fundamental problem of the specific control of the synthesis or repression of different proteins (different hemoglobins) within the same cell. We can accept the thesis that the so-called structural genes control the primary structure of peptide chains and proteins; but how does the cell determine whether to make, for example, β-peptide chains or γ chains?

ACKNOWLEDGMENTS

The author wishes to acknowledge the support of grants from the National Science Foundation and the National Institutes of Health, United States Public Health Service.

REFERENCES

Atwater, J., I. R. Schwartz, and L. M. Tocantins. 1960. A Variety of Human Hemoglobin With 4 Distinct Electrophoretic Components. *Blood, The Journal of Hematology*, 15:901–908.

Baglioni, C. 1961. Chemistry of Hemoglobin-Norfolk, A Rare Variant of Human Hemoglobin. *Federation Proceedings*, 20:254, and *Journal of Biological Chemistry*, in press.

Baglioni, C., and V. M. Ingram. 1961. Four Adult Haemoglobin Types in One Person. *Nature, London*, 189:465–467.

Benzer, S., V. M. Ingram, and H. Lehmann. 1958. Three Varieties of Human Haemoglobin D. *Nature, London*, 182:852–854.

Bowman, B., and V. M. Ingram. (1961). Abnormal Human Haemoglobins. VII. The Comparison of Normal Human Haemoglobin and Haemoglobin D CHICAGO. *Biochimica et biophysica acta*, 53:569–573.

Braunitzer, G., R. Gehring-Müller, N. Hilschmann, K. Hilse, G. Hobom, V. Rudloff, and B. Wittmann-Liebold. 1961a. Konstitution des normalen adulten Humanhämoglobins. *Zeitschrift für Physiologische Chemie*, 325:283–286.

Braunitzer, G., N. Hilschmann, V. Rudloff, K. Hilse, B. Liebold, and R. Müller. 1961b. The Haemoglobin Particles. *Nature, London*, 190:482–482.

Cepellini, R. 1959. "Physiological Genetics of Human Blood Factors," *Biochemistry of Human Genetics*, G. E. W. Wolstenholme and C. M. O'Connor, Eds., p. 242. London, England: J. & A. Churchill, Ltd.

Crick, F. H. C. 1958. "On Protein Synthesis," *Symposium for Society of Experimental Biology*, Vol. 12, p. 138.

Gerald, P. S., and V. M. Ingram. 1961. Recommendations for the Nomenclature of Hemoglobins. *Journal of Biological Chemistry*, 236:2155–2156.

Hill, R. L. Unpublished data.

Hill, R. L., and H. C. Schwartz. 1959. A Chemical Abnormality in Haemoglobin G. *Nature, London*, 184(Supplement 9):641–642.

Hunt, J. A., and V. M. Ingram. 1958. Allelomorphism and the Chemical Differences of the Human Haemoglobins A, S and C. *Nature, London*, 181:1062–1063.

Hunt, J. A., and V. M. Ingram. 1959a. A Terminal Peptide Sequence of Human Haemoglobin? *Nature, London*, 184(Supplement 9):640–641.

Hunt, J. A., and V. M. Ingram. 1959b. Human Haemoglobin E: the Chemical Effect of Gene Mutation. *Nature, London*, 184:870–872.

Hunt, J. A., and V. M. Ingram. 1960. Abnormal Human Haemoglobins: IV. The Chemical Difference Between Normal Human Haemoglobin and Haemoglobin C. *Biochimica et biophysica acta*, 42:409–421.

Hunt, J. A., and H. Lehmann. 1959. Haemoglobin "Barts": A Foetal Haemoglobin Without α Chains. *Nature, London*, 184:872–873.

Ingram, V. M. Unpublished data.

———. 1957. Gene Mutations in Human Haemoglobin: The Chemical Difference Between Normal and Sickle Cell Haemoglobin. *Nature, London*, 180:326–328.

———. 1959. Abnormal Human Haemoglobin III: The Chemical Difference Between Normal and Sickle Cell Haemoglobins. *Biochimica et biophysica acta*, 36:402–411.

———. 1960. "The Genetic Control of Protein Structure," *Genetics*, H. E. Sutton, Ed., pp. 65–176. New York, New York: Josiah Macy, Jr., Foundation.

———. 1961. Evolution of the Haemoglobin Genes. *Nature, London,* 189: 704–708.

Ingram, V. M., and A. O. W. Stretton. 1961. Human Haemoglobin A_2. *Nature, London,* 190:1079–1084.

Jones, R. T., W. A. Schroeder, J. E. Balog, and J. R. Vinograd. 1959. Gross Structure of Hemoglobin H. *Journal of the American Chemical Society,* 81:3161.

Konigsberg, W., G. Guidotti, and R. J. Hill. 1961. Amino Acid Sequence of the α Chain of Human Hemoglobin. *Journal of Biological Chemistry,* 236: PC55–56.

Meyering, C. A., A. L. M. Israels, T. Sebens, and T. H. J. Huisman. 1960. Studies on the Heterogeneity of Hemoglobin. II. The Heterogeneity of Different Human Hemoglobin Types in Carboxymethylcellulose and in Amberlite IRC-50 Chromatography; Quantitative Aspects. *Clinica chimica acta,* 5:208–222.

Murayama, M. 1960. The Chemical Difference Between Normal Human Hemoglobin and Hemoglobin I. *Federation Proceedings,* 19:78.

Murayama, M., and V. M. Ingram. 1959. Comparison of Normal Adult Human Haemoglobin with Haemoglobin I by Fingerprinting. *Nature, London,* 183:1798–1799.

Naughton, M. A. Unpublished data.

Perutz, M. F., M. G. Rossmann, A. F. Cullis, H. Muirhead, G. Will, and A. C. T. North. 1960. Structure of Haemoglobin. *Nature, London,* 185: 416–422.

Schroeder, W. A. 1959. "The Chemical Structure of the Normal Human Hemoglobins," *Progress in Chemistry of Organic Natural Products,* L. Zechmeister, Ed., Vol. 17, pp. 371–378. Vienna, Austria: Springer-Verlag.

Schroeder, W. A., R. T. Jones, J. R. Shelton, J. B. Shelton, J. Cormick, and K. McCalla. 1961. A Partial Sequence of the Amino Acid Residues in the γ Chain of Human Hemoglobin F. *Proceedings of the National Academy of Sciences of the U.S.A.,* 47:811–818.

Stretton, A. O. W., and V. M. Ingram. 1960. An Amino Acid Difference Between Human Hemoglobins A and A_2. *Federation Proceedings,* 19:343.

CONTROLLING MECHANISM AND ENZYME SYNTHESIS

Mutationally Altered Tryptophan Synthetase in *Neurospora crassa*

SIGMUND R. SUSKIND, PH.D., DOROTHY S. LIGON, A.B., AND MICHAEL CARSIOTIS,* PH.D.

McCollum-Pratt Institute,
The Johns Hopkins University,
Baltimore, Maryland

Current molecular genetic studies suggest that genetic control of enzyme formation and function is exerted by two classes of genes, the structural and the regulatory genes (Jacob, Shaeffer, and Wollman, 1960). It has been proposed that the structural genes are polynucleotide segments which control the primary structure or amino acid sequence of specific proteins. The regulatory genes, conversely, would function in a manner not concerned with denoting primary structure. Regulatory genes might play a role at some other stage in protein synthesis or in controlling the function of fully formed proteins. They may also provide a mechanism for controlling the expression of activity of adjacent genetic material (Jacob, Shaeffer, and Wollman, 1960; Vogel, 1961).

If one genetic function is to control the primary structure of protein and if the major responsibility for specifying the correct amino acid in a protein resides in a specific sequence of nucleotides in deoxyribonucleic acid (DNA), then modifications in nucleotide sequence might elicit the formation of mutationally altered proteins. These altered proteins could have unique physical or chemical properties that reflect changed amino acid sequence in the molecule.

---

* Postdoctoral Fellow, United States Public Health Service.

It has been suggested that the mutation which causes an incorrect amino acid to be substituted in a protein be called a "mis-sense" mutation, as opposed to a "non-sense" mutation, in which no amino acid is specified (Crick, 1959). This latter class of mutations, the non-sense type, might conceivably result in the formation of fragments of a protein, or perhaps no protein at all, since a necessary linking amino acid may be missing.

The specific question we would like to discuss in this paper, therefore, can be simply stated, though it is rather more difficult to answer. How are mutations of the "structural" and "regulatory" genes concerned with *Neurospora* tryptophan synthetase formation and function expressed in terms of the properties of the enzyme?

The Tryptophan Synthetase System

Figure 1 shows the three reactions in *Neurospora crassa* catalyzed by wild type tryptophan synthetase (Tsase), a single protein having a molecular weight of about 140,000 (Yanofsky, 1960; Bonner, Suyama, and DeMoss, 1960; Mohler and Suskind, 1960). The same reactions are catalyzed by tryptophan synthetase of *Escherichia coli*, but the *E. coli* enzyme can be readily dissociated into two

Reactions Catalyzed by Tryptophan Synthetase and Certain CRM Proteins

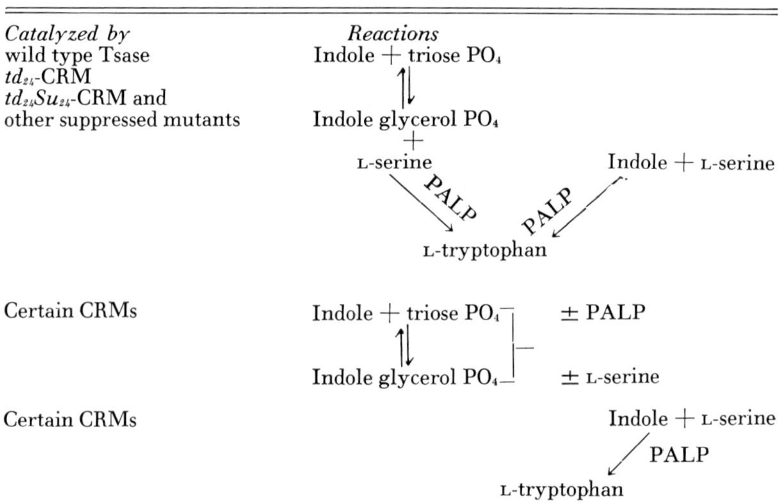

Fig. 1. Diagramatic representation of reactions catalyzed by tryptophan synthetase and certain cross-reactive proteins (CRM). (PALP = pyridoxal phosphate.)

protein components (called A and B), each having catalytic activity for part of the tryptophan synthetase reaction (Crawford and Yanofsky, 1958).

Many tryptophan-requiring mutants of *Neurospora* which are unable to form normal Tsase have been isolated (Bonner, 1959; Yanofsky, 1960). These mutants all appear to be damaged within a restricted genetic region of chromosome number two called the *td* locus. By genetic, precursor accumulation studies, enzymatic, and immunological methods, differences between many of these mutants have been established (Yanofsky and Bonner, 1955a; Suskind, Yanofsky, and Bonner, 1955; Suskind, 1957; Suyama, 1960; Lacy and Bonner, 1961). Employing rabbit antienzyme prepared against highly purified tryptophan synthetase, it is possible to demonstrate the presence, in certain mutants, of mutationally altered proteins called CRMs (cross-reactive material). These proteins retain sufficient structural similarity to normal Tsase to exhibit serological cross reaction with it. Interestingly enough, not all of the *td* mutants produce such defective proteins. All *td* mutants can be readily divided into two classes, CRM-positive and CRM-less, the latter class forming no protein recognizable by the standard method of CRM-determination (Suskind, Yanofsky, and Bonner, 1955; Suskind, 1957). It is to the CRM-positive mutants and to the types of defective proteins they produce that we will initially direct our attention.

Considerable evidence is now available to justify the statement that the CRM proteins in *Neurospora* represent mutationally altered tryptophan synthetase molecules. These studies include the detailed comparison of the normal enzyme and several of the CRM proteins by methods which include purification, column chromatography, sedimentation, antigenic and immunogenic characteristics, and residual enzymatic activities (DeMoss and Bonner, 1959; Mohler and Suskind, 1960; Carsiotis and Suskind, 1960; Suyama, 1960; Yanofsky, 1960). It is also clear that when a sufficient number of criteria are available for comparison, one finds that genetially distinct mutants form characteristic CRM proteins. Thus, it seems that different types of mutationally altered enzymes are formed as a consequence of damage to specific sites within the *td* genetic region. Furthermore, it appears that mutants which form similar types of altered Tsase molecules are all damaged in certain well-defined regions of the Tsase gene. On this basis, it is possible to envisage the Tsase gene as possessing a definite organization (Bonner, Suyama, and DeMoss, 1960) and, most interestingly, there are several striking similarities found between the Tsase genetic regions of *Neurospora* and *E. coli* (Yanofsky, 1960; Bonner, Suyama, and De Moss, 1960).

Certain *td* mutants of *Neurospora* can regain enzymatic activity when they form a heterocaryon, a mycelium containing nuclei of the two mutant types (Lacy and Bonner, 1961; Yanofsky, 1960). The detailed mechanism of this interaction, called "intragenic complementation," is not known, but one fact has become apparent: namely, CRM formation by both contributing mutants is a prerequisite (Lacy and Bonner, 1961). This suggests the possibility that protein-protein interactions of some sort may be involved in the complementation phenomenon (Woodward, 1960). As seen in Table 1, there appear to be five to six complementation groups among the *td* mutants (Lacy and Bonner, 1961). Hopefully, some information on the structure of Tsase may be available soon, so that the question of whether complementation represents a reaggregation of protein subunits of the enzyme or a reuniting of polypeptide chains may be investigated.

The mutational events discussed thus far all occur within the Tsase genetic region and might be thought of as alterations in the structural gene. Other genes are known in *Neurospora* (Yanofsky and Bonner, 1955a) which affect tryptophan synthetase activity, but whose locations are distant from the Tsase genetic region. Mutations of these genes, which are called suppressor genes, phenotypically reverse (suppress) the effect of primary mutations within the Tsase genetic region, permitting the mutant to form low levels of functional Tsase. These suppressor genes show a high degree of

TABLE 1

The Relationship Between CRM Formation, Complementation, and Suppression in Certain td Mutants of N. crassa

Mutational site map: 71 2 16 6 3 7 24 1 A-78

Mutant	CRM	Complements with mutants	Suppressed by *Su* gene
1	0	None	No known *Su* gene
16	0	None	No known *Su* gene
7	+	2, 71, A-78	No known *Su* gene
71	+	7, 3, 24, A-78	Su_3
2	+	7, 3, 24, A-78	Su_2, Su_6
6	+	3, 24, A-78	Su_6
3	+	2, 71, 6, A-78	Su_3, Su_{24}
24	+	2, 71, 6, A-78	Su_3, Su_{24}
A-78	+	2, 71, 6, 7, 3, 24	Information unavailable

Abbreviations: CRM, cross-reactive material.

specificity and are able to function only in conjunction with specific *td* mutants (Yanofsky and Bonner, 1955a). Conversely, there appear to be many different genetic sites which are able to function as specific suppressors of a given *td* mutant (Yanofsky and Bonner, 1955b). Hence, we find strict specificity of action and also a multiplicity of such specifically functioning genetic regions. A further word should be said about the requirements for such genetic interaction. In *Neurospora*, CRM formation appears to be a necessary but insufficient requirement for suppression (Bonner, personal communication). No CRM-less mutants are suppressible. More will be said subsequently about the nature of the CRM in suppressed and unsuppressed mutants.

Clearly, the CRM proteins can provide a clue to our eventual understanding of several fundamental problems. How are the CRM proteins made functional in certain "leaky" *td* mutants? What role do the CRM proteins play, at the molecular level, in the complementation and suppression phenomena? Do these "repair" mechanisms involve the formation of a fully normal enzyme, or simply the reactivation of specific CRM proteins? It was in the hope of answering some of these questions that the following work was pursued.

The Conversion of CRM to Tsase in a Temperature-Sensitive Mutant

A temperature-sensitive mutant of *Neurospora* was isolated (strain td_{24}) which forms little or no active Tsase at 25° C and which requires tryptophan at this temperature (Yanofsky and Bonner, 1955a). The slow growth of the organism on minimal medium can be initiated by elevating the growth temperature to 30° to 33°C. Does the increase in temperature effect the formation or the function of Tsase in this mutant?

It was found that crude extracts of mutant td_{24} contain considerable quantities of CRM, although the Tsase activity of such preparations is negligible compared to that of the wild type organism. On fractionation of these extracts, considerable Tsase activity can be recovered, ranging from 30 to 90 per cent of the normal level (Suskind and Kurek, 1957; Suskind and Ligon, unpublished data). When the enzyme and antigen units of the crude and fractionated samples are compared (Table 2), it can be seen that fractionation results in about a fivefold increase in the enzyme/antigen ratio of the extract. These results suggested that Tsase was activated by

TABLE 2

The Effect of Fractionation on the Enzyme/Antigen Ratio of Mutant td_{24} *and Suppressed Mutant* $td_{24}Su_{24}$

Mutant	Crude extract	Fractionated extract
td_{24}	$\frac{2.8\ TSU}{42.0\ AgU} = 0.067$	$\frac{128\ TSU}{380\ AgU} = 0.327$
$td_{24}Su_{24}$	$\frac{6.8\ TSU}{35.0\ AgU} = 0.194$	$\frac{145\ TSU}{197\ AgU} = 0.737$

Abbreviations: TSU, tryptophan synthetase unit; AgU, antigen unit.

fractionation and that this most likely involved the conversion of CRM to active enzyme.

The presence of residual CRM in these fractionated samples can be readily demonstrated by comparing the inhibitory effect of a calibrated antienzyme on the activity of normal Tsase and on the Tsase of fractionated td_{24}. As seen in the lower half of Table 3, an antiserum which has 243 antienzyme units/ml., when tested against normal Tsase, has an apparent value of only 21.7 units/ml. when standardized with fractionated td_{24}. Clearly these td_{24} samples contain an antigen, in addition to active Tsase, which competes with Tsase for the available antibody.

Further studies on the nature of the conversion of CRM to active Tsase indicated that the td_{24} extracts contained an inhibitor which

TABLE 3

A Comparison of the Antigenic Properties of Normal Tryptophan Synthetase and CRM from Mutants td_{24} *and* td_3 *and from Suppressed Mutant* $td_{24}Su_{24}$

	Antigen units/ml.	
Tsase or CRM	Calculation based on reaction with anti-Tsase (C-84)	Calculation based on reaction with anti-CRM (td_{24})
Tsase (C-84)	195	180
Tsase (5297)	182	174
td_{24}-CRM	345	175
$td_{24}Su_{24}$-CRM	231	150
td_3-CRM	247	165
	Antibody units (anti-enzyme units/ml. serum)	
Antiserum	Calculation based on reaction with Tsase (C-84)	Calculation based on reaction with td_{24}-CRM
Anti-Tsase (C-84)	243.0	21.7
Anti-CRM (td_{24})	40.6	6.4

Abbreviations: CRM, cross-reactive material; Tsase, tryptophan synthetase.

inactivated the td_{24} enzyme, but which had no effect on normal Tsase at equivalent concentrations (Suskind and Kurek, 1957). It was subsequently found that all wild type and *td* extracts contained a factor which would inhibit td_{24} Tsase, and that the substrates and coenzyme for the Tsase reaction did not reduce the inhibition. Studies with the inhibitory ammonium sulphate fraction of td_{24} extracts indicated that the factor was heat stable, dialyzable, precipitable by trichloroacetic acid, and eluted with 0.1 M phosphate buffer, pH 7.8. Inhibitor was recovered after ashing the sample and after refluxing in hydrochloric acid, supporting the view that the inhibitor was a metal (Suskind and Kurek, 1957). It has not been possible to effect a conversion of td_{24}-CRM to active Tsase by salt dissociation or by dialysis, but extraction of lyophilized mycelia with a solution containing pyridoxal phosphate, L-serine and ethylenediamine tetraacetic acid (EDTA) gives some increase in Tsase activity.

The components of the trace element mixture used in *Neurospora* minimal medium were screened against td_{24} Tsase to determine their inhibitory effect. The most effective inhibitor in the mixture was zinc, at a concentration (10^{-5}M) which did not inhibit normal Tsase. While this suggests that the inhibitor in *Neurospora* extracts may be zinc, no metal analyses on inhibitor preparations have been carried out. However, the effect on td_{24} enzymatic activity of both the inhibitor and of zinc can be reversed by EDTA (10^{-3} M) and the enzyme can be protected against both inhibitor and zinc by EDTA-containing solutions.

It should be noted that neither zinc, the inhibitor, nor EDTA have any effect on td_{24} antigenic activity. Furthermore, antisera prepared against inhibitor-containing fractions of *Neurospora* do not block the reaction of inhibitor with td_{24} Tsase.

Properties of td_{24}-CRM

On the basis of the inhibitor studies, it was suggested that the CRM in td_{24} actually represented a mutationally altered, metal-sensitive Tsase molecule (Suskind and Kurek, 1957). In order to further understand the nature of this alteration, and to relate it to the *in vivo* behavior of the mutant, a study of the properties of the td_{24} protein was undertaken and a comparison made with the normal enzyme. The results of these experiments are summarized in Table 4 and experimental details will appear elsewhere (Suskind

TABLE 4

A Summary of the Properties of Normal Tryptophan Synthetase and Mutationally Altered Tryptophan Synthetase from Mutant td_{24} *and Suppressed Mutant* $td_{24}Su_{24}$

Criterion	Normal	td_{24}	$td_{24}Su_{24}$
In vitro			
1. Sensitivity to zinc (10^{-5} M)	resistant	sensitive	sensitive
2. Lability to overnight dialysis (4°C)	stable	labile	labile
3. Lability to 55°C (5 minutes)	stable	labile	labile
4. Apparent energy of activation (range 25°C to 45°C)	9 to 10 kilocalories	30 to 50 kilocalories	30 to 50 kilocalories
5. Immunological properties	normal	altered	altered
6. Enzyme/antigen ratio following fractionation	not increased	increased	increased
7. Ratio of activities: indole glycerol phosphate + L-serine → L-tryptophan / indole + L-serine → L-tryptophan	0.38	0.31	0.45
In vivo			
8. Effect of zinc deficiency on growth	inhibitory	little effect	little effect
9. EDTA stimulation of resting cell tryptophan synthetase activity	not known	increased	not known
10. Tryptophan repression of Tsase or CRM formation	slight	slight	not known
11. Effect of temperature on growth	growth on minimal medium at 25°C	no growth on minimal medium at 25°C, but slow growth at 30° to 33°C	growth on minimal medium at 25°C

Abbreviations: EDTA, ethylenediaminetetraacetic acid; Tsase, tryptophan synthetase; CRM, cross-reactive material.

and Ligon, unpublished data). Several points should be made concerning these results. The dialysis lability of td_{24} enzymatic and antigenic activities is evident in the presence of EDTA (10^{-2} M), pyridoxal phosphate (10^{-4} M), L-serine (10^{-4} M), and phosphate buffer. Under these conditions normal Tsase is stable. The antigenic activity of td_{24} is much more stable to dialysis against phosphate buffer in the absence of EDTA, pryidoxal phosphate, and L-serine, conditions in which normal Tsase is inactivated. Hence, it appears that dialysis against EDTA-containing solutions may be converting CRM to enzymatically active Tsase, as suggested by the EDTA results mentioned earlier, but that the active td_{24} Tsase is highly labile. Additional evidence supports this view. For example, both the enzymatic and antigenic activities of the td_{24} protein are extremely heat labile, as contrasted with the normal enzyme.

Of considerable importance is the apparent energy of activation of the td_{24} Tsase for the indole + L-serine → L-tryptophan reaction. This inordinately high value of 30 to 50 kilocalories, measured in the range 25° to 45° C, provides an explanation for the *in vivo* temperature-growth response of the mutant between 30° to 33° C. It should be noted that mixtures of normal and td_{24} Tsase give the intermediate energy of activation expected for a system exhibiting no interaction. In addition, td_{24} Tsase preincubated at 37° C returns to its inactive form when the temperature is reduced to 25° C, in agreement with *in vivo* results; e.g., 30° C-grown cells (minimal medium) cease growing when transferred to 25° C. As seen in Table 4, the ratio of two of the tryptophan synthetase reactions of fractionated td_{24} does not differ significantly from the normal value.

As indicated in Tables 3, 4, and 5, there are distinct serological differences between normal Tsase (strains C-84 and 5297) and the

TABLE 5

*Molecular Combining Ratios of Anti-Tsase/Tsase and Anti-Tsase/CRM**

Antigen	Antibody	Ab/Ag molecular ratio at equivalence
C-84 Tsase	anti-Tsase	2.5
td_{24}-CRM	anti-Tsase	8
$td_{24}Su_{24}$-CRM	anti-Tsase	9

* Based on: Tsase molecular weight = 140,000; assumed molecular weight = 140,000 of td_{24}-CRM and $td_{24}Su_{24}$-CRM; rabbit γ-globulin molecular weight = 188,000.

Abbreviations: Tsase, tryptophan synthetase; CRM, cross-reactive material; Ab/Ag, antibody/antigen.

td_{24} protein. However, in contrast to the effect of temperature on td_{24} enzymatic activity, differences in the antigen-antibody neutralization reactions are not apparent if the system is preincubated at 30° C *versus* 0° C or if the antienzyme is assayed at 25° C *versus* 37° C. Hence, whatever subtle structural changes occur as a function of temperature are not discernible by an immunochemical test.

As summarized in Table 5, one can conclude either that the td_{24} protein has three to four times the number of combining sites per molecule of 140,000 molecular weight, or that the td_{24} molecule is composed of three to four subunits each of molecular weight 30,000 to 40,000. In either case, it is quite clear that a major configurational difference exists between the normal and the mutant molecule, and it is hoped that additional experiments will clarify this point. It should be emphasized that similar experiments conducted with mutant td_2 failed to resolve any immunochemical difference between normal Tsase and td_2-CRM (Carsiotis and Suskind, 1960).

On the Action of Suppressor Genes

As mentioned, several important points are known about suppressor genes which affect certain *td* mutants. These include: (1) their location at genetic sites distinct from the *td* locus; (2) their function only in conjunction with specific *td* alleles; (3) the recurrence of nonallelic suppressor genes exhibiting the same *td*-allele specificity; and finally, (4) the requirement of CRM formation for effective genetic suppression of the *Neurospora td* mutants. Some of these relationships are summarized in Table 1.

The prerequisite for CRM formation suggests that a protein of a certain type or size may be needed for effective supressor-gene action. One exception to this generalization has been found in mutant td_7. This mutant forms considerable quantities of CRM, as judged by neutralization tests, but no suppressor gene has yet been isolated in this mutant which will restore Tsase function (Bonner, personal communication). Recently some evidence has been obtained at our laboratory which indicates that td_7-CRM is unlike any of the CRMs formed by the suppressible *td* mutants. When td_7-CRM was tested for precipitation with anti-enzyme in agar diffusion or tube precipitin tests, it proved to be inactive. However, if td_7-CRM is mixed with normal Tsase at increasing ratios of td_7-CRM to Tsase, it blocks precipitation of the homologous Tsase/anti-Tsase reaction. These preliminary results would support the view that there is a minimum of genetic information which must be present in the *Neurospora td* region before a suppressor gene can function, and that CRM-less mutants and mutants of the td_7 type fall below this minimum requirement. From this, it would follow that a potentially functional protein must be present before a suppressor gene can be effective.

In all of the suppressed Tsase mutants, one characteristically finds a low enzyme/antigen ratio as compared to the wild type organism (Suskind, Yanofsky, and Bonner, 1955). This low Tsase activity suggests: (1) that the primary mutation at the *td* locus is is still being expressed (in terms of CRM formation) and that some of the CRM is now functioning enzymatically; or (2) that a structurally new enzyme of low turnover number is being formed; or (3) that a small amount of normal Tsase is being formed in addition to CRM.

These possibilities introduce several important considerations bearing on the nature of the suppressed mutant enzyme. If the *td* region does, in fact, represent the structural gene responsible for the amino acid sequence of the Tsase molecule, how do the several unlinked suppressor genes act to restore some Tsase function? Do the suppressor genes function as regulatory genes, or do they possess some structural component? In an attempt to answer, critically, some of these questions in one suppressed mutant system, mutant td_{24} was selected. This mutant is suppressible by suppressor genes which affect either td_{24} or td_3 (Table 1) (Yanofsky and Bonner, 1955a). Furthermore, as indicated earlier, many properties of the td_{24}-CRM have been studied, and there are several known means of activating the CRM to functional Tsase, both *in vivo* and *in vitro*. Consequently, a comparison of the properties of Tsase from the unsuppressed mutant (td_{24}), the suppressed mutant (td_{24} Su_{24}) and the wild type organism should be most informative. A summary of the properties of the respective enzymes can be seen in Table 4 (Suskind and Ligon, unpublished data). Clearly the enzyme formed in suppressed mutant td_{24} Su_{24} has all of the properties of td_{24}-CRM and none of the properties of normal Tsase.

Consequently, in the case of td_{24} Su_{24}, it would seem that the mutant protein is still being formed and that the suppressor gene acts *in vivo* in some manner that permits this CRM, which is indistinguishable from the mutant protein, to function as an active enzyme (Suskind and Kurek, 1959). An alternative suggestion, the presence of low levels of newly synthesized normal Tsase, would appear to be ruled out by reconstitution experiments. If a mixture of td_{24} Su_{24} Tsase and normal Tsase are heat-treated (55° C for five minutes), the normal Tsase component can be recovered, while the suppressed mutant Tsase is inactivated. Under the conditions of this experiment, a 1 per cent contamination of normal Tsase in the suppressed mutant preparation could have been detected.

Hence, one is faced with little alternative except to conclude that the suppressor-24 gene is serving in some regulatory capacity. It is of interest that mutant td_3, which is genetically distinct from td_{24}, but which is sensitive to the same suppressor genes (Yanofsky and Bonner, 1955a), appears to have serological properties which are similar to td_{24} (Table 3). However, it has not yet been possible to demonstrate any enzymatic activity (tryptophan synthesis) in td_3 extracts. Certainly, it is unwarranted to suggest that all suppressors act as regulatory genes, but it is not unreasonable to assume that in many instances, mutationally altered proteins, which are enzymatically inactive under certain intracellular conditions, can be converted to a functional state under conditions initiated by a specific suppressor gene. The results of experiments designed to examine certain factors which might influence Tsase formation and *in vivo* enzyme function are summarized in Table 4. First, repeated washing of whole cells of mutant td_{24} with EDTA (10^{-2} M) significantly stimulates indole uptake in the presence of L-serine. This is in agreement with the *in vitro* effect of EDTA observed with td_{24}. Unfortunately, EDTA is quite toxic in growth experiments, even in the presence of tryptophan, so that the tryptophan growth requirement of td_{24} could not be spared by EDTA. Second, growth of wild type *Neurospora* on zinc-deficient medium normally results in a 30 to 50 per cent inhibition of growth and a concomitant 90 to 95 per cent loss of Tsase enzymatic (Nason, Kaplan, and Colowick, 1951) and antigenic activity. However, if strains td_{24} or $td_{24}Su_{24}$ are grown on minimual medium at 30 to 37° C, zinc deficiency does not cause marked growth inhibition. However, two other *td* mutants, td_1 and td_2, are quite sensitive to zinc deficiency. Increasing the zinc concentration in the medium to 50 times the usual trace element concentration (10^{-3} M) caused no inhibition of growth of any of the strains which were examined. In view of the known zinc sensitivity of the td_{24} and $td_{24}Su_{24}$ Tsases, these differences are of some interest. Finally, it appears that the initial exogenous tryptophan concentration in the medium may control the specific activity of the CRM formed in mutant td_{24}. The highest specific activity is found in cells grown on low tryptophan, suggesting that tryptophan in *Neurospora* as well as in *E. coli* (Lester and Yanofsky, 1961) may be acting as a repressor of CRM formation.

CRM Proteins From Other *td* Mutants and Their Relation to the Structure and Function of Tsase

As mentioned previously, the CRMs from a number of *td* mutants still retain some enzymatic activity; i. e., they are still able to catalyze part of the Tsase reaction (Figure 1). The fact that some CRMs are completely inactive enzymatically while others have some enzymatic activity would appear to be a priori evidence for a structural difference between the molecules. But what of other lines of evidence?

Studies on the tryptophan synthetase system of *E. coli* indicate that the CRMs may differ in a number of ways, such as acid, urea, and temperature stability (Yanofsky, 1960). Furthermore, work on the A component of *E. coli* Tsase (molecular weight of A is about 29,500) has reached the point where fine structure analysis of peptide and amino acid differences in A-CRMs are being investigated (Helinski and Yanofsky, personal communication).

The relatively large molecular weight of *Neurospora* Tsase makes such a direct approach difficult, if not impossible, at the present time. Certain other methods are being examined, including the use of the Edman stepwise degradation technique (Fraenkel-Conrat, Harris, and Levy, 1955) to determine the number of N-terminal amino acids and, consequently, the number of polypeptide chains in the Tsase molecule. In addition, successful differential inactivation of the enzymatic and antigenic activities of Tsase by trypsin may permit the separation and identification of immunologically active fragments. As mentioned, growth of *Neurospora* on zinc-deficient medium markedly reduces the enzymatic and antigenic activity of Tsase in wild-type cells and of CRM in certain *td* mutants. If zinc plays any role in the formation of this protein, such zinc-deficient cells could conceivably be forming fragments of the Tsase molecule that might be recognized by suitable methods. A somewhat similar approach is suggested by preliminary work on two CRM-less mutants, td_1 and td_{16}. Crude extracts and fractions of these mutants contain no CRM, as judged by neutralization or precipitation tests. However, such CRM-less preparations do contain some component which can block the precipitation of normal Tsase by antienzyme in the Ouchterlony agar diffusion test. Perhaps these CRM-less mutants are forming fragments or dissociated subunits of the enzyme which lack sufficient functional sites to form a precipitable antigen-antibody complex, and which are of a haptenic nature. To date, no preparation from a CRM-less *td* mutant has been capable of eliciting the formation of anti-Tsase in rabbits.

Conclusion

It would appear that many types of mutationally altered Tsase proteins may be formed. These range from proteins having aberrant enzymatic activity, but possessing immunological and physical properties very similar to Tsase, to those proteins having no enzymatic activity and aberrant immunological activity. It remains to be seen what role these mutationally altered proteins play at the molecular level in such complex cell functions as intragenic complementation and suppression, and what value they may possess in helping to unravel the mysteries of genetic control of protein structure and function.

ACKNOWLEDGMENT

Contribution No. 343 of the McCollum-Pratt Institute, The John Hopkins University, Baltimore, Maryland. This research is supported by Grant C-3080, The National Cancer Institute, National Institutes of Health.

REFERENCES

Bonner, D. M. Personal Communication.

———. 1959. "Gene Action," *Genetics and Cancer* (The University of Texas M. D. Anderson Hospital and Tumor Institute, 13th Annual Symposium on Fundamental Cancer Research), pp. 207–225. Austin, Texas: The University of Texas Press.

Bonner, D. M., Y. Suyama, and J. A. DeMoss. 1960. Genetic Fine Structure and Enzyme Formation. *Federation Proceedings*, 19:926–930.

Carsiotis, M., and S. R. Suskind. 1960. Immunochemistry of Normal and Genetically Altered Tryptophan Synthetase from *Neurospora crassa. Federation Proceedings*, 19:206.

Crawford, I. P., and C. Yanofsky. 1958. On the Separation of the Tryptophan Synthetase of *Escherichia coli* into Two Protein Components. *Proceedings of the National Academy of Sciences of the U.S.A.*, 44:1161–1170.

Crick, F. H. C. 1959. "The Present Position of the Coding Problem," *Structure and Function of Genetic Elements* (Brookhaven Symposium in Biology, No. 12), pp. 35–39. Upton, New York: Brookhaven National Laboratory.

DeMoss, J. A., and D. M. Bonner. 1959. Studies on Normal and Genetically Altered Tryptophan Synthetase from *Neurospora crassa. Proceedings of the National Academy of Sciences of the U.S.A.*, 45:1405–1412.

Fraenkel-Conrat, H., J. I. Harris, and A. L. Levy. 1955. Recent Developments in Techniques for Terminal and Sequence Studies in Peptides and Proteins. *Methods of Biochemical Analysis*, 2:359–425.

Helinski, D., and C. Yanofsky. Personal Communication.

Jacob, F., P. Shaeffer, and E. L. Wollman. 1960. "Episomic Elements in Bacteria," *Microbial Genetics* (10th Symposium of the Society for General Microbiology), pp. 67–91. Cambridge, England: The University of Cambridge Press.

Lacy, A., and D. M. Bonner. 1961. Complementation Between Alleles of the *td* Locus in *Neurospora crassa. Proceedings of the National Academy of Sciences of the U.S.A.*, 47:72–77.

Lester, G., and C. Yanofsky. 1961. Influence of 3-Methylanthranilic and Anthranilic Acids on the Formation of Tryptophan Synthetase in *Escherichia coli. Journal of Bacteriology*, 81:81–90.

Mohler, W. C., and S. R. Suskind. 1960. The Similar Properties of Tryptophan Synthetase and a Mutationally Altered Enzyme in *Neurospora crassa. Biochimica et biophysica acta*, 43:288–299.

Nason, A., N. O. Kaplan, and S. P. Colowick. 1951. Changes in Enzymatic Constitution in Zinc-Deficient *Neurospora. Journal of Biological Chemistry*, 188:397–406.

Suskind, S. R. 1957. Properties of a Protein Antigenically Related to Tryptophan Synthetase in *Neurospora crassa. Journal of Bacteriology*, 74:308–318.

Suskind, S. R., and L. I. Kurek. 1957. Enzyme-Inhibitor Complex in a Tryptophan-Requiring Mutant of *Neurospora crassa. Science*, 126:1068–1069.

———. 1959. On a Mechanism of Suppressor Gene Regulation of Tryptophan Synthetase Activity in *Neurospora crassa. Proceedings of the National Academy of Sciences of the U.S.A.*, 45:193–196.

Suskind, S. R., and D. S. Ligon. Unpublished data.

Suskind, S. R., C. Yanofsky, and D. M. Bonner. 1955. Allelic Strains of *Neurospora* Lacking Tryptophan Synthetase: A Preliminary Immunochemical Characterization. *Proceedings of the National Academy of Sciences of the U.S.A.*, 41:577–582.

Suyama, Y. 1960. Effects of Pyridoxal Phosphate and Serine in Conversion of Indole Glycerol Phosphate to Indole by Extracts from Tryptophan Mutants of *Neurospora crassa. Biochemical and Biophysical Research Communications*, 3:493–496.

Vogel, H. (1961). "Control by Repression," *Control Mechanisms in Cellular Processes.* (Symposium of the Society of General Physiologists), D. M. Bonner, Ed. pp. 23–65. New York, New York: The Ronald Press Company.

Woodward, D. O. 1960. A Gene Concept Based on Genetic and Chemical Studies in *Neurospora. Quarterly Review of Biology*, 35:313–323.

Yanofsky, C. 1960. The Tryptophan Synthetase System. *Bacteriological Reviews*, 24:221–245.

Yanofsky, C., and D. M. Bonner. 1955a. Gene Interaction in Tryptophan Synthetase Formation. *Genetics*, 40:761–769.

———. 1955b. Non-Allelic Suppressor Genes Affecting a Single *td* Allele. *Genetics*, 40:602.

Genes, Enzymes, and Control Mechanisms in Histidine Biosynthesis

Bruce N. Ames, Ph.D.
and
Philip E. Hartman, Ph.D.

National Institutes of Health, Bethesda, Maryland
and
The Johns Hopkins University, Baltimore, Maryland

The gene-enzyme relationships in histidine biosynthesis in *Salmonella typhimurium* have been examined.

A cluster of eight genes controlling histidine biosynthesis has been mapped in detail. These genes are linked on the chromosome in the order E, F, A, H, B, C, D, G, as described in the section on Genetic Analysis. There appear to be nine enzymes in the biochemical pathway and most of these are discussed in detail in the section on Biochemical Pathway. The genes have been correlated with the enzymes and the sequence has been analyzed in the section on Gene Sequence and Enzyme Sequence. The first step of the pathway has been characterized (PRPP + ATP $\rightleftarrows$ N-1-(5′-phosphoribosyl)-ATP + PP); the enzyme has been purified and shown to be strongly inhibited by histidine as discussed in the sections on Biochemical Pathway and Control Mechanisms.

Several observations support a unified control of the expression of the histidine cluster of genes. Five of the enzymes of the pathway have been examined in detail and their synthesis has been shown to be repressed by histidine coordinately, i.e., all to the same extent.

Several mutations which appear to involve a region at the end of the histidine cluster (next to the *G* gene) prevent all the other histidine genes from being functional, even though these genes are undamaged, as discussed in the sections on Control Mechanisms and Control Region of the Chromosome.

Two control mechanisms, histidine inhibition of the first enzyme and histidine repression of the synthesis of all the histidine biosynthetic enzymes, appear to regulate histidine production in *Salmonella typhimurium*. This will be discussed in the section on Control Mechanisms.

The *B* gene has four complementation groups and controls two nonsequential enzymes which appear to be the same protein. The work of Loper showing *in vitro* complementation and the implications of that work for the understanding of intragenic complementation are discussed in the section on Complementation.

The length of the histidine cluster appears to be about 15,000 nucleotide pairs, and this is discussed in connection with the molecular weight of a number of the enzymes in the section on Genetic Analysis.

In general, the genetic analysis presented is due to the work of Hartman and associates, and the biochemical analysis is due to the work of Ames and coworkers. Each of these analyses was greatly facilitated by the results of the parallel analysis.

Biochemical Pathway

The pathway of histidine biosynthesis involves the conversion of the 5-carbon chain of ribose to the 5-carbon chain of histidine. There seem to be nine enzymes involved in this transformation, five of which have been investigated in detail. The pathway of histidine biosynthesis does not have any branches giving rise to other essential metabolites: mutants lacking all nine enzymes require only histidine as a growth supplement. The pathway is presented in Figure 1.

The first enzyme, phosphoribosyl-ATP pyrophosphorylase (Ames, Martin, and Garry, 1961) condenses phosphoribosylpyrophosphate (the source of the 5-carbon backbone of histidine) with adenosine triphosphate (ATP) (the donor of a carbon atom and a nitrogen atom of the imidazole ring [Moyed and Magasanik, 1960]). The products of the reaction have been characterized (Ames, Martin, and Garry, 1961) as N-1-(5′-phosphoribosyl)-ATP and pyrophosphate, and the reaction has been shown to be reversible (Figure 2). The enzyme has been purified and its molecular weight

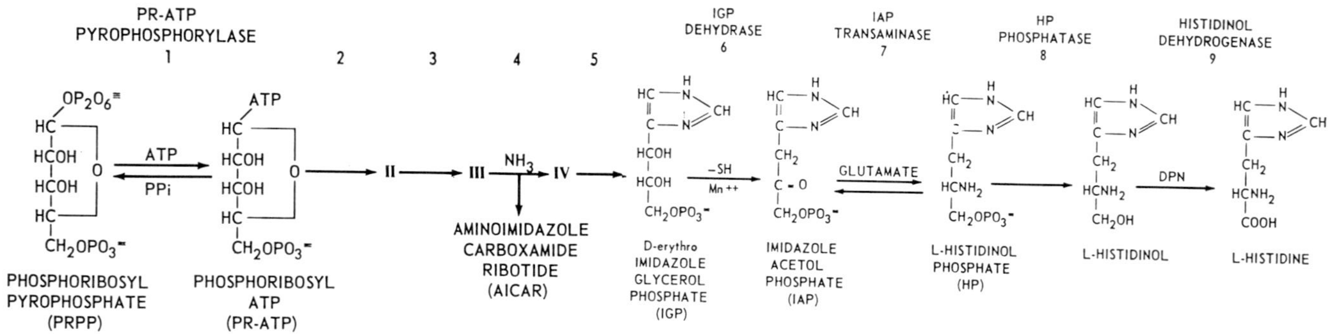

FIG. 1. The pathway of L-histidine biosynthesis in *Salmonella typhimurium*.

has been found to be approximately 170,000 (Martin and Ames, 1961). The inhibition of the action of this enzyme by histidine will be discussed under Control Mechanisms. The evidence that this is actually the first enzyme of the pathway (and the criteria for defining a first enzyme) has been presented (Ames, Martin, Garry, 1961).

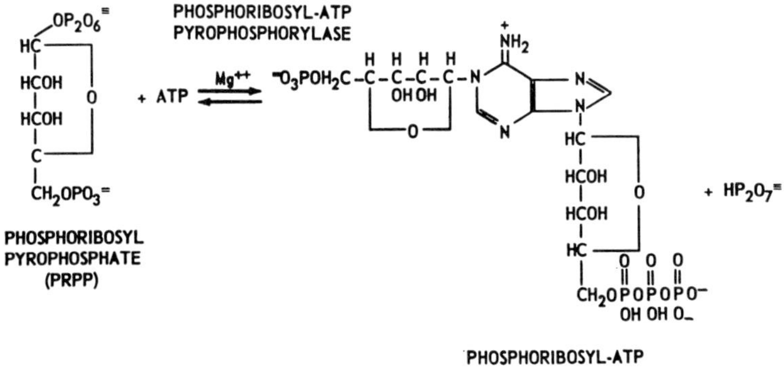

FIG. 2. The first step of histidine biosynthesis.

The second, third, fourth, and fifth enzymes are involved in the conversion of phosphoribosyl-ATP to imidazoleglycerol phosphate. The exact biochemistry is unclear, though several aspects of the over-all reaction are known (Moyed and Magasanik, 1960; Ames, Martin, and Garry, 1961). There are four classes of mutants, each blocked in one of these steps. Extracts of any two of these mutants in combination will make imidazoleglycerol phosphate from phosphoribosyl-ATP (Martin, Garry, and Ames, unpublished data). Some evidence has been obtained indicating that the second enzyme opens the pyrimidine ring of the phosphoribosyl-ATP. The fourth step requires ammonia and releases amino-imidazole-carboxamide ribotide, a side product which is then converted back to regenerate the adenine nucleotide (Moyed and Magasanik, 1960).

The sixth enzyme, imidazoleglycerol phosphate dehydrase (Ames, 1957a; Ames, Garry, and Herzenberg, 1960) removes a water molecule from D-*erythro*-imidazoleglycerol phosphate to form imidazoleacetol phosphate.

The seventh enzyme, imidazoleacetol phosphate transaminase (Ames and Horecker, 1956; Ames, Garry, and Herzenberg, 1960), converts imidazoleacetol phosphate and L-glutamate to L-histidinol phosphate and α-ketoglutarate. The molecular weight of this enzyme in *S. typhimurium* is approximately 68,000 (Martin and Ames, 1961).

The eighth enzyme, histidinol phosphate phosphatase (Ames, 1957b; Ames, Garry and Herzenberg, 1960), hydrolyzes L-histidinol phosphate to form histidinol and inorganic phosphate. Evidence that this enzyme and the sixth enzyme may be a single bifunctional protein, will be discussed after presentation of the genetic data.

The ninth enzyme, L-histidinol dehydrogenase (Adams, 1954, 1955; Ames, Garry, and Herzenberg, 1960) converts L-histidinol and diphosphopyridine nucleotide (DPN) to L-histidine and DPNH (the reduced form of DPN). This enzyme has a molecular weight of approximately 75,000 (Martin and Ames, 1961). It has been highly purified by Loper and Adams (1961) from *S. typhimurium*. Their preparation has a specific activity 2,000 to 3,000 times that of the wild-type extract.

Control Mechanisms

Two control mechanisms appear to regulate the rate of histidine production in *S. typhimurium*. When excess histidine accumulates in the cell the biosynthetic production of histidine is stopped. Histidine can inhibit the action of the first enzyme of the pathway (*feedback inhibition*). Histidine can inhibit the synthesis of the nine biosynthethic enzymes (enzyme repression).

Feedback Inhibition

The inhibitory effect of the end product of a pathway on the activity of an early enzyme in the pathway has been called *feedback inhibition*, and has been described by a number of investigators (Adelberg and Umbarger, 1953; Brooke, Ushiba, and Magasanik, 1954; Umbarger, 1956; Yates and Pardee, 1956) in a variety of organisms. Some evidence had been presented (Moyed and Friedman, 1959; Moyed and Magasanik, 1960) that in *Escherichia coli* and in *S. typhimurium* one of the early enzymes in histidine biosynthesis is inhibited *in vitro* by low amounts of histidine. Recently the first enzyme of histidine biosynthesis has been characterized in *S. typhimurium* (Ames, Martin, and Garry, 1961) and shown to be extremely sensitive to inhibition by L-histidine. The other enzymes of the pathway are insensitive to L-histidine. There is evidence that histidine does shut off the biosynthesis of histidine *in vivo* (Moyed and Friedman, 1959; Magasanik and Karibian, 1960).

Enzyme Repression

The size of the pool of the end product of a biosynthetic pathway also regulates the rate of synthesis of the enzymes of that pathway (Cohn, Cohen, and Monod, 1953; Vogel, 1957; Yates and Pardee, 1957; Gorini and Maas, 1957). This control mechanism (enzyme repression) appears to be one of coarse adjustment as compared to the fine adjustment of the feedback inhibition mechanism. Both controls together presumably regulate histidine production with a minimum energy expenditure.

We have investigated repression of the histidine biosynthetic enzymes by histidine in *S. typhimurium* (Ames and Garry, 1959). The level of these enzymes was low (specific activity defined as 1) in wild-type cells grown on minimal medium or on minimal medium plus histidine. Histidine-requiring mutants, grown on minimal medium plus excess histidine, also had low levels (specific activity of 1) of those of the histidine enzymes that were present. When the growth of a mutant was limited by the amount of histidine available, the cellular concentration of the histidine biosynthetic enzymes increased to a specific activity of about 30. This high level appears to result from a relief of repression when the size of the histidine pool is made smaller. What then, one might ask, is the use in Nature of this latent capacity to make histidine enzymes? It appears as if an increased level of the histidine enzymes would be needed when the bacteria are growing much faster than they do on a minimal medium, e.g., on a complex medium lacking histidine (see discussion in Ames and Garry, 1959). The enzyme levels were not repressed below a specific activity of 1, even by adding large amounts of histidine to the minimal growth medium.

Histidine repression affected to the same extent each of the five histidine enzymes that have been examined (Ames and Garry, 1959; Ames, Martin, and Garry, 1961). There was a parallel increase in the specific activity of each of the enzymes following a decrease in the histidine pool. In any extract, no matter how the cells were grown, there was a constant ratio of the activity of one histidine enzyme to another. This phenomenon was called *coordinate repression.* The hypothesis that such coordinate control represents the effect of the repression of enzyme synthesis at the gene level (Ames and Garry, 1959) will be discussed after the genetic data have been presented.

Histidine-Activating Enzyme

In order to extend the studies on enzyme repression, we have investigated the histidine-activating enzyme, which links histidine with a specific soluble ribonucleic acid (S RNA), presumably the first step in the incorporation of histidine into protein. It has been found (Ames and Garry, unpublished data) that the histidine-activating enzyme was not repressed by histidine: the level of this enzyme was not affected by the level of histidine in the cell, unlike the histidine biosynthetic enzymes. The gene for the histidine-activating enzyme did not appear to be within the cluster of the histidine biosynthetic genes: all histidine-requiring mutants tested, including those containing multisite mutations for the entire histidine region of the chromosome (e.g., *his-63* + *his-712*) contained normal amounts of activating enzyme.

L-Histidinol was found to be a very potent inhibitor of the activating enzyme: the K_i for L-histidinol is 5×10^{-5} M and the K_m for L-histidine is 1.4×10^{-4} M.

Genetic Analyses

A General Map of the Histidine Region

Approximately 600 independently derived histidine-requiring mutants have been mapped by complete transduction (Hartman, Loper, and Šerman, 1960) and abortive transduction (Hartman, Hartman, and Šerman, 1960). In transduction, phage grown on one bacterial histidine mutant is used to transfer the bacterial genetic material to another bacterial histidine mutant. The transduced bacteria are then plated on a medium lacking histidine. In complete transduction the fragment is integrated into the bacterial chromosome resulting in a cross between the two bacterial mutants; only the wild-type recombinants grow to form a colony. The number of these colonies in a cross is a measure of the distance apart of the two mutations involved in the cross. A genetic map can be constructed in this way. In abortive transduction, the transduced fragment is not integrated, and appears to exist in a nonreplicating form, passing unilinearly from the recipient cell to only one of the daughter cells at each cell division. If the two mutations are in different functional units, then complementation will occur and the cell containing the fragment will be able to grow and give rise to a microcolony. This test is useful for determining functional relationships between mutants. Figure 3 shows a simplified procedure used for rough mapping.

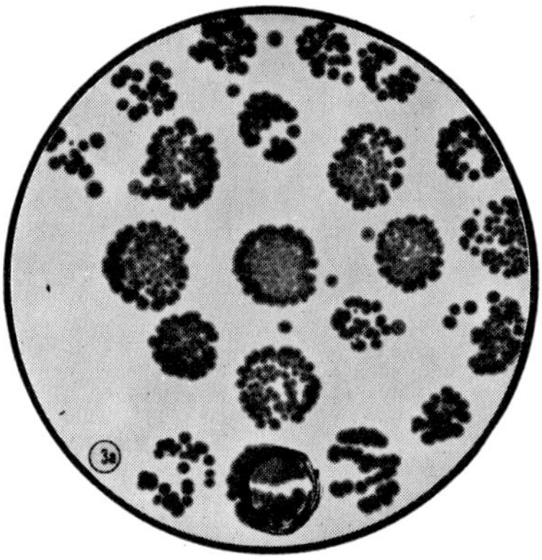

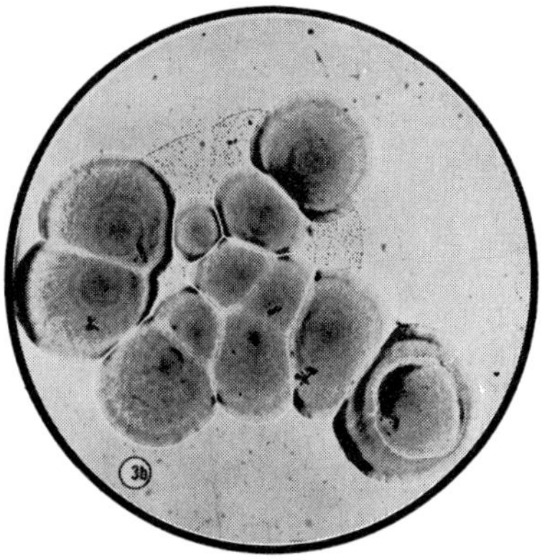

Fig. 3a. Spot test mapping of mutant *his*-539. Mutant *his*-539 was grown overnight in nutrient broth with aeration, centrifuged, resuspended in T2 buffer, and then about 5×10^8 bacteria were spread on a plate of minimal medium supplemented with 20 μg./ml. of each of the amino acids except histidine. This plate was spotted with 24 small drops of phage suspension (1×10^{10}/ml.), using an Accu-Drop machine (Wolfson and Ghitter, 1960). Each phage suspension had been prepared by growing phage on one of the 24 histidine mutants that are used to divide the histidine region into segments. This plate was then incubated for 18 hours at 37° C. The circled spot at the bottom of the figure is from phage grown on wild-type bacteria. Each black dot is a clone of bacteria deriving from a nonhistidine-requiring recombinant. Clockwise from the wild-type spot are: *E-145*, *EFAHBCD-712*, *EF-135*, blank, *F-41*, *FA-703*, *A-517*, *A-481*, *A-484*, *AH-134*, *H-107*, *B-22*, *B-29*, *B-206*, *B-116* (above wild-type), *B-40*, *C-43*, *C-8*, *DG-63*, *D-208*, *D-113*, *D-216*, and *G-255* (center). The blank between *EF-135* and *F-41* is because a preparation of phage from *FA-55* was not available at the time of this test.

The absence of wild-type recombinants is seen in the crosses with *EFAHBCD-712* and with *EF-135*. This indicates that *his-539* lies in the region covered by *EF-135*. The location of *his-539* is narrowed down to the IVb region by the production of recombinants with *F-41*. As expected, all mutants not in the IVb region recombine with *his-539*, the number of wild-type recombinants is a rough measure of how far from *his-539* any marker is located. A few spontaneous revertants of *his-539* are located outside of the spots.

Fig. 3b. Enlargement of the *his-539* $\times$ *F-41* spot. Examination of the plate for abortive transductions (microcolonies) showed that *his-539* gave rise to abortive transductions in all crosses except those with *E-145*, *EFAHBCD-712*, *EF-135*, and *DG-63*, thus placing the mutant in gene *E*. The anomalous result with *DG-63* is of great interest in connection with the peculiarity of *DG-63* in not complementing other mutants, and this mutant will be discussed in Section VII.

Figure 4 shows some general aspects of the histidine region of the chromosome. All of the genes for histidine biosynthesis are clustered in this small region of the chromosome; all histidine mutants, examined to date, map within this cluster. The division into

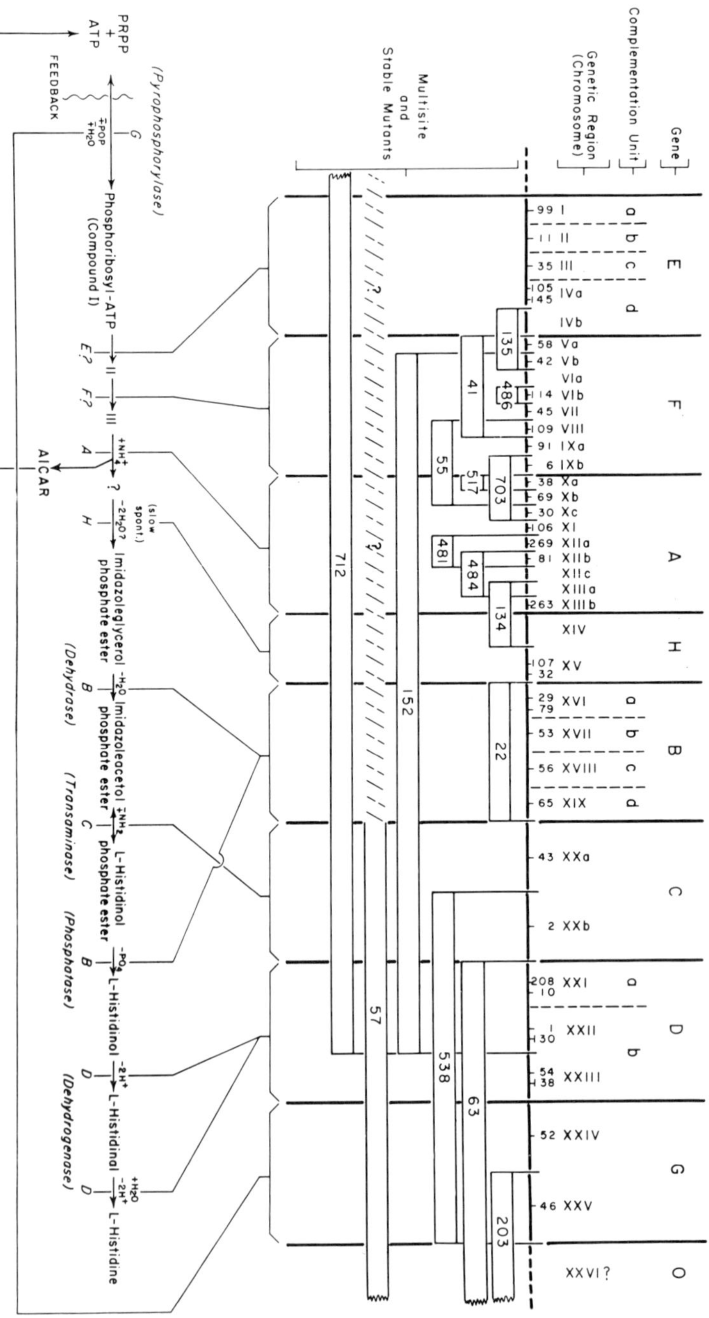

See legend on page 331.

functional units was established by complementation tests. The association of these functional units with the histidine biosynthetic enzymes will be presented in the next section. The mutants mapped in Figure 4 include single site, or "point" mutants, as well as multisite, or "deletion" mutants. The multisite mutants are especially valuable in mapping. It is interesting that two of the rare multisite mutants (*his-152*, *his-712*) terminate at identical positions as determined by crosses to more than 100 *D* mutants. A similar situation occurring with high frequency has been detected in the *cysC* region by Demerec *et al.* (1960). The single site mutants that have been mapped are distributed over the whole histidine cluster. Even though several independently occurring mutations are inseparable by recombination, there are no "hot spots" of spontaneous mutations comparable in size to the two described by Benzer (1957). The map in Figure 4 incorporates a fundamental change from that published previously (Hartman, Loper, and Šerman, 1960) in that the *his-G* gene is shown differently. The reason for this change will be discussed in the last section. Mapping by two-point tests is particularly inadequate at the terminal portions of the *his* region. The precise structure must await the isolation of double mutants (so that three-point tests can be carried out) or the isolation of more overlapping deletions in this region. Both approaches are being undertaken.

Recombination data indicate that each of the genes is of approximately the same size, except for locus *H* which may be smaller (Fig. 4). These approximations strikingly bear no relation to the number of complementation units per locus (See Complementation).

Comparisons of abortive and complete transduction frequencies indicate that the entire *his* region is contained in most, if not all, phage particles carrying transducing activity for any one *his* marker, i.e., the transducing pieces are relatively uniform in their size and composition (cf. Ozeki, 1959). Furthermore, it is highly possible that other bacterial genes of unknown function extend to the right and to the left of the *his* region for a distance allowing normal recombination frequencies with, for example, multisite mutants *his-712* and *his-63*.

FIG. 4. A map of the *S. typhimurium* histidine region of the chromosome. The dark horizontal line represents the chromosome. Multisite (deletion) mutants are represented by bars beneath the chromosome. The location of a few of the single site mutants is shown immediately above the chromosome. Roman numerals refer to segments of the *his* region defined by the various multisite mutants or by complementation studies.

Inactivation of Abortive and Complete Transduction

Four agents have been utilized in inactivation studies on transducing and on plaque-forming activities of *P22* phage suspensions: ultraviolet irradiation (Benzinger and Kosch, unpublished data), X-rays (Takebe and Hartman, 1961), P^{32} decay experiments (Kozinski and Hartman, unpublished data), and nitrous acid (Adye, 1961). The effects of ultraviolet irradiation, nitrous acid, and indirect effects of X-rays, though not identical, are similar. The effects of P^{32} decay and direct X-ray effects also may be classed together. Data obtained in the inactivation studies, as well as in studies of dissociation of linkage, indicate that the *his* region of the chromosome constitutes one third to one fifth of the genetic material contained in an infective phage particle. These experiments are complicated and the details and the assumptions involved in this estimate will be published elsewhere.

A Coding Ratio for the his *Region*

Each *P22* phage particle carries an amount of deoxyribonucleic acid (DNA) containing about 7×10^4 nucleotide pairs (Garen and Zinder, 1955) and since transducing particles carrying the whole histidine region are essentially of the same density as infectious particles (Sheppard, unpublished data), we assume that they contain about the same amount of DNA. Taking into account results of inactivation studies (see the previous section), we conclude that the *his* region is probably between 1.3×10^4 and 2×10^4 nucleotide pairs in length. If it is assumed that the region elicits the production of eight proteins and that there are no long "nonsense" sections in the nucleotide sequence (Crick, 1959), it follows that each of the genes is about 2,000 nucleotide pairs in length. Genetic studies have indicated that the *his* genes appear to be truly adjacent (Hartman, Loper, and Šerman, 1960).

One can make the assumption that an average molecular weight for one of the eight protein monomers controlled by this region would be about 75,000 (the molecular weight of three of the enzymes has been determined as 68,000, 75,000 and 170,000, although some of these may be polymers of identical subunits; Martin and Ames, 1961). A 75,000 molecular weight protein would have about 700 amino acids. Based on the above assumptions the coding ratio (nucleotide pairs per amino acid residues) appears to be about 3:1. As the assumptions must be supported by further experimental evidence, this ratio should not be taken too seriously.

Mutation and the Nature of the Sites Constituting the his *Genes*

Procedures are now available for the induction in bacteria of single site mutants with chemical mutagens. Such techniques promise to provide, after simplified penicillin screening procedures, practically unlimited numbers of mutants for fine structure analysis. In addition, transduction fragments contained in phage particles can be mutated directly with nitrous acid, and selected for, with relatively little regard for leakiness of the genetic block, thus allowing ready isolation of leaky mutants, which are strongly selected against in the penicillin procedure (Adye, 1961).

Back mutation tests by Kirchner (1960) indicate that base analogues and the mutator gene of *LT-7* induce single site histidine mutants, which probably involve single base pairs and seem to be of the transition type, i.e., one purine-pyrimidine base pair has been substituted for the other purine-pyrimidine base pair (Freese, 1960; Demerec, 1960). Kirchner's studies also indicate that as many as four different states may exist at a single site: the wild type and three different mutant types.

Location of the his *Region on the Enteric Chromosome*

The location of histidine markers on the circular map of the *E. coli* chromosome has been established (Wollman and Jacob, 1958; Taylor and Adelberg, 1960) and is the same as that described for the location of *his* markers in *S. typhimurium* as shown by *E. coli - S. typhimurium* crosses (Demerec *et al.*, 1960). The *his* region is located between the serine *A* locus and a cluster of genes controlling cysteine and tryptophan synthesis (*cysB, tryA,B,C,D*). The *H-1* (phage antigen) locus of *E. coli* probably lies between serine *A* and *his* (Makela, personal communication) as does an adenine locus (Taylor and Adelberg, 1960) and a locus of phage *424* (Jacob and Wollman, 1958). The prophage locus of phage *21* has been mapped between the *his* region and the cluster of tryptophan loci (Jacob and Wollman, 1958). None of these loci appear to be very intimately linked with the *his* region and the nature of the genetic material immediately adjacent to the *his* region remains obscure.

Gene Sequence and Enzyme Sequence

The genes controlling histidine biosynthesis have been shown to be in a cluster on the *S. typhimurium* chromosome (Hartman, Loper, and Šerman, 1960). The fact that the genes are in a cluster is remarkable. One explanation of this clustering of related genes is that this region of the chromosome functions as a unit. (This is discussed under Control Region of the Chromosome). It is also of interest to compare the sequence of the genes in the cluster with the sequence of the biosynthetic enzymes they control. The histidine genes are linked in the order *E,F,A,H,B,C,D,G*. Mutants from these various classes have been examined for the histidine enzymes (Ames, Garry, and Herzenberg, 1960; Ames and Garry, 1959; Ames, Martin, and Garry, 1961).

Gene *G* controls the first enzyme (PR-ATP pyrophosphorylase). Gene *D* controls the ninth enzyme (histidinol dehydrogenase). Gene *C* controls the seventh enzyme (imidazoleacetol phosphate transaminase). Gene *B* controls the sixth enzyme (imidazoleglycerol phosphate dehydrase). Loper (1960) has evidence that gene *B* also controls the eighth enzyme (histidinol phosphate phosphatase). Genes *E*, *F*, *A*, and *H* are associated with the enzymes between phosphoribosyl-ATP and imidazoleglycerol phosphate (second, third, fourth, and fifth enzymes [Ames, Martin, and Garry, 1961; Moyed and Magasanik, 1960]), though the exact sequence is not known (Figures 1 and 4). The sequence of the genes on the chromosome seems to correspond in general with the sequence of the enzymes they control, with the striking exception of the gene for the first enzyme, which is next to the gene for the last enzyme. The exact sequence of the enzymes of genes *E*, *F*, *A*, *H* will have to be determined before any generalization can be made.

What significance this gene sequence has is not clear. The general correspondence between the sequences of the histidine genes and enzymes has been pointed out (Hartman, 1956), and discussed (Hartman, Loper, and Šerman, 1960). In other biosynthetic pathways where the genes are clustered (see examples in Hartman, 1957; Demerec *et al.*, 1960) it will be of interest to see whether there is a comparable ordering of genes and, if there is, whether the sequences all run in one direction along the circular chromosome (e.g., clockwise). It will also be of interest to see whether the genes for the first and last enzymes of a pathway are together in other systems.

Complementation

Intragenic Complementation

The division of the chromosome map into units by complementational analysis is consistent with the division into units by the enzyme analysis (i.e., into genes). But, the analyses show that a number of genes (or enzyme specificity units) have several subunits.

The *B* gene has been analyzed in detail and is particularly interesting because of its complexity: it is composed of four subunits, and controls two enzyme activities. At first the *B* gene appeared to be only the dehydrase gene: all mutants of the *his-B* gene accumulated imidazoleglycerol phosphate and its derivative imidazoleglycerol (Hartman, Loper, and Šerman, 1960). Extracts of a number of these mutants were tested and were found to be lacking only the dehydrase (Ames, Garry, and Herzenberg, 1960). Complementation analysis (by abortive transduction) demonstrated that the gene was divisible into four subunits: *Ba*, *Bb*, *Bc* and *Bd* (Hartman, Hartman, and Šerman, 1960). Multisite mutant *his-22* covers the entire *B* region. Surprisingly, it was also found to lack the phosphatase (Ames, Garry, and Herzenberg, 1960). Loper (1960, 1961) has analyzed the *B* gene in more detail and found that 23 mutants in *Bc* are lacking both the dehydrase and the phosphatase; but a large number of *Ba*, *Bb* and *Bd* mutants were lacking only the dehydrase. His immunological and enzyme purification studies supported the idea that these two activities were associated with one protein. The two activities run exactly together on a diethylamino ethylcellulose column (Ames and Garry, 1959). If, as seems likely, these two activities actually reside in one protein, it will be especially remarkable, as they are not consecutive steps on the pathway.

The *B* gene is composed of four subunits, as has been shown by complementation analysis. The meaning of complementation subunits within a gene has aroused considerable controversy. The complementation map of the *B* gene is shown in Figure 5. Two overlapping lines indicate that two mutations cannot cooperate with each other to form active enzyme, when present in the same cell (in abortive transduction). All the mutants shown map as points on the genetic map. Loper (1960, 1961), studying this system, has been able to show *in vitro* complementation. Extracts of mutants in different subgroups (all lacking dehydrase) will give active dehydrase upon mixed incubation. His results suggest that a protein-protein interaction is involved in complementation. Many of the mutants isolated in the *B* gene are revertible, single site mutants, which do not complement any other mutant in *Ba*, *Bb*, *Bc* or *Bd* (Figure 5). This would argue that the whole *B* region produces one single protein.

FIGURE 5

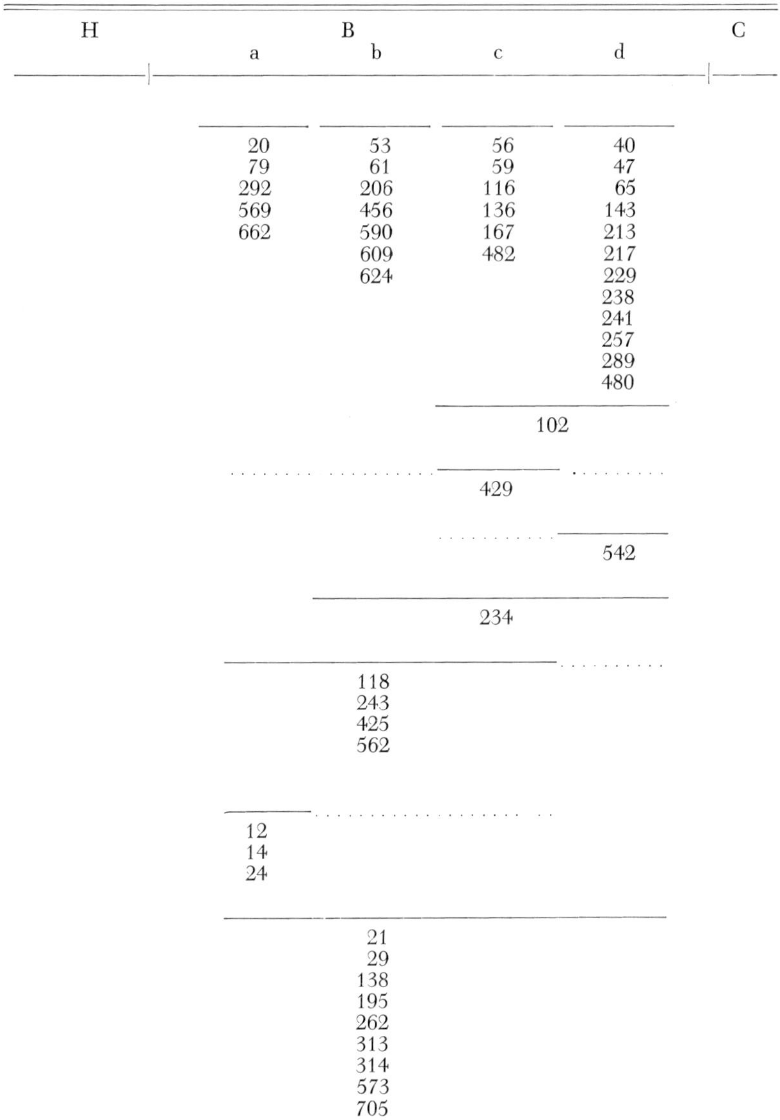

H
B
C
a
b
c
d
20 79 292 569 662
53 61 206 456 590 609 624
56 59 116 136 167 482
40 47 65 143 213 217 229 238 241 257 289 480
102
429
542
234
118 243 425 562
12 14 24
21 29 138 195 262 313 314 573 705

FIG. 5. A revised complementation map of the *his-B* locus. Mutants have been tested for complementation by abortive transduction tests. The results are represented above in the following way: The numbers indicate the mutants. Each mutant is represented by a solid line. Mutants having the same complementation characteristics are represented by the same line, and listed below it (they do not complement each other). Overlapping lines indicate failure to complement. Dotted

Brenner (1959) and Crick and Orgel (in preparation) have presented a theory which holds that complementation may be explained in terms of protein-protein interactions among identical polypeptide chains, which form a polymer enzyme. They have discussed this subject in detail. Loper's data are consistent with their general theory. Sucrose density gradient centrifugation indicates that the phosphatase-dehydrase protein has a complex aggregation picture (possibly a monomer-tetramer) (Martin and Ames, 1961), under conditions that Loper has shown to stimulate *in vitro* complementation (presence of Mg^{++} and mercaptoethanol).

The *a, b, c,* and *d* complementation units in *B,* differ markedly from the cistrons of Benzer (1957) in that point mutants are common in *his-B* which do not complement with *a, b, c,* or *d,* while this situation is not true in the r_{II} A or B cistrons. The whole *his-B* gene then appears to be a unit comparable to r_{II}A or r_{II}B.

The above results and Crick and Orgel's interpretation suggest that this type of complementation unit, while interesting from the standpoint of protein chemistry, is not so relevant genetically (as a meaningful unit of function) as commonly assumed.

The *D* gene (histidinol dehydrogenase) also contains complementation subunits. Tests in which over 100 histidinol dehydrogenase mutants have been crossed in all possible combinations show a higher degree of complexity that was originally reported by Hartman, Hartman, and Šerman (1960). About half of these *D* mutants fail to complement within the locus. There are now 11 *Da* mutants which complement 48 *Db* mutants, though it is impossible to predict with which *Da* mutant a new *Db* mutant will complement. Furthermore, *his-D-130* complements some *Da* and some *Db* mutants, creating a new class, *Dc.* In the map (based on recombination) previously presented (Hartman, Loper, and Šerman, 1960) *his-D-130* maps to the right of all *Da* and *Db* mutants. Construction of a meaningful complementation map, analogous to that of the *B* gene (Figure 5) is impossible. We conclude that this analysis may be measuring some structural peculiarities of the dehydrogenase protein, and the answer to the problem probably lies in a study of the enzyme itself.

---

lines indicate weak complementation (i.e., the abortive transductional clones are smaller than those obtained in combination with phage grown on wild-type bacteria).

These data are from a scheme by Hartman, Hartman, and Šerman (1960) with more recent additions by Loper (1960) and Hartman (unpublished).

Some genes do not appear to have complementation subunits. The transaminase gene (C) has been analyzed in great detail and no complementation has been observed.

Intergenic Complementation

In the abortive transduction test, most mutants complement mutants of other genes as adequately as does wild-type phage. In a minority of cases, however, complementation by the mutant-mutant combination is distinctly inferior to complementation by the wild type. For example, a very high proportion of interactions between *B* and *H* mutants has been detected. This has been interpreted in terms of a position effect (Hartman, Hartman, and Šerman, 1960), since its analysis was not extended beyond the level of genetic analysis. When point mutants show this effect (Hartman, Hartman, and Šerman, 1960) (and new isolates) it is possible that in some cases protein-protein interactions at the physiological level are responsible for the effect. It is possible that enzyme-enzyme interactions play a role in the intracellular coordination and efficient functioning of this sequence of enzymes. The depression of intergenic complementation in the cases noted above is slight, however, when compared with the extremely weak *in vivo* complementation noted with multisite mutants *his-63* and *his-203* and complete absence in *his-57*. This is particularly evident when plating is performed on rich growth medium containing a histidine-free amino acid pool. The enriched medium stimulates the growth of the minute colonies (resulting from abortive transduction), except those formed in combinations involving the above three mutants. These three mutants are of particular interest, and are discussed in the section on Control Region of the Chromosome.

Some Effects of Histidine Analogues

The E Gene

E, but not *F*, *A*, *B*, *C*, or *D* mutants use DL-1,2,4-triazole-3-alanine as a histidine substitute; it is clear that triazolealanine is not substituting for histidine in proteins or being converted to it. *E* mutants do no grow on 2-thiazolealanine, which is another histidine analogue. Presumably the *E* reaction can proceed in the cell to some extent without the actual *E* enzyme (all the *E* mutants will grow slowly on minimal medium; Hartman, Loper and Šerman, 1960), and the rapid growth on triazolealanine could be due to an effect on some control mechanism. The elucidation of the biochemistry of the *E* step is necessary before any definite theory can be put forward. It has been established, however, that triazolealanine does not act in feedback inhibition (Ames, Martin, and Garry, 1961), and that it does catalyze a pyrophosphate exchange reaction with ATP (an assay for amino acid-activating enzyme) (Ames and Garry, unpublished data).

E mutants are also unique in forming small colonies at the periphery of regions of growth surrounding crystals of histidine placed on minimal medium. It is possible, but remains to be demonstrated, that the intermediate accumulated by *E* mutants (presumably phosphoribosyl-ATP) has mutagenic properties.

Leaky Mutants

Some histidine mutants grow very slowly on minimal media lacking histidine; such mutants are termed "leaky" mutants. Most histidine leaky mutants are not stimulated by adenine (or adenosine) or by the histidine analogue, DL-2-thiazolealanine. However, a number of leaky mutants are stimulated by both these compounds, or will mutate with high frequency to a form that is stimulated by them. Some of these mutants are: *his F-58, F-147, F-440, A-81, A-106, A-423, H-32, H-107, C-62, C-212,* and *D-214*. Indeed, all *H* mutants fall into this category. Shedlovsky and Magasanik (1960) first observed this stimulation in an *A* mutant of *E. coli*.

Thiazolealanine is a very effective inhibitor of pyrophosphorylase (Ames, Martin, and Garry, 1961; Moyed and Friedman, 1959); it may be that the leaky mutants result in an adenine drain because of the accumulation of precursors. Thiazolealanine, by inhibiting the first enzyme, could somewhat overcome such an effect (cf., Shedlovsky and Magasanik, 1960), though it is not quite clear why a block at a later enzyme would result in any adenine drain. Triazolealanine is ineffective in stimulating *E* mutants; therefore, the two cases seem quite different.

A number of mutants (e.g., *his-6*) readily mutate to the utilization of purines for growth. The ability to grow on adenine is linked with the histidine genetic block in a number of cases so far examined (Hartman, 1956, and unpublished data). However, the ability to grow on adenine may not be "an inherent property resulting from mutation at the histidine locus," as originally believed (Hartman, 1956). The nature of the crosses used in the original tests did not take into account that this ability might reside in two mutations within the histidine region, one being very closely linked with gene *D* (e.g., in gene *G*). Therefore, further analysis by genetic and biochemical techniques is required to resolve this question.

Control Region of the Chromosome

The observations that the histidine genes are in a cluster on the chromosome and that all the histidine enzymes are coordinately repressed, led us to suggest (Ames and Garry, 1959) that the repressor might act at a single control point on the chromosome, thus determining the functionality of the whole group of genes as a unit. In support of the existence of a small region of the chromosome which does control all the histidine genes, are studies on three unusual histidine mutants that differ from the other 600 histidine mutants examined.

These multisite mutants, *G-203*, *DG-63*, and *CDG-57* are unusual in two respects: 1) They lack all the histidine biosynthetic enzymes (Ames, Garry, and Herzenberg, 1960; Ames, Martin, and Garry, 1961), even though almost all of the histidine genes are outside of the mutated region (Hartman, Loper, and Šerman, 1960) (Figure 4). 2) They show extremely weak, or absent, complementation in abortive transduction tests with mutants localized in genes outside this mutated region (Hartman, Hartman, and Šerman, 1960). Thus, in these three mutants, even though most of the histidine genes are undamaged, none of the histidine genes function. The three mutants have in common damage in part of the *G* gene. The damage may extend into the region to the right of the *G* gene (referred to as the *O* region). At least part of this mutated region appears necessary for the functioning of all the histidine biosynthetic genes. Only the histidine genes appear to be controlled by this region, as these mutants do not require supplements other than histidine for growth. Multisite mutations of other parts of the histidine cluster do not destroy the functioning of all histidine genes; e.g., deletion mutant *EFAHBCD-712* contains pyrophosphorylase, despite damage at every other gene. Thus this one region appears to have a specific importance in the histidine cluster. It is not clear whether it is a region in *G* that is important, or the *O* region (Figure 4). Mutant *CDG-538* is a new mutant which seems similar to the three mutants just discussed.

Jacob, Perrin, Sanchez, and Monod (1960) have postulated, as a result of their intensive investigation of the β-galactosidase system in *E. coli*, that the repression is effected at the gene level, through an *operator* site which controls a cluster of genes, the *operon*. Our data are consistent with this hypothesis and the three unusual deletion mutants are very similar to their 0° operator mutants.

Of over 600 histidine-requiring mutants examined by complementation tests, no single site mutants have been found that appear to be operator mutants. Single site mutants in *G* (e.g., *G-46*, *G-200*) contain, as one would expect in an ordinary mutant, all the histidine enzymes except the pyrophosphorylase (Ames, Martin, and Garry, 1961). This failure to detect single site operator mutants could be due to a number of factors: 1) the small size of the operator region; 2) failure of the region to be grossly affected in function by a single site mutation; 3) a single site mutation in the *O* region, if leading to high levels of enzymes (due to the failure of the repressor to control enzyme production), could result in semilethality or a bacterium that would not be a histidine mutant. A multisite mutant lacking both *G* and *O* would be a histidine mutant. Some evidence might indicate that the operator mutants do not completely destroy the functioning of all the histidine genes, but that a trace of enzymes might be made. Hartman, Hartman, and Šerman (1960) noted that *his-57* would not complement with any *his* mutant, that *his-63* failed to complement only in genes *D* and *G*, while *his-203* failed to complement in gene *G*, but complemented extremely weakly with *D* and more strongly with the region *E* through *C*. All these complementation reactions were extremely weak compared to normal complementation, though they do seem to be real. Even though no enzymes were detected in extracts, this weak complementation may be significant, as a complementation test seems considerably more sensitive than enzyme assay (see the case of *his-22* and imidazoleacetol phosphate transaminase, [Hartman, Hartman, and Šerman, 1960; Ames, Garry, and Herzenberg, 1960]). In view of the complementation reactions, it is possible that these mutants do have extremely low levels of enzyme activities. Furthermore, the complementation reactions indicate that there may be a gradient in this very slight residual activity, the activity increasing in those genes further away from the operator region. If this observation is supported by further analysis, it might be important in understanding the way the operator works and the meaning of the sequence of genes in relation to the operator.

In connection with this operator, the case of a cluster of two genes in *Neurospora crassa* might be mentioned. The histidine genes are scattered on the chromosomes in *Neurospora* except for this group of two genes (Haas, Mitchell, Ames, and Mitchell, 1952; Webber and Case, 1960; Webber, 1960; Catcheside, 1960). This cluster, the histidine *3* group, consists of the gene for the last enzyme and the gene for an early enzyme (Ames, 1957b; Webber, 1960; Ames, unpublished data). Mutations in histidine *3* which inactivate both genes are common. It is not clear whether this case involves an operator, or a bifunctional protein similar to the dehydrase-phosphatase gene in *Salmonella.*

ACKNOWLEDGMENTS

The portion of this work contributed by Dr. Hartman was supported in part by Research Grant E1650 from the National Institute of Arthritis and Metabolic Diseases, United States Public Health Service.

We extend our thanks to our associates cited in the text. Their experimental results and stimulating discussions have both intellectually and materially contributed to the progress of the research presented in this report.

REFERENCES

Adams, E. 1954. The Enzymatic Synthesis of Histidine from Histidinol. *Journal of Biological Chemistry*, 209:829–846.

———. 1955. L-Histidinol, a Biosynthetic Precursor of Histidine. *Journal of Biological Chemistry*, 217:344.

Adelberg, E. A., and H. E. Umbarger. 1953. Isoleucine and Valine Metabolism in *Escherichia coli. Journal of Biological Chemistry*, 205:475–482.

Adye, J. 1961. Effect of Nitrous Acid in Transduction by *P22* Phage in *S. typhimurium.* (Abstract) *Bacteriological Proceedings*, p. 80.

Ames, B. N. 1957a. The Biosynthesis of Histidine: Imidazoleglycerol Phosphate Dehydrase. *Journal of Biological Chemistry*, 228:131–143.

———. 1957b. The Biosynthesis of Histidine: L-Histidinol Phosphate Phosphatase. *Journal of Biological Chemistry*, 226:583–593.

———. Unpublished data.

Ames, B. N., and B. Garry. 1959. Coordinate Repression of the Synthesis of Four Histidine Biosynthetic Enzymes by Histidine. *Proceedings of the National Academy of Sciences of the U.S.A.*, 45:1453–1461.

Ames, B. N., B. Garry, and L. A. Herzenberg. 1960. The Genetic Control of the Enzymes of Histidine Biosynthesis in *Salmonella typhimurium. The Journal of General Microbiology*, 22:369–378.

Ames, B. N., and B. L. Horecker. 1956. The Biosynthesis of Histidine: Imidazoleacetol Phosphate Transaminase. *Journal of Biological Chemistry*, 220:113–128.

Ames, B. N., R. G. Martin, and B. J. Garry. 1961. The First Step of Histidine Biosynthesis. *Journal of Biological Chemistry*, 236:2019–2026.

Benzer, S. 1957. "The Elementary Units of Heredity," *Symposium on the Chemical Basis of Heredity*, W. D. McElroy and B. Glass, Eds., pp. 70–93. Baltimore, Maryland: Johns Hopkins Press.

Benzinger, R., and W. E. Kosch. Unpublished data.

Brenner, S. 1959. "The Mechanism of Gene Action," *Ciba Foundation Symposium on Biochemistry of Human Genetics*, G. E. W. Wolstenholme and C. M. O'Connor, Eds., pp. 304–317. Boston, Massachusetts: Little, Brown and Company.

Brooke, M. S., D. Ushiba, and B. Magasanik. 1954. Some Factors Affecting the Excretion of Orotic Acid by Mutants of *Aerobacter aerogenes. Journal of Biological Chemistry*, 68:534–540.

Catcheside, D. G. 1960. "Relation of Genotype to Enzyme Content," *Microbial Genetics*, pp. 181–207. Cambridge, England: Cambridge University Press.

Cohn, M., G. N. Cohen, and J. Monod. 1953. L'effet inhibiteur specifique de la methionine dans la formation de la methionine-synthase chez *Escherichia coli. Comptes rendus hebdomadaires des séances de l'Académie des sciences*, 236:746–748.

Crick, F. H. C. 1959. "The Present Position of the Coding Problem," *Brookhaven Symposia in Biology* (Brookhaven Symposium, 12), pp. 35–38. Long Island, New York: Brookhaven National Laboratory.

Crick, F. H. C., and L. E. Orgel. (In preparation). Complementation: The Protein-Protein Interaction Theory.

Demerec, M. 1960. Frequency of Deletions Among Spontaneous and Induced Mutations in *Salmonella. Proceedings of the National Academy of Sciences of the U.S.A.*, 46:1075–1079.

Demerec, M., E. L. Lahr, E. Balbinder, T. Miyake, J. Ishidsu, K. Mizobuchi, and B. Mahler. 1960. Bacterial Genetics, in "Department of Genetics," *Carnegie Institution of Washington Year Book 59*, pp. 426–441. Baltimore, Maryland: The Lord Baltimore Press, Inc.

Freese, E. 1960. "On The Molecular Explanation of Spontaneous and Induced Mutations," *Brookhaven Symposia in Biology* (Brookhaven Symposium, 12), pp. 63–75. Long Island, New York: Brookhaven National Laboratory.

Garen, A., and N. D. Zinder. 1955. Radiological Evidence for Partial Genetic Homology Between Bacteriophage and Host Bacteria. *Virology*, 1:347–376.

Gorini, L., and W. K. Maas. 1957. The Potential for the Formation of a Biosynthetic Enzyme in *E. coli. Biochimica et biophysica acta*, 25:208–209.

Haas, F., M. B. Mitchell, B. N. Ames, and H. K. Mitchell. 1952. A Series of Histidineless Mutants of *Neurospora crassa. Genetics*, 37:217–226.

Hartman, P. E. 1956. "Linked Loci in the Control of Consecutive Steps in the Primary Pathway of Histidine Synthesis in *Salmonella typhimurium*," *Genetic Studies with Bacteria*, (Carnegie Institution Publication No. 612), p. 35. Washington, D. C.: The Carnegie Institution.

———. 1957. "Transduction: A Comparative Review," *The Chemical Basis of Heredity*, W. D. McElroy and B. Glass, Eds., pp. 408–462. Baltimore, Maryland: Johns Hopkins Press.

———. Unpublished data.

Hartman, P. E., J. C. Loper, and D. Šerman. 1960. Fine Structure Mapping by Complete Transduction Between Histidine-Requiring *Salmonella* Mutants. *The Journal of General Microbiology*, 22:323–353.

Hartman, P. E., and S. H. Goodgal. 1959. Bacterial Genetics. *Annual Review of Microbiology*, 13:465–504.

Hartman, P. E., Z. Hartman, and D. Šerman. 1960. Complementation Mapping by Abortive Transduction of Histidine-Requiring *Salmonella* Mutants. *The Journal of General Microbiology*, 22:354–368.

Jacob, F., D. Perrin, C. Sanchez, and J. Monod. 1960. L'Opéron: Group de Gènes à éxpression coordonnée par un opérateur. *Comptes rendus hebdomadaires des séances de l'Académie des sciences*, 250:1727–1729.

Jacob, F., and E. L. Wollman. 1958. Sur les processus de conjugaison et de recombinaison génétique chez *Escherichia coli*. IV. Prophages inductibles et mesure des segments génétiques transférés au cours de la conjugaison. *Annales de l'Institut Pasteur*, 95:497–519.

Kirchner, C. E. J. 1960. The Effects of the Mutator Gene on Molecular Changes and Mutation in *Salmonella typhimurium*. *Journal of Molecular Biology*, 2:331–338.

Kozinski, A., and P. E. Hartman. Unpublished data.

Loper, J. C. 1960. Gene-Enzyme Relationships in Histidine Biosynthesis in *Salmonella*. Ph.D. Dissertation. Johns Hopkins University, Baltimore, Maryland.

———. 1961. Enzyme Complementation in Mixed Extracts of Mutants from the *Salmonella histidine B*. *Proceedings of the National Academy of Sciences of the U.S.A.*, 47:1440–1450.

Loper, J., and E. Adams. 1961. Purification of Histidinol Dehydrogenase from *Salmonella*. (Abstract) *Federation Proceedings*, 20(1, Pt 1): 254.

Magasanik, B., and D. Karibian. 1960. Purine Nucleotide Cycles and Their Metabolic Role. *Journal of Biological Chemistry*, 235:2672–2681.

Makela, H. Personal Communication.

Martin, R. G., and B. N. Ames. 1961. A Method for Determining the Sedimentation Behavior of Enzymes: Application to Protein Mixtures. *Journal of Biological Chemistry*, 236:1372–1379.

Martin, R. G., B. Garry, and B. N. Ames. Unpublished data.

Moyed, H. S., and M. Friedman. 1959. Interference with Feedback Control: A Mechanism of Antimetabolite Action. *Science*, 129:968–969.

Moyed, H. S., and B. Magasanik. 1960. The Biosynthesis of the Imidazole Ring of Histidine. *Journal of Biological Chemistry*, 235:149–153.

Ozeki, H. 1959. Chromosome Fragments Participating in Transduction in *Salmonella typhimurium*. *Genetics*, 44:457.

Shedlovsky, A., and B. Magasanik. 1960. Adenine Deficiency in a Histidine Auxotroph. (Abstract) *Federation Proceedings*, 19(1, Pt. 1)51.

Sheppard, D. E. Unpublished data.

Takebe, H., and P. E. Hartman. 1961. Effects of X-Rays on Transduction by *S. typhimurium* Phage P22. (Abstract) *Bacteriological Proceedings*, p.80.

Taylor, A. L., and E. A. Adelberg. 1960. Linkage Analysis with Very High Frequency Males of *Escherichia coli*. *Genetics*, 45:1233–1243.

Umbarger, H. E. 1956. Evidence for a Negative-Feedback Mechanism in the Biosynthesis of Isoleucine. *Science*, 123:848.

Vogel, H. J. 1957. "Repression and Induction as Control Mechanisms of Enzyme Biogenesis," *The Chemical Basis of Heredity*, p. 276, Baltimore, Maryland: Johns Hopkins Press.

Webber, B. 1960. Genetic and Biochemical Studies of Histidine-Requiring Mutants of *Neurospora crassa*. II. Evidence Concerning Heterogeneity among *hist-3* Mutants. *Genetics*, 45:1617–1626.

Webber, B., and M. Case. 1960. Genetic and Biochemical Studies of Histidine-Requiring Mutants of *Neurospora crassa*. I. Classification of Mutants and Characterizations of Mutant Groups. *Genetics*, 45:1605–1616.

Wolfson, S. W., and L. R. Ghitter. 1960. A Simplified Approach to the Phage Typing of *Staphylococcus aureus*. II. A Mechanical Adjunct to the Typing Procedure. *American Journal of Clinical Pathology*, 34:92–94.

Wollman, E. L., and F. Jacob. 1958. Sur les processus deconjugaison et de recombinaison chez *Escherichia coli*. V. Le mécanisme du transfert de materiel génétique. *Annales de l'Institut Pasteur*, 95:641–66.

Yates, R. A., and A. B. Pardee. 1956. Control of Pyrimidine Biosynthesis in *E. coli* by a Feedback Mechanism. *Journal of Biological Chemistry*, 221:757–770.

———. 1957. Control by Uracil of Formation of Enzymes Required for Orotate Synthesis. *Journal of Biological Chemistry*, 227:677–692.

Gene-Enzyme Relationships in Isoleucine-Valine Biosynthesis

R. P. Wagner, Ph.D., Kazuyoshi Kiritani,* Ph.D.,
and Arloa Bergquist, B.A.

*The Genetics Laboratory, Department of Zoology,
The University of Texas, Austin, Texas*

The realization of the close relationship between the genotype and the specific protein constitution of the organism has been one of the great scientific advances of this century. By the application of this knowledge it has been possible to formulate significant hypotheses for the role of the nucleic acids in cell function and to form the first significant bridge between genotype and phenotype with a molecular basis.

Prior to the recognition of this relationship, the role of the genotype in producing a given phenotype had been described only in vague terms, but it was recognized that chromosomes were organized into units of action, called genes, each of which appeared to have a rather specific role to play in the production of the final phenotype. However, when closer scrutiny was made of the concept of the gene as both a functional and physical entity, it became evident that a clear one to one relationship could not be demonstrated. This conclusion is reflected in the results of work done on a number of organisms, varying from corn and *Drosophila* to viruses. The results are not always clear and do not easily lend themselves to interpretation, but they do show that it is not yet possible to

* Present address: Institute of Applied Microbiology, University of Tokyo, Tokyo, Japan.

translate such organization as can be detected by recombination and complementation analysis of the fine structure of the chromosome to the protein level with any degree of confidence. This is tantamount to saying that, assuming that deoxyribonucleic acid (DNA) is the genetic stuff, its organization in the chromosome is yet to be related to the presumed end product of its activity. It should be recognized that this is a significant omission in our knowledge, and noble attempts to bridge the gap by ignoring the problem, or by making vague references to a code and its transmission, do not remove the necessity for experimental work.

The experimental attack on the gene-protein problem is being made in a number of closely related ways. First is the direct method of correlating intrinsic protein differences as reflected in physical properties and amino acid sequences with the occurrence of mutant genes. It is work of this type which has confirmed the undoubted relation between genes and protein specificity, and led to the search for the code in DNA. The second approach is dependent on knowledge gained from the first, and seeks to determine the nature of the synthetic mechanisms extrinsic to the gene which cause a specific protein to be produced. These studies involve investigating the relationship between DNA, ribonucleic acid (RNA), and protein synthesis. Third are the very important studies of the built-in controlling mechanisms which regulate the cellular environment in such a way as to regulate protein synthesis or activity. The fourth approach is most directly related to the first. It seeks to analyze genetic organization by recombination or complementation, and to relate such findings as are made to what is found in the proteins. In a sense, this approach constitutes one of the last stands of the geneticist. At stake is the most fundamental of the genetic concepts —the gene concept.

In order to utilize the genetic approach, the experimental organism must be one that has an easily manipulated sexual cycle, and which enables one to screen easily up to millions of meiotic products for phenotype and genotype. Furthermore, the mutants must show some readily determined association with a specific protein difference or differences. These requirements limit one primarily to microorganisms, such as fungi and bacteria, in which a sufficient amount of preliminary work has already been done to establish linkage relationships. For, as will be seen in the following, this type of approach requires an analysis of the relationship between certain apparent small segments of chromosomes and the quantitative and qualitative condition of certain enzymes.

It is the purpose of this communication to present a summary of some findings made in our laboratory by utilizing genetic analysis in combination with the application of biochemical techniques on mutants of *Neurospora crassa* requiring isoleucine and valine.

Biochemical Description of the Isoleucine-valine Mutants of *Neurospora*

A number of nutritional mutants of *N. crassa* have been described in the literature which require both isoleucine and valine for growth (Adelberg, Bonner, and Tatum, 1951; Wagner, Bergquist, and Forrest, 1959; Wagner, Somers, and Bergquist, 1960). The requirement for two amino acids simultaneously is easily understood when it is recognized that isoleucine and valine are structurally very closely related (Figure 1), and apparently share the same enzymes in their four terminal biosynthetic steps (Figure 2) (Wagner, Radhakrishnan, and Snell, 1958; Radhakrishnan, and Snell, 1960; Radhakrishnan, Wagner, and Snell, 1960).

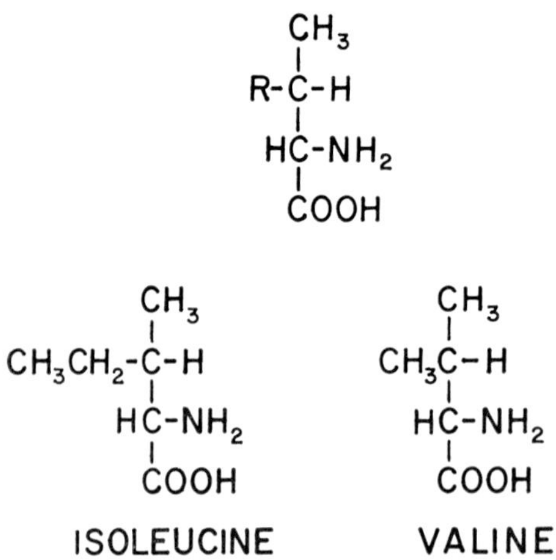

Fig. 1. The structure of isoleucine and valine.

In the work described here, only the two intermediate steps diagramed in Figure 2 are considered. In these reactions the β-keto acids, α-acetolactate (AL) and α-aceto-α-hydroxybutyrate (AHB) are converted in the presence of the reduced triphospyridino-nucleotide (TPNH) requiring enzyme, reductoisomerase, to their respective derivatives, α, β-dihydroxyisovaleric acid (DHV) and α, β-dihy-

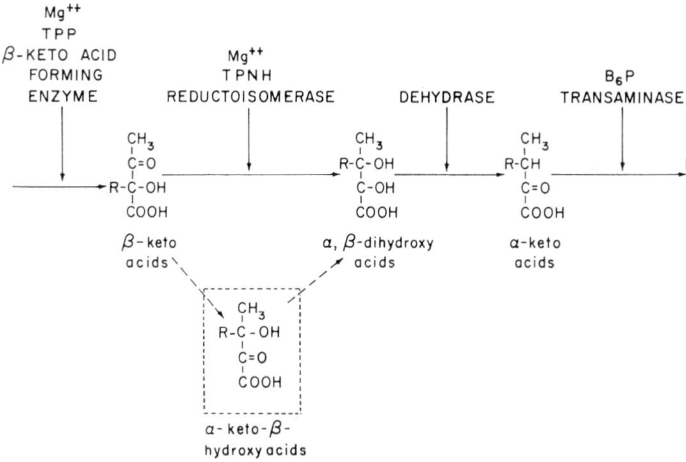

FIG. 2. The biosynthesis of isoleucine and valine. The α-keto-β-hydroxy acids are hypothetical intermediates.

droxy-β-methylvaleric acid (DHI). This reaction is a complex one, since it involves two steps, a rearrangement to situate the side chain (R in Figure 2) β to the carboxyl group, and a reduction to form the dihydroxy acids from the hypothetical α-keto-β-hydroxyl intermediates. Nonetheless, despite the necessity for two steps, the evidence indicates only a single enzyme or complex which accepts only the β-keto acids as substrates when it is partially purified, and converts them directly to the dihydroxy acids without any detectable accumulation of the possible intermediate α-keto-β-hydroxy acids.

The dihydroxy acids are converted to the α-keto acids, α-ketoisovaleric acid and α-keto-β-methylvaleric acid, in the presence of a dehydrase. This enzyme is very unstable even in crude extracts, and it has not been found possible to purify it from a *Neurospora* source up to the present time. The two other steps indicated in Figure 2 are not considered here, because they do not appear to be involved directly in the analysis of the mutants to be described.

In our laboratory, we have isolated a series of 19 mutants of *Neurospora*, all of which require both isoleucine and valine for growth at maximal rates. These have been previously described by Wagner, Somers, and Bergquist (1960) as *Tiv* mutants. They have been divided into three major groups, I, II, and III, based on their genetic and biochemical differences. Their biochemical and physiological differences and similarities are summarized in Table 1. Methods for determining the enzyme activities and the accumula-

TABLE 1

Characteristics of Neurospora Tiv *Mutants*

Group	Enzyme activity µmoles/hour/mg. Reductoiso-merase	Dehy-drase	Accumulations Carbinols µg./mg.	Dihydroxy acids	Growth at pH 7.5
I (7)Δ	0.0– 1.3	1.0–1.9	206–850	0*	0
II (3)Δ	6.5–16.2	0.6–1.6	10.4(311)	++(311)	0 (304)
			200(304)	DHV(304)	+(318)
			385(318)	0 (318)	+(311)
IIIb (2)Δ	2.4– 4.8	0.8–1.6	233–374	++	0
IIIa (7)Δ	4.8–11.8	0.25–0.45	0.9–5.5	++	+
Wild type	3.7	0.70	0.2	0	+

* Two of the mutants in this group may accumulate α, β-dihydroxyisovaleric acid (DHV).
Δ The number of mutants in each group.

tions have been published earlier (Wagner, Bergquist, and Forrest, 1959; Wagner, Bergquist, and Karp, 1958; Radhakrishnan, Wagner, and Snell, 1960). The enzyme activities given in Table 1 are for crude extracts, and the enzyme activities and carbinol accumulations are indicated as ranges. These represent the highest and the lowest values found for the members of each of the indicated groups. The numbers in parentheses are strain numbers, except as indicated. The wild type used was KJT 1960, a strain arising from a cross between the Emerson wild types 5256A and 5297a. It was from these latter two strains that the *Tiv* mutants were originally derived (Wagner, Somers, and Bergquist, 1960).

Group I mutants are similar in their dehydrase activities, in the accumulation of large amounts of carbinols in the medium, and in their inability to grow on supplemented medium at pH 7.5 or above. Furthermore, they are not leaky, i.e., they have an absolute requirement for isoleucine and valine. The members of this group have low to undetectable reductoisomerase activity. In all cases the activities are significantly lower than wild type, as can be seen from the ranges given in Table 1. One member of this group, 313, has considerable reductoisomerase activity when raised at 25°C, but undetectable reductoisomerase when raised at 37°C. This finding is in agreement with 313 being a temperature mutant with a requirement for isoleucine and valine above 30°C only.

The Group II mutants are heterogeneous and intermediate in their characteristics. Both enzymes are present at or above wild type levels of activity, and the mutants accumulate low to high levels of carbinols. One accumulates both dihydroxy acids, one apparently accumulates DHV, and one neither.

Group III mutants are all characterized by being leaky, and by the accumulation of large amounts of both dihydroxy acids, DHV and DHI, during growth on supplemented media. From 1 to 3 μmoles of dihydroxy acids are accumulated per milligram of mycelium in three days. These mutants are divided into two classes, IIIa and IIIb. Group IIIa mutants have a low dehydrase activity and do not accumulate appreciable amounts of carbinols. Furthermore, they do not grow at pH 7.5 or above. The two mutants in Group IIIb, however, show no enzyme activity deficiency for dehydrase or reductoisomerase; they accumulate large amounts of carbinols, and, like the Group I mutants, do not grow at or above pH 7.5.

The accumulation of dihydroxy acids is understandable considering that these mutants are isoleucine-valine requiring, and DHV and DHI are precursors. The accumulation of the carbinols, acetylmethylcarbinol (AMC) and acetylethylcarbinol (AEC), is undoubtedly the result of preaccumulation of the β-keto acids, AHB and AL. It has been shown previously that *Neurospora* possesses an active decarboxylase which decarboxylates AHB and AL with the formation of AEC and AMC, respectively (Wagner, Bergquist, and Forrest, 1959).

From these facts, it follows that the Group I mutants are blocked at the reductoisomerase step, since they are low in reductoisomerase activity and accumulate large amounts of the carbinols, AMC and AEC, and do not accumulate dihydroxy acids, (with the possible exception of DHV accumulation by 313 and 324). In the same way, it can also be postulated that the Group IIIa mutants are blocked at the dehydrase step, since they are low in dehydrase, accumulate dihydroxy acids, and do not accumulate significant amounts of carbinols.

Where the other mutants are blocked, if they are blocked, is difficult to say on the basis of the presently available data. They are not blocked prior to the reductoisomerase steps, since all accumulate either AEC + AMC or dihydroxy acids or both, nor are they blocked at the transaminase step, for all possess transaminase activity for ketovaline and ketoisoleucine conversion to valine and isoleucine in the presence of the appropriate donors. Furthermore, none of the mutants accumulate detectable quantities of the α-keto acids, α-keto-β-methylvaleric acid, ketoisoleucine (KI) or α-ketoisovaleric acid, ketovaline (KV).

Genetic Analysis of the Mutants

The 19 *Tiv* mutants were crossed to two marker stocks carrying the mutant genes, lysine-1 (*lys*-1), and spray (*sp*), on the Vth chromosome about 25 map units apart (Strickland, Perkins, and Veatch, 1959). All of the *Tiv* mutants were found to be linked to these markers and located between them. In Figure 3 are shown the calculated average crossover values with their standard deviations. These values were calculated from the pooled data from each of the three groups, I, II, and III, for reasons that will be apparent below. It is evident from the standard deviations that the differences are not significant, and that all mutants, on the basis of these data, can be considered for practical purposes to be about 10 units to the left of *sp* and about 15 units to the right of *lys*-1.

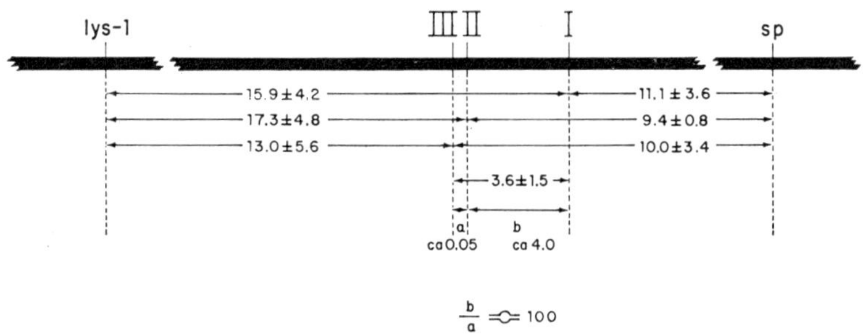

Fig. 3. The linkage map of the *Tiv* mutants indicating their positions relative to the outside markers spray and lysine-1, and their positions relative to one another.

After establishing the approximate position of each of the *Tiv* mutants on the Vth chromosome, they were crossed to one another. The crosses were carried out in such a way that a *Tiv* mutant carrying *lys*-1 was generally crossed to one carrying *sp*. The ascospores resulting from the cross were then germinated on Petri dishes containing minimal medium supplemented with lysine according to the method of Newmeyer (1954). Under these conditions, all those segregants which are wild type or prototrophic for isoleucine-valine should grow. By determining the total number of germinating ascospores for each cross on control plates containing isoleucine, valine and lysine, and those which germinate and grow on the plates with lysine only, one may estimate the per cent recombination between the different mutant genes resulting from interchanges between the genes. In addition, by determining the distribution of the outside markers in the wild-type segregants, the order of the mutant genes relative to spray and lysine may be found (Figure 4). If mutant gene *a* is to the left of *b*, then the predominant wild type segregant should also be lys^+ and sp^+. Those which have *lys* or *sp*, only, and are iv^+, should occur in a frequency of about 10 per cent, and presumably be the result of double crossovers. Those resulting from a triple crossover should carry both *lys* and *sp* and occur at a frequency of about 1 per cent. If, however, *a* is to the right of *b*, then the expected segregants are as listed on the right side of Figure 4, with the *lys* iv^+ *sp* segregants being predominant and the lys^+ iv^+ sp^+ segregants being least dominant.

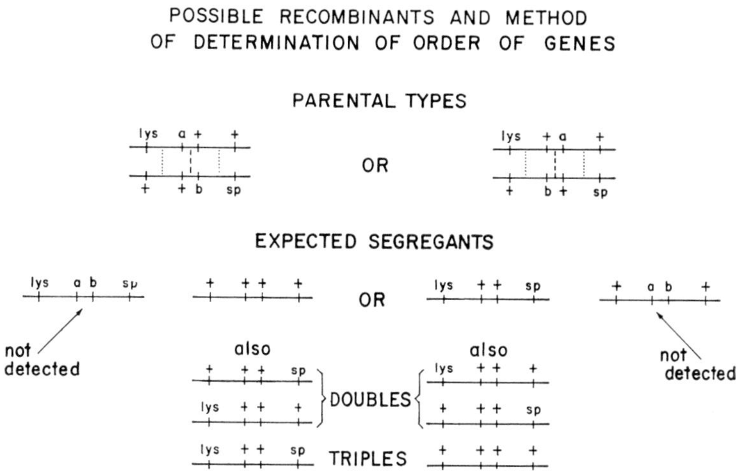

FIG. 4. The types of recombinants expected from the crosses depending upon the order of the mutant genes.

All the possible crosses were made between the different *Tiv* mutants. Not all crosses produced ascospores in sufficient numbers, but 140 different combinations did. About 100,000 germinatable ascospores were tested for each cross. These gave sufficient data to establish that the 19 *Tiv* mutants occur in three clusters or groups designated above as Groups I, II, and III. Group I includes mutants T 325, 322, 320, 319, 305, 313 and 324. No wild type recombinants occur out of about 100,000 germinated spores when these are crossed together, except that 313 × 324 gave in one trial 0.88 per cent recombination. (The per cent recombination is calculated as twice the actual percentage of the observed wild types.) These two mutants did not produce wild type recombinants when crossed to the other members of the Group I mutants, however. The Group II mutants include T 318, 304, and 311. These showed 0.000 to 0.009 per cent recombination when crossed together. Group II mutants include strains T 331, 321, 326, 327, 328, 329, 323, 332, and 330. These gave 0.00 to 0.05 per cent recombination. Intergroup crosses established that the groups are arranged as shown in Figure 3, between *sp* and *lys* with I to the right of III, and II in the middle. The average recombination values found were 3.6 per cent between I and III, 4.2 per cent between I and II, and 0.05 per cent between III and II. The small indicated distance between III and II raises the question of whether they should be considered the same group. These have been separated because all three members of Group II can be unequivocally located to the right of III, and they possess certain peculiarities not found in III. (On the basis of the present data, it is impossible to arrange the members of III in any order because insufficient segregants were obtained to determine the genotypes of the segregants with highest frequency, i.e., whether lys^+ iv^+ sp^+ or *lys* iv^+ *sp* predominated.)

The genetic data make it apparent that there is a segment of the Vth chromosome which has some control over a series of two successive reactions leading to isoleucine and valine. The actual physical length of this segment cannot be estimated at present. But the map distance between Group I and Group III mutants is estimated at about four, as established by the appearance of iv^+ ascospores, all of which are assumed in the above discussion to be the result of recombination within this segment. If this value is taken as a correct reflection of random crossover within this segment, which we further assume is no different from crossover incidence in other parts of the Vth chromosome, then this segment may be assumed to occupy about 16 per cent of the interval between *sp* and *lys*-1. This could be true, for the standard deviations for the distances to the outside markers and for the distance between Groups I and III are such that a segment as long as this may exist between *sp* and *lys* with the indicated functions. Conversely, it is just as likely that the segment is shorter than indicated. In many of the crosses, an unexpectedly large number of wild type segregants were obtained which were lys^+ iv^+ *sp*. As will be seen from Figure 4 these may be interpreted as being the result of double crossovers. About 10 to 15 per cent double crossovers are expected among the wild type segregants. However, in a small number of the crosses, up to 50 per cent or more of the tested wild-type segregants were apparently double recombinants. Furthermore, the frequency of triple crossovers was significantly higher than the expected 1.5 per cent in a few crosses. These results indicate that a phenomenon other than standard crossover is occurring. If so, the map distance of 4 per cent, as calculated from the occurrence of total wild segregants, should be reduced, but there is no way of determining what it should be reduced to. A partial resolution of this problem is dependent upon making analysis of the various crosses to establish whether orthodox crossover or gene conversion or both is occurring to produce the wild type segregants. Tetrad analysis with mutants would be difficult and laborious, however, since most of them show low recombination, and all of them produce ascospores in crosses which mature only after the ascus sacs in which they develop have disintegrated.

The possibility of back mutation to wild type must also be considered as an explanation for the occurrence of the wild type segregants. This cannot be eliminated entirely as a possible mechanism, but it is unlikely to be important since, in general, there was definite asymmetry in the distribution of the segregants, i.e., they were either lys^{+} iv^{+} sp^{+} or lys iv^{+} sp. If mutation were important, the segregants expected to predominate would be lys^{+} iv^{+} sp and lys iv^{+} sp^{+}.

Whatever the situation is, regarding the origin of the segregants with no requirement for isoleucine and valine, it is clear that a relatively short segment of the Vth chromosome is being dealt with here. The data are unambiguous in placing the Group III and Group I mutants at the opposite extremes of the known limits of this segment. This being so, it is of interest to note that all the mutants with a detectable reduction in enzyme activity and a single type of accumulation are in these two groups. Hence, Group IIIa contains all mutants which accumulate only dihydroxy acids and have a low dehydrase activity, and Group I includes all those which have a high carbinol accumulation and low reductoisomerase activity. These are precisely the accumulations expected when these enzymes are absent or low in activity. With these data alone, this would be a demonstration of only moderate interest showing that two successive steps in the biosynthesis of isoleucine and valine are controlled by genes fairly closely linked to one another. This has been well established to be the general rule in *Salmonella typhimurium* (Demerec and Hartman, 1959; Glanville and Demerec, 1960; Wagner and Bergquist, 1960). In addition, it has been shown that a number of genes involved in the biosynthesis of the aromatic amino acids in *Neurospora* are closely linked (Gross and Fein, 1960).

It is of more than passing interest, however, that a number of the mutants, those in Groups II, and IIIb, show wild type or higher activity for the reductoisomerase and dehydrase, yet accumulate known precursors of isoleucine and valine and require these amino acids for maximum growth. All of these mutants are leaky, showing that they can function with whatever deficiency they possess, albeit not as efficiently as the wild type. The location of the mutations, causing these phenotypes within the general area to have a close relationship to dehydrase and reductoisomerase activity, would not appear to be fortuitous. That these mutants bear some relationship to isoleucine and valine biosynthesis would seem likely, not only because they require these compounds, but because they accumulate precursors identical to those accumulated by the IIIa and I mutants.

Of seven mutants in this group, the three in Group II are of particular interest because of their intermediate position and their intermediate characteristics. The three show considerable differences in biochemical characteristics but have one interesting property in common in addition to close linkage. When they are crossed to one another they demonstrate an extremely low frequency of recombination, but in certain crosses to Group III and I mutants, they produce extremely high numbers of wild type spores. Up to 19 per cent iv^+ spores have been produced by crossing to members of other groups. One should question, then, placing Group II in this area. The reasons for doing so are (1) they only show this high reversion in occasional crosses, and (2) when these mutants are selfed, they also produce wild type segregants, but again only in occasional crosses. We have established that this reversion is generally associated with a crossover between the outside markers *lys*-1 and *sp*. Hence, it is a most peculiar phenomenon, not to be described as a typical reverse mutation from mutant to wild type. Its occurrence, however, in the company of apparent crossovers suggests that the region between III and I may include a duplication or duplications. Unequal crossover under these circumstances might produce wild type segregants. But why these segregants should occur in large numbers both in the selfing and intergroup crosses, we are unable to explain at present. The phenomenon we are observing here may well be related to what is called negative interference in the other lower organisms and viruses (Pateman, 1960; Pritchard, 1960; Chase and Doermann, 1958), but manifested in a very peculiar fashion.

Reactions Between Mutant Genes In Heterocaryotic Combinations

Besides genetic and biochemical analyses, one other method of analysis of complex loci is available to observe the effects of incorporating two kinds of nuclei into one mycelium. This is not the same as heterozygosity, but an approximation to it. One may take, for example, *Tiv* mutants 305 and 323, and inoculate them together in the same spot on a minimal agar plate. Appropriate controls will show that the mutants will not grow alone to any significant extent on minimal agar, but from a mixture of the two, a strain may be derived which contains nuclei of both mutants and is capable of growing on minimal agar better than either of the pure strains alone. If two mutants grow together under these conditions, they are said to complement one another or show complementation. It would appear that, in combination, the nuclei are in some way able to make up each other's deficiency. Therefore, one assumes that two mutants which show complementation are different, i.e., they are mutant at different sites.

All of the *Tiv* mutants described above have been tested together in pairs to determine which will complement. Figure 5 is a complementation map which supersedes an earlier map published by Wagner, Somers, and Bergquist (1960), but differs from it only in details. The mutants have been arranged in the previously established Groups I, II, and III and their subgroups. Those mutants do not complement in heterocaryons, which show overlapping bars in Figure 5. All the others do.

Several interesting points are brought out by the complementation data. First, it will be seen that some of the mutants, notably those in Group I which give no recombinants in intergroups crosses and have almost identical biochemical characteristics, can actually be separated into five different types on the basis of what they complement. T 313, which is not represented in the map, is also different because it is a temperature mutant. Only 325 and 319 appear to be identical. Indeed, no other two mutants, except these, appear to be identical in any of the groups. Second, if we assume that complementation between two mutants indicates that they are mutant at different sites and produce a functional enzyme from the

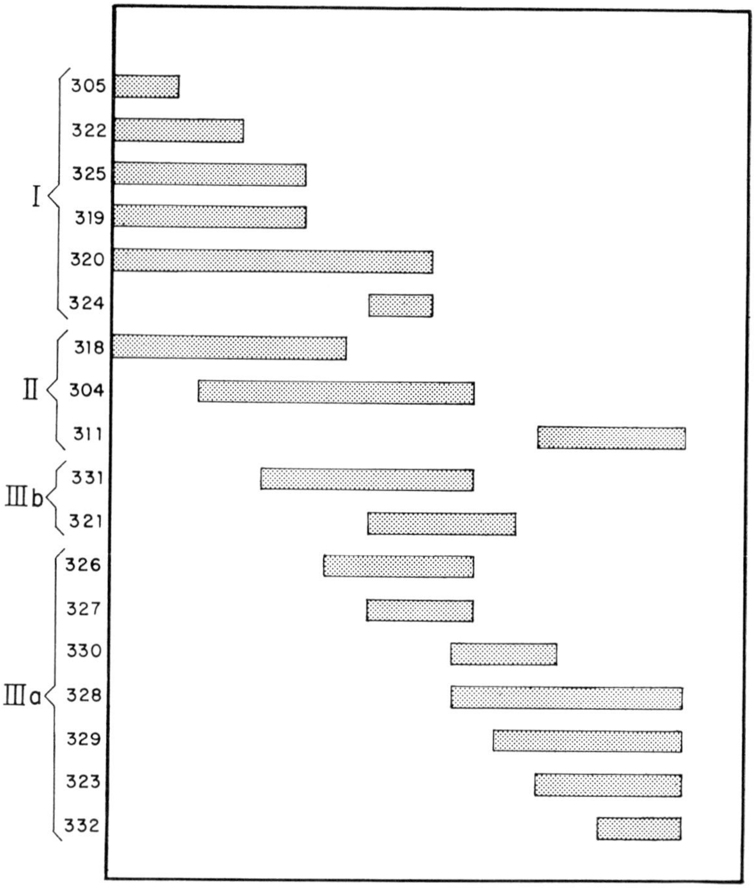

FIG. 5. Complementation map for the *Tiv* mutants.

nonmutant parts of each, it follows that the complementation map may indicate that the mutants in Group I are partially separated from those in Group IIIb. The others occupy a more or less intermediate position, with the exception of 318, 311 and 321.

The complementation relationships show that we appear to be dealing with possibly 18 different mutation sites, and that the arrangement of these sites is in more or less general agreement with the recombination data, i.e., I and III mutants are linearly separated and the II mutants are intermediate with the exception of 311. This is not to say that there is a one to one proved relation between complementation and recombination, however, for mutants which do not complement may recombine readily, and those which do complement may not recombine with sufficient frequency to be observed. Such a relationship is approximated, and may exist, but our data at present do not decisively demonstrate it. A negative result from a complementation test may only indicate that the strains are carrying incompatibility factors for heterocaryon formation. The inability of two strains to complement, which otherwise recombine, has been found at other loci in *Neurospora* (de Serres, 1960).

Discussion and Conclusions

Perhaps the primary fact established for this group of isoleucine-valine mutants is that despite their apparent location within a short segment of chromosome, they show a considerable degree of heterogeneity. Indeed, out of 19 mutants studied, only two seem identical by biochemical, recombination, and complementation criteria. Therefore, we are seemingly dealing with at least 18 different mutants, and, if each is assumed to be mutant at a single site, with 18 different mutational sites. From this it may be estimated that this region consists of at least 171 sites capable of mutating, following the reasoning previously used by Roman (1956) in his analysis of the adenineless mutants of *Saccharomyces*.

This finding is not surprising, but is, in fact, expected. Every reported investigation in the last 15 years designed to analyze large numbers of "alleles" with similar phenotypic effects in organisms as diverse as *Drosophila*, maize, bacteria, phage, and fungi has demonstrated a similar genetic heterogeneity by the various recombination tests employed. It is possible that every locus is complex, i.e., it is capable of mutating at a number of different sites and these sites are separable by recombination.

The second fact of significance established for these mutants is that, heterogeneous as they are, they are not distributed at random, but are localized according to function. This is particularly evident for I and IIIa mutants. Intragroup homogeneity for apparent function and recombination frequency is high for members of both groups, which also show low to zero complementation in heterocaryons. Intergroup complementation incidence is high, functional differences are distinct and nonoverlapping, and recombination between the groups is high in frequency. These facts alone might be taken to indicate that we are dealing here with two separate loci or genes, with no relationship other than that they happen to be fairly close together on the same chromosome. But the fact that they control sequential reactions, and that between them exists a region containing Group II mutants which have wild type or higher activity for both enzymes but yet accumulate precursors, indicates a functional relationship.

It is quite possible that the whole segment functions as a unit in producing a complex possessing reductoisomerase activity and dehydrase activity *in vivo.* When the complex is destroyed or modified, each of the fragments may show activity *in vitro,* but be unable to function adequately *in vivo.* We hypothesize, then, that the role of the area occupied by the Group II and Group IIIb mutants is to produce a substance, assume it is a protein, which binds together the two enzymes produced by the areas occupied by I and IIIa. Figure 6 illustrates this hypothesis. In this diagram, the II and IIIb area product is designated as the G factor. It is considered to have no catalytic activity other than transport, or it may only hold the two enzymes closely together so the dihydroxy acids produced by the reductoisomerase will be formed in proximity to the dehydrase and be readily converted to the keto acids. In either case, its nonfunctioning would cause the accumulation of the dihydroxy acids, DHI and DHV, as in mutant 311.

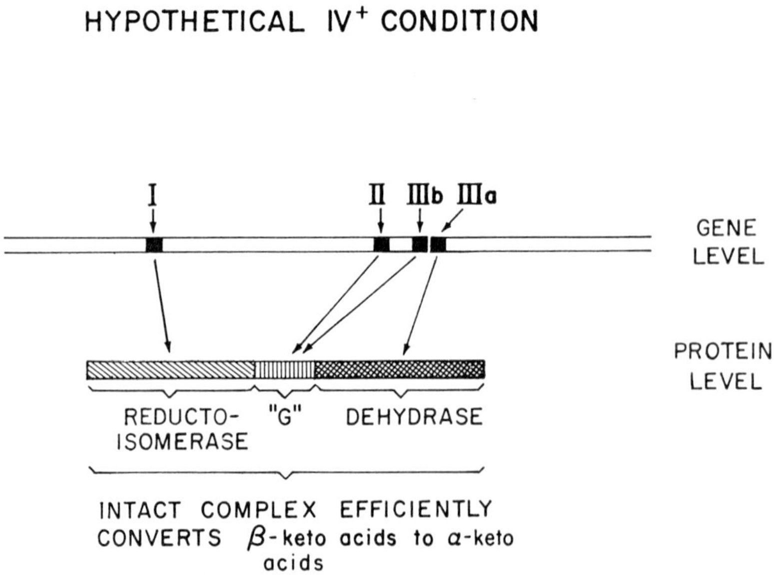

FIG. 6. Hypothetical products of the *Tiv* area and their relationship.

Somewhat harder to explain is the high accumulation of carbinols only by 318, and the accumulation of both carbinols and dihydroxy acids by IIIb mutants, 331, 321 and possible also by 304 and the I mutants. The joint accumulation of carbinols and dihydroxy acids being the result of a pile-up of dihydroxy acids followed by a forced accumulation of the β-keto acids does not seem reasonable, since the IIIa mutants accumulate only the dihydroxy acids, presumably due to a deficiency of the dehydrase. If we assume that the G factor acts in the transport of the dihydroxy acids from the reductoisomerase to the dehydrase, then it seems reasonable to assume that its severe malfunctioning could, under certain circumstances, result in an accumulation of β-keto acids, and hence carbinols only, as in 318, and its partial nonfunctioning in the accumulation of both carbinols and dihydroxy acids, as in 331 and 321. Severe malfunctioning of G might be expected to make it impossible for a product to detach from the reductoisomerase surface causing a pile-up of β-keto acids. A partial malfunctioning might result in dihydroxy acid removal, but a slow or inefficient transport to the active sites on the dehydrase, thus causing an accumulation of dihydroxy acids. An intermediate condition could be expected to cause the accumulation of both, particularly if free dihydroxy acids inhibit the reductoisomerase when a certain concentration is reached in the mutants. We have found definite evidence that the dihydroxy acids inhibit the reductoisomerase activity *in vitro*.

A further factor enters which must be recognized. We are presumably dealing with at least two enzymes and at least four substrates. AHB and AL are both competing for reductoisomerase and DHI and DHV for the dehydrase. It is quite possible that an efficient production of both α-keto acids and hence amino acids will not be maintained so long as there is an overproduction of one of the precursors relative to the other. The G factor may be functioning, therefore, in part, to maintain a balance to insure that both AL and AHB are metabolized at equivalent rates despite their initial rate of production.

These speculations have no direct support in the data we have presented. However, adequate precedent exists for postulating a cementing or transporting factor. For example, Wadkins and Lehninger (1960) have recently discovered a protein factor in mitochondria which affects the activity of the adenosine triphosphate (ATP)-adenosine diphosphate (ADP) exchange reaction in oxidative phosphorylation by digitonin particles. They postulate that this factor may act either as a transferring enzyme, or as a specific cement binding ATP-ADP exchange enzyme on specific sites on digitonin particles, so that an adjacent enzyme catalyzing an earlier stage of energy coupling may act more readily with the exchange enzyme.

ACKNOWLEDGMENTS

The authors wish to acknowledge the excellent technical assistance of Francis Wadill, Linda Myers, and Barbara Ehrlich.

This work was supported by grants from the National Institutes of Health, United States Public Health Service, and the Robert A. Welch Foundation, Houston, Texas.

REFERENCES

Adelberg, E. A., D. M. Bonner, and E. L. Tatum. 1951. A Precursor of Isoleucine Obtained from a Mutant Strain of *Neurospora crassa*. *Journal of Biological Chemistry*, 190:837–841.

Chase, M., and A. H. Doermann. 1958. High Negative Interference Over Short Segments of the Genetic Structure of Bacteriophage T4. *Genetics*, 43:332–353.

Demerec, M., and P. E. Hartman. 1959. Complex Loci in Microorganisms. *Annual Review of Microbiology*, 13:377–406.

de Serres, F. J. 1960. Studies with Purple Adenine Mutants in *Neurospora crassa*. IV. Lack of Complementation Between Different ad-3A Mutants in Heterocaryons and Pseudowild Types. *Genetics*, 45:555–566.

Glanville, E. V., and M. Demerec. 1960. Threonine, Isoleucine, and Isoleucine-Valine Mutants of *Salmonella typhimurium*. *Genetics*, 45:1359–1374.

Gross, S. R., and A. Fein. 1960. Linkage and Function in *Neurospora*. *Genetics*, 45:885–904.

Newmeyer, D. 1954. A Plating Method for Genetic Analysis in *Neurospora*. *Genetics*, 39:604–618.

Pateman, J. A. 1960. High Negative Interference at the AM Locus in *Neurospora crassa*. *Genetics*, 45:839–846.

Pritchard, R. H. 1960. Localized Negative Interference and Its Bearing on Models of Gene Recombination. *Genetical Research*, 1:1–24.

Radhakrishnan, A. N., and E. E. Snell. 1960. Biosynthesis of Valine and Isoleucine. II. Formation of α-Acetolactate and α-Aceto-α-hydroxybutyrate in *Neurospora crassa* and *Escherichia coli*. *Journal of Biological Chemistry*, 235:2316–2321.

Radhakrishnan, A. N., R. P. Wagner, and E. E. Snell. 1960. Biosynthesis of Valine and Isoleucine. III. α-Keto-β-hydroxy Acid Reductase and α-Hydroxy-β-keto Acid Reductoisomerase. *Journal of Biological Chemistry*, 235:2322–2331.

Roman, H. 1956. "Studies of Gene Mutation in *Saccharomyces*," *Genetic Mechanisms: Structure and Function* (Cold Spring Harbor Symposia on Quantitative Biology, Vol. 21), pp. 175–186, Cold Spring Harbor, New York: Long Island Biological Association.

Strickland, W. N., D. D. Perkins, and C. C. Veatch. 1959. Linkage Data for Group V Markers in *Neurospora*. *Genetics*, 44:1221–1226.

Wadkins, C. L., and A. L. Lehninger, 1960. A Factor Which Increases the Dinitrophenol Sensitivity of the ATP-ADP Exchange Reaction of Oxidative Phosphorylation. *Proceedings of the National Academy of Sciences of the U.S.A.*, 46:1582–1585.

Wagner, R. P., and A. Bergquist. 1960. Nature of the Genetic Blocks in the Isoleucine-Valine Mutants of *Salmonella*. *Genetics*, 45:1375–1386.

Wagner, R. P., A. Bergquist, and H. S. Forrest. 1959. The Accumulation of Acetylmethylcarbinol and Acetylethylcarbinol by a Mutant of *Neurospora crassa* and Its Significance in the Biosynthesis of Isoleucine and Valine. *Journal of Biological Chemistry*, 234:99–104.

Wagner, R. P., A. Bergquist, and G. W. Karp. 1958. Some Factors Influencing Valine and Isoleucine Activity in *Neurospora crassa*. *Archives of Biochemistry and Biophysics*, 74:182–197.

Wagner, R. P., A. N. Radhakrishnan, and E. E. Snell. 1958. The Biosynthesis of Isoleucine and Valine in *Neurospora crassa*. *Proceedings of the National Academy of Sciences of the U.S.A.*, 44:1047–1053.

Wagner, R. P., C. E. Somers, and A. Bergquist. 1960. Gene Structure and Function in *Neurospora*. *Proceedings of the National Academy of Sciences of the U.S.A.*, 46:708–717.

BERTNER FOUNDATION LECTURE

Enzyme Studies on the Deletion Hypothesis of Carcinogenesis

VAN R. POTTER, PH.D., SC.D. (HON.)

McArdle Memorial Laboratory,
University of Wisconsin Medical School,
Madison, Wisconsin

The present report will have as its substantive content some recent findings on a new transplantable rat hepatoma that we regard as representative of a very early stage in carcinogenesis. The new findings have permitted us to evaluate some of the older data from a fresh vantage point. For the purposes of the present occasion, the new findings will be preceded by some background discussion.

The molecular basis of neoplasia is something that we all believe in but know very little about. By this time we are all aware of the broad principles of molecular biology and are accustomed to thinking in terms of genes as deoxyribonucleic acid (DNA) molecules, enzyme-forming systems as ribonucleic acid (RNA) protein complexes, and enzymes as proteins with specified sequences of amino acids. We are also aware of the fact that the enzyme content of cells is not dictated once and for all by the genes, but the pattern of enzymes varies according to the balance of substrates, inhibitors, inducers, and repressors in the chemical environment (Figure 1). Moreover, within these broad principles, which are still being challenged and perfected, as we are witnessing in this symposium, much latitude is permitted in working out the details of life processes. Owing to the occurrence of alternative metabolic pathways for synthesis and degradation, various individual types of cells

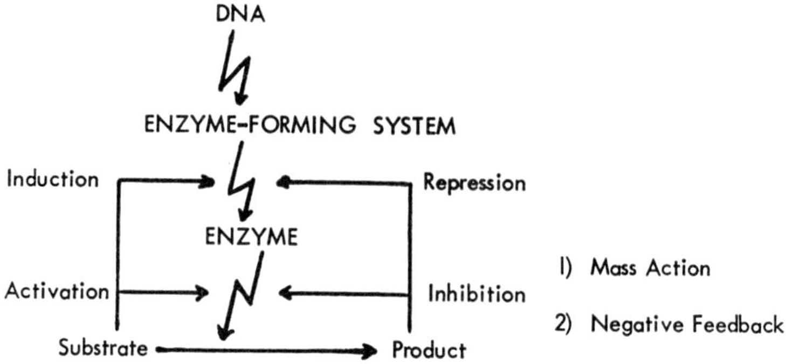

FIG. 1. Diagramatic representation of the factors modifying the relationship between deoxyribonucleic acid (DNA) and the corresponding enzyme.

solve their individual problems in a variety of ways, using metabolic pathways that show amazing similarities in all living cells, but combining them in all sorts of permutations and combinations of enzyme quality and quantity, with survival and reproduction the only test that a new variant has to meet (Potter, 1958a).

When we come to multicellular organisms, we find the same broad principles that apply to the microorganisms. However, the management and spatial organization of enzymes in higher organisms are much more involved than they are in bacteria. If we assume that DNA molecules form the basis of the entire response of the organism to its environment in terms of enzymatic and structural development, it is interesting to note that a bacterial cell contains about 2,000 molecules of DNA (assuming a molecular weight of 8×10^6) while the human cell contains about 450,000 molecules of DNA (Potter, 1960). If we assume that the varieties of enzymes in a human cell are about as numerous as in a bacterial cell, we are confronted with the possibility that in human cells there are 2,000 molecules of DNA telling the cells what enzymes to make and 448,000 molecules telling the cells when to make them, where to keep them, and how to use them. Such a situation would be quite in line with the normal tendency of administrative organizations to expand disproportionately with respect to the number of individuals engaged in production, a corollary to the well-known Parkinson's Law.

Although it is quite conceivable that the study of enzymes in normal and cancer cells will eventually turn out to involve the function of the 448,000 DNA molecules, it is nevertheless necessary to see what can be done in terms of measurements of enzyme amount. We should be aware of the possibility that the differences between normal and cancer cells may involve factors other than enzyme amount, such as:

1. Differences in enzyme distribution within cell compartments.
2. Differences in communication between cell compartments.
3. Differences in the affinity of enzymes for normal feedback inhibitors.
4. Differences in rate of production of enzymes by enzyme-forming systems.
5. Differences in response of the enzyme-forming systems to products responsible for regulation by repression.

However, the advantage of the enzyme approach is that it can be pushed to limits that extend further and further into genetic and morphological territory. The function of enzyme-forming systems can be studied by measuring the amount of enzyme as a function of time and of the chemical environment, and it is this approach which I will later emphasize.

The Enzyme Approach

For the past 20 years I have been trying to find out how cancer cells differ from normal cells in terms of the enzymes that they contain. There are some important considerations that have not always been explicitly stated, and perhaps now is a proper time to list them.

The Deletion Hypothesis

The general hypothesis under which we have operated has come to be known as the deletion hypothesis, and in its simplest form it is intended to mean that a cancer cell lacks some enzyme that is present in the normal cell from which it was derived (Figure 2). This simple idea was based, first, on the fact that different varieties of cells do not have to have the same enzyme pattern in order to live and reproduce: vast differences have been observed in different cell types and the commonest (perhaps most readily observed) difference between a wild-type microorganism and a mutant is a loss of a specific kind of enzyme capability. Second, it has become clear that alternative metabolic pathways exist for a great many individual metabolites (Potter and Heidelberger, 1950) and thus it was possible to conceive that the loss of one enzyme could stimulate an alternative metabolic pathway for the corresponding substrate.

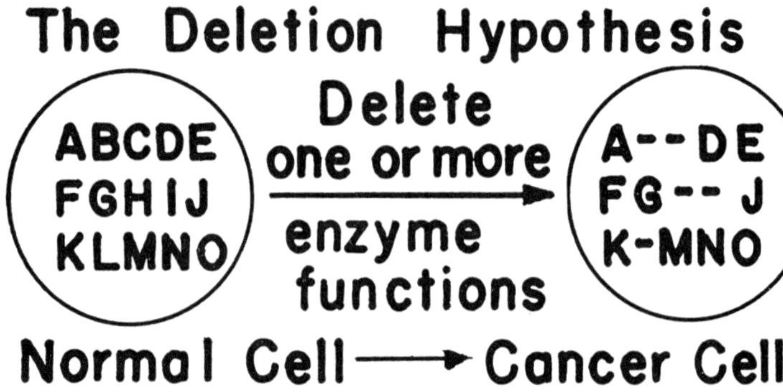

FIG. 2. Diagramatic representation of the deletion hypothesis of cancer formation in its enzymatic form.

If a given compound could be used as a building block by one enzyme and degraded by another, it seemed reasonable that a loss of the catabolic enzyme could increase the flow over the other pathway merely by decreased competition. This idea is illustrated in Figure 3. For me, this concept goes back to the spring of 1939 when E. E. Lockhart and I were postdoctoral fellows in the laboratory of Prof. H. von Euler in Stockholm, where we carried out some experiments on the aerobic oxidation of reduced diphosphopyridine nucleotide (DPNH) by extracts of normal and tumor tissue. In the abstract for the 98th meeting of the American Chemical Society in 1939, we reported that extracts of tumors were incapable of oxidizing DPNH unless cytochrome *c* was added, and raised the question of whether this might explain the aerobic glycolysis of tumors (cf. Lockhart and Potter, 1941, footnote 2). While the mechanism of aerobic glycolysis in tumors is still unsettled, here at least was an experimental result that was able to focus my attention on the concept of alternative metabolic pathways, and many years were spent trying to find a qualitative difference between normal and tumor catabolism. The most promising results came from studies on hepatomas

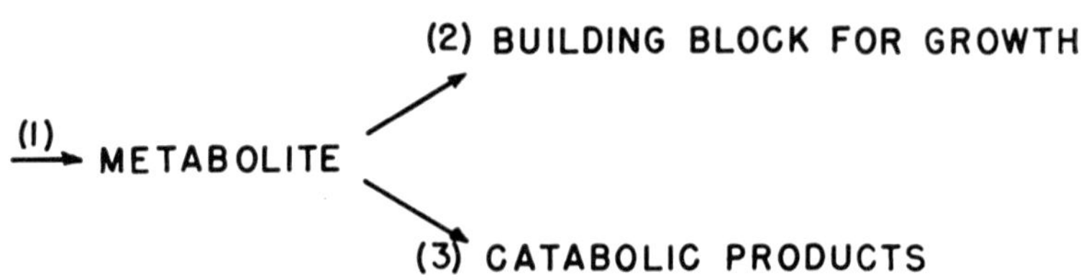

FIG. 3. Diagramatic representation of deletion hypothesis of cancer formation in terms of alternative metabolic pathways.

in other laboratories, and these were summarized in 1958 (Potter, 1958a). By this time several enzymes had been found missing in both primary and transplanted hepatomas, especially the Novikoff hepatoma, and a list of "deleted" catabolic enzymes could be presented.

I think the deletion idea might not have persisted had it not been for the important work of the Millers, who obtained independent lines of evidence that supported the concept of a protein deletion in connection with the conversion of normal liver cells to hepatoma cells by the feeding of various azo dyes (Miller and Miller, 1947). It strongly appeared that the hepatoma cells lacked the type of protein that could bind the dye, and arguments to connect the finding with carcinogenesis appeared convincing. We collaborated on attempts to identify the deleted protein as an enzyme (Potter, Price, Miller, and Miller, 1950) and were able to demonstrate decreases in succinoxidase and mitochondria in the livers during carcinogenesis and in the tumors produced. However, there have never been in any laboratory studies that could be said to have identified the enzyme or enzymes that are present in liver and absent from hepatomas and which account for the dye binding in normal liver and the lack of it in hepatomas. Moreover, it now appears that the new transplantable hepatoma referred to earlier (Morris hepatoma 5123) has been found to have measurable carcinogen-binding capacity (Morris, personal communication; Miller and Miller, personal communication).

It is my present opinion that most primary tumors and nearly all transplantable tumors are unsuitable for enzyme studies on the mechanism of carcinogenesis. I should like to enlarge on this point, making a distinction between the problem of carcinogenesis and the problem of chemotherapy.

Carcinogenesis or Chemotherapy

The study of the enzyme pattern (amount, activity, and localization) in normal and cancer tissues has to be carried out with different materials depending upon whether we are concerned with *carcinogenesis* or with *chemotherapy*.

If we are concerned with chemotherapy, we are not concerned about how many changes have occurred since the original malignant cell was formed, we are not concerned with the cell of origin, we are not concerned about whether a given enzyme deletion is relevant to carcinogenesis. We are concerned with the *de facto* enzyme pattern and whether it differs sufficiently from the pattern in the most sensitive normal tissue to permit the use of a chemotherapeutic agent that will stop the growth of the tumor cells or kill them without destroying the most sensitive normal tissue and thereby killing the host. If we are concerned with chemotherapy, we must seek the explanation of why some cancers respond to a drug and others do not, and we are concerned with why some cancers respond at first and then become drug resistant. We are concerned primarily with the enzymes that attack the drugs, and with enzymes that are attacked by the drugs. We are concerned with how enzymes can be rendered more vulnerable to attack by the drugs, and this has been approached in terms of sequential blocking and all the theoretical considerations of enzyme inhibitions (Potter, 1951). We are interested in the enzyme patterns of transplantable animal tumors if we have data on enzymes that help to explain the resistance or sensitivity of the tumor to a given drug *in vivo*. We should be concerned with the enzyme patterns of human tumors, but mainly insofar as the enzyme patterns can be related to given drugs. It is folly for us to think that we can learn the fundamental nature of cancer or of carcinogenesis by studying tumors that represent far advanced stages of cancer evolution, or tumors that represent a single stage variation from a normal cell that cannot be identified and used as a basis for comparison.

Conversely, if we are concerned with carcinogenesis, we want to know what are the minimal deviations that must be effected in a normal cell to make it a malignant cell? We must be able to define malignancy and to test for it, and at present this can only be done in terms of a tumor-host relationship. Biological malignancy may be defined as a cell:host relationship in which there are: uncontrolled DNA synthesis, mitosis, and cell division; invasion of normal tissues; and metastasis to distant sites in the host. We must be aware of the many biological studies that indicate the ability of cancer cells to lie dormant for weeks or years without increasing exponentially. The phenomenon of carcinoma *in situ* indicated that normal cells may undergo a transition to cancer cells in stages, and the experimental studies of Berenblum (1954), of Rusch (1954), and of Boutwell (1961), among others, strongly suggest that there are stages in carcinogenesis. What is beginning to emerge are the ideas that in the over-all transition from normal cells to cancer cells there is an accumulation of changes, that evolution by selection occurs throughout the life of a neoplastic cell population, and that the intervals between the successive steps may vary from days to years. We know that drug-sensitive cell populations can undergo evolution into drug-resistant populations and indeed the most commonly reported change according to Heidelberger and co-workers (Heidelberger, Kaldor, Mukherjee, and Danneberg, 1960) is a deletion of an enzyme that converts a purine or pyrimidine analogue into the corresponding ribotide, which is the active form of the drug. It seems likely that successive changes occur in the conversion of normal cells to cancer cells and that many of the observed differences between cancer cells and normal cells may be completely irrelevant to the transformation. Once a normal cell has been converted to a cancer cell, the increased occurrence of cell division will permit the expression of additional mutations, and the only test that any mutation has to meet is the test of survival. Here we might note that, in the case of the normal animal cells that are rapidly dividing, certain daughter cells survive for one or a few generations and then die without further offspring, while every neoplastic daughter cell is potentially immortal, and can perpetuate any mutation that is not lethal. Thus, the life history of a cancer cell is pictured as beginning with a normal cell accumulating one or

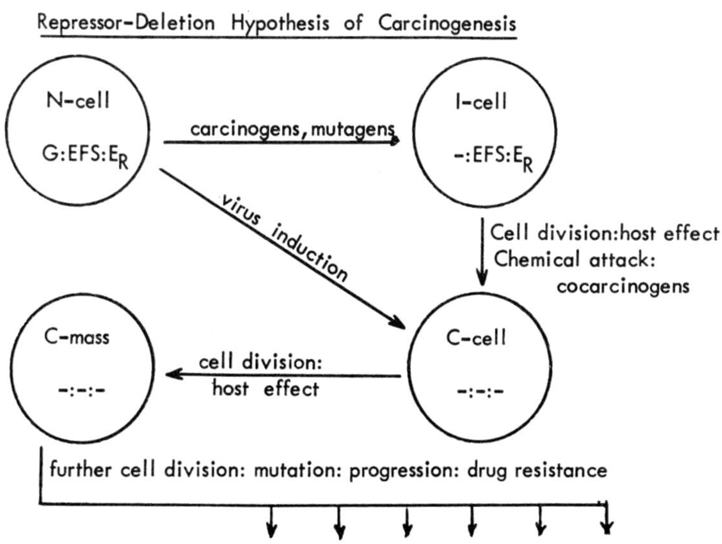

FIG. 4. Diagramatic representation of the concept of stages of carcinogenesis. N, normal; I, intermediate; C, cancer; G, gene; EFS, enzyme forming system; E_R, enzyme that forms a repressor substance (see Figures 1, 2, 3, 20). (Evolved from Boutwell, 1961.)

more changes (Figure 4) that make it potentially capable of escaping the restraints that apply to normal cells, and then entering a period of DNA synthesis and cell division with or without further change or through a change in the host, followed by further changes that make it independent of restraint by the host. (This view is not incompatible with the rapid induction of neoplastic growth by various viruses, which I would assume to be capable of bringing about the several needed changes from the moment of infection and would no doubt be able to bring in several irrelevant changes at the same time.) Following the conversion, with or without virus, additional changes occur spontaneously and under the selective pressures of various forms of therapy, until the total number of possible enzyme patterns in cancer cells is probably as great as in the *Neurospora* mutants (Figure 4).

Thus, we emphasize that there are two aspects to the biochemistry of cancer cells: One is the definition of the strategic changes that are able to result in carcinogenesis, and the other is the definition of the most commonly evolved end results of cancer evolution, i.e., the most frequently encountered chemotherapeutic problems.

In the biochemical attack on the cancer problem, previous investigators including myself have not always clearly distinguished between the two aspects of cancer biochemistry, and I think it is probably the recent advances with 5-fluorouracil and similar compounds (Heidelberger, Kaldor, Mukherjee, and Danneberg, 1960) that have helped to crystallize my own ideas in this area.

Earlier work on the biochemistry of cancer did not have the benefit of the more recent data. Warburg certainly was in an overextended position when he based his conclusions on tumors that surely represented advanced stages of cancer evolution. Even when these tumors have become biologically stable, they are capable of evolving into new strains under the selective pressure of new chemotherapeutic regimens. The aerobic glycolysis of tumors is undoubtedly a property of the evolved tumor, but it would indeed be an act of fate if the first biochemical property to be found in tumors were to be also the first change to occur in the transition of a normal cell to a tumor cell, as Warburg maintained. It may be mentioned here that aerobic and anaerobic glycolysis in the Morris hepatoma 5123 appears to be essentially the same as in normal liver on the basis of preliminary results in this laboratory (Pitot, personal communication) and elsewhere (Burk, personal communication; Aisenberg, personal communication) and a similar lack of aerobic glycolysis has been reported in a new transplantable mouse hepatoma (Albert and Orlowski, 1960).

Weinhouse, who has always played a keen role as antagonist in the forum of cancer biochemistry, has continuously denied the Warburg concept of a defective respiration (Weinhouse, 1956) and on many occasions denied the existence of qualitative or quantitative differences between the enzymes of carbon or electron transport in normal and tumor tissues. Meanwhile, Greenstein had enunciated the hypothesis of convergence and I had also published several papers (Potter, 1956) showing differences between normal and tumor tissues and it seemed that we were at odds with the Weinhouse view. However, it turned out that Weinhouse did not deny the existence of differences but that he now raised questions as to their significance. His conclusions were based on observations that ranges of values for tumor tissues overlapped the ranges for normal tissues so much that critical differences could not be described. He questioned whether the differences occurred before carcinogenesis, or whether they were a result of carcinogenesis: "If it is a normal liver cell which becomes neoplastic, is the metabolism altered before cell division occurs, or does cell division bring about the altered metabolism? . . . Are all of the biochemical activities which are absent [*sic*] in the fully grown tumor lost [*sic*] with the first cell division, or are they lost gradually with successive cell divisions?" (Weinhouse, 1956).

The answer to these questions has been our principal concern for the past four or five years, and it hinges on the problem of identifying the normal cell that is the immediate precursor of the first biologically malignant cell, and on the availability of both types of cells in adequate quantities. It may be emphasized that most if not all of the neoplastic cells previously studied by Warburg, Greenstein, Weinhouse, Potter, and others may be so far removed from their cell of origin that little confidence can be placed in any comparisons made up to now. In short, we don't know what normal cells to compare them with. The Greenstein hypothesis of convergence may be useful for indicating the most probable enzyme patterns that tumors converge to, and as such may have a bearing on chemotherapy problems; but the findings add little to our knowledge of carcinogenesis. It may also be repeated that the distinction between transplantable and primary tumors is no assurance of meaningful data. Except for the original 5123 hepatoma, there have been no enzyme studies on primary hepatomas that resemble liver as closely as does the transplantable hepatoma 5123 that will be described in the present report, and several studies indicate that the primary hepatomas usually seen are either only infrequently derived from parenchymal liver cells or very far removed from them (see below).

The Problem of Normal Tissue Controls

The problem of normal tissue controls is basic to any attempt to unravel the sequence of events that occur during carcinogenesis. During the period 1956–1958, there were many indications that the Novikoff hepatoma lacked many enzymes that were present in normal adult liver (Potter, 1958a); but in 1957 and on subsequent occasions (Potter, 1958a,b) we emphasized the need for identifying the cell of origin. For example, it was stated "Thus the Novikoff hepatoma exhibits an enzyme pattern that is lacking in certain catabolic enzymes for purines, pyrimidines, amino acids, and a specific type of hydrogen transport. The upshot of these studies is that either the Novikoff hepatoma cell is a liver cell that has undergone profound alteration or it is a descendant of a cell that never was a liver cell" (Potter, 1957). By 1960 it was possible to make the suggestion (Pitot and Potter, 1960) that the Novikoff hepatoma was more closely related to bile duct epithelial cells than to parenchymal liver cells on the basis of the fact that it is rich in deoxycytidylic deaminase, an enzyme that is low or missing from normal adult rat liver but present in high amounts when proliferating bile ducts are present.

The old approach to the problem of controls was to study a so-called "homologous" tissue, or to pick a tissue that contained dividing cells, or simply to analyze tissue from several different organs and hope something would come of it. Of course it was always known that organs contain different tissues and that the tissues are composed of similar cells, but it is now possible to comment on differences in the enzyme patterns of normal cells as follows:

1. Each type of normal cell in a multicellular organism has a different and characteristic enzyme pattern, with variations that are both quantitative and qualitative (qualitative within experimental error).
2. The enzyme pattern of normal cells is not constant but varies widely as age, physiological condition, and environment alter the rate of enzyme synthesis, activation, and destruction.
3. The enzyme pattern of a given normal cell type varies even

with its position in a tissue and in an organ. Thus, individual parenchymal liver cells in a single lobule of the liver contain different amounts of certain enzymes (Novikoff, 1959).

4. Cancer cells do not necessarily have uniform enzyme patterns even when they are morphologically similar.

5. Cancer cell populations with a given enzyme pattern evolve into populations with a different enzyme pattern when chemotherapeutic agents are given.

With the above considerations in mind, it is apparent that comparisons between the enzyme patterns of normal cells and cancer cells involve crucial problems of selection in the case of both the normal and the cancer cells. Since there are so many enzyme patterns in different types of cancer cells, it would appear that if we wish to identify the strategic alteration that is carcinogenic in any given variety, we will have to pick a highly favorable situation for study. It may be suggested that we will need a type of cancer in which (1) the cells are readily and reproducibly available, (2) the enzyme pattern is stable, (3) the enzyme pattern deviates as little as possible from that of the normal cell of origin, (4) the cell of origin can be identified, and (5) the cell of origin is available in adequate amounts. In addition, the normal cells and the tumor cells should be available for study in the host and preferably also in tissue cultures cloned from single cells and repeatedly challenged in the original host strains. With this background discussion, I will briefly mention some recent studies with a new hepatoma that we believe meets many of the above requirements.

Studies of Hepatomas

The Search for the Cell of Origin

In 1958 in Philadelphia we presented a list of the enzymes that had been reported to be "deleted," i.e., low or missing in the Novikoff hepatoma in comparison with rat liver (Table 1), and I may point out that in every discussion of the deletion problem we emphasized the need for greater assurance that the hepatoma cells were actually being compared with the normal cells from which they were derived (Potter, 1957, 1958a,b). These reports have been followed by numerous other studies from other laboratories showing that still other enzymes are missing from the Novikoff hepatoma or that other differences can be detected. But by this time, so many enzymes were missing from the Novikoff hepatoma that we no

TABLE 1

Enzymes Reported to be Deleted in the Novikoff Hepatoma

Enzyme
Glucose-6-phosphatase
Xanthine oxidase
Uricase
Esterase
Glutamic dehydrogenase
Transhydrogenase
TPN cytochrome *c* reductase
Tryptophan peroxidase*
Tyrosine transaminase*
Threonine dehydrase*
Phenylalanine hydroxylase
Cysteine desulfurase
p-OH phenylpyruvic acid oxidase
Arginase

* The enzymes marked by asterisk were reported to be not only missing but also noninducible. (Based on tabulation by Potter, 1958a)

longer had any enzymatic clues to prove that the cells were related to liver cells or descended from them.

Two courses were open to us: we could attempt to discover what cells the Novikoff hepatoma did come from, or we could attempt to discover "a cancer cell that differs from a normal prototype as little as possible and try to narrow the spectrum of enzymatic differences that exist in order to decide what differences are definitive" (DeVerdier and Potter, 1960). In the period since 1958, both courses have in fact been pursued with some success, with the element of luck playing a positive role in the outcome.

At the time of the Philadelphia meeting there were already several transplantable hepatomas available although none had received the wide dissemination that was given to the Novikoff, and none had received much biochemical study. Thus, the Novikoff was the only one that had been the subject of a symposium (Novikoff, 1957). Another hepatoma, the Dunning LC 18, had been available since 1950 (Dunning, Curtis, and Maun, 1950) but had not been utilized by many investigators, probably for two reasons: its availability was not generally known, plus the fact that it was carried in a special inbred strain (Fischer Line 344).

Following the 1958 symposium, we learned of the existence of the Dunning hepatoma and of the fact that several "deletions" seen in the Novikoff did not occur in the Dunning hepatoma (Pitot, personal communication; Pitot, Fohn, Clark, and Farber, 1959). The Dunning was accordingly brought to the McArdle Laboratory, and it was shown to contain extremely low levels of deoxycytidylic deaminase resembling normal rat liver (Brumm and Potter, unpublished data), in contrast to the Novikoff hepatoma, which had been shown by G. F. Maley and F. Maley (1959) to contain high levels of the enzyme.

When Dr. Pitot joined our group in 1959, these results were confirmed, and in addition a clue to the origin of the Novikoff hepatoma was obtained. By providing rats with a diet containing 3′-methyl-4-dimethylaminoazobenzene (3′-MeDAB) (furnished by E. C. Miller and J. A. Miller), it was possible to obtain liver with a high proportion of proliferating bile duct cells (Price, Harman, Miller, and Miller, 1952) and to show that such livers contain high levels of deoxycytidylic deaminase. The time course of the enzyme appearance is shown in Figure 5, which also shows the rapid disappearance of the enzyme when the dye is withdrawn (Pitot and Potter, unpublished data). A summary of the studies shows the comparative values for liver, regenerating liver, embryonic liver, and the two

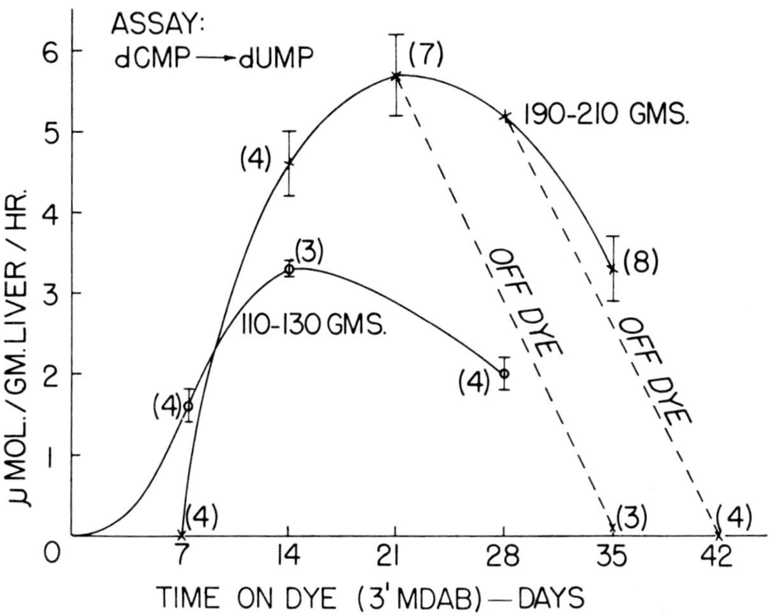

FIG. 5. Deoxycytidylate deaminase activity in rat liver after various periods of time on a diet containing 3′-methyl-4-dimethylaminoazobenzene and after being taken off the dye-containing diet. The weight ranges of two groups of animals are shown, with numbers of animals at each point shown in parentheses. dCMP, deoxycytidine monophosphate: dUMP, deoxyuridine monophosphate; 3′-MeDAB, 3′-methyl-4-dimethylaminoazobenzene.

TABLE 2

Deoxycytidylic Deaminase Assays in Rat Livers and in Hepatomas

Tissue	Enzyme activity, μmoles of product/Gm. of tissue/hour
Normal liver	0, 0, 0
Embryonic liver (17–20 days)	58, 20
Regenerating liver (48 hours)	0, 1, 5
Dunning LC 18 hepatoma	0, 0, 0, 0
Novikoff hepatoma	70, 59, 66, 41
Liver, 3′-MeDAB diet—22 days	11, 11, 11, 8
Liver, 3′-MeDAB diet—36 days	7, 5, 8, 5
Liver, 3′-MeDAB diet—27 days—followed by 15 days of Laboratory Chow diet	0, 0, 0, 0.4

(Data from Pitot and Potter, 1960)

hepatomas (Table 2) (Pitot and Potter, 1960). It will be recalled that this enzyme was reported by the Maleys to occur in thymus, bone marrow, and in HeLa cells in tissue culture but to be low or absent in other normal tissues. The Maleys have subsequently shown that measurable increases in the enzyme occur in regenerating liver (F. Maley and G. F. Maley, 1960), but it is not yet clear whether the increases occur in bile duct or in parenchymal cells. The data in Figure 5 and Table 2 might be taken as an indication that the Maley's results with regenerating liver could be explained if the bile duct cells produce the enzyme and feed the regenerating parenchymal cells deoxyuridine, without the occurrence of the enzyme in the parenchymal cells. In any case, a pronounced difference between the Novikoff and the Dunning hepatomas was seen, and there seemed to be a possibility that the Dunning was derived from parenchymal liver cells and the Novikoff from bile duct epithelium. Histological studies of the hepatomas were compatible with this view. These data contributed to the first course of action, which was to try to identify the cell of origin for the Novikoff hepatoma.

At this point we decided to pursue the second course of action, which was to look for a hepatoma more closely related to parenchymal liver cells than either the Novikoff or the Dunning. By writing to various laboratories we obtained additional hepatomas, and Dr. H. P. Morris of the National Cancer Institute was especially helpful. A series of 10 hepatoma strains was surveyed for the deoxycytidine monophosphate (dCMP) deaminase, and it was found that a graduation between "zero," the amount in normal liver, and the level in the Novikoff could be shown to occur, but none had values higher than the Novikoff (Figure 6), and only the Dunning and Morris 5123 had low values approaching those found in normal liver.

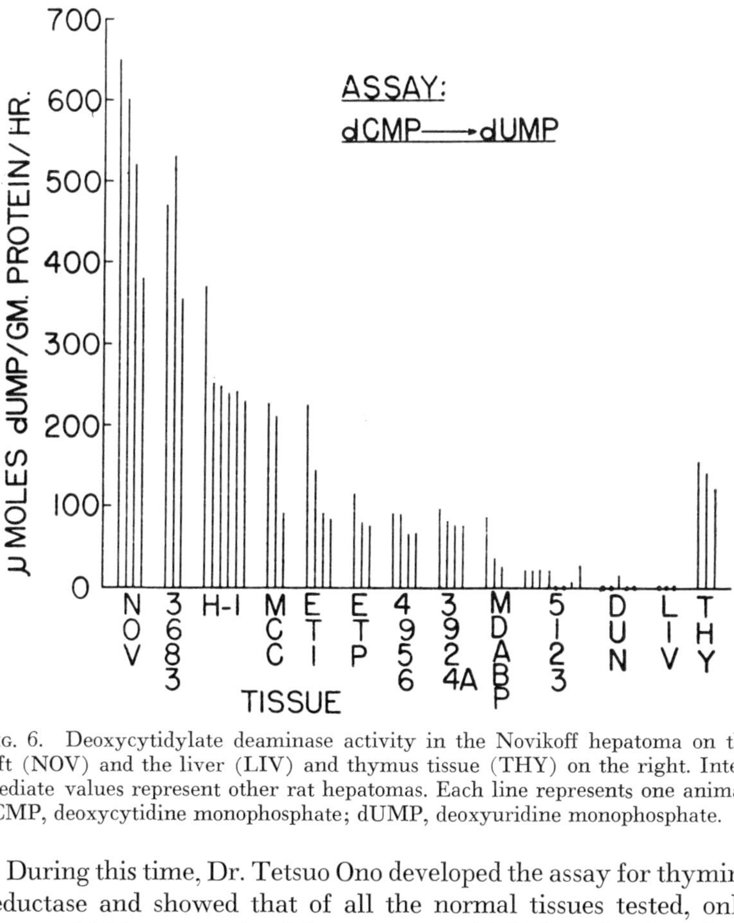

FIG. 6. Deoxycytidylate deaminase activity in the Novikoff hepatoma on the left (NOV) and the liver (LIV) and thymus tissue (THY) on the right. Intermediate values represent other rat hepatomas. Each line represents one animal. dCMP, deoxycytidine monophosphate; dUMP, deoxyuridine monophosphate.

During this time, Dr. Tetsuo Ono developed the assay for thymine reductase and showed that of all the normal tissues tested, only liver and kidney contained the enzyme, with kidney having about one tenth the amount in liver. When the Dunning, Novikoff, and Morris 5123 were assayed for this enzyme, only the Morris contained it, and the levels were similar to the amounts in normal liver (Figure 7). Regenerating liver and embryonic liver also contain thymine reductase, and tabulation of results with the two enzymes shows how clearly the three hepatomas are distinguished from each other (Table 3). On the basis of these results, the relationship between the enzyme patterns of the three hepatomas

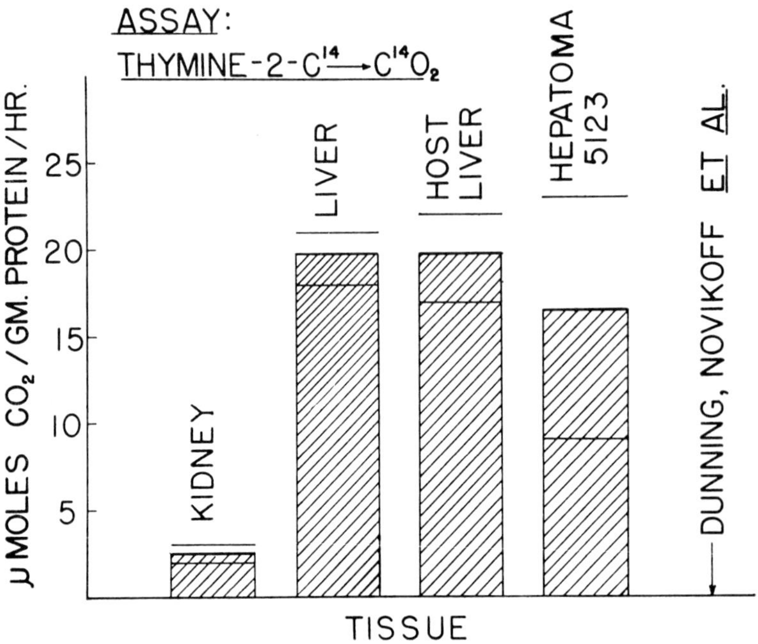

FIG. 7. Thymine reductase activity in rat kidney, rat liver, host liver from rats bearing Morris hepatoma 5123, hepatoma 5123, and the Dunning and Novikoff hepatomas. Normal tissues other than kidney and liver do not contain the enzyme.

could be used to indicate possible cells of origin (Figure 8), but no difference between liver and the Morris hepatoma could be shown (Potter, Pitot, Ono, and Morris, 1960). It was concluded that the Morris hepatoma 5123 is more closely related to parenchymal liver cells than any hepatoma seen thus far and that further studies were

TABLE 3

Enzymatic Markers for Rat Liver and Hepatoma Strains

Tissue	dCMP deaminase	Thymine reductase
Embryonic rat liver	+	+
Normal adult rat liver	—	+
Adult rat liver with proliferating bile duct epithelium	+	+
Morris hepatoma 5123	—	+
Novikoff hepatoma	+	—
Dunning hepatoma LC 18	—	—
Thymus	+	—
Most other normal tissues	—	—

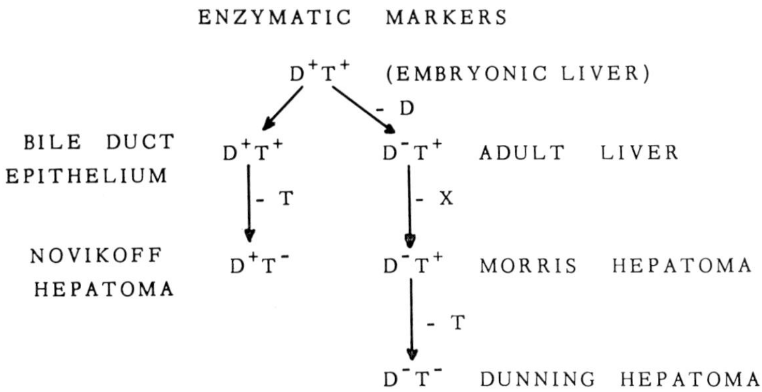

FIG. 8. Enzymatic markers in rat liver and hepatomas. D and T represent the deoxycytidylate deaminase and thymine reductase, respectively. The chart suggests possible cell origins of the hepatomas, but single step conversions are not meant to be implied by the arrows.

justified. The histological characteristics of the tumor support the idea of parenchymal cell origin, and although the tumor grows slowly, it kills the host and is capable of both metastasis and invasion (Morris, Sidransky, Wagner, and Dyer, 1960). As soon as the Morris hepatoma 5123 was found to possess thymine reductase, it was decided to begin carrying the hepatoma in four separate transplant lines, so that in case of a mutation to rapid growth, the original line might be preserved.

Enzymes Present in Liver and in Morris Hepatoma 5123

During and after the above studies, additional enzyme assays were applied to the hepatoma series. The Morris hepatoma contains higher levels of glucose-6-phosphate dehydrogenase than normal liver, but less than reported for the Novikoff by Weber and Cantero (1955). However, glucose-6-phosphatase, which these workers reported to be missing in the Novikoff, is present in the Morris hepatoma at approximately normal liver levels (Figure 9) (Pitot, 1960), while the other hepatomas resembled the Novikoff or contained intermediate levels. In the paper just referred to, Dr. Pitot also demonstrated that three other enzymes that had been reported missing from the Novikoff were present in the Morris, while other hepatomas contained intermediate levels. Figure 10 shows glutamic dehydrogenase at normal levels, Figure 11 shows choline oxidase somewhat reduced, and Figure 12 shows tryptophan pyrrolase present but in lowered amounts equivalent to about 20 per cent of

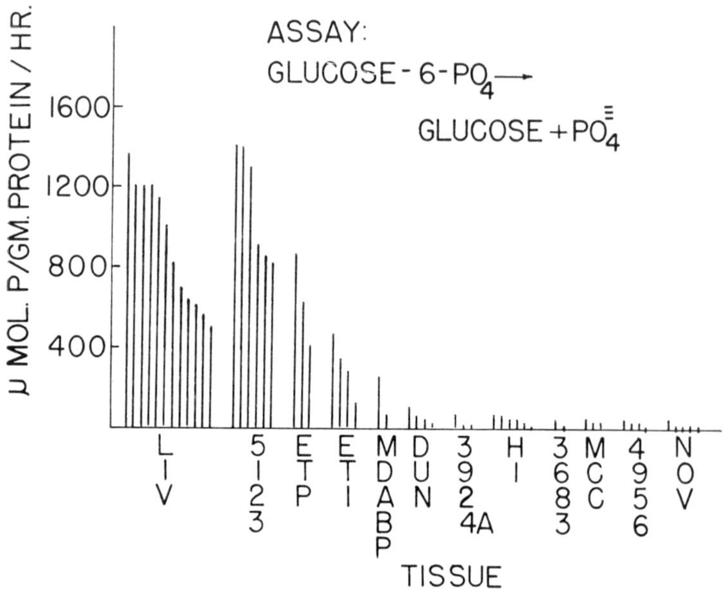

Figure 9. See legend on page 385.

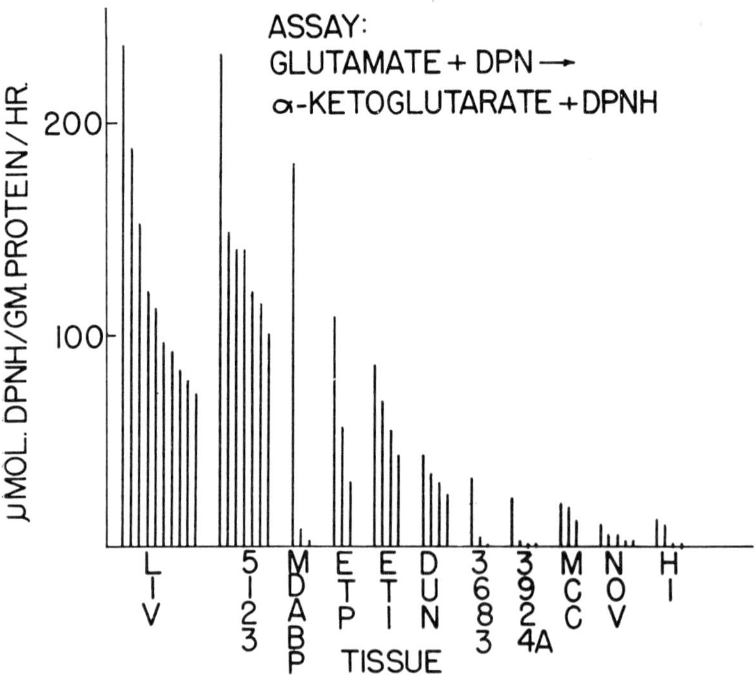

Figure 10. See legend page 385.

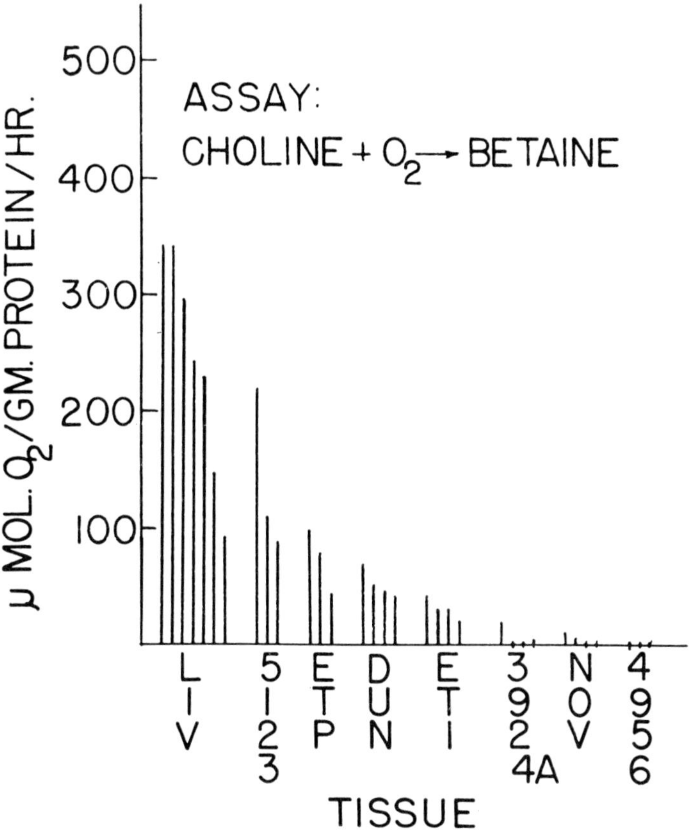

Figure 11. See legend below.

Fig. 9. Glucose-6-phosphatase activity in rat liver and in rat hepatomas. Liver (LIV) and the 5123, shown on the left, contain high amounts of the enzyme, and the Novikoff hepatoma (NOV), on the right, contains little if any of the enzyme. Intermediate values represent other rat hepatomas. Each line represents one animal.

Fig. 10. Glutamic dehydrogenase activity in rat liver (LIV), and in rat hepatomas. Each line represents one animal.

Fig. 11. Choline oxidase activity in rat liver (LIV) and in hepatomas. Each line represents one animal.

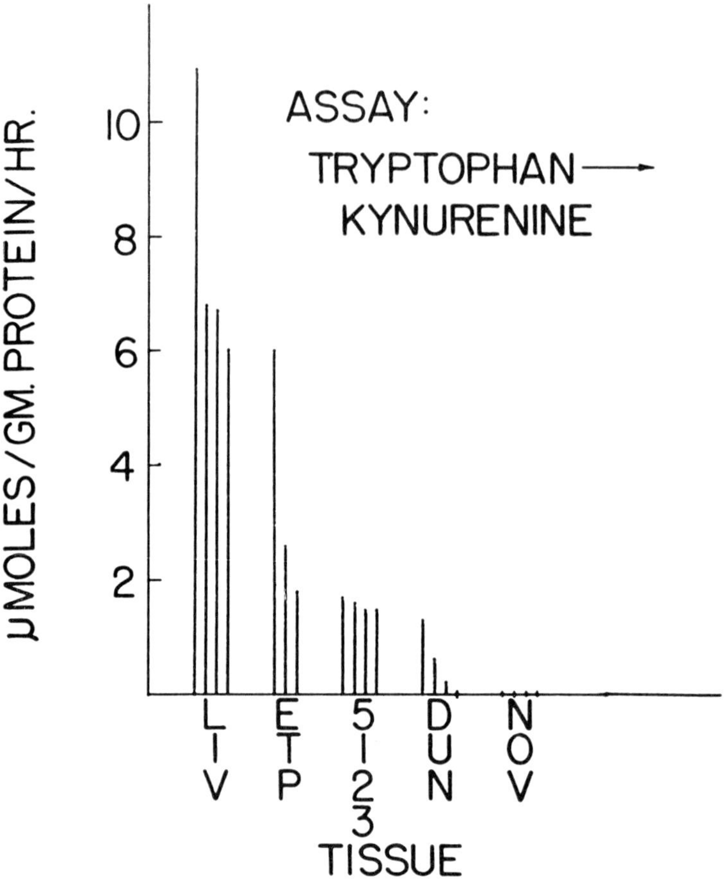

FIG. 12. Tryptophan pyrrolase activity in rat liver (LIV) and in hepatomas. Each line represents one animal.

the liver values, but readily demonstrable, which was not the case with the Novikoff hepatoma.

By this time the Morris 5123 hepatoma was clearly a remarkable tumor in that it had been transplanted for over 18 generations and had maintained an enzyme pattern remarkably similar to that of normal liver. It began to look as if the deletion theory was about to be deleted. It may be mentioned that the tumor is carried in a highly inbred strain of rats called the Buffalo strain, and this may account for its ability to live with the host without undergoing rapid change. In order to hasten the finding of a difference between the new hepatoma and liver, we enlisted the interest of as many biochemists as

TABLE 4

*Enzymes Present in Morris Hepatoma 5123 and in Normal or Regenerating Rat Liver**

Glucose-6-phosphatase	Glutamic dehydrogenase
Glucose-6-phosphate dehydrogenase	Threonine dehydrase
Glycerophosphate dehydrogenase (Boxer)	Serine dehydrase
Choline oxidase	Tryptophan peroxidase
Aspartic transcarbamylase	Tyrosine transaminase
Succinoxidase	Proline oxidase
Catalase (V. Price)	Phenylalanine hydroxylase (Freedland *et al.*)
Uricase (Novikoff)	Arginase (Cohen *et al*)
Thymine reductase	Arginosuccinase (Cohen *et al.*)
Uracil reductase	Ornithine transcarbamylase
Thymidylic synthetase (Maleys)	
Thymidine kinase	

* Parentheses indicate personal communications.

possible, and Dr. Morris has kindly supplied tumor-bearing animals to all who have asked for them.

In general, the enzyme assays have shown a pattern remarkably similar to liver, and by this time it has become obviously necessary to compare the hepatoma with regenerating liver rather than adult liver, since the tumor is producing new DNA. In Table 4 are listed some of the enzymes present in the Morris hepatoma 5123 and in normal or regenerating liver. Unless otherwise indicated, the assays were carried out by Dr. Pitot, Dr. Ono, or Dr. Ives in our laboratory. Dr. George Weber (personal communication) has shown fructose-diphosphatase to be present at about 40 per cent of the normal liver level on the nitrogen basis in contrast to the Novikoff hepatoma, which appeared to lack the enzyme.

The hepatoma appears to have destroyed a series of previous generalizations about tumors, and among these, perhaps one of the most interesting is Warburg's generalization that aerobic glycolysis is a characteristic of tumors and is the first change to occur when a normal cell is converted to a cancer cell (cf. Quastel and Bickis, 1959). Further experiments are in progress (Aisenberg, personal communication), and so much is unpublished that I will not attempt to describe the positive findings or possible deletions found in other laboratories. Instead I will emphasize the direction of the present research undertaken by Dr. Pitot and by my group.

Studies on Enzyme Induction in Morris Hepatoma 5123

It was mentioned earlier that Dr. Pitot found tryptophan pyrrolase present at only about one fifth the activity found in normal rat liver (Figure 12). One of the main reasons for assaying for this enzyme, aside from the fact that it was absent from the Novikoff hepatoma, was the fact that it is an inducible enzyme and it therefore provides an opportunity to see whether there is a difference between the tumor and liver at the level of the enzyme-forming system. Figure 13 shows the results of an attempt to induce tryptophan pyrrolase in the hepatoma and in the host liver (Pitot, unpublished data). Both cortisone and tryptophan were effective inducers in the host liver and gave responses similar to control liver, but the tumors showed no response. It had been shown earlier by Pitot (1959) that regenerating liver responds to tryptophan injections with a six- or sevenfold increase in the enzyme; thus, the results with the hepatoma cannot be ascribed solely to the occurrence of cell division. This finding is the most distinctive difference between the hepatoma and normal liver that has been found so far, but it is not the only difference.

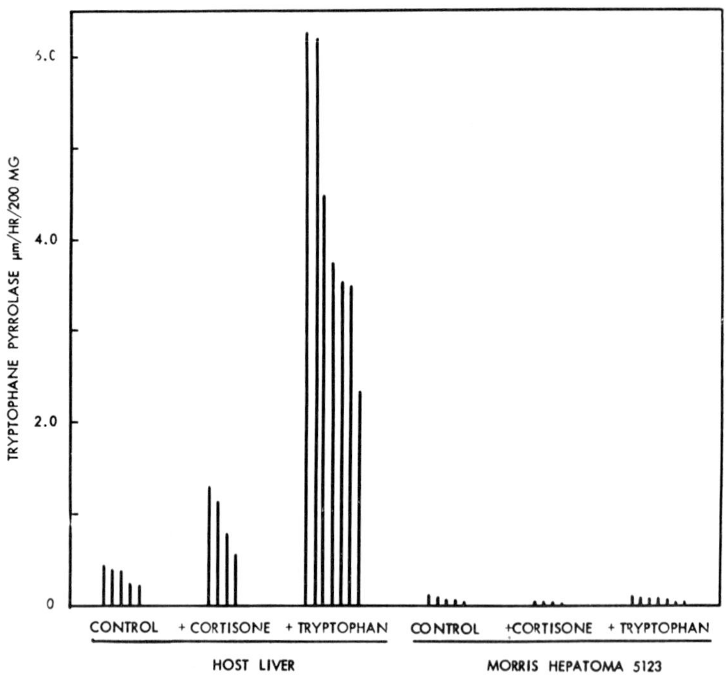

FIG. 13. Induction of tryptophan pyrrolase in host liver of rats bearing Morris hepatoma 5123 and failure to induce the enzyme in hepatomas in the same animals, using cortisone or tryptophan injections. Each line represents one animal.

The question might be raised as to whether the tryptophan reached the hepatomas. It was shown by means of labeled tryptophan that radioactivity was incorporated into protein and was present in the acid-soluble fraction at four hours and at eight hours in amounts similar to those found in liver. Although tryptophan pyrrolase could not be induced in the hepatoma, it has not yet been possible to explain the finding. Various approaches indicate that the enzyme-forming system is present, and several enzymes necessary for enzyme formation also appear to be present (Pitot, Potter, and Ono, 1961).

The failure to produce an adaptive enzyme is not a general

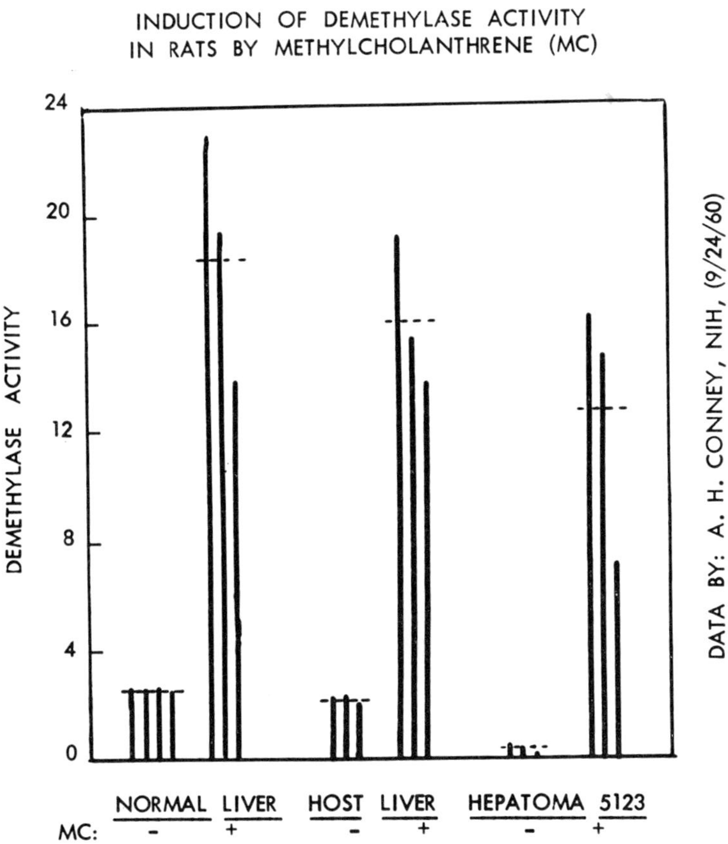

FIG. 14. Induction of demethylase activity in normal rat liver, in host liver, and in Morris hepatoma 5123 by injection of methylcholanthrene. Each line represents one animal. (Data by A. H. Conney.)

phenomenon. Demethylase that can be induced in rat liver by injecting methylcholanthrene (Conney *et al.*, 1959) can be raised to the same high levels seen in the host liver following induction (Figure 14) (Conney, personal communication). It is interesting to note the low level of the enzyme in animals in which the enzyme was not induced. It appears that in these animals the metabolic balance is such that the net rate of enzyme synthesis is greatly lowered even though the genome and the capacity for synthesis are present. This case provides a control for the previous case in terms of the effect of blood supply and nutrient.

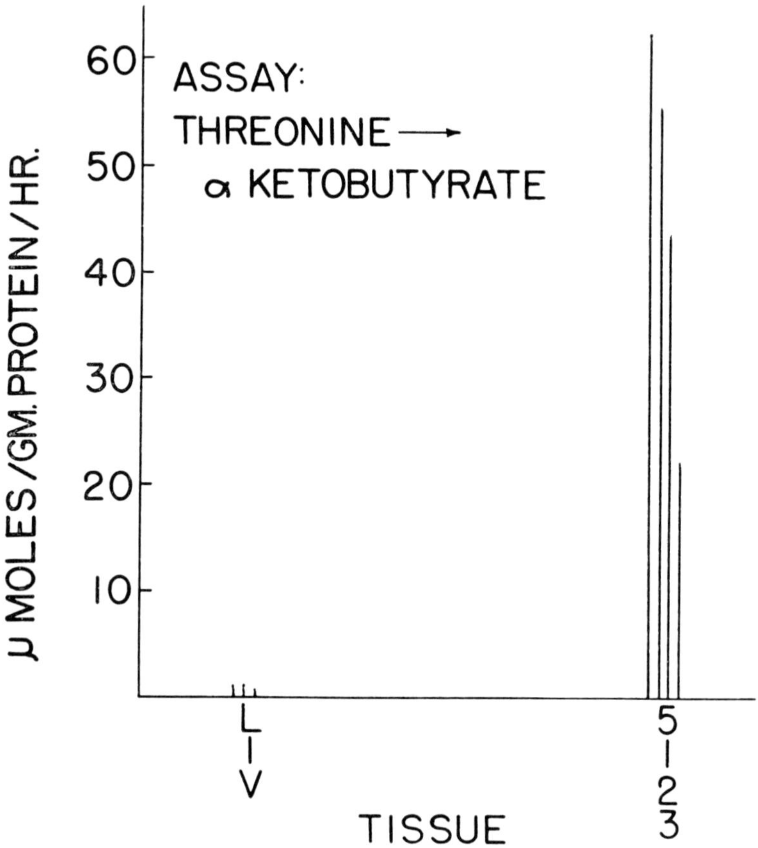

FIG. 15. Example of a "derepressed" enzyme in Morris hepatoma 5123. Threonine dehydrase in hepatoma (5123) and in host liver (LIV) of rats on 16 per cent protein diet. The host liver behaves as if on a 2 per cent protein diet, and the hepatoma has values resembling liver from rats on 91 per cent protein diet. Each line represents one animal.

Enzymes That Appear Derepressed in Morris Hepatoma 5123

Tryptophan pyrrolase and demethylase were cited as two enzymes that are present in the Morris hepatoma in low amounts in the nonadapted animals, the former being noninducible and the latter being inducible.

Certain other enzymes are present in high amounts in the hepatoma and appear to be what the microbiologists would call derepressed. Threonine dehydrase is an enzyme that was reported missing in the Novikoff hepatoma (Table 1). When the Morris hepatoma was assayed for the enzyme, it was found to contain high levels comparable to what was previously seen only in the livers of animals on high protein diets (Figure 15), and the host livers were almost devoid of the enzyme, as seen in livers of animals on 2 per cent protein diets (Pitot, 1959). Animals with and without hepatomas were fed various levels of protein, and it was shown that control liver showed rapid changes in enzyme level, that host liver contained low levels of enzyme in all cases, and that Morris hepatoma contained high levels in female rats (Figure 16). A number of other enzymes were assayed in the same animals, and serine dehydrase behaved in a similar manner. (Pitot, Potter, and Morris, 1961).

Another example of a high noninduced enzyme level is tyrosine transaminase. The Morris hepatoma contains about the same level in the saline-injected animals as in the tyrosine-injected animals, and this level is approximately that in the host liver of the animal in which the enzyme is induced (Figure 17) (Pitot and Morris, 1961).

At the present time, the meaning of the above data in terms of uncontrolled growth is not known, but it is clear that both noninducible and derepressed enzymes can be demonstrated, suggesting that the control mechanisms of the cell are not working as they do in normal liver. Since the cells are unable to stop making DNA, it is assumed that the enzymes that are peculiar to DNA synthesis are somehow not responsive to the normal shut-off mechanism. The most valuable system for comparison with the hepatoma is the system of regenerating liver, in which DNA synthesis is turned on when it's needed and shut off when the job is done, as shown in slice experiments (Figure 18) (Hecht and Potter, 1958).

These experiments were followed by studies in which we showed the occurrence of the DNA polymerase, thymidine kinase, and

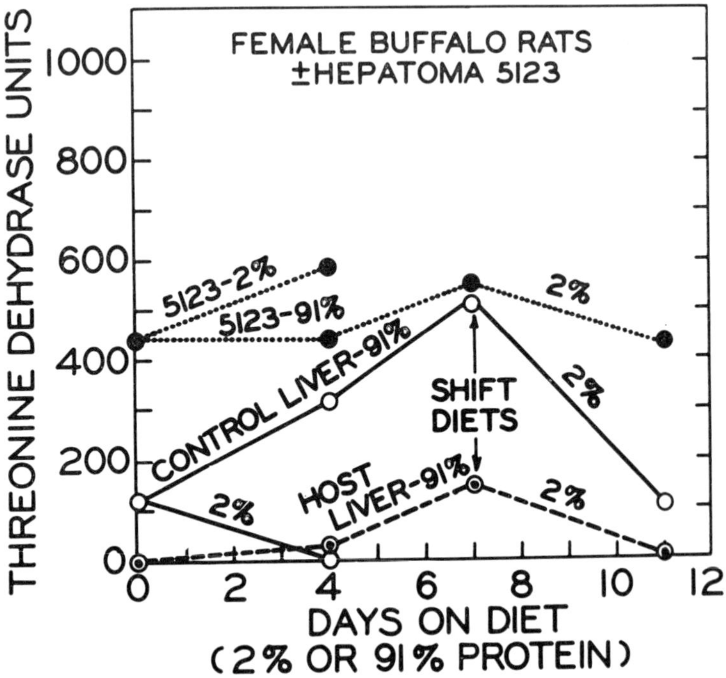

Figure 16. See legend page 393.

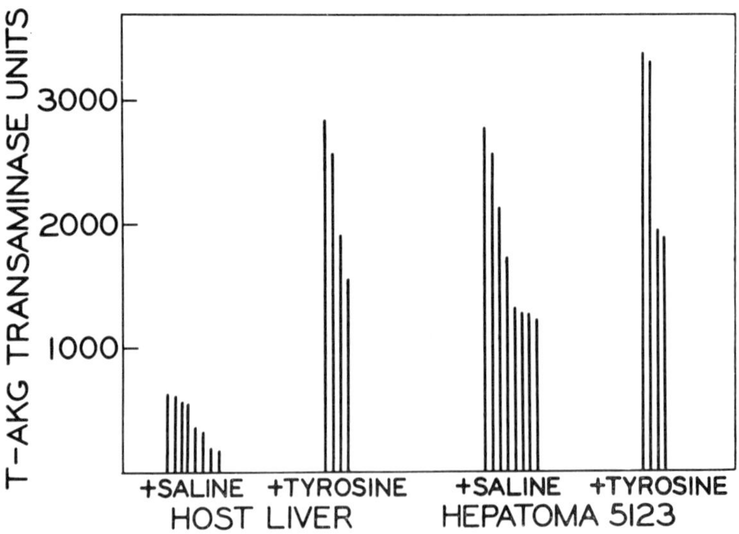

Figure 17. See legend page 393.

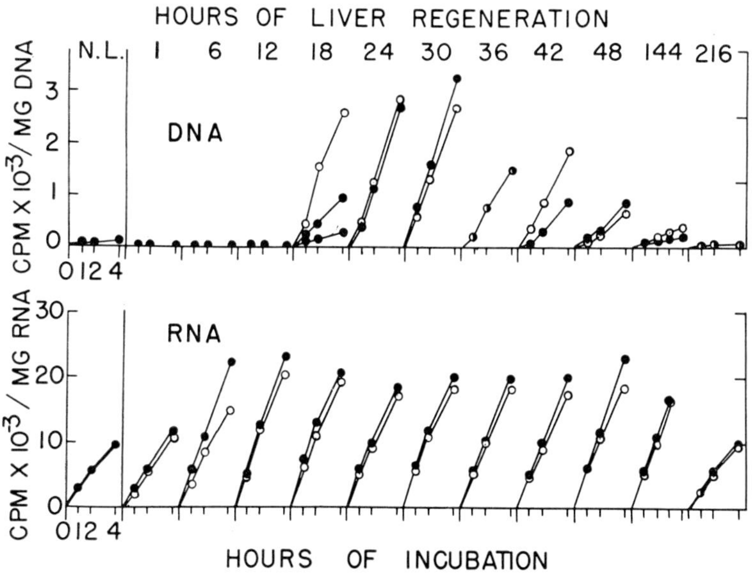

FIG. 18. Induction and disappearance of enzymes for DNA synthesis in regenerating liver, as indicated by incorporation of orotic acid-6-C^{14} into DNA and RNA in rat liver slices incubated *in vitro* for four hours, at various intervals after partial hepatectomy. CPM, counts per minute; DNA, deoxyribonucleic acid; RNA, ribonucleic acid.

thymidylic kinase in regenerating liver and demonstrated that the enzymes appear at the time DNA synthesis begins and disappear when the job is done (Figure 19) (Bollum and Potter, 1959). Much more penetrating studies have subsequently been carried out by Prof. Davidson and his colleagues, who have suggested sequential induction of these enzymes (Weissman, Smellie, and Paul, 1960; Gray *et al.*, 1960), and we look forward to a detailed presentation of their results later in this symposium (see pages 420 to 434, this volume). Similar studies on other enzymes in this series have been carried out by the Maleys (F. Maley and G. F. Maley, 1960), who

---

FIG. 16. Threonine dehydrase in normal rat liver, host liver, and 5123 hepatoma of rats maintained on 16 per cent protein and shifted to 2 per cent or 91 per cent protein as indicated.

FIG. 17. Induction of tyrosine-α-ketoglutarate (T-AKG) transaminase in host liver by the injection of tyrosine, and demonstration of "derepressed" levels of the enzyme in hepatomas from both injected and uninjected animals.

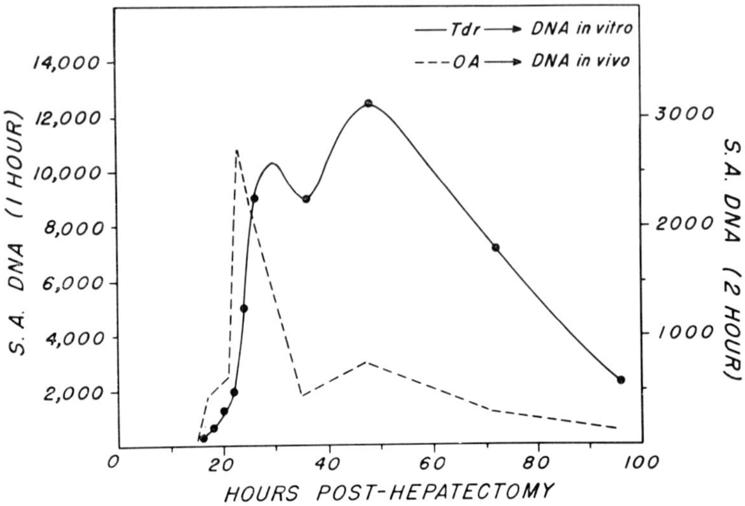

FIG. 19. Induction and disappearance of enzymes for DNA synthesis measured *in vitro* using the same livers that were used to measure DNA labeling *in vivo* at various intervals after partial hepatectomy. Tdr, thymidine; OA, orotic acid; DNA, deoxyribonucleic acid; S.A., specific activity, counts per minute per mg. DNA.

showed that thymidylic synthetase and dCMP deaminase appear and disappear in a similar manner, with the deaminase appearing several hours sooner. Sköld has shown similar data for uridine monophosphate (UMP) synthesis and for deoxyuridine (Udr) phosphokinase (Sköld, 1960). It seems clear that these enzymes appear and disappear according to a controlled time schedule in the regenerating liver and in other dividing cells, and that, whatever the controls may be in regenerating liver, it would seem that they are diminished in the case of the hepatomas.

Some hints as to possible negative feedback or repression on these enzymes or their synthesis have already appeared in the literature. A number of papers on the inhibitory effect of deoxyadenosine have appeared (cf. G. F. Maley and F. Maley, 1960), and a block on the reduction of cytidylic to deoxycytidylic acid by a product of thymidine has been suggested (Morris and Fischer, 1960). Negative feedback by deoxyuridine monophosphate (dUMP) and thymidine monophosphate (TMP) on dCMP deaminase was reported by the Maleys (G. F. Maley and F. Maley, 1959). We can confidently expect that each case of feedback or repression will ultimately be documented and examined in both normal and neoplastic cells.

A Revised Deletion Hypothesis

We believe that the above data plus the available knowledge of feedback mechanisms permit us to suggest that the simple deletion of catabolic enzymes, such as thymine reductase, may be preceded by deletions that operate in a manner that will derepress the enzymes associated with DNA synthesis and cell division and thereby produce cancer cells. These may be indicated as in Figure 20. The

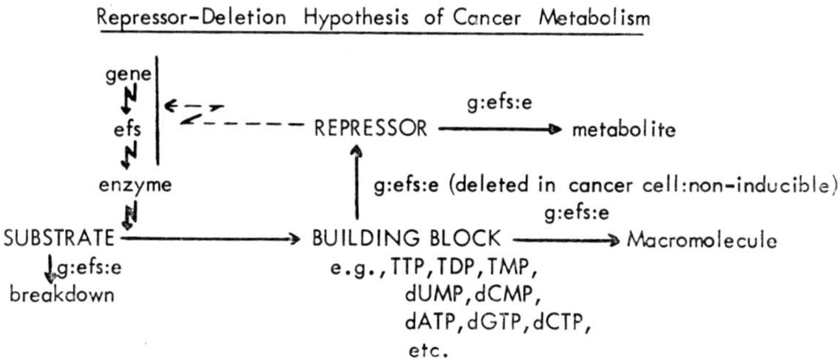

FIG. 20. Revised deletion hypothesis based on experimental demonstration of noninducible and depressed enzymes in the 5123 hepatoma. The conversion of a building block to a repressor represents an alternative metabolic pathway as in Figure 3. Deletion of any part of the enzyme-forming system (EFS) for repressor formation should make this enzyme noninducible and the target of the repressor that is not formed should become derepressed. TTP, 5′-thymidine triphosphate; TDP, 5′-thymidine diphosphate; TMP, thymidine monophosphate; dUMP, deoxyuridine monophosphate; dCMP, deoxycytidine monophosphate; dATP, deoxyadenosine triphosphate; dGTP, deoxyguanine triphosphate; dCTP, deoxycytidine triphosphate.

basic idea is that one enzyme may produce a product (repressor) that will repress the formation of another enzyme. If this enzyme-forming system or some component of it is lost, the former enzyme will be noninducible, and the other one will be derepressed. Since we have seen examples of both in the Morris hepatoma and since the enzymes of DNA synthesis are active in this tumor and appear to be repressed in adult liver and derepressed in regenerating liver, we are hopeful that further studies along this line, stimulated by the findings of many participants in the present symposium, may lead to an understanding of the carcinogenic mechanism in the Morris hepatoma, and perhaps contribute something to the cancer problem in general.

ACKNOWLEDGMENTS

It is fitting that on this occasion I should recall the pleasant memories of 22 years of association with students and postdoctoral fellows who have gone on to take their place in the world of science. In Table 5 are given the names of those with whom I have had the good fortune to be associated over the years. I should also like to mention the names of the McArdle faculty, several of whom I have known for almost the entire period: H. P. Rusch, G. A. LePage, J. A. Miller, E. C. Miller, G. C. Mueller, C. Heidelberger, R. K. Boutwell, H. C. Pitot, W. Szybalski, and Howard Temin. I am indebted to all of these people for a pleasant life, for fruitful discussions, and friendly cooperation. In particular, I wish to acknowledge the productive and intellectually stimulating collaboration with Dr. H. C. Pitot since 1959.

TABLE 5

Students and Postdoctoral Fellows with V. R. Potter

1940–1955		1955–1960	
1942	K. C. DuBois	1955	Y. Takagi*
1943	H. G. Albaum*	1955	A. C. Aisenberg
1945	W. C. Schneider	1956	L. I. Hecht
1946	G. A. LePage*	1956	J. E. Stone*
1947	H. L. Klug	1956	J. H. Schneider
1948	A. B. Novikoff*	1957	F. J. Bollum*
1948	A. B. Pardee*	1958	C. Scholtissek*
1949	W. W. Ackermann*	1959	C. H. DeVerdier*
1951	R. O. Recknagel*	1959	J. W. Anderegg*
1952	R. B. Hurlbert	1959	Robert Logan*
1952	A. E. Reif*	1960	H. C. Pitot*
1952	H. Busch	1960	T. Ono*
1953	P. Siekevitz*	1960	D. Ives*
1954	H. Schmitz*	1960	G. Gentry*
1955	E. Herbert*	1960	D. Blair

* Postdoctoral.

Supported in part by Grant C-646 from the National Cancer Institute, National Institutes of Health, United States Public Health Service.

REFERENCES

Aisenberg, A. C., and H. P. Morris. 1961. Personal Communication.

Albert, Z., and M. Orlowski. 1960. Some Peculiar Biological and Biochemical Properties of a Mouse Hepatoma Induced by Chrysaidin: II. Metabolic Properties of the Hepatoma. *Journal of the National Cancer Institute*, 25:455–460.

Berenblum, I. 1954. A Speculative Review: The Probable Nature of Promoting Action and its Significance in the Understanding of the Mechanism of Carcinogenesis. *Cancer Research*, 14:471–477.

Bollum, F. J., and V. R. Potter. 1959. Nucleic Acid Metabolism in Regenerating Rat Liver: VI. Soluble Enzymes Which Convert Thymidine to Thymidine Phosphates and DNA. *Cancer Research*, 19:561–565.

Boutwell, R. K. 1961. Further Dissection of the Process of Skin Tumor Formation in Mice. *Proceedings of the American Association for Cancer Research*, 6:211.

Brumm, A. F., and V. R. Potter. Unpublished data.

Burk, D. Personal Communication.

Conney, A. H. Personal Communication.

Conney, A. H., J. R. Gillette, J. K. Onscoe, E. R. Trams, and H. S. Posner. 1959. Induced Synthesis of Liver Microsomal Enzymes Which Metabolize Foreign Compounds. *Science*, 130:1478–1479.

DeVerdier, C. H., and V. R. Potter. 1960. Alternative Pathways of Thymine and Uracil Metabolism in the Liver and Hepatoma. *Journal of the National Cancer Institute*, 24:13–29.

Dunning, W. F., M. R. Curtis, and M. E. Maun. 1950. The Effect of Added Dietary Tryptophane on the Occurrence of 2-Acetylaminofluorene-Induced Liver and Bladder Cancer in Rats. *Cancer Research*, 10:454–459.

Gray, E. D., S. M. Weissman, J. Richards, D. Bell, H. M. Keir, R. M. S. Smellie, and J. N. Davidson. 1960. Studies on the Biosynthesis of Deoxyribonucleic Acid by Extracts of Mammalian Cells. V. Factors Interfering with Biosynthesis. *Biochimica et biophysica acta*, 45:111–120.

Hecht, L. I., and V. R. Potter. 1958. Nucleic Acid Metabolism in Regenerating Rat Liver. V. Comparison of Results *in vivo* and in Tissue Slices. *Cancer Research*, 18:186–192.

Heidelberger, C., G. Kaldor, K. L. Mukherjee, and P. B. Danneberg. 1960. Studies on Fluorinated Pyrimidines. XI. *In vitro* Studies on Tumor Resistance. *Cancer Research*, 20:903–909.

Lockhart, E. E., and V. R. Potter. 1941. Studies on the Mechanism of Hydrogen Transport in Animal Tissues. II. Reaction Involving Cytochrome c. *Journal of Biological Chemistry*, 137:1–12.

Maley, F., and G. F. Maley. 1960. Nucleotide Interconversions. II. Elevation of Deoxycytidylate Deaminase and Thymidylate Synthetase in Regenerating Rat Liver. *Journal of Biological Chemistry*, 235:2968–2970.

Maley, G. F., and F. Maley. 1959. Nucleotide Interconversions in Embryonic and Neoplastic Tissues. I. The Conversion of Deoxycytidylic Acid to Deoxyuridylic Acid and Thymidylic Acid. *Journal of Biological Chemistry*, 234: 2975–2980.

———. 1960. Inhibition of Deoxyribonucleic Acid Synthesis in Chick Embryos by Deoxyadenosine. *Journal of Biological Chemistry*, 235:2964–2967.

Miller, E. C., and J. A. Miller. 1947. The Presence and Significance of Bound Aminoazo Dyes in the Livers of Rats Fed *p*-Dimethylaminoazobenzene. *Cancer Research*, 7:468–480.

Miller, J. A., and E. C. Miller. Personal Communication.

Morris, H. P. Personal Communication.

Morris, H. P., H. Sidransky, B. P. Wagner, and H. M. Dyer. 1960. Some Characteristics of Transplantable Rat Hepatoma No. 5123 Induced by Ingestion of N-(2 fluorenyl) phthalamic Acid. *Cancer Research*, 20:1252–1254.

Morris, N. R., and G. A. Fischer. 1960. Studies Concerning Inhibition of the Synthesis of Deoxycytidine by Phosphorylated Derivatives of Thymidine.

Biochimica et biophysica acta, 42:183–184.

Novikoff, A. B. 1957. A Transplantable Liver Tumor Induced by 4-Dimethylaminoazobenzene. *Cancer Research,* 17:1010–1027.

———. 1959. Cell Heterogeneity Within the Hepatic Lobule of the Rat. *Journal of Histochemistry and Cytochemistry,* 7:240–244.

Pitot, H. C. 1959. *Studies on the Control of Protein Synthesis in Normal and Neoplastic Rat Liver.* Ph.D. Dissertation. Tulane University, New Orleans, Louisiana.

———. 1960. The Comparative Enzymology and Cell Origin. II. Glutamate Dehydrogenase, Choline Oxidase, and Glucose-6-phosphatase. *Cancer Research,* 20:1262–1268.

———. Personal Communication.

———. Unpublished data.

Pitot, H. C., C. H. Fohn, W. H. Clark, and E. H. Farber. 1959. A Comparative Biochemical and Morphologic Study of Some Transplanted and Primary Rat Hepatomas. *Proceedings of the American Association for Cancer Research,* 3:52.

Pitot, H. C., and H. P. Morris. 1961. Metabolic Adaptations in Rat Hepatomas. II. Tryptophane Pyrrolase and Tyrosine α-Keto-glutarate Transaminase. *Cancer Research,* 21:1009–1014.

Pitot, H. C., and V. R. Potter. 1960. An Enzymic Study on the Cellular Origin of the Dunning and the Novikoff Hepatomas in the Rat. *Biochimica et biophysica acta,* 40:537–539.

———. Unpublished data.

Pitot, H. C., V. R. Potter, and H. P. Morris. 1961. Metabolic Adaptations in Rat Hepatomas. I. The Effect of Dietary Protein on Some Inducible Enzymes in Liver and Hepatoma 5123. *Cancer Research,* 21:1001–1008.

Pitot, H. C., V. R. Potter, and T. Ono. 1961. Defective Control of Enzyme Synthesis in Hepatoma 5123. *Proceedings of the American Association for Cancer Research,* 3:259.

Potter, V. R. 1951. Sequential Blocking of Metabolic Pathways *in vivo. Proceedings of the Society for Experimental Biology and Medicine,* 76:41–46.

———. 1956. Biochemical Uniformity and Heterogeneity in Cancer Tissue (Further Discussion). *Cancer Research,* 16:658–667.

———. 1957. The Present Status of the Deletion Hypothesis. *University of Michigan Medical Bulletin,* 23:401–412.

———. 1958a. The Biochemical Approach to the Cancer Problem. *Federation Proceedings,* 17:691–697.

———. 1958b. Deletion of Catabolic Enzymes in Relation to the Cause and Nature of Cancer. *Acta Unio internationalis contra cancrum,* 16:27–31.

———. 1960. *Nucleic Acid Outlines.* Vol. 1. Minneapolis, Minnesota: Burgess Publishing Company, 292 pp.

Potter, V. R., and C. Heidelberger. 1950. Alternative Metabolic Pathways. *Physiological Reviews,* 30:487–512.

Potter, V. R., H. C. Pitot, T. Ono, and H. P. Morris. 1960. The Comparative Enzymology and Cell Origin of Rat Hepatoma. I. Deoxycytidylate Deaminase and Thymine Degradation. *Cancer Research,* 20:1255–1261.

Potter, V. R., J. M. Price, E. C. Miller, and J. A. Miller. 1950. Studies on the Intracellular Composition of Livers from Rats Fed Various Aminoazo Dyes. III. Effects of Succinoxidase and Oxalacetic Acid Oxidase. *Cancer Research*, 10:28–35.

Price, J. M., J. W. Harman, E. C. Miller, and J. A. Miller. 1952. Progressive Microscopic Alterations in the Livers of Rats Fed the Hepatic Carcinogens 3′-Methyl-4-dimethylaminoazobenzene. *Cancer Research*, 12:192–200.

Quastel, J. H., and I. J. Bickis. 1959. Metabolism of Normal Tissue and Neoplasms *in vitro*. *Nature, London*, 183:281–286.

Rusch, H. P. 1954. Carcinogenesis: A Facet of Living Processes. *Cancer Research*, 14:407–417.

Sköld, Ola. 1960. Enzymes of Uracil Metabolism in Tissues with Different Growth Characteristics. *Biochimica et biophysica acta*, 44:1–12.

Weber, G. Personal Communication.

Weber, G., and Cantero, A. 1955. Glucose-6-phosphatase Activity in Normal, Precancerous, and Neoplastic Tissues. *Cancer Research*, 15:105–108.

Weinhouse, S. 1956. Discussion of Doctor Greenstein's Paper. *Cancer Research*, 16:654–658.

Weissman, S. M., R. M. S. Smellie, and J. Paul. 1960. Studies on the Biosynthesis of Deoxyribonucleic Acid by Extracts of Mammalian Cells: IV. The Phosphorylation of Thymidine. *Biochimica et biophysica acta*, 45:101–110.

CONTROLLING MECHANISMS AND BIOCHEMICAL ALTERATIONS INDUCED BY VIRAL NUCLEIC ACIDS

Feedback Control of Enzyme Levels in Higher Animals

JAMES B. WALKER, PH.D.

Department of Biochemistry,
Baylor University College of Medicine,
Houston, Texas

In the past investigators in the life sciences have tacitly assumed that many of the homeostatic systems in higher animals involve negative feedback mechanisms, in which input is regulated by output (Figure 1). However, nothing was known of the mechanisms of these controls at the molecular level. Recent breakthroughs in our knowledge of metabolic controls operative in bacteria, stimulated in part by the isotopic studies of the Carnegie group (Roberts *et al.*, 1955), have provided guideposts for investigators concerned with metabolic control mechanisms in higher animals. In bacteria, two types of negative feedback control have been described which operate at the enzyme level. In the first type of control, the end product of a biosynthetic sequence inhibits the catalytic action of an early enzyme in that sequence, whereas in the second type of control, the end product controls the concentration of catalytically active protein (enzyme repression). Feedback controls in bacteria have been the subject of several reviews (Magasanik, 1957; Pardee, 1959), which describe the investigations of Umbarger, Pardee, Magasanik, Vogel, Gorini, Maas, Ames, Cohn, Jacob, Monod, Gots, and others.

Corresponding studies on negative feedback controls in higher animals have understandably lagged behind studies on the more easily manipulated bacterial systems. But, significant investigations

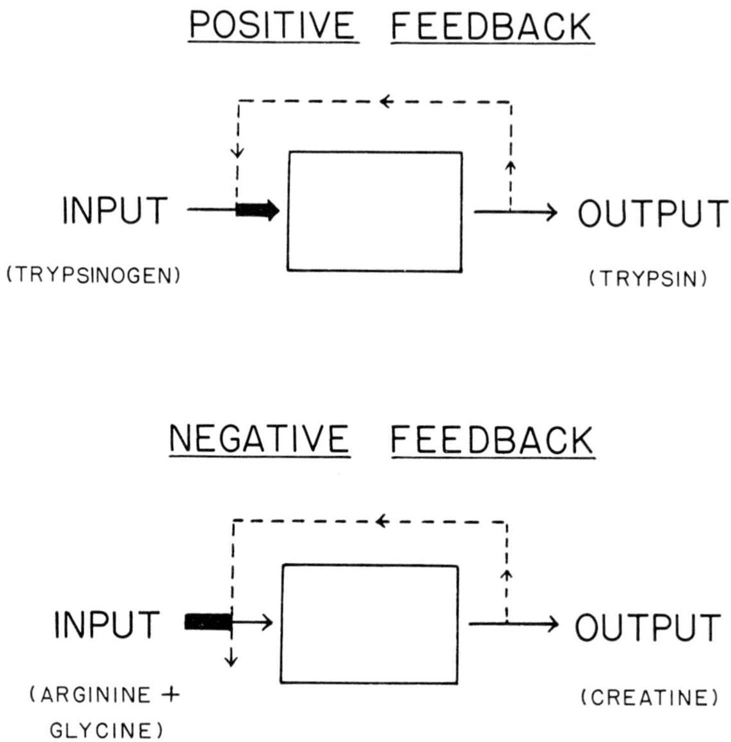

FIG. 1. Feedback systems in higher animals. The trypsin-catalyzed conversion of trypsinogen to trypsin is an example of positive feedback. Rapid, unidirectional responses are characteristic of positive feedback systems. One of the purposes of negative feedback systems is to equate supply with demand to maintain homeostatic conditions. For example, an increase in tissue creatine acts to lower the concentration of an enzyme involved in its synthesis, so that proportionately less arginine and glycine are converted into creatine.

have been carried out in this area. For example, DeMars, who is in Eagle's laboratory, has described a glutamine repression of glutamine synthetase in HeLa cells growing in tissue culture (DeMars, 1958). Unfortunately, when the compound involved is the immediate product of the enzyme whose concentration is lowered, as is the case with glutamine synthetase, the situation is not clear-cut. Indeed, Eagle interprets the same data as indicating induction of glutamine synthetase by its substrate, glutamic acid, rather than repression by its enzymic product, glutamine. Negative feedback systems have recently been implicated in the synthesis of purines in pigeon liver (Wyngaarden and Ashton, 1959) and in cultured

Ehrlich ascites cells (McFall and Magasanik, 1960); synthesis of cholesterol in rat liver (Tomkins, Sheppard, and Chaikoff, 1953; Bucher, 1959; Beher and Baker, 1959; Siperstein, 1960); and the synthesis of pyrimidines in man (Huguley, Bain, Rivers, and Scoggins, 1959). Undoubtedly other feedback systems also occur in higher animals (cf. Potter and Auerbach, 1959). For example, one might predict that where end product inhibition of the catalytic action of an enzyme occurs in bacteria, a similar inhibition of activity might occur at the same site in higher animals, since the active catalytic sites should be somewhat similar in both instances. A case in point is end product inhibition of the initial step in pyrimidine biosynthesis in *Escherichia coli* (Yates and Pardee, 1956) and in Ehrlich ascites cells (Bresnick and Hitchings, 1961). Analogous predictions concerning the comparative biochemistry of enzyme repressions would be less reliable, inasmuch as even among bacteria the same enzyme is repressible in some strains and not in others.

Recently a particularly clear-cut example of negative feedback in higher animals, which has no analogue in bacteria, has been discovered in our laboratory: a negative feedback control of the steady-state tissue concentration of the enzyme, arginine-glycine transamidinase, by its remote biosynthetic end product, creatine (Walker, 1959, 1960, 1961). A description of this experimental system will be the subject of this report.

We had been interested for some time in the metabolic mechanisms responsible for the control of creatine biosynthesis. Precise metabolic control of creatine biosynthesis may be inferred from the known constancy of creatine plus creatinine excretion by individuals on a creatine- and creatinine-free diet. We reasoned that, since creatine is synthesized only by the metazoa, and only in specific differentiated tissues of the metazoa, controls which regulate the rate of creatine biosynthesis might well have evolved after attainment of the multicellular stage. If this were the case, the control system might conceivably have characteristics somewhat different from systems which control reaction sequences common to both unicellular and multicellular forms. Since creatine is synthesized only by certain tissues, we hoped that our investigations might also contribute to an understanding of the mechanisms responsible for the establishment and maintenance of the characteristic enzyme patterns of differentiated tissues in higher animals. The experimental material used for most of these studies was the chick; our discussion here will be confined to that organism. It should be noted that some of our previously published studies on repression of rat kidney transamidinase by dietary creatine (Walker, 1959) have been confirmed by other workers (Fitch, Hsu, and Dinning, 1960).

Creatine Biosynthesis in the Chick

At this point we should perhaps review the enzymic reactions involved in the biosynthesis of creatine. Reaction 1 is catalyzed by the enzyme arginine-glycine transamidinase, and reaction 2 is catalyzed by guanidinoacetate methylferase. Both enzymes are present in the liver of chicks (Walker, 1960),

$$\text{Arginine} + \text{Glycine} \xrightarrow{1} \text{Ornithine} + \text{Guanidinoacetate}$$

$$\text{Guanidinoacetate} + \text{S-Adenosylmethionine} \xrightarrow{2} \text{Creatine} + \text{S-Adenosylhomocysteine}$$

and it would appear that this organ is the physiological site of creatine biosynthesis in birds, amphibians, and reptiles.

It is of interest that all three of the amino acid precursors of creatine; arginine, glycine, and methionine, are dietary essential amino acids for the chick (cf. Almquist, 1959). Since transamidinase is the first enzyme of the biosynthetic pathway which leads

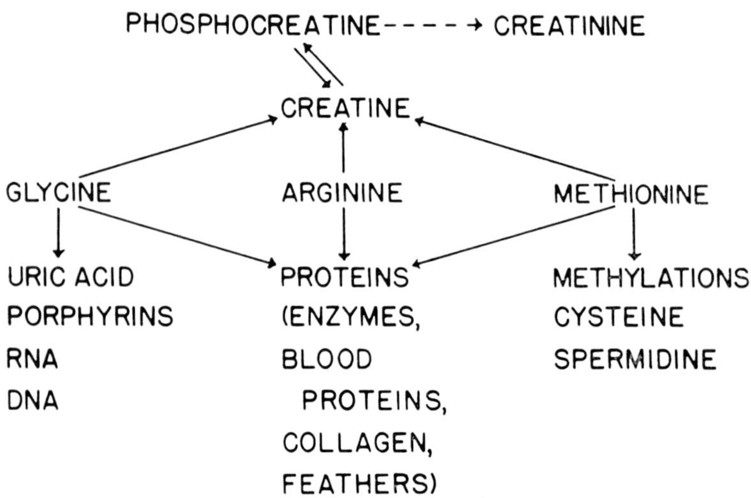

Fig. 2. Scheme showing the diverse biosynthetic responsibilities of creatine precursors in the chick. An increased concentration of liver creatine, whether of endogenous or exogenous origin, lowers the concentration of arginine-glycine transamidinase so that the amino acid precursors of creatine can be diverted into more essential metabolic pathways.

exclusively to creatine, variations in concentration of this enzyme can function as a valve for controlling the relative proportions of these essential amino acids which are utilized for creatine biosynthesis, as opposed to the competing reactions involved in the synthesis of proteins, purines, porphyrins, etc. (Figure 2). From nutritional studies with chicks it has been known for some time that, whereas a dietary deficiency of methionine does not affect creatine synthesis, a dietary deficiency of either arginine or glycine markedly lowers creatine synthesis (Almquist, Mecchi, and Kratzer, 1941). It also has been established that dietary creatine can spare a portion of the arginine and glycine requirements of chicks (Hegsted, Briggs, Elvehjem, and Hart, 1941; Almquist, Mecchi, and Kratzer, 1941; Savage and O'Dell, 1960). These observations suggest a pre-eminent controlling role for the reaction catalyzed by arginine-glycine transamidinase. Consequently, we are interested in determining what factors might influence the level of this enzyme in the chick.

Dietary Factors Influencing Transamidinase Level

Effect of Dietary Guanidinoacetate

When we first addressed ourselves to this problem in 1958, we were well indoctrinated in the concept of enzyme induction (cf. Halvorson, 1960), so we tested as potential inducers compounds for which transamidinase has a high affinity. Neither dietary ornithine, for which we had high hopes, nor arginine or glycine had marked effects. Conversely, dietary guanidinoacetate, for which the enzyme has only a low affinity, was found to affect drastically the level of chick liver transamidinase. However, instead of increasing the enzyme level, as would an inducer, dietary guanidinoacetate markedly lowered the transamidinase level. At this point we recalled the then recent experiments of Yates and Pardee (1957) and of Vogel (1957a) on end product repression in bacteria. Perhaps a similar mechanism was operative here. It was also possible that we were inhibiting protein synthesis in general by bleeding off methionine for the biosynthesis of excessive amounts of creatine from the exogenous guanidinoacetate (cf. reaction 2). Therefore, our next step was to determine the effect of dietary creatine on the transamidinase level (Figure 3). It can be seen that dietary creatine is equally as effective as guanidinoacetate in lowering the steady-state level of chick liver transamidinase. By employing creatine in

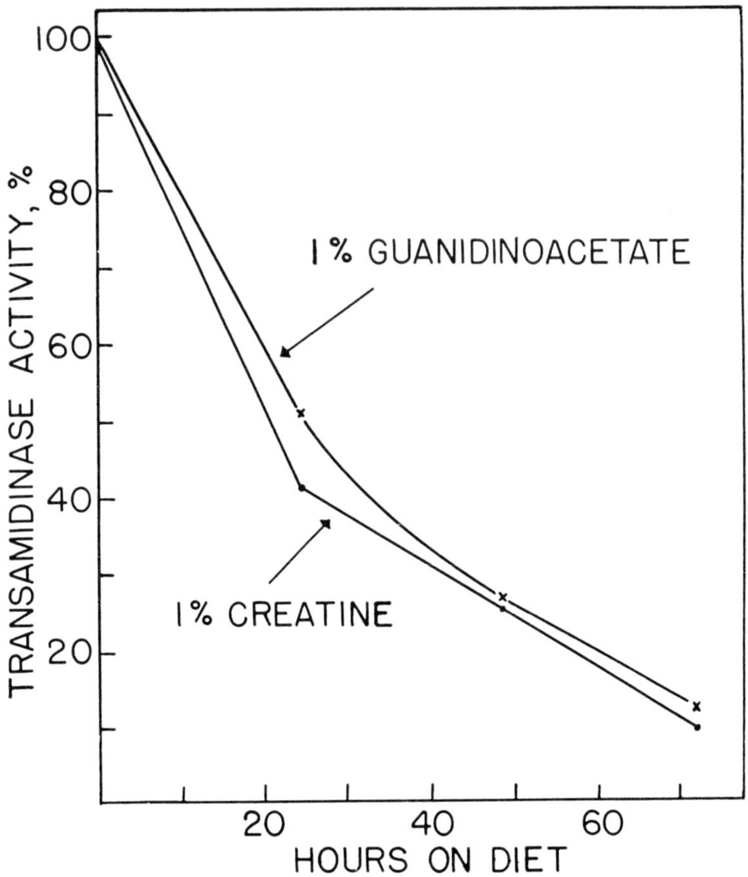

FIG. 3. Time course of repression of chick liver transamidinase by dietary guanidinoacetate and by creatine. The basal diet employed in our experiments was Purina Chick Startena. Transamidinase activity was assayed as the rate of arginine-NH_2OH transamidination, and is expressed as micromoles of hydroxyguanidine formed/hour/Gm. of liver (wet weight). The question posed by this experiment is whether guanidinoacetate is an independent repressor, or must first be converted to creatine. (Redrawn from Walker, 1961).

our subsequent studies, we have eliminated the uncertainties involved in the use of guanidinoacetate.

Effect of Dietary Creatine

Figure 4 illustrates the effect of various concentrations of dietary creatine on the steady-state level of chick liver arginine-glycine transamidinase. The basal diet consisted of ground Purina Chick

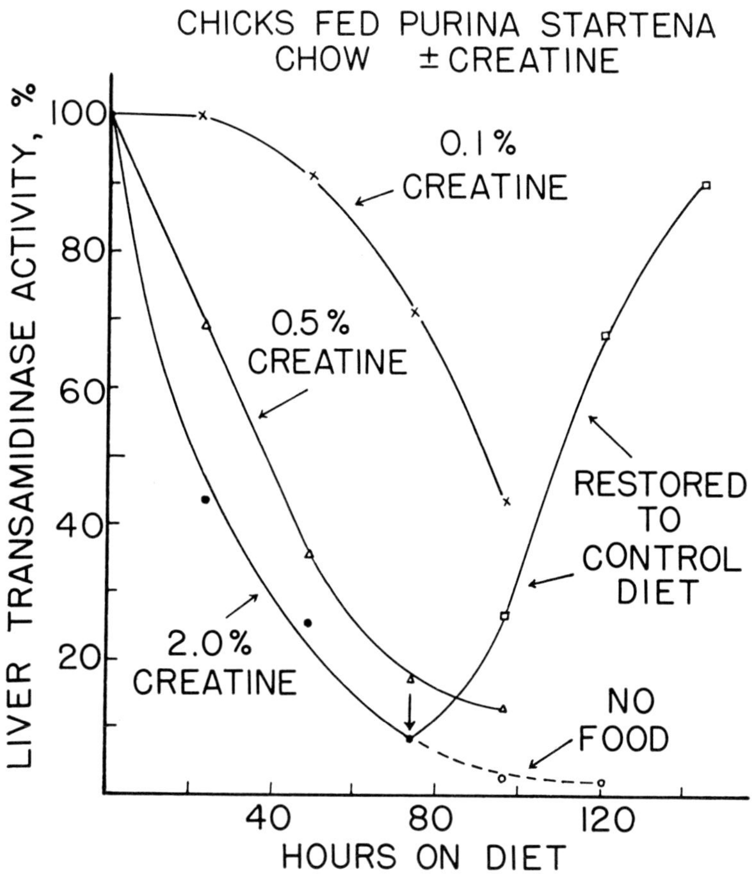

FIG. 4. Time course of repression of chick liver transamidinase by various concentrations of dietary creatine. At the time indicated, creatine was removed from the diet, and the time course of recovery of enzyme activity was followed in the presence and absence of food. (Redrawn from Walker, 1960).

Startena, admixed with creatine as indicated. Removal of creatine from the diet resulted in prompt recovery of the transamidinase level. It might be noted that the time courses of repression and recovery are reasonably symmetrical, which suggests, but does not prove, that the two processes represent different sides of the same coin. When the chicks are fasted following creatine repression, no recovery occurs. The absence of dietary creatine is thus necessary but not sufficient for restoration of the transamidinase level. Dietary creatine at a concentration approximating that in skeletal muscle

(0.5 per cent) was included to show that the transamidinase level can be lowered under conditions which would be physiological for carnivorous birds. Creatine at the 0.1 per cent level lowers the enzyme concentration to approximately 40 per cent that of control chicks.

Specificity of Target Enzyme

The next question which arises concerns the specificity of enzyme repression by dietary creatine. While administration of toxic compounds or fasting lowers chick liver transamidinase, numerous other enzymes also are lowered under these conditions. However, we believe that creatine repression markedly affects only transamidinase, out of the hundreds of enzymes present in chick liver. It is particularly significant that the levels of guanidinoacetate methylferase and arginase are unaffected by dietary creatine (Walker, 1960), since these enzymes are related metabolically or mechanistically to transamidinase. Arginase, for example, is the hydrolytic enzymic counterpart of the transferring enzyme, transamidinase. Other chick liver enzymes whose levels are not altered on creatine feeding include glutamic dehydrogenase and succinic dehydrogenase. Since chicks continue to grow and thrive on diets containing creatine, it would appear that widespread enzyme changes are unlikely.

It is of interest that creatine added to the growth medium does not repress the enzyme arginine-X transamidinase from *Streptomyces griseus*, even though this enzyme is assayed in the same manner as arginine-glycine transamidinase from chick liver, i.e., by measuring the hydroxyguanidine formed from arginine-NH_2OH transamidination (Walker, 1958).

Mechanism of Dietary Creatine Effect

The results of our initial experiments were compatible with the gross mechanism shown in Figure 5, a mechanism analogous to that proposed for end product repression of biosynthetic enzymes in bacteria (Yates and Pardee, 1957; Vogel, 1957b). In this scheme, dietary creatine serves to exaggerate a normal physiological control mechanism. Our subsequent experiments have been concerned with exploring the alternative possibilities indicated by the more sophisticated scheme shown in Figure 6. The reactions indicated by dash lines represent hypothetical alternative possibilities which must be

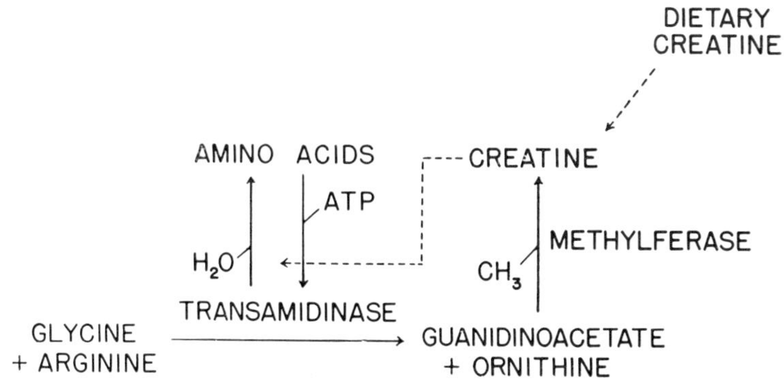

FIG. 5. Gross mechanism of creatine repression first proposed by author (Walker, 1960). Analogous mechanisms have been proposed for repressions in bacterial systems. (Vogel, 1957b; Yates and Pardee, 1957).

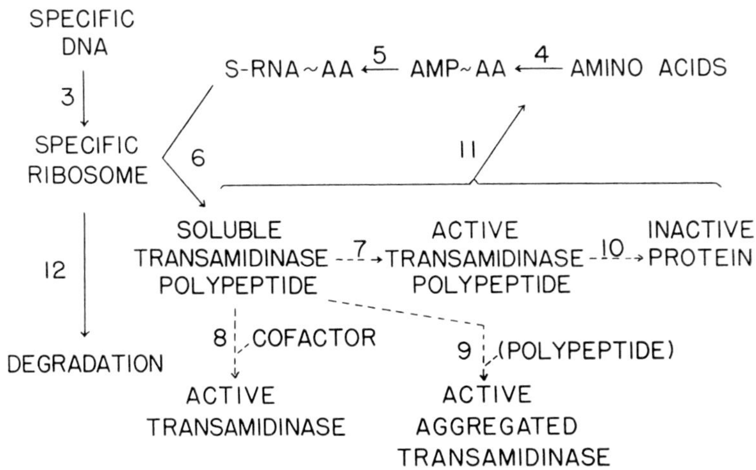

FIG. 6. Scheme showing potential sites of creatine repression currently under consideration. Broken lines indicate hypothetical alternative reactions. The repressor might act by inhibiting one of the reactions numbered 3 through 9, or by stimulating one of the reactions numbered 10 through 12.

considered in any careful study of repression mechanisms. Presumably the active repressing agent acts on one of the reactions numbered 3 through 12. If the actual repressing agent turns out to be a derivative of creatine (Szilard, 1960), for completeness the over-all scheme might include reactions 13 and 14:

$$\text{Creatine} + \text{X} + \text{ATP} \xrightarrow{13} \text{Creatine-X}$$

$$\text{Creatine-X} + H_2O \xrightarrow{14} \text{Creatine} + \text{X}$$

The repressor might act by inhibiting one of the reactions 3 through 9, or by stimulating one of reactions 10 through 12. If reaction 13 occurs, excess creatine might cause the formation of more creatine-X, which, in turn, would act on one of the above-mentioned reactions. Inasmuch as transamidinase repression has thus far been observed only in the intact animal, the possibility that repression is mediated via neural or humoral mechanisms must also be considered.

Comments on Potential Sites of Repression

Reaction 3. For this site to be considered, it is necessary that the rate of turnover of this particular species of ribosome be high enough to account for the time-course of repression. Recent results of the Carnegie group (Cowie, Spiegelman, Roberts, and Duerksen, 1961), which indicate that after induction a greater number of a particular species of ribosome is present, suggest that creatine repression might act upon reactions 3 or 12. Techniques similar to those employed by these investigators should prove valuable for testing this hypothesis. Moreover, if recent work with bacteria can be extrapolated to animal tissues, the following relationship should be considered: nonspecific ribosome plus messenger RNA equals specific ribosome.

Reactions 4 and 5. Specificity of repression would appear to rule out these sites, but it is possible that chick tissues synthesize an RNA-creatine molecule which could be adsorbed only by a transamidinase-synthesizing ribosome, and thus block enzyme synthesis.

Reaction 6. This is the site of repression in bacterial systems favored by many investigators. The repressor is visualized as hindering release of newly formed polypeptide from the template (Vogel, 1957b; Brenner, 1959; Szilard, 1960). Brenner has suggested that during protein synthesis there is a certain probability that folding of a partially completed polypeptide will block addition of the next amino acid; the rate of synthesis of the complete protein depends on the probability with which the system can escape from this self-inhibiting configuration (Brenner, 1959). Repression would favor an inhibiting configuration, while inducers would favor a configuration which allows addition of the next amino acid. Brenner's mechanism accounts for the characteristic rates of synthesis of constitutive, as well as inducible and repressible, enzymes. It is obvious that we need to know much more about the factors which operate *in vivo* to facilitate the release of ribosome-bound enzyme after the complete polypeptide chain is formed on the template.

Reaction 7. The repressor might modify the tertiary structure of the enzyme during a critical phase in its formation, either while still partially attached to the ribosome, or after detachment (cf. Vogel, 1957b). In the presence of repressor, inactive or less active enzyme would be formed. Immunological studies would prove helpful here. We have ascertained experimentally that, if the structure of the catalytically active site of transamidinase is altered during creatine repression, the site specific for arginine is affected to the same degree as is the site specific for guanidinoacetate (Walker, 1961).

Reaction 8. M. S. Walker, in unpublished experiments, has partially purified transamidinases from dog pancreas (35-fold), chick liver (eightfold), and *Streptomyces griseus* (fourfold), and thus far has obtained no evidence for the presence of a readily dissociable cofactor. However, recent work on the role of cofactor availability on the substrate induction of tryptophan pyrrolase (Greengard and Feigelson, 1961) emphasizes the fact that such a site of repressor action remains a real possibility.

Reaction 9. Interference with the aggregation of constituent polypeptides of multichain enzymes remains an intriguing potential site for repressor action. The complex structures of muscle phosphorlyase (Madsen and Cori, 1956; Krebs, Kent, and Fischer, 1958), tryptophan synthetase (Crawford and Yanofsky, 1958), glutamic dehydrogenase (Frieden, 1959), hemoglobin (Ingram, 1959), and perhaps certain mechanoenzymes attest to the possible importance of this site. However, our experimental results in this area thus far have been negative.

Reaction 10. This site is perhaps the one most amenable to experimentation. To test this possibility, we have performed the following experiments: (1) Homogenates from liver, skeletal muscle, pancreas, and spleen from creatine-fed birds were mixed with liver homogenates from control birds; no effect on the controls was observed. Apparently an excess of inhibitor is not formed in these tissues as a result of creatine feeding. (2) Incubation of control chick liver slices with creatine for several hours likewise had no marked differential effect. (3) The essential sulfhydryl group of transamidinase might be considered as a particularly vulnerable site of inhibition (Walker and Walker, 1960); but, incubation of liver homogenates from creatine-fed chicks with cysteine had no significant effect. (4) Dialysis or incubation of repressed homogenates with ribonuclease, trypsin, or deoxycholate did not restore transamidinase activity. Since the possibility remains that a suitable experimental design will be rewarded with positive results, the reaction 10 site will continue to be investigated in our laboratory. It is evident that immunological experiments will prove useful here also; such experiments can be performed when purified enzyme becomes available in quantity.

Reactions 11 and 12. In animal systems, the term "repression" in its broader concept (Walker, 1961) would embrace negative feedback control of the steady-state level of an enzyme, by whatever mechanism this might occur. Stimulation of degradation would produce the same end result as inhibition of enzyme synthesis; both processes occur at the same rate under homeostatic conditions. It should be noted that an increased vulnerability of transamidinase to degradation might accompany participation of the repressor in reactions 7, 8, 9, or 10, as well as at site 11 alone.

Conclusions. It is evident that much work remains to be done in this area. This is not surprising, if one considers the long history of the phenomenon of enzyme induction, which many consider to be an antagonism of an endogenous repression (Vogel, 1957b; Cohen and Gros, 1960). In spite of countless investigations over a period of many years, the precise mechanism of inducer action is not yet known with certainty.

Recovery from Creatine Repression

It will be recalled that transamidinase recovery following creatine repression does not occur in the absence of food (Figure 4). As a matter of fact, during fasting the differential rate of decrease in transamidinase activity is similar to that observed on a high creatine diet (Figure 7). We believe that this similarity in rates may be more than coincidental. With the thought that perhaps, by studying the mechanism of restoration of transamidinase activity following creatine repression, we might throw some light on the mechanism of repression itself, we undertook to determine the minimal dietary requirements for recovery. We have found that significant recovery could occur after 46 hours on a diet of 40 sucrose-10 alphacel-50 casein (Walker, 1961). Both carbohydrate and a protein of high biological value were required, and in the proper proportions; zein or hemoglobin could not substitute for casein. Acid-hydrolyzed casein could substitute for casein if sup-

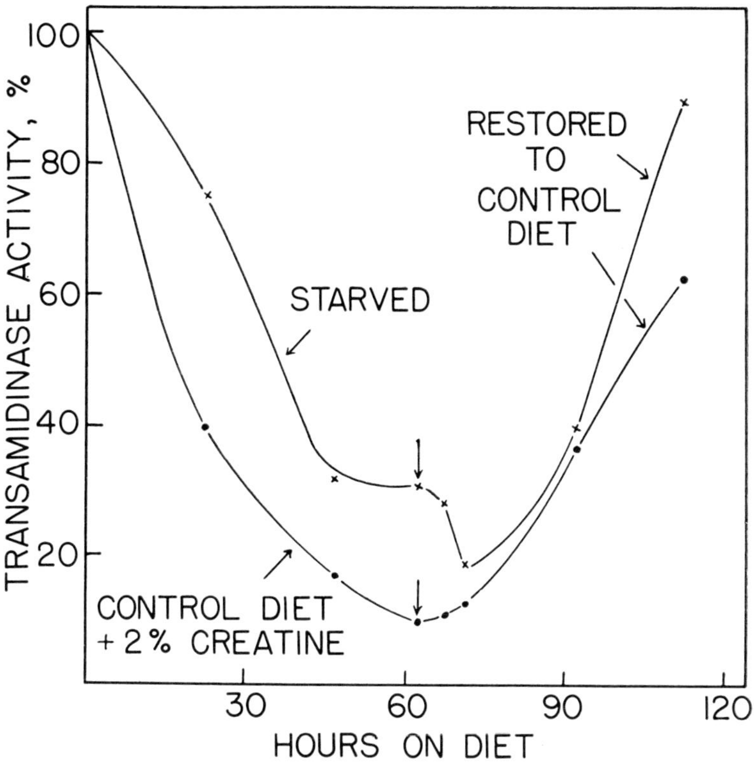

FIG. 7. Time course of differential decrease in chick liver transamidinase activity during fasting, as compared with decrease resulting from creatine feeding. It is of interest that both fasting and creatine feeding give rise to an increased concentration of liver creatine. It is suggested that differential repression of transamidinase by endogenous creatine occurs during fasting and in many pathological conditions. (Redrawn from Walker, 1961).

plemented with tryptophan. Furthermore, on a complete diet, ethionine inhibited restoration of transamidinase, and this inhibition could be reversed by methionine (Walker, 1961). These experiments are all compatible with the concept that recovery involves synthesis *de novo* of transamidinase molecules. One should keep in mind, however, that some of these results may reflect decreased food intake by the chicks. In view of recent work with tryptophan pyrrolase (Greengard and Feigelson, 1961), it is of interest that Harper has noted no effect of dietary amino acid imbalance upon the induction of tryptophan pyrrolase (Harper and Kumta, 1959). In any event, immunological and radioactive tracer studies like those recently reported for carbamyl phosphate synthetase synthesis

(Metzenberg, Marshall, Paik, and Cohen, 1961) are necessary before the matter can be regarded as settled.

Physiological Significance of Creatine Repression of Transamidinase

Special Significance for the Chick

End product control of the tissue concentration of transamidinase would enable carnivorous birds, such as the vulture or seagull, to utilize the dietary essential amino acids, arginine, glycine, and methionine, for the various functions depicted in Figure 2 when creatine is present in their diet. We have enough quantitative data to predict that a diet of raw meat would contain enough creatine to make the transamidinase level a limiting factor in the rate of creatine biosynthesis for such birds (Walker, 1960). As for the chicken, it has been mentioned earlier that dietary creatine spares a portion of the arginine (and hence glycine and methionine) requirement of chicks, and we believe that our findings furnish a biochemical basis for this sparing action. But the question remains whether this feedback mechanism is only a vestigial control which has survived the evolutionary process, or actually functions in a chick ingesting a creatine-free diet of grains and insects. Experiments showing a decrease of transamidinase during fasting (Figure 7) may provide an answer. Fasting is known to result in creatinuria and an increase in the creatine content of liver and kidneys; presumably the excess creatine represents creatine released from muscle or newly synthesized creatine not utilized by muscle. This increased level of tissue creatine during fasting would differentially repress transamidinase relative to many of the other chick liver proteins, and thus tend to conserve the dietary essential amino acids which are precursors of creatine for the more essential syntheses indicated in Figure 2.

General Significance

The fact that repression of a biosynthetic enzyme by its remote end product has now been found to occur in higher animals, as well as in unicellular forms, is of general significance in that it encourages a search for similar control systems in more critical biosynthetic pathways, e.g., in pathways involved in the initiation and cessation of cell division (cf. Potter, 1958). Meanwhile, since such systems might be difficult to study because of the participation of repressors which cannot penetrate cell membranes, more intensive study of the creatine-transamidinase system should be undertaken. The long range goal of such research would be to elucidate at the molecular level the homeostatic mechanisms responsible for establishing and maintaining the characteristic enzyme patterns of differentiated metazoon tissues.

ACKNOWLEDGMENTS

This work has been supported by Senior Research Fellowship SF-26 and Grant RG-4898 from the United States Public Health Service, and by a grant from the Robert A. Welch Foundation, Houston, Texas. The generous grants of Mrs. Alice Nicholson Hanszen to the Department of Biochemistry have greatly facilitated these investigations.

The help of Margaret Skorvaga Walker in certain phases of this work is gratefully acknowledged.

REFERENCES

Almquist, H. J. 1959. "The Amino Acid Requirements of Animals," *Protein and Amino Acid Nutrition*, A. A. Albanese, Ed., pp. 349–380. New York, New York: Academic Press, Inc.

Almquist, H. J., E. Mecchi, and F. H. Kratzer. 1941. Creatine Formation in the Chick. *Journal of Biological Chemistry*, 141:365–373.

Beher, W. T., and G. D. Baker. 1959. Build-up and Regression of Inhibitory Effects of Cholic Acid on *in vivo* Liver Cholesterol Synthesis. *Proceedings of the Society for Experimental Biology and Medicine*, 101:214–217.

Brenner, S. 1959. "The Mechanism of Gene Action," *Ciba Foundation Symposium on Biochemistry of Human Genetics*, G. E. W. Wolstenholme and C. M. O'Connor, Eds., pp. 304–317. Boston, Massachusetts: Little, Brown and Company.

Bresnick, E., and G. H. Hitchings. 1961. Feedback Control in Ehrlich Ascites Cells. *Cancer Research*, 21:105–109.

Bucher, N. R. L. 1959. "Alterations of Cholesterol Biosynthesis in Liver Cell Fractions from Rats in Various Experimental Conditions," *Ciba Foundation Symposium on Biosynthesis of Terpenes and Sterols*, G. E. W. Wolstenholme and C. M. O'Connor, Eds., pp. 46–60. Boston, Massachusetts: Little, Brown and Company.

Cohen, G. N., and F. Gros. 1960. Protein Biosynthesis. *Annual Review of Biochemistry*, 29:525–546.

Cowie, D. B., S. Spiegelman, R. B. Roberts, and J. D. Duerksen. 1961. Ribosome-Bound β-Galactosidase. *Proceedings of the National Academy of Sciences of the U.S.A.*, 47:114–122.

Crawford, I. P., and C. Yanofsky. 1958. On the Separation of the Tryptophan Synthetase of *Escherichia coli* into Two Protein Components. *Proceedings of the National Academy of Sciences of the U.S.A.*, 44:1161–1170.

DeMars, R. 1958. The Inhibition by Glutamine of Glutamyl Transferase Formation in Cultures of Human Cells. *Biochimica et biophysica acta*, 27:435–436.

Fitch, C. D., C. Hsu, and J. S. Dinning. 1960. Some Factors Affecting Kidney Transamidinase Activity in Rats. *Journal of Biological Chemistry*, 235:2362–2364.

Frieden, C. 1959. Glutamic Dehydrogenase. I. The Effect of Coenzyme on the Sedimentation Velocity and Kinetic Behavior. *Journal of Biological Chemistry*, 234:809–814.

Greengard, O., and P. Feigelson. 1961. The Activation and Induction of Rat Liver Tryptophan Pyrrolase *in vivo* by Its Substrate. *Journal of Biological Chemistry*, 236:158–161.

Halvorson, H. O. 1960. The Induced Synthesis of Proteins. *Advances in Enzymology*, 22:99–156.

Harper, A. E., and U. S. Kumta. 1959. Amino Acid Balance and Protein Requirement. *Federation Proceedings*, 18:1136–1142.

Hegsted, D. M., G. M. Briggs, C. A. Elvehjem, and E. B. Hart. 1941. *Journal of Biological Chemistry*, 140:191–200.

Huguley, C. M., Jr., J. A. Bain, S. L. Rivers, and R. B. Scoggins. 1959. Refractory Megablastic Anemia Associated with Excretion of Orotic Acid. *Blood, The Journal of Hematology*, 14:615–634.

Ingram, V. M. 1959. Separation of the Peptide Chains of Human Globin. *Nature, London*, 183:1795–1798.

Krebs, E. G., A. B. Kent, and E. H. Fischer. 1958. The Muscle Phosphorylase b Kinase Reaction. *Journal of Biological Chemistry*, 231:73–83.

Madsen, N. B., and C. F. Cori. 1956. The Interaction of Muscle Phosphorylase with *p*-Chloromercuribenzoate. I. Inhibition of Activity and Effect on the Molecular Weight. *Journal of Biological Chemistry*, 223:1055–1065.

Magasanik, B. 1957. Nutrition of Bacteria and Fungi. *Annual Review of Microbiology*, 11:221–252.

McFall, E., and B. Magasanik. 1960. The Control of Purine Biosynthesis in Cultured Mammalian Cells. *Journal of Biological Chemistry*, 235:2103–2108.

Metzenberg, R. L., M. Marshall, W. K. Paik, and P. P. Cohen. 1961. The Synthesis of Carbamyl Phosphate Synthetase in Thyroxin-Treated Tadpoles. *Journal of Biological Chemistry*, 236:162–165.

Pardee, A. B. 1959. "The Control of Enzyme Activity," *The Enzymes*, P. D. Boyer, H. Lardy, and K. Myrback, Eds., Vol. 1, pp. 681–716. New York, New York: Academic Press, Inc.

Potter, V. R. 1958. The Biochemical Approach to the Cancer Problem. *Federation Proceedings*, 17:691–697.

Potter, V. R., and V. H. Auerbach. 1959. Adaptive Enzymes and Feedback Mechanisms. *Laboratory Investigation*, 8:495–509.

Roberts, R. B., P. H. Abelson, D. B. Cowie, E. T. Bolton, and R. J. Britten. 1955. Studies of Biosynthesis in *Escherichia coli*. (Carnegie Institution of Washington Publication 607.) Washington, D.C.

Savage, J. E., and B. L. O'Dell. 1960. Arginine Requirement of the Chick and the Arginine-Sparing Value of Related Compounds. *Journal of Nutrition*, 70:129–134.

Siperstein, M. D. 1960. The Homeostatic Control of Cholesterol Synthesis in Liver. *American Journal of Clinical Nutrition*, 8:645–649.

Szilard, L. 1960. The Control of the Formation of Specific Proteins in Bacteria and in Animal Cells. *Proceedings of the National Academy of Sciences of the U.S.A.*, 46:277–292.

Tomkins, G. M., H. Sheppard, and I. L. Chaikoff. 1953. Cholesterol Synthesis by Liver. III. Its Regulation by Ingested Cholesterol. *Journal of Biological Chemistry*, 201:137–141.

Vogel, H. J. 1957a. "Repression and Induction as Control Mechanisms of Enzyme Biogenesis: The Adaptive Formation of Acetylornithinase," *Symposium on the Chemical Basis of Heredity*, W. D. McElroy and B. Glass, Eds., pp. 276–289. Baltimore, Maryland: Johns Hopkins Press.

———. 1957b. Repressed and Induced Enzyme Formaion: A Unified Hypothesis. *Proceedings of the National Academy of Sciences of the U.S.A.*, 43:491–496.

Walker, J. B. 1958. Further Studies on the Mechanism of Transamidinase Action: Transamidination in *Streptomyces griseus*. *Journal of Biological Chemistry*, 231:1–9.

———. 1959. Repression of Arginine-Glycine Transamidinase Activity by Dietary Creatine. *Biochimica et biophysica acta*, 36:574–575.

———. 1960. Metabolic Control of Creatine Biosynthesis. I. Effect of Dietary Creatine. *Journal of Biological Chemistry*, 235:2357–2361.

———. 1961. Metabolic Control of Creatine Biosynthesis. II. Restoration of Transamidinase Activity Following Creatine Repression. *Journal of Biological Chemistry*, 236:493–498.

Walker, J. B., and M. S. Walker. 1960. Inhibition of Sulfhydryl Enzymes by Formamidine Disulfide. *Archives of Biochemistry and Biophysics*, 86:80–84.

Wyngaarden, J. B., and D. M. Ashton. 1959. The Regulation of Activity of Phosphoribosylpyrophosphate Amidotransferase by Purine Ribonucleotides: A Potential Feedback Control of Purine Biosynthesis. *Journal of Biological Chemistry*, 234:1492–1496.

Yates, R. A., and A. B. Pardee. 1956. Control of Pyrimidine Biosynthesis in *Escherichia coli* by a Feedback Mechanism. *Journal of Biological Chemistry*, 221:757–770.

———. 1957. Control by Uracil of Formation of Enzymes Required for Orotate Synthesis. *Journal of Biological Chemistry*, 227:677–692.

The Control of DNA Biosynthesis

J. N. Davidson, M.D., D.Sc.

Department of Biochemistry,
The University of Glasgow, Glasgow, Scotland

The biosynthesis of deoxyribonucleic acid (DNA) (Kornberg, 1960; Davidson, 1961) can be considered as taking place in four main stages: (1) the biosynthesis of purine and pyrimidine ribonucleoside monophosphates, (2) the conversion of these ribonucleotides to the corresponding deoxyribonucleotides, (3) the phosphorylation of the deoxyribonucleoside monophosphates to the triphosphate stage, and (4) the polymerization of the deoxyribonucleoside triphosphates to yield deoxyribopolynucleotide in the presence of an appropriate DNA primer (Figure 1).

In this paper an attempt will be made to give a brief general survey of the factors controlling these reactions as described in the literature by a large number of authors, and to add to it a few original observations made by a group of colleagues including Drs. R. M. S. Smellie, H. M. Keir, S. M. Weissman, E. D. Gray, and J. Paul.

The formation of purine and pyrimidine ribonucleotides is controlled by well-known feedback mechanisms which need be mentioned only briefly (Figure 2). Both adenosine monophosphate (AMP) and guanosine monophosphate (GMP) inhibit the first specific enzyme in the purine biosynthetic pathway, phosphoribosylpyrophosphate- (PRPP) aminotransferase (Wyngaarden and Ashton, 1959), and are involved in other control mechanisms (Magasanik, 1959). The cytidine monophosphate (CMP) exercises a

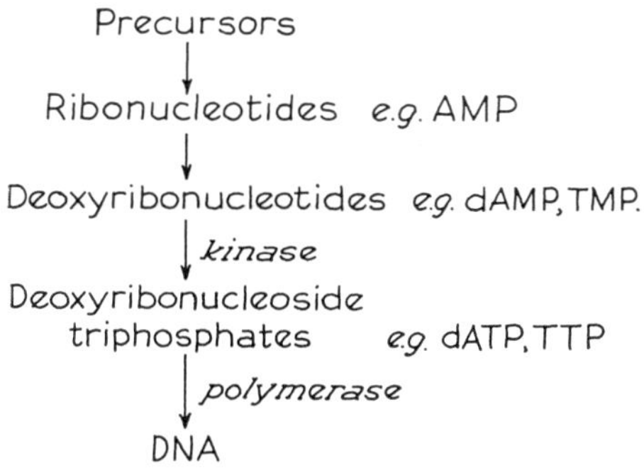

FIG. 1. Stages in the biosynthesis of DNA.

controlling influence on pyrimidine biosynthesis by directly inhibiting the first specific enzyme in the biosynthetic pathway, aspartic carbamyl transferase, which catalyzes the condensation of carbamyl phosphate and aspartate to yield ureidosuccinate (Yates and Pardee, 1956a,b). The activity of this enzyme is increased in regenerating rat liver and in Novikoff hepatoma (Calva, Lowenstein, and Cohen, 1959).

It is well known that the conversion of ribose derivatives to deoxyribose derivatives takes place at nucleotide level with the glycosidic linkage between sugar and base intact. The recent work of Reichard and Rutberg (1960) has shown that, when the base is cytosine, the reduction takes place at the diphosphate level; for the guanosine series, the conversion probably also occurs at the

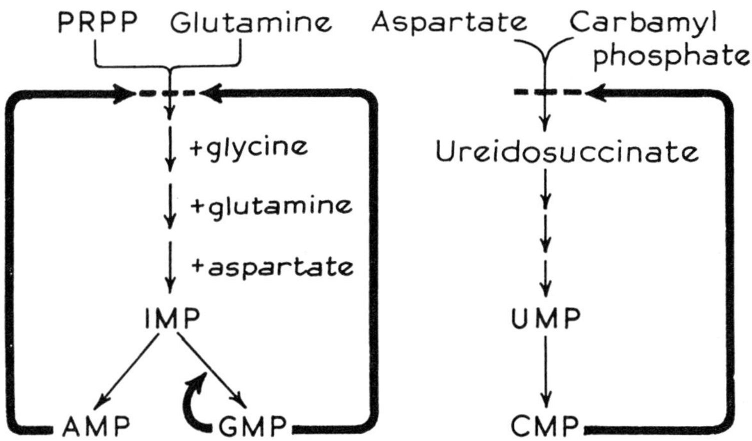

FIG. 2. Feedback mechanisms operating in the biosynthesis of purine pyrimidine nucleotides.

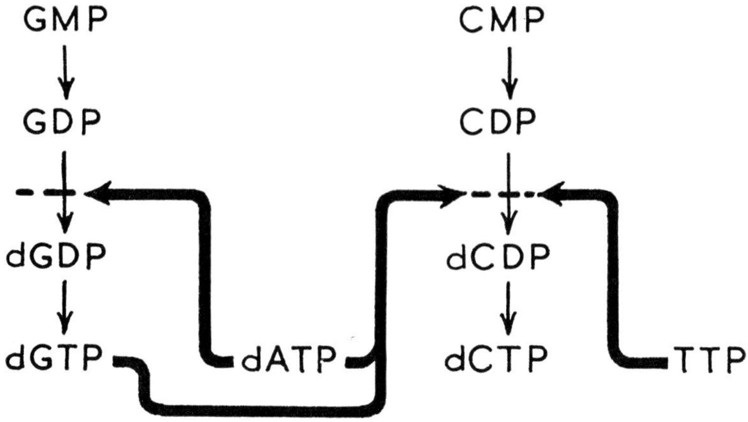

FIG. 3. Inhibition of reduction of ribonucleotides to deoxyribonucleotides by deoxyribonucleotide triphosphates.

diphosphate level with the production of deoxyguanosine diphosphate (dGDP) (Reichard, 1960).

The conversion of CMP to deoxycytidine monophosphate (dCMP), or rather of cytidine diphosphate (CDP), to deoxycytidine diphosphate (dCDP), in extracts of chick embryos, and hence, ultimately, the biosynthesis of DNA, has been shown by Reichard, Canellakis, and Canellakis (1960) to be inhibited by very low (5×10^{-5} M) concentrations of deoxyadenosine triphosphate (dATP), deoxyguanosine triphosphate (dGTP), and, to a lesser extent, of thymidine triphosphate (TTP). This effect of TTP can also be demonstrated in cultures of mammalian cells (Morris and Fischer, 1960).

In Ehrlich ascites cells, a similar inhibitory effect of dATP on the reduction of guanosine nucleotide to deoxyguanosine nucleotide has been recorded (Munch-Petersen, 1960), and this is almost certainly the explanation of the observation by Klenow (1959) that DNA synthesis in such cells, and also in chick embryos (Maley and Maley, 1960a), is inhibited by deoxyadenosine which is readily converted to its triphosphate.

It would appear, therefore, that DNA synthesis takes place most readily at critical concentrations of the deoxyribonucleoside triphosphates, and that these compounds are components of a homeostatic mechanism (Reichard, Canellakis, and Canellakis, 1960; Figure 3).

A third regulating mechanism operates in relation to the formation of deoxyuridine monophosphate (dUMP) which is the immediate precursor of the thymidine series of nucleotides. There is evidence both from *Salmonella typhimurium* (Grossman and Hawkins, 1957) and from chick embryos (Reichard, 1958) that uridine monophosphate (UMP) may be a direct precursor of dUMP. But in certain tissues this conversion also takes place by a more indirect route involving the cytidine nucleotides (Figure 4; Hecht and Potter, 1956; Potter, Pitot, McElya, and Morse, 1960), the amination of the uridine series to the cytidine series probably taking place at ribonucleoside triphosphate level (Liebermann, 1956; Hurlbert and Kammen, 1960). The enzyme deoxycytidylate deaminase then brings about the conversion of dCMP to dUMP. This enzyme is very low in most adult mammalian tissues except thymus and bone marrow (Potter, Pitot, McElya, and Morse, 1960) which synthesize DNA readily, but is active in such rapidly growing tissues as rat and chick embryos and regenerating rat liver (Maley and Maley, 1959, 1960b; Scarano, Talarico, Bonaduce, and de Petrocellis, 1960) and may be involved in a rate-limiting step in DNA biosynthesis (Maley and Maley, 1959). It is abundant in certain tumors such as the Novikoff hepatoma, but not in other hepatomas, i.e., Morris 5123 and Dunning L-C18 (Potter.

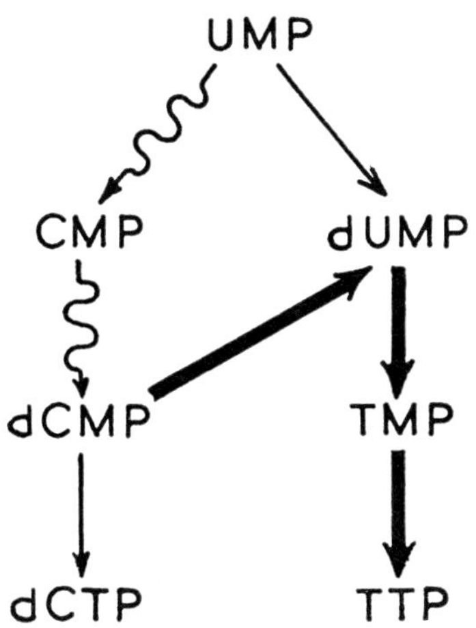

FIG. 4. Conversion of UMP to dUMP and TMP. Undulating arrows indicate that the level of phosphorylation has not been taken into account. Heavy arrows denote reactions catalyzed by enzymes which are increased in such rapidly growing tissues as regenerating rat liver.

Pitot, Ono, and Morris, 1960). The significance of these observations has been discussed by Potter and his colleagues in relation to the deletion hypothesis (Potter, Pitot, Ono, and Morris, 1960).

Deoxycytidylate deaminase is present in small amounts in normal rat liver (Maley and Maley, 1961) but increases in regenerating rat liver about 12 hours after partial hepatectomy, reaches a maximum at about 48 hours, and then declines. Maley and Maley (1960b) have concluded that its elevation before that of the other enzymes involved in thymidine monophosphate (TMP) formation and phosphorylation is consistent with a sequential induction of the enzymes concerned in DNA biosynthesis. The first of these other enzymes is thymidylate synthetase, which converts dUMP to TMP and which also rises in regenerating rat liver shortly after the deaminase. It has been suggested that dUMP may activate or induce the formation of thymidylate synthetase which, in turn, through its product TMP, may induce the formation of TMP kinase (Maley and Maley, 1960b). This kinase and related enzymes

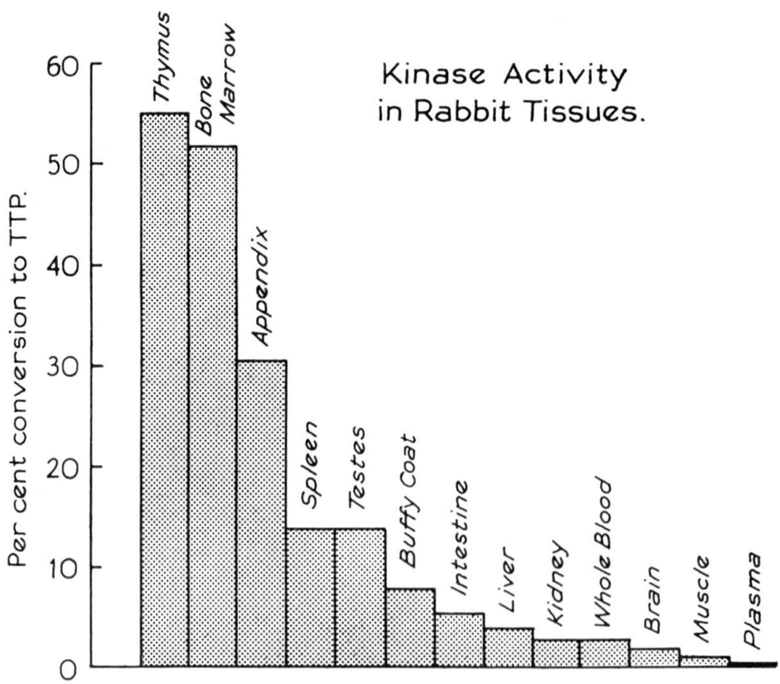

FIG. 5. Kinase activities in extracts of various rabbit tissues capable of phosphorylating thymidine to thymidine triphosphate (TTP).

must now be considered.

The over-all activity of the kinases phosphorylating the thymidine nucleotides to TTP in a series of rabbit tissues is illustrated in Figure 5. As might be expected, they are active in such tissues as thymus and bone marrow in which DNA synthesis is pronounced, and low in nonproliferating tissues such as liver. In liver regenerating after partial hepatectomy, however, kinase activity is high, especially at about 48 hours after operation (Bollum and Potter, 1958, 1959; Mantsavinos and Canellakis, 1959a; Canellakis, Jaffe, Mantsavinos, and Krakow, 1959; Hiatt and Bojarski, 1960; Weissman, Paul, Thomson, Smellie, and Davidson, 1960; Weissman, Smellie, and Paul, 1960). In this respect the thymine nucleotide kinase system differs from the kinases involved in the phosphorylation of deoxyadenosine monophosphate (dAMP), deoxyguanosine monophosphate (dGMP), and dCMP (Figure 6), which are of comparable activity in normal and regenerating liver (Bollum and Potter, 1959; Weissman, Smellie, and Paul, 1960; Table 1).

A study of the kinases in regenerating rat liver at various times after partial hepatectomy shows that the appearance of the enzymes tends to be sequential (Weissman, Smellie, and Paul, 1960; Figure 7). By 24 hours the thymidine (TdR) kinase has begun to increase sharply, reaching maximum activity in about 30 hours. It is followed closely by the TMP kinase, while the peak of the over-all reaction for the incorporation of H^3-TdR is at about 48 hours. Subsequently, all kinases decline in activity.

A similar sequential pattern of kinase appearance is also found in cultures of the L strain of mouse subcutaneous fibroblasts (Weissman, Smellie, and Paul, 1960). Such cells in the resting phase after

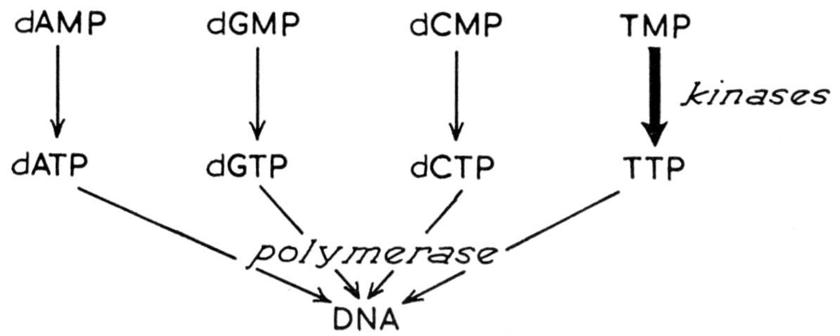

FIG. 6. Action of kinases in the formation of deoxyribonucleoside triphosphates. The heavy arrow denotes a reaction catalyzed by enzymes which are increased in regenerating rat liver.

TABLE 1

Phosphorylation of P^{32} Deoxycytidine Monophosphate by Kinases in Extracts of Ehrlich Ascites Cells, Normal Liver Tissue, and Regenerating Liver Tissue (48 Hours After Partial Hepatectomy)

Material tested		Per cent applied counts recovered		
		Total	Mono-phosphate	Di + triphosphate
A	Control	100	92	8
	Normal liver	88	59	29
	Regenerating liver	96	65	31
B	Control	100	95	5
	Ascites	85	69	16
	Normal liver	85	65	20
	Ascites + liver	87	59	28

The reaction mixture (1 ml.) contained 50 μmoles tris buffer pH 7.4, 80 μmoles KCl, 25 μmoles $MgCl_2$, 25 μmoles adenosine triphosphate (Na salt), 5 μmoles P^{32} deoxycytidine monophosphate; and in A, either 0.4 ml. liver extract or 0.4 ml. water (control); in B, two of the following: 0.2 ml. ascites extract, 0.2 ml. liver extract, or 0.2 ml. water.

Incubation time, 90 minutes. Temperature, 37°C.

(After Weissman, Smellie, and Paul, 1960)

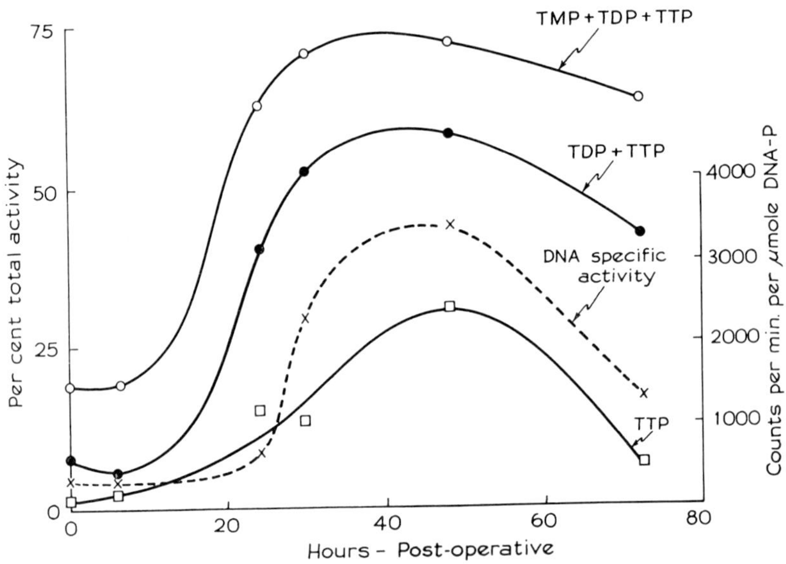

FIG. 7. The phosphorylation of H^3-TdR and its incorporation into DNA by extracts of rat liver regenerating for various times following partial hepatectomy. The reaction vessels contained 0.6 ml. of extracts of regenerating liver. The results are expressed as per cent total counts/minute recovered in TTP, TDP + TTP, and TMP + TDP + TTP, and represent TDP, TMP, and TdR kinase activities, respectively. (After Weissman, Smellie, and Paul, 1960.)

exhaustion of the medium show either no kinase activity or only TdR kinase activity. On inoculation into fresh medium, a period of rapid growth occurs after a lag phase (Figure 8). The TdR kinase appears early, rises sharply, and remains elevated. The TMP kinase activity rises later, reaches its peak of activity during the early part of the growth phase, and declines before growth (increase in cell number) has stopped. This pattern can be greatly modified by adding thymidine to the cultures, without affecting the growth rates. While there is little effect on the enzymes during the early period of growth, the TdR kinase activity remains elevated for a much longer period in the test cultures, and TMP kinase rises to a second peak during the period when its activity in the control culture declines. These elevations in the kinase activities can be produced only during the growth phase, and are apparently due to true enzyme induction, although it must be kept in mind that TMP kinase is a very labile enzyme which is stabilized in the presence

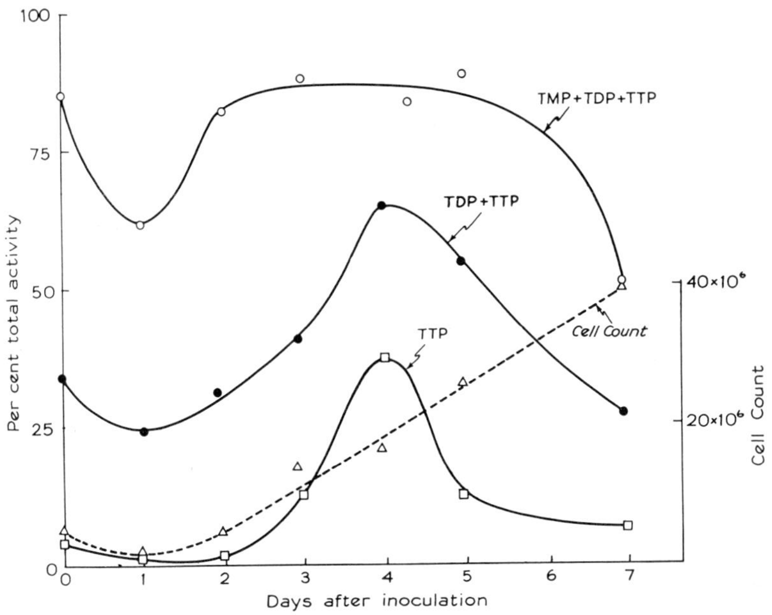

FIG. 8. The phosphorylation of H^3-TdR by disrupted preparations of L strain mouse fibroblasts at various times during growth. Each reaction vessel contained 1.0 mg. total protein. Results are expressed as per cent total counts/minute recovered in TTP, TDP + TTP, and TMP + TDP + TTP, representing TDP, TMP, and TdR kinases, respectively. (After Weissman, Smellie, and Paul, 1960.)

of thymidine or thymidylate (Bojarski and Hiatt, 1960).

While normal liver is lacking in the kinases for phosphorylating the thymine nucleotides, it contains the enzymes required for the reductive catabolism of thymine. In hepatomas such as the Novikoff and the Dunning, the catabolic enzymes are lacking (Potter, Pitot, Ono, and Morris, 1960) and thymine derivatives can, therefore, be diverted along the anabolic pathway to TTP. The importance of the absence of catabolic enzymes in rapidly proliferating tissues which are active in DNA biosynthesis has been fully discussed by Potter in the exposition of the deletion hypothesis (Potter, 1957, 1958; Potter and Auerbach, 1959; Potter, Pitot, Ono, and Morris, 1960).

The DNA polymerase which Kornberg and his co-workers have studied so extensively in extracts of *Escherichia coli* is also present in mammalian cells, and its activity in a series of rabbit tissues is shown in Figure 9. Again, as might be expected, it is most active

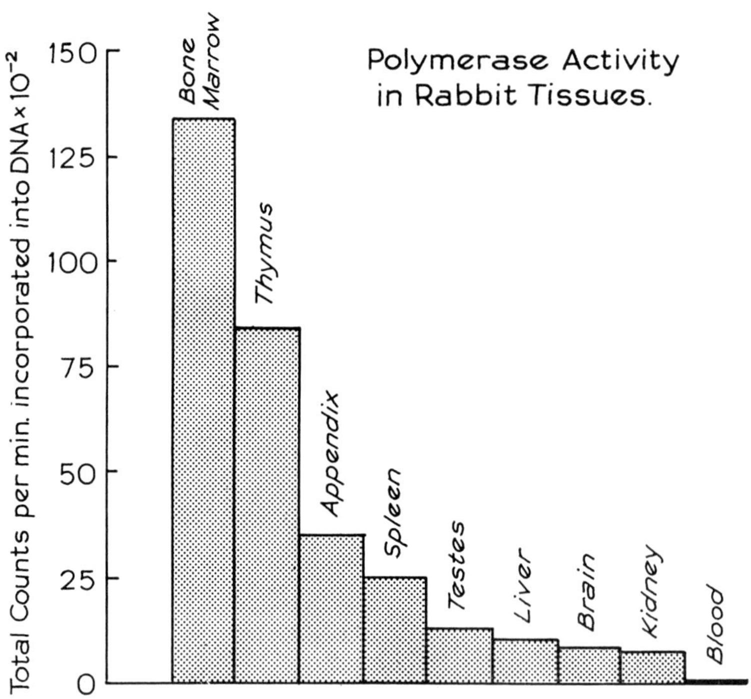

FIG. 9. Incorporation of P^{32}-TTP into DNA in the presence of the deoxyribonucleoside triphosphates of adenine, guanine, and cytosine by extracts of rabbit tissues containing the same concentration of protein. (After Smellie, 1961.)

in rapidly proliferating tissues such as thymus and bone marrow, and it has been studied in some detail in extracts of regenerating rat liver (Bollum and Potter, 1958, 1959; Mantsavinos and Canellakis, 1959a), of Ehrlich ascites cells (Davidson, Smellie, Keir, and McArdle, 1958; Smellie, Keir, and Davidson, 1959; Smellie, 1960), of calf thymus (Bollum, 1960), of HeLa cells (Harford and Kornberg, 1958), of mouse leukemic cells (Mantsavinos and Canellakis, 1959b) and of Novikoff hepatoma (Furlong, 1960; Furlong and Griffin, 1960). Like the kinases for the thymine series, it also is increased in regenerating rat liver (Bollum and Potter, 1959; Weissman, Smellie, and Paul, 1960). The polymerase is very sensitive to increases in ionic strength of the medium, and roughly 50 per cent inhibition is produced by salt concentrations greater than 0.1 M (Bollum, 1960; Walwick and Main, 1959).

A good example of the appearance of enzymes involved in DNA biosynthesis is found in cells of *E. coli* infected with phage. The subject has been reviewed by Kozloff (1960), and will not be further discussed here.

Although crude extracts of normal liver tissue show little polymerase activity, they nevertheless contain an active polymerase which can be separated by ammonium sulphate fractionation (Gray *et al.*, 1960). The low activity of whole extracts of liver suggests that they might contain factors which interfere with polymerase or kinase action, and this has, indeed, been found to be the case. Addition of extract of normal rat liver to partially purified polymerase and kinases for the thymidine system prepared from extracts of Ehrlich ascites cells causes a very pronounced drop in activity (Table 2). Similarly, the addition of extract of normal liver to extract of regenerating liver or of bone marrow greatly reduces the polymerase and kinase activity.

The presence of factors interfering with polymerase and kinase activity is not confined to liver tissue. Factors inhibiting polymerase are pronounced in liver, kidney, and serum, but not in brain or muscle. The phosphorylation of thymidine is strongly inhibited by liver extracts but not by extracts of other tissues so far tested, while the formation of thymidine diphosphate (TDP) and TTP is inhibited by liver and kidney extracts, by serum, and, to a much less pronounced extent, by muscle extracts. The polymerase used in most of these tests has been purified from Ehrlich ascites tumor cells, but polymerases from spleen, thymus, and bone marrow are likewise affected.

The interfering factors are thermolabile, nondialysable, and precipitable with ammonium sulphate, but so far have not been identified with any known enzyme or enzymes. The distribution of the interfering substances in various tissues suggests that different factors are involved in the inhibition of the various enzymes, and this has been confirmed by fractionation of liver extract with purification and separation from each other of the factors inhibiting TdR kinase, TMP kinase, and the polymerase.

Kinase inhibitions so far discussed have referred to the system producing TTP. The pattern of results obtained with the kinases for dAMP, deoxyguanosine monophosphate (dGMP), and dCMP is quite different in that these enzymes in ascites cell extracts are not inhibited by extracts of normal liver (Table 1). The kinase system for producing TTP would accordingly appear to be unique, both in its tendency to vary with the state of proliferation of the tissue and its susceptibility to the action of the interfering factors present in extracts of normal resting liver. This system obviously exercises a profound effect in the regulation of DNA biosynthesis. Such a conclusion would be in agreement with the well-known views of Potter (1957, 1958).

TABLE 2

Polymerase and Kinase Activity in Extracts of Different Tissues

Tissue	Polymerase*	Kinases** Thymidine monophosphate	Thymidine diphosphate	Thymidine triphosphate
Ascites tumor	4.7	430	830	2130
Ascites tumor + rat liver	0.4	14	12	0
Rat liver	1.2	10	3	1
Regenerating rat liver	7.3	30	70	50
Normal + regenerating rat liver	0.6	40	20	7
Rabbit liver	0.4	10	2	1
Rabbit bone marrow	5.3	20	80	130
Rabbit liver + bone marrow	0.2	20	20	20

* mμmoles TTP^{32} incorporated in 2 hours/mg. protein.

** μμmoles formed in 1.5 hours/mg. protein.

Polymerase assay. Reaction mixtures contained 25 μmoles tris buffer pH 7.9, 62.5 mμmoles DPN, 1.25 μmoles $MgCl_2$, 1 μmole 2-mercaptoethanol, 50 μg. DNA (previously heated for 10 minutes at 100°C and cooled quickly), generally 50 mμmoles each of dATP, dGTP, dCTP, and P^{32}-TTP, and 0.075 ml. of the polymerase preparation, all in a total volume of 0.25 ml. The mixtures were incubated with shaking in 10×1 cm. test tubes for two hours at 37°C.

Kinase assay. Reaction mixtures contained 5.5 μmoles $MgCl_2$, 5.5 μmoles ATP, 110 μmoles tris buffer pH 7.9, 0.5 μc H^3-TdR and 0.35 ml. of kinase preparation, all in a total volume of 1.1 ml. The mixtures were incubated with shaking in 25 ml. conical flasks for 90 minutes at 37°C. For inhibition effects, incubation mixtures contained equal volumes of enzyme and inhibitor preparations. These were 0.075 ml. and 0.35 ml. for polymerase and kinase respectively.

For liver and bone marrow assays, whole extracts were employed. For ascites cells, fraction AS 4.5 was used for kinase assays, and fraction AP 4.5 for polymerase assays.

(After Gray *et al.*, 1960)

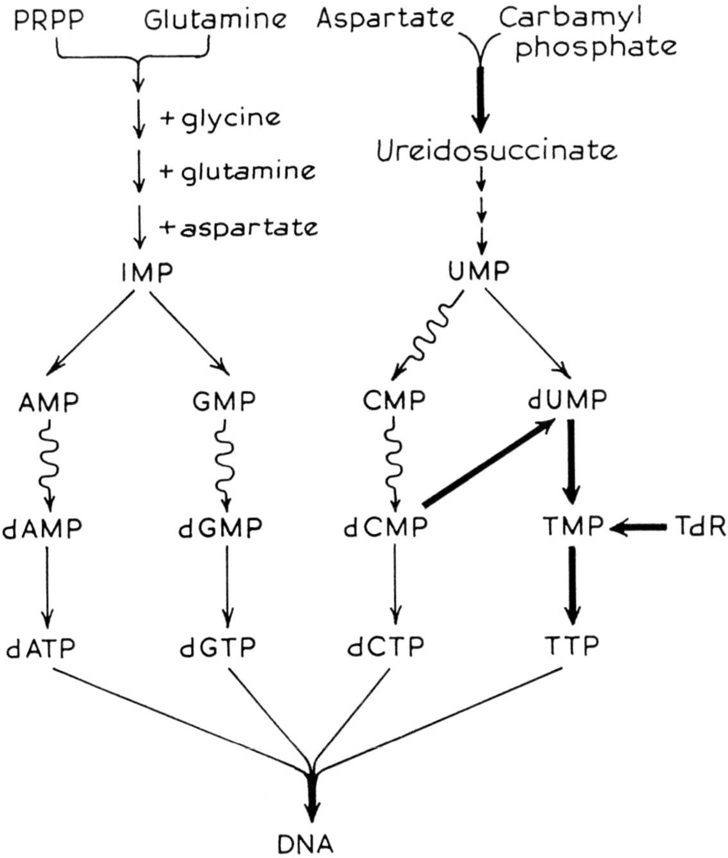

FIG. 10. Pathways involved in DNA biosynthesis. Undulating arrows indicate that the level of phosphorylation has not been taken into account. Heavy arrows denote reactions catalyzed by enzymes which are increased in such rapidly growing tissues as regenerating rat liver.

The final pattern is shown in Figure 10, and emphasizes the large number of points at which control can be exercised, especially in relation to the thymine nucleotide series. The importance of further knowledge about these control systems, especially in relation to the control of cancer, cannot be overemphasized.

REFERENCES

Bojarski, T. B., and H. H. Hiatt. 1960. Stabilization of Thymidylate Kinase Activity by Thymidylate and by Thymidine. *Nature, London*, 188:1112–1114.

Bollum, F. J. 1960. Calf Thymus Polymerase. *Journal of Biological Chemistry*, 235:2399–2403.

Bollum, F. J., and V. R. Potter. 1958. Incorporation of Thymidine into Deoxyribonucleic Acid by Enzymes from Rat Tissues. *Journal of Biological Chemistry*, 233:478–482.

———. 1959. Nucleic Acid Metabolism in Regenerating Rat Liver. VI. Soluble Enzymes which Convert Thymidine to Thymidine Phosphates and DNA. *Cancer Research*, 19:561–565.

Calva, E., J. M. Lowenstein, and P. P. Cohen. 1959. Carbamyl Phosphate-Aspartate Transcarbamylase Activity in Tumors. *Cancer Research*, 19:101–103.

Canellakis, E. S., J. J. Jaffe, R. Mantsavinos, and J. S. Krakow. 1959. Pyrimidine Metabolism. IV. A Comparison of Normal and Regenerating Rat Liver. *Journal of Biological Chemistry*, 234:2096–2099.

Davidson, J. N. 1961. The Biosynthesis of Nucleic Acids. *Annual Reports of the Chemical Society* (London), 57:352–366.

Davidson, J. N., R. M. S. Smellie, H. M. Keir, and A. H. McArdle. 1958. Synthesis of Deoxyribonucleic Acid in Extracts of Mammalian Cells. *Nature, London*, 182:589–590.

Furlong, N. Burr. 1960. Incorporation of Thymidine-2-C^{14} into Deoxyribonucleic Acid Catalyzed by Extracts of Novikoff Tumor Tissue. *Archives of Biochemistry and Biophysics*, 87:154–155.

Furlong, N. Burr, and A. C. Griffin. 1960. Deoxyribonucleic Acid Polymerase Activity in Extracts of Novikoff Hepatoma Tissue. (Abstract) *Federation Proceedings*, 19:306.

Gray, E. D., W. M. Weissman, J. Richards, D. Bell, H. M. Keir, R. M. S. Smellie, and J. N. Davidson. 1960. Studies on the Biosynthesis of Deoxyribonucleic Acid by Extracts of Mammalian Cells. V. Factors Interfering with Biosynthesis. *Biochimica et biophysica acta*, 45:111–120.

Grossman, L., and G. R. Hawkins. 1957. The Formation of Deoxyribonucleosides from Ribonucleosides in Extracts of *Salmonella typhimurium*. *Biochimica et biophysica acta*, 26:657–658.

Harford, C. G., and A. Kornberg. 1958. Enzymatic Synthesis of Deoxyribonucleic Acid (DNA) in Extracts of Mammalian Cells. (Abstract) *Federation Proceedings*, 17:515.

Hecht, L. I., and V. R. Potter. 1956. Nucleic Acid Metabolism in Regenerating Rat Liver. III. Intermediates in the Synthesis of DNA Pyrimidine Nucleotides. *Cancer Research*, 16:999–1004.

Hiatt, H. H., and T. B. Bojarski. 1960. Stimulation of Thymidylate Kinase Activity in Rat Tissues by Thymidine Administration. *Biochemical and Biophysical Research Communications*, 2:35–39.

Hurlbert, R. B., and H. O. Kammen. 1960. Formation of Cytidine Nucleotides from Uridine Nucleotides by Soluble Mammalian Enzymes: Requirements for Glutamine and Guanosine Nucleotides. *Journal of Biological Chemistry*, 235:443–449.

Klenow, H. 1959. On the Effect of Some Adenine Derivatives on the Incorporation *in vitro* of Isotopically Labelled Compounds into the Nucleic Acids of Ehrlich Ascites Tumor Cells. *Biochimica et biophysica acta*, 35:412–421.

Kornberg, A. 1960. Biologic Synthesis of Deoxyribonucleic Acid. *Science*, 131:1503–1508.

Kozloff, L. M. 1960. Biochemistry of Viruses. *Annual Review of Biochemistry*, 29:475–502.

Lieberman, I. 1956. Enzymatic Amination of Uridine Triphosphate to Cytidine Triphosphate. *Journal of Biological Chemistry*, 222:765–775.

Magasanik, B. 1959. "Mechanisms for Control of Enzyme Synthesis and Enzyme Activity in Bacteria," *The Regulation of Cell Metabolism*, G. E. W. Wolstenholme and C. M. O'Connor, Eds., pp. 305–307. London, England: J. & A. Churchill, Ltd.

Maley, G. F., and F. Maley. 1959. Nucleotide Interconversions in Embryonic and Neoplastic Tissues. I. The Conversion of Deoxycytidylic Acid to Deoxyuridylic Acid and Thymidylic Acid. *Journal of Biological Chemistry*, 234: 2975–2980.

———. 1960a. Inhibition of Deoxyribonucleic Acid Synthesis in Chick Embryos by Deoxyadenosine. *Journal of Biological Chemistry*, 235:2964–2967.

———. 1960b. Nucleotide Interconversions. II. Elevation of Deoxycytidylate Deaminase and Thymidylate Synthetase in Regenerating Rat Liver. *Journal of Biological Chemistry*, 235:2968–2970.

———. 1961. The Presence of Deoxycytidylate Deaminase in Normal Adult Rat Liver. *Biochimica et biophysica acta*, 47:181–183.

Mantsavinos, R., and E. S. Canellakis. 1959a. Studies on the Biosynthesis of Deoxyribonucleic Acid by Soluble Mammalian Enzymes. *Journal of Biological Chemistry*, 234:628–635.

———. 1959b. Studies on the Biosynthesis of DNA by Cell-free Extracts of Mouse Leukemic Cells. *Cancer Research*, 19:1239–1243.

Morris, N. R., and G. A. Fischer. 1960. Studies Concerning Inhibition of the Synthesis of Deoxycytidine by Phosphorylated Derivatives of Thymidine. *Biochimica et biophysica acta*, 42:183–184.

Munch-Petersen, A. 1960. Formation *in vitro* of Deoxyadenosine Triphosphate from Deoxyadenosine in Ehrlich Ascites Cells. *Biochemical and Biophysical Research Communications*, 3:392–396.

Potter, V. R. 1957. The Present Status of the Deletion Hypothesis. *University of Michigan Medical Bulletin*, 23:401–512.

———. 1958. The Biochemical Approach to the Cancer Problem. *Federation Proceedings*, 17:691–697.

Potter, V. R., and V. H. Auerbach. 1959. Adaptive Enzymes and Feedback Mechanisms. *Laboratory Investigation*, 8:495–500.

Potter, V. R., H. C. Pitot, A. B. McElya, and P. A. Morse. 1960. Alternative Pathways for Biosynthesis of Thymidylic Acid. (Abstract) *Federation Proceedings*, 19:312.

Potter, V. R., H. C. Pitot, T. Ono, and H. P. Morris. 1960. The Comparative Enzymology and Cell Origin of Rat Hepatomas. I. Deoxycytidylate Deaminase and Thymine Degradation. *Cancer Research*, 20:1255–1261.

Reichard, P. 1958. The Synthesis of Deoxyribose by the Chick Embryo. *Biochimica et biophysica acta*, 27:434–435.

———. 1960. Formation of Deoxyguanosine 5′-Phosphate from Guanosine 5′-Phosphate with Enzymes from Chick Embryos. *Biochimica et biophysica acta*, 41:368–369.

Reichard, P., Z. N. Canellakis, and E. S. Canellakis. 1960. Regulatory Mechanism in the Synthesis of Deoxyribonucleic Acid *in vitro*. *Biochimica et biophysica acta*, 41:558–559.

Reichard, P., and L. Rutberg. 1960. Formation of Deoxycytidine 5′-Phosphate from Cytidine 5′-Phosphate with Enzymes from *E. coli*. *Biochimica et biophysica acta*, 37:554–555.

Scarano, E., M. Talarico, L. Bonaduce, and B. de Petrocellis. 1960. Enzymatic Deamination of 5-Deoxycytidylic Acid and 5-Methyl 5′-Deoxycytidylic Acid in Growing and Non-Growing Tissues. *Nature, London*, 186:237–238.

Smellie, R. M. S. 1961. Studies on the Biosynthesis of Deoxyribonucleic Acid by Extracts of Mammalian Cells. *Proceedings of the 5th International Congress of Biochemistry*, Moscow, U.S.S.R.

Smellie, R. M. S., E. D. Gray, H. M. Keir, J. Richards, D. Bell, and J. N. Davidson. 1960. Studies on the Biosynthesis of Deoxyribonucleic Acid by Extracts of Mammalian Cells. III. Net Synthesis of Polynucleotides. *Biochimica et biophysica acta*, 37:243–250.

Smellie, R. M. S., H. M. Keir, and J. N. Davidson. 1959. Studies on the Biosynthesis of Deoxyribonucleic Acid by Extracts of Mammalian Cells. I. Incorporation of (^{3}H) Thymidine. *Biochimica et biophysica acta*, 35:389–404.

Walwick, E. R., and R. R. Main. 1959. Inhibition of DNA Synthesis by Sodium Ions. *Technical Report USNRDL-TR-319 NM-62-03-60 OCDM*. 8 pp. San Francisco, U. S. Naval Radiological Defense Laboratory. May 12, 1959.

Weissman, S. M., J. Paul, R. Y. Thomson, R. M. S. Smellie, and J. N. Davidson. 1960. Thymidine Kinases in Mammalian Tissues. (Abstract) *Biochemical Journal*, 76:1P.

Weissman, S. M., R. M. S. Smellie, and J. Paul. 1960. Studies on the Biosynthesis of Deoxyribonucleic Acid by Extracts of Mammalian Cells. IV. The Phosphorylation of Thymidine. *Biochimica et biophysica acta*, 45:101–110.

Wyngaarden, J. B., and D. M. Ashton. 1959. Feedback Control of Purine Biosynthesis by Purine Ribonucleotides. *Nature, London*, 183:747–748.

Yates, R. A., and A. B. Pardee. 1956a. Pyrimidine Biosynthesis in *Escherichia coli*. *Journal of Biological Chemistry*, 221:743–756.

———. 1956b. Control of Pyrimidine Biosynthesis in *Escherichia coli* by a Feed-Back Mechanism. *Journal of Biological Chemistry*, 221:757–770.

Mechanisms Involved in the Control of Enzyme Synthesis

G. DAVID NOVELLI, PH.D.

*Biology Division, Oak Ridge National Laboratory,
Oak Ridge, Tennessee**

It had been my original intention to survey types of control mechanisms utilized by various cells to control enzyme synthesis. Since several of the speakers in this symposium will describe a number of different control mechanisms, I will confine my remarks to a comparison of enzyme induction with the phenomenon of derepressed enzyme synthesis. Specifically, the systems to be considered will be the induced synthesis of β-galactosidase and the synthesis of ornithine transcarbamylase (OTC) by *Escherichia coli*. These are two enzymes for which we have developed cell-free systems that can carry out enzyme synthesis (Kameyama and Novelli, 1960b; Rogers and Novelli, 1960), thus permitting a closer analysis of the mechanisms involved in control.

ENZYME INDUCTION

Enzyme induction was defined by Stanier (1951) as an increase in the activity of aspecific enzyme brought about by a specific substance, usually the substrate or a close derivative, without change in genotype. A detailed discussion of enzyme induction will not be considered here, since a number of excellent reviews of this phenomenon, as well as considerations of the various theories proposed

* Operated by Union Carbide Corporation for the United States Atomic Energy Commission.

to explain it, have been published (Mandelstam, 1956; Spiegelman and Campbell, 1956; Cohn, 1957; Monod, 1958; Chantrenne, 1958; Pollock, 1959; Hogness, 1959; Halverson, 1960). From this vast literature a few pertinent generalizations can be made:

1. Induction involves the *de novo* synthesis of enzyme molecules from free amino acids.

2. Shortly after the addition of inducer, enzyme synthesis proceeds at a maximal rate and represents a constant fraction of new protein synthesis.

3. The capacity to make the specific enzyme as well as the property of inducibility is genetically determined, but by different genes (Pardee, Jacob, and Monod, 1959).

4. The inducer acts catalytically and brings about the synthesis of the same enzyme as is made by constitutive mutants.

We will confine ourselves to a discussion of the role of the inducer in controlling enzyme synthesis. The many theories proposed to account for the action of the inducer can be generalized into two classes: those that view the inducer as initiating the formation of a specific enzyme-forming system (templates), and those that hold the inducer functions to permit a preformed enzyme-forming system to act catalytically. If we assume that the specific enzyme-forming system is the template and has a specific ribonucleic acid as part of the machinery, we can restate the foregoing proposals as follows:

1. The inducer triggers the formation of specific ribonucleic acid (RNA).

2. The inducer permits specific RNA to act.

It would seem that decisive experiments to choose between these alternates could easily be designed, since the first proposition states that new RNA synthesis must precede or attend induced enzyme formation, but the second proposition implies that induced enzyme synthesis can proceed in the absence of RNA synthesis. Chantrenne (1958) reviewed the literature on the role of a linkage between RNA synthesis and enzyme induction and was unable to reach a firm conclusion one way or another.

Repression and Derepression

In 1953, investigators in several laboratories observed that the addition of certain amino acids to the culture medium resulted in lowered levels of some of the intracellular enzymes involved in the synthesis of the added amino acid (Vogel, 1953; Monod and Cohen-Bazire, 1953; Cohn, Cohen, and Monod, 1953; Adelberg and Umbarger, 1953; Wijesundera and Woods, 1953). The observations led to the discovery of a new mechanism for the control of enzyme synthesis. This concept was formulated and elaborated by Vogel (1957, 1958, in press) and called repression and depression of enzyme synthesis. Repression is defined as "a relative decrease, resulting from the exposure of cells to a given substance, in the rate of synthesis of a particular apoenzyme." Repression applies specifically to enzyme formation, and is distinct from effects that involve enzyme function. Therefore, enzyme synthesis following removal of repressor (derepression) implies the *de novo* synthesis of enzyme molecules from free amino acids.

We will be concerned here with asking certain questions regarding the function of the inducer and can thus restate the propositions concerning the role of the inducer, somewhat inversely, as follows:

1. Does the repressor prevent the formation of specific RNA-containing, enzyme-forming systems?

2. Does the repressor prevent the catalytic activity of pre-existing enzyme-forming systems?

Recently Pardee, Jacob, and Monod (1959) obtained genetic evidence suggesting that inducibility can be viewed as a derepression, i.e., the inducible strain is capable of making an internal repressor that prevents β-galactosidase synthesis. When the inducer enters the cell, the system is then derepressed and enzyme formation proceeds at a maximal rate. The constitutive strain is one that lacks the gene for making internal repressor, and is thus in a perpetual state of derepression. Therefore, the phenomenon of induction and derepression can be viewed as exhibiting identical mechanisms.

Experiments were conducted on these two systems that may allow some interpretations concerning the control mechanisms.

Comparative Behavior of the Synthesis of OTC and β-galactosidase Under Various Conditions

In 1957 Rogers and I had elected to study the biosynthesis of OTC in *E. coli* with the hope of eventually developing a cell-free system that would permit a closer analysis of the events leading to the formation of the specific enzyme. Gorini and Maas (1957) had recently discovered that the synthesis of this enzyme that is involved in the formation of arginine could be severely repressed when cells are grown on arginine. Upon removal of arginine, an explosive synthesis of enzyme occurred.

Figure 1 is a scheme illustrating the pathway of synthesis of arginine in *E. coli.* The enzyme OTC brings about a reaction between ornithine and carbamyl phosphate leading to the formation of citrulline. Figure 2 shows the kinetics of the derepressed synthesis of OTC. Its theoretical curve is derived from the assumption that at the moment of derepression, enzyme synthesis starts immediately and at a constant rate per cell. These kinetics had been worked out for β-galactosidase (Monod, Pappenheimer, and Cohen-Bazire, 1952) in which the maximum level of enzyme per cell is not attained until after about four generations.

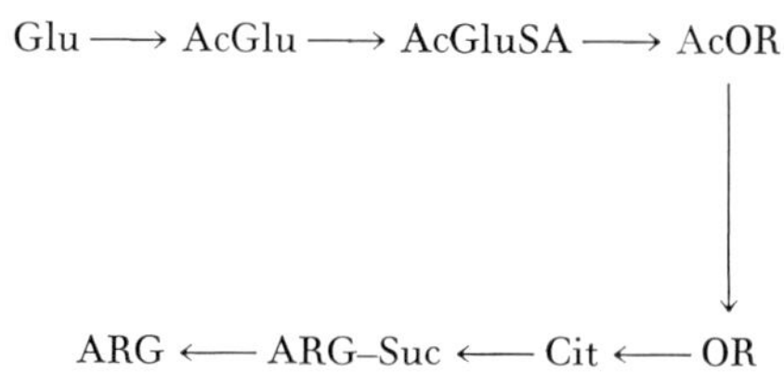

FIG. 1. Pathway of the biosynthesis of arginine by *Escherichia coli.*

Figure 3 depicts another experiment from the work of Gorini and Maas (1957) that holds the explanation for these kinetics. In this case an arginine auxotroph was used, and thus the organism needed to be supplied with low levels of arginine in order to grow. Here the experimental curve and the theoretical curve are very nearly the same. The kinetics in Figure 2 suggest that when sufficient OTC had been made to open the arginine biosynthetic pathway, internal arginine now began to act as a repressor inhibiting all further enzyme synthesis and the enzyme molecules in the population were thus distributed among the progeny. These experiments illustrate the striking capacity these cells have for altering enzyme synthesis as a function of available arginine. One interpretation of the rapid response of these cells to derepression is that when they grow in the presence of arginine, they manufacture the enzyme-forming system or templates but these cannot function in enzyme synthesis owing to the presence of the repressor arginine. Upon removal of the repressor, all the enzyme-forming sites are ready to act and do so, thus accounting for the explosive synthesis of enzyme. Viewed in connection with the two propositions to describe

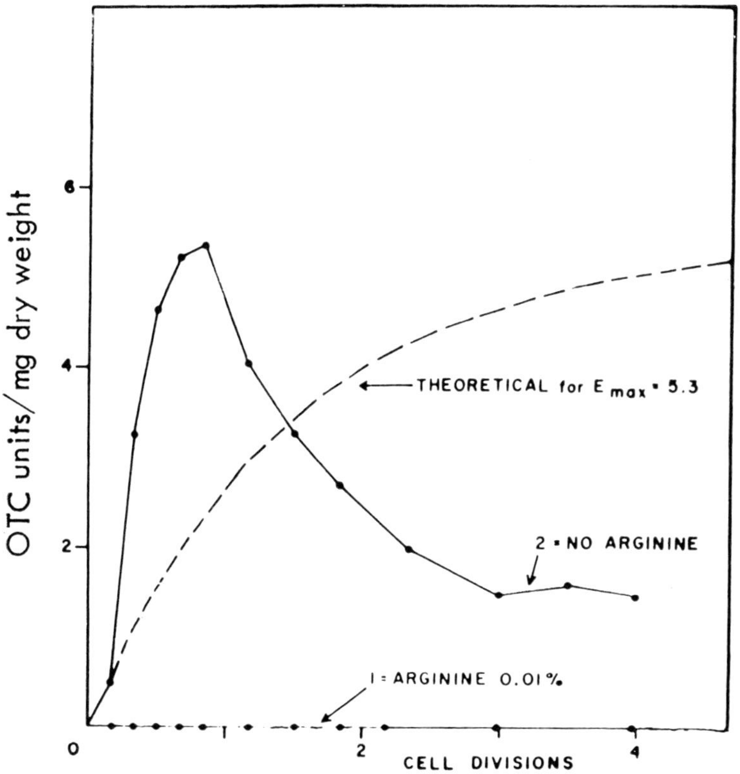

FIG. 2. Kinetics of ornithine transcarbamylase (OTC) synthesis by *Escherichia coli w*. (Adapted from Gorini and Maas, 1957.)

the action of the repressor mentioned earlier, one would be inclined to think that the derepressed synthesis of OTC should take place in the absence of concomitant RNA synthesis.

Uracil Deprivation

During a study of OTC synthesis in cells and protoplasts of *E. coli w*, Rogers and I (1959) found that OTC synthesis in protoplasts was inhibited by treatment with ribonuclease (RNase). With whole cells, the addition of 6-mercaptopurine caused a 30 per cent inhibition of OTC synthesis, although high concentrations of 8-azaguanine or 5-bromouracil had little or no effect. These data suggested that some components of the OTC system depend on either net synthesis

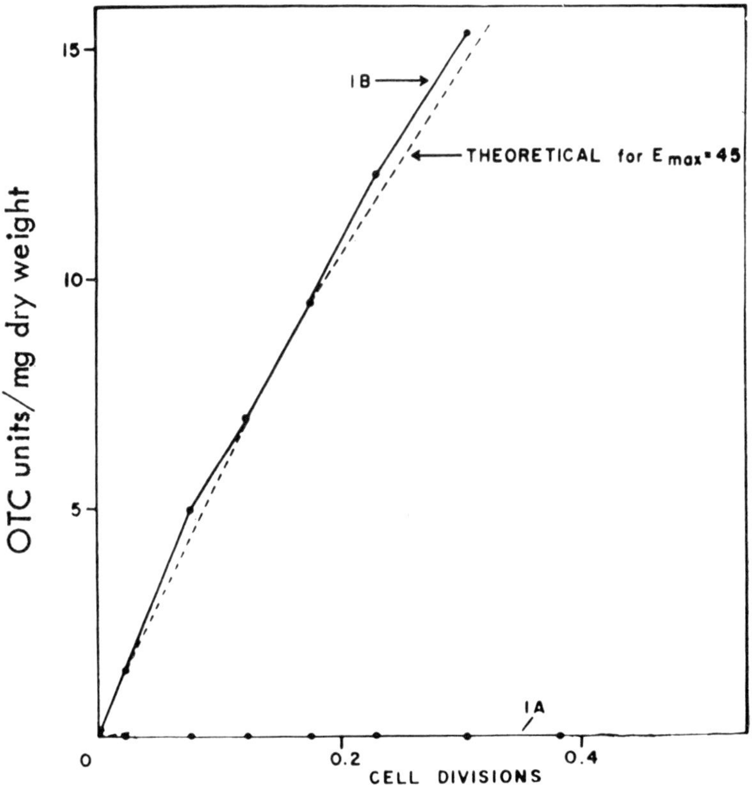

FIG. 3. Kinetics of ornithine transcarbamylase (OTC) synthesis by an arginine-requiring mutant of *Escherichia coli*. (Adapted from Gorini and Maas. 1957.)

or turnover of RNA. In order to clarify a possible involvement of RNA in OTC synthesis, we turned to a uracil auxotroph. Since Pardee (1954) had reported that purine and pyrimidine auxotrophs of *E. coli* could not form the induced β-galactosidase unless supplied with the required nucleic acid precursor, we tested simultaneously the induced synthesis of β-galactosidase and the derepressed synthesis of OTC in the presence and absence of uracil.

Figure 4 illustrates that little or no β-galactosidase was formed unless the cells were supplied with uracil. With OTC, however, almost as much enzyme was made in the absence of uracil as was made in the supplemented culture. The results of this experiment suggest that induction of β-galactosidase requires simultaneous RNA synthesis, but OTC synthesis can proceed under conditions

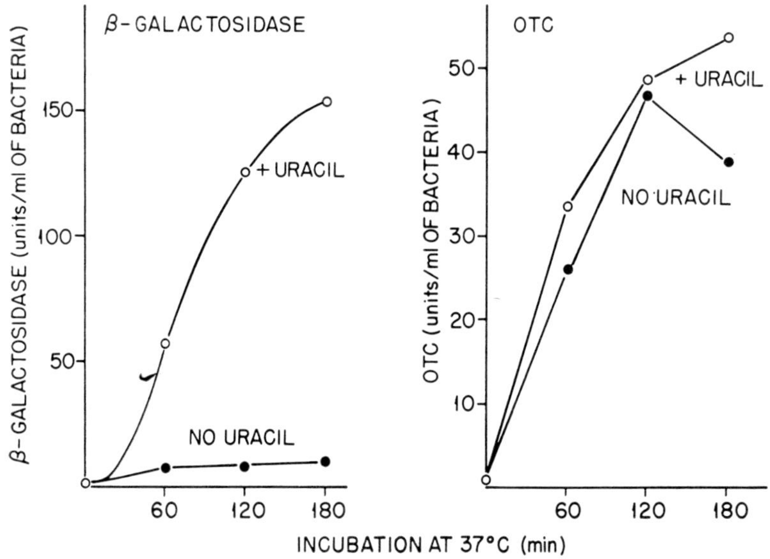

FIG. 4. Simultaneous synthesis of β-galactosidase and ornithine transcarbamylase (OTC) by a uracil-requiring mutant of *Escherichia coli*. (Adapted from Rogers and Novelli, 1959.)

where new synthesis of RNA is not possible. However, a detailed discussion by Chantrenne (1958) on the possible role of RNA in induced enzyme synthesis points out a number of pitfalls in generalizations from data such as these. Turnover of RNA in the absence of uracil might account for OTC synthesis. We attempted to test this possibility by studying OTC synthesis and P^{32} incorporation into RNA in the presence and absence of uracil (Rogers and Novelli, 1959). The data obtained, although favoring the idea that possible turnover of RNA could not account for the observed enzyme synthesis in the absence of uracil, were not definitive in this respect.

Magasanik (personal communication) gives another possible interpretation of these results, based on a theory that the well-known effect of glucose in inhibition of induced enzyme formation can be explained by the rapid formation from glucose of an internal repressor of the enzyme-forming system (Neidhardt and Magasanik, 1956). In Figure 4, succinate or glycerol was used as the carbon source. Under normal circumstances it can be argued that the rate of metabolism of these compounds is too slow to permit the accumulation of internal repressor. Under conditions of uracil deprivation, however, many reactions that would ordinarily utilize metabolites of these carbon sources are inhibited, thereby allowing the accumulation of internal repressor. Thus the failure of the cells to form β-galactosidase in the absence of uracil could be ascribed to conditions that favor accumulation of internal repressor rather than a requirement for simultaneous RNA synthesis.

The information available at the present time does not permit a clear choice between these alternate interpretations.

Effect of Ultraviolet Irradiation and Photoreactivation

In connection with experiments to determine the nature of the aberration in nucleic acid metabolism following exposure of cells to heavy doses of ultraviolet (UV) irradiation, Kameyama and Novelli (1960a) observed that UV irradiation prevented subsequent induction of β-galactosidase synthesis. Figure 5 shows the effect of UV irradiation on the induced synthesis of β-galactosidase in media containing two different carbon sources. It is evident that the synthesis of this enzyme is much more sensitive to UV if the cells are grown with glycerol as the carbon source rather than succinate.

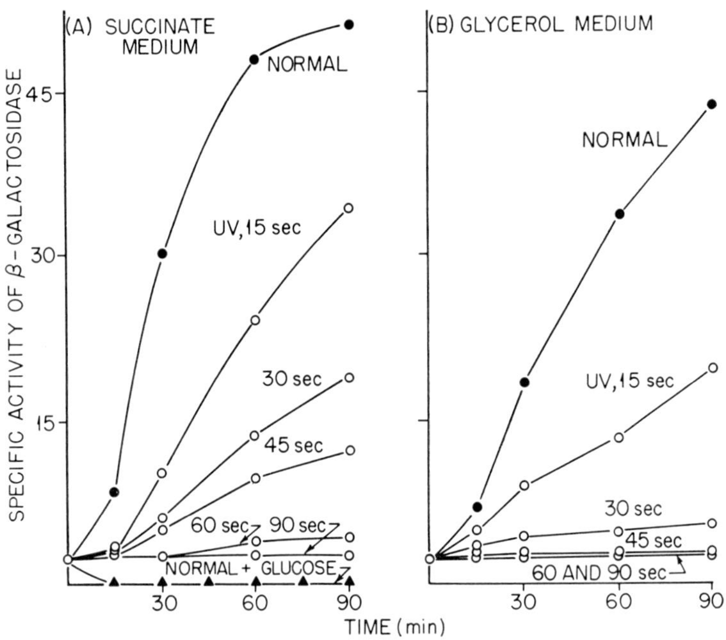

FIG. 5. Ultraviolet-(UV) dose effect on induced synthesis of β-galactosidase (Kameyama and Novelli, in preparation a).

The explanation for this phenomenon is not presently known, and may reside in the different modes of metabolism of the two compounds. Data shown in Figure 6 demonstrate that the effect of UV on induced enzyme formation can be reversed by exposure of the cells to white light, a process called photoreactivation (PR). That the photoreactivation of enzyme induction is preferential is seen by comparing the effect on specific enzyme formation with the same effect on general protein synthesis.

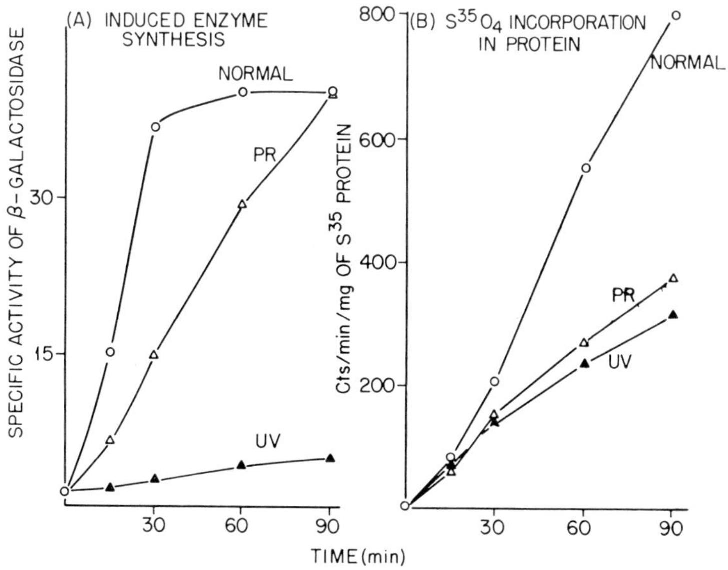

FIG. 6. Differential effect of photoreactivation on enzyme formation (Novelli, Kameyama and Eisenstadt, 1961).

Because of the well-documented effect of UV irradiation on nucleic acid metabolism and the dramatic effect of UV and PR on the induction of β-galactosidase synthesis, we decided to compare the behavior of β-galactosidase induction and derepression of OTC under these two sets of conditions.

The curves in Figure 7 illustrate this comparison. Once again, the difference in behavior of these two systems is unmistakable. Induction of β-galactosidase is almost completely eliminated by exposure to UV irradiation, whereas synthesis of OTC is hardly affected. This experiment can also be interpreted as indicating a requirement for nucleic acid metabolism in order to support β-galactosidase synthesis and the lack of such a requirement for OTC

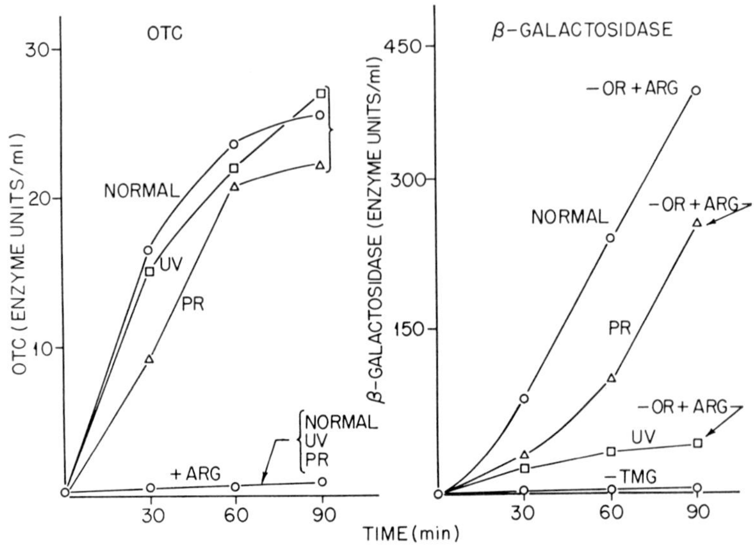

FIG. 7. Simultaneous biosynthesis of ornithine transcarbamylase and β-galactosidase by normal ultraviolet (UV) and photoreactivation (PR) *Escherichia coli* B. (From Novelli, Kameyama and Eisenstadt, 1961.)

synthesis. Here again, however, it is difficult to rule out possible metabolic derangements caused by UV exposure that result in the accumulation of internal repressors of the β-galactosidase system.

Effect of Phage Infection

The metabolism of nucleic acids in bacteria can be profoundly altered by infection with bacteriophages, especially those of the T-even series. When *E. coli* is infected with T_2 phage, deoxyribonucleic acid (DNA) and protein synthesis proceed at a vigorous rate, although net synthesis of RNA ceases abruptly (Hershey, 1953). Volkin and Astrachan (1956) observed that when *E. coli* is infected with T_2 there is a rapid turnover of a small part of the RNA, and the calculated base composition of this RNA is similar to the composition of the analogous nucleotides in phage DNA. Because of these alterations in nucleic acid metabolism as a consequence of phage infection, it became of interest to compare the behavior of these two enzyme-forming systems when the cells were infected with phage T_2.

It is evident (Figure 8) that in induced synthesis of β-galactosidase, infection with T_2 simultaneously with initiation of induction

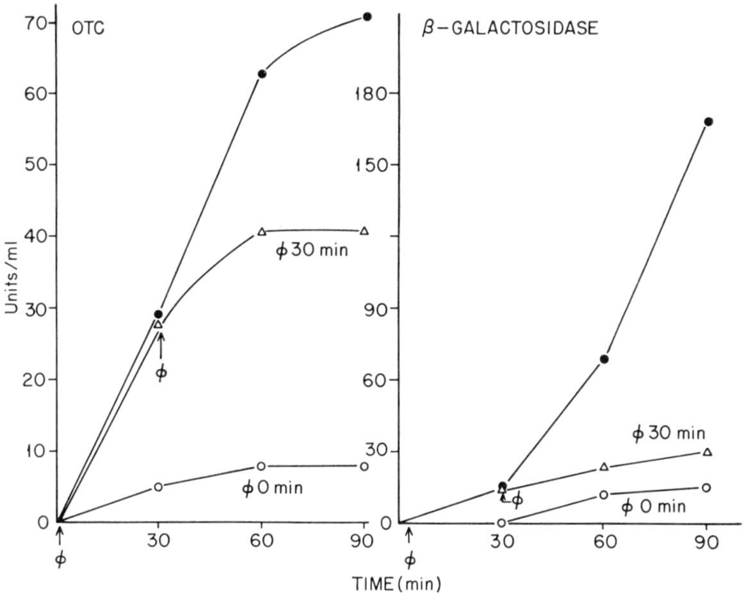

FIG. 8. Effect of phage T_2 infection on synthesis of β-galactosidase and ornithine transcarbamylase (OTC). (From Kameyama and Novelli, unpublished observations.)

or after 30 minutes of induction leads to an abrupt cessation of enzyme synthesis. This is somewhat similar to the results reported by Fry and Gros (1959) in which introduction of the phage λ stopped β-galactosidase synthesis. With the OTC system, infection with T_2 after derepression allowed a considerable synthesis of enzyme to occur until the cells lysed. Here again a striking difference between the behavior of these two enzyme systems is evident, and the difference is consistent with the postulate that β-galactosidase synthesis requires simultaneous RNA synthesis, whereas limited OTC synthesis may occur in the absence of RNA synthesis.

Effect of X-Irradiation

X-irradiation has long been known to damage DNA, and seems like a good reagent to distinguish between the nucleic acid requirements of these two enzyme systems. However, Baron, Spiegelman, and Quastler (1953) have shown that high doses of X-rays that completely suppress DNA synthesis do not inhibit the induced formation of galactozymase and maltozymase in yeast, and Chantrenne (1958) reports that 200,000 r of the X-rays induced some catalase formation in yeast and stimulated oxygen-induced formation of the enzyme. Clayton and Adler (in preparation), however, found that induction of catalase synthesis in *Rhodopseudomonas spheroides* exhibited the same sensitivity to X-irradiation as did cell viability. We, therefore, compared the effect of X-irradiation on the synthesis of β-galactosidase and OTC. The results of these experiments are shown in Figures 9 and 10. In Figure 9 the data are shown

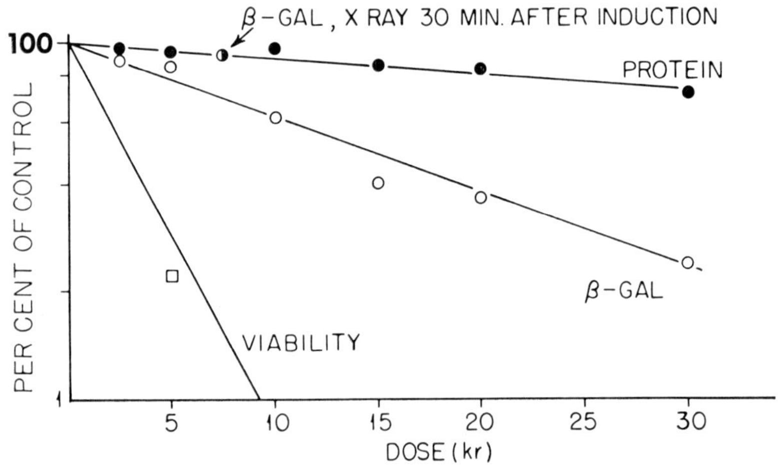

Fig. 9. Dose effect of X-ray inactivation of β-galactosidase synthesis in *Escherichia coli*. (From Novelli, Kameyama and Eisenstadt, 1961)

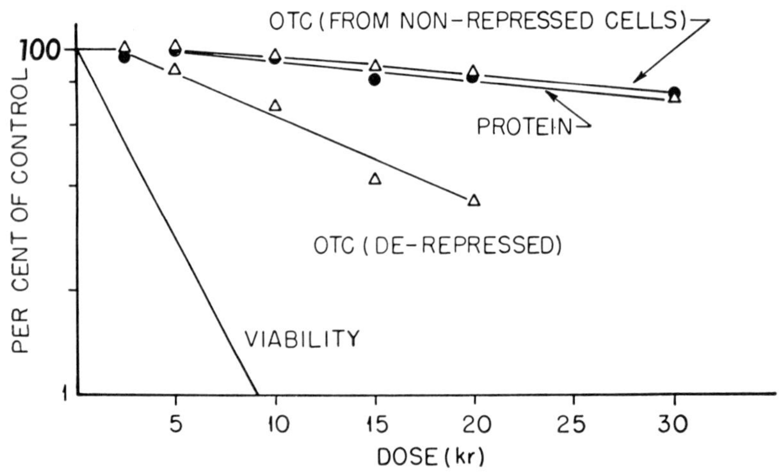

Fig. 10. Dose effect of X-ray inactivation of ornithine transcarbamylase (OTC) synthesis. (From Eisenstadt and Novelli, unpublished observation.)

for the β-galactosidase system. The data are plotted in terms of loss of synthetic activity or viability as a function of radiation dose in kiloroentgens. If X-irradiation is applied 30 minutes after induction, enzyme synthesis is inhibited along a curve of inactivation that is identical with inhibition of general protein synthesis. When X-irradiation is applied before induction, the ability to synthesize the induced enzyme is now much more sensitive than is general protein synthesis. The X-ray sensitivity of induced β-galactosidase synthesis is less than and independent of the sensitivity of cell multiplication, since superimposable curves of β-galactosidase sensitivity are obtained with *E. coli* B/r and *E. coli* BS Hill that differ in sensitivity as measured by viability by a factor of 1,000 or more.

In Figure 10, similar data for the behavior of the OTC system are shown. The X-ray sensitivity of derepressed cells is not quite as marked as the β-galactosidase system, but is considerably more sensitive than general protein synthesis. The nonrepressed cells, however, like the preinduced cells, show a greater resistance to X-rays. This is the first of the various comparative tests applied to the two systems in which the behavior is so similar and is not easily compatible with our working hypothesis that β-galactosidase synthesis requires simultaneous RNA synthesis, whereas derepressed OTC synthesis can occur in its absence. Nevertheless, the data discussed so far illustrate some striking differences in the behavior of these two enzyme systems that will eventually require a rational explanation.

Occurrence of Particle-Bound β-Galactosidase

I mentioned earlier that the investigation of β-galactosidase synthesis began with experiments on ultraviolet inactivation of the system and its photoreactivation (Figure 6). During the course of these experiments, we had occasion to electrophorese crude cell extracts on Geon. In such experiments, we observed a form of β-galactosidase that did not migrate in the electric field, which was later identified as a particle-bound enzyme (Kameyama and Novelli, 1960a; in preparation). This form of the enzyme, as well as the soluble form, did not appear if the cells were treated with UV before induction. The particle-bound enzyme became a larger fraction of the total enzyme if the UV-treated cells were photoreactivated before induction. An example of this phenomenon is illustrated in Figure 11. Cowie, Spiegelman, Roberts, and Duerksen

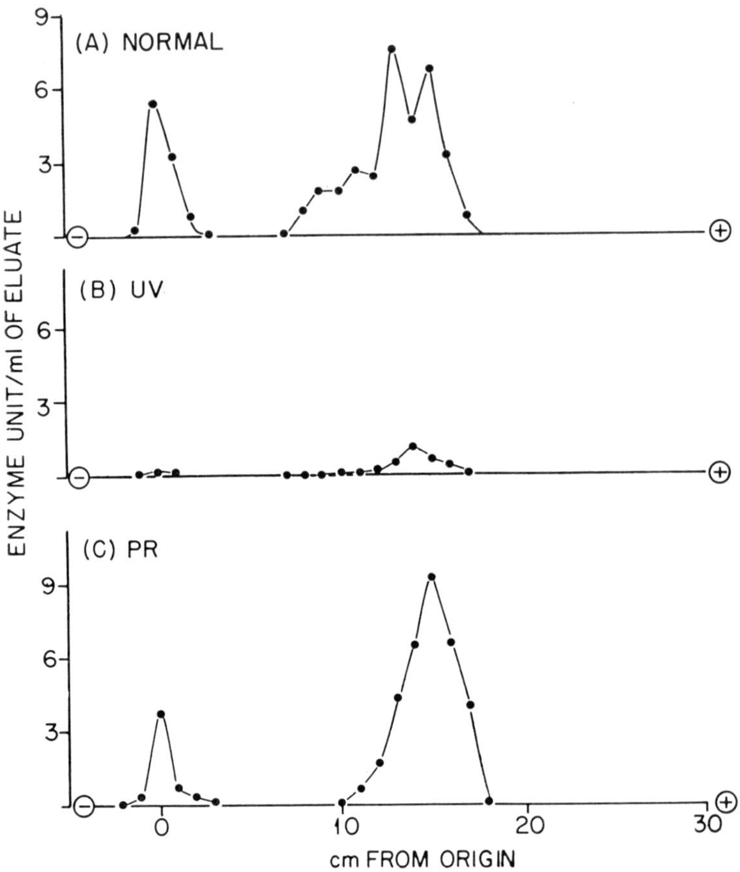

FIG. 11. Geon fractionation of normal ultraviolet (UV) and photoreactivation (PR) cell extracts. (From Kameyama and Novelli, in press.)

(1961), in the meantime, also observed a particle-bound form of β-galactosidase by ultracentrifugation techniques. They report much lower values for the fraction of β-galactosidase observed to be particle-bound. Their particles, however, were subjected to extreme washing procedures, and it is therefore possible that they may have fortuitously washed out a small molecule responsible for the binding of the enzyme to the particle.

Since it was well known that removal of inducer led to the abrupt cessation of further enzyme synthesis, we wondered what would happen if the cells were subjected to further incubation in the

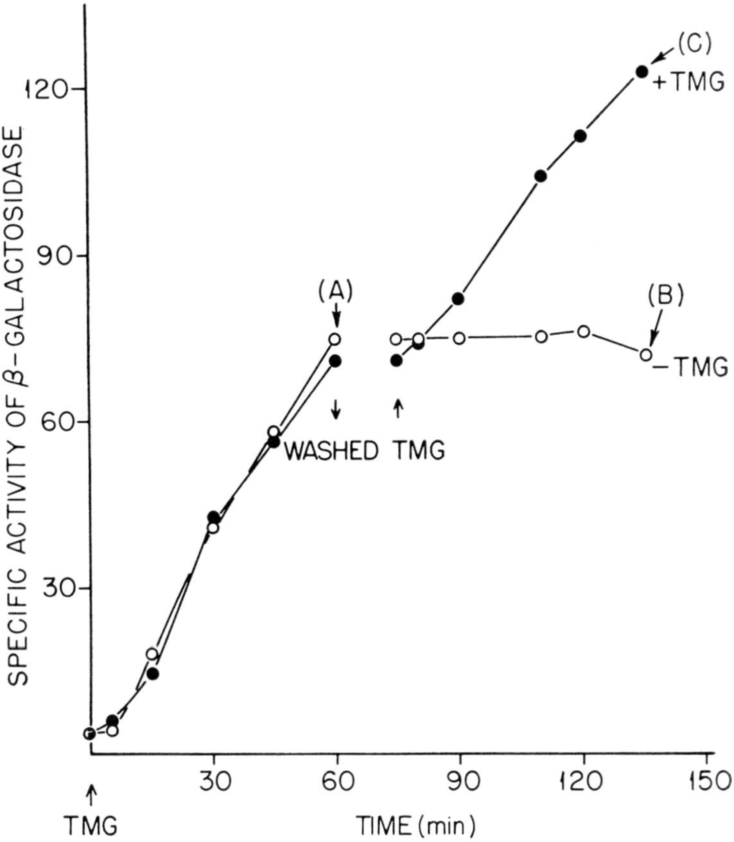

FIG. 12. Effect of removal of inducer on β-galactosidase synthesis. (From Kameyama and Novelli, in press.)
Abbreviations: TMG, thiomethyl β-galactoside.

absence of inducer. Figure 12 illustrates the time course of induction of β-galactosidase and the failure to observe further enzyme synthesis upon removal of inducer. The cells removed from the culture at the times indicated on Figure 12 were broken open, centrifugated at 6,000 $\times$ g to remove cellular debris, and the crude extracts were subjected to electrophoresis on Geon with the results indicated in Figure 13. It is evident that a period of metabolism in the absence of inducer resulted in a loss of the particle-bound enzyme and its transfer to the soluble pool. Thus it is clear that inducer is not required to convert the particle-bound enzyme to the soluble form. If the particle-bound enzyme really represents the

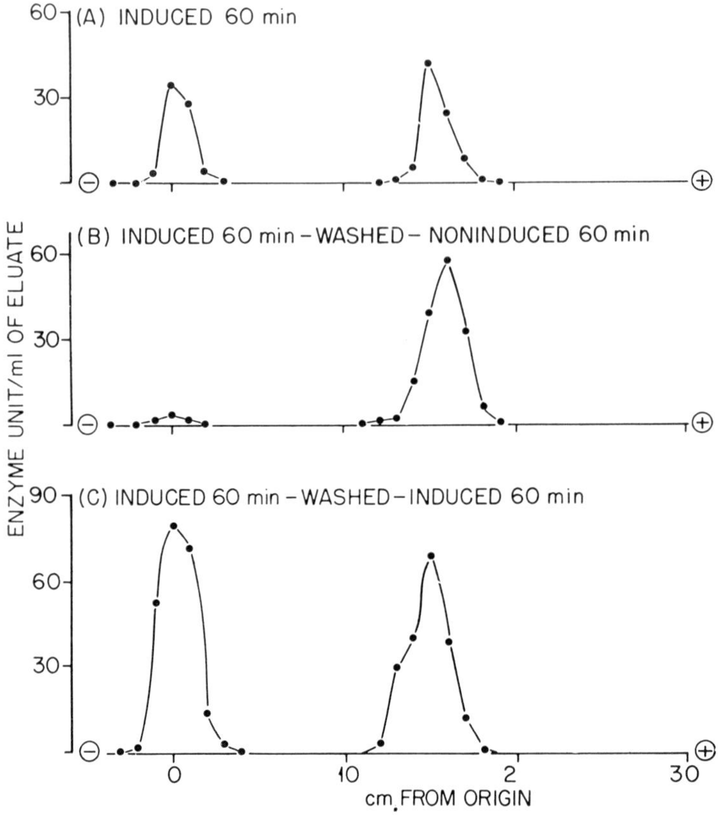

FIG. 13. Effect of removal of an inducer on particle-bound enzyme. (From Kameyama and Novelli, in press.)

template-bound enzyme, an original theory relating to the role of the inducer, i.e., that the inducer is required to remove template-bound enzyme, is no longer tenable.

Cell-Free Synthesis of β-Galactosidase

Because of the behavior of the particle-bound enzyme upon removal of inducer, we suspected that the particle might be involved in enzyme synthesis. Accordingly, we prepared particles and supernatant from preinduced cells by first disintegrating the cells by passage through a French pressure cell and subsequent centrifugal fractionation of the extract (Kameyama and Novelli, 1960b). With washed particles and dialyzed supernatant, we proceeded to set up a cell-free system that might be capable of *de novo* enzyme synthesis. Representative data from such an experiment are shown in Table 1. It seems clear that in order to observe an increase in enzyme activity during incubation, the particles and supernatant must be supplemented with a source of energy, a complete mixture of amino acids, nucleoside di- and triphosphates, and the specific inducer. The observed increase in enzyme activity is inhibited by chloramphenicol, RNase, and deoxyribonuclease (DNase). These data are consistent with the idea that the properly supplemented cell-free system is capable of synthesizing the enzyme β-galactosidase. However, we were painfully aware that an increase in enzyme synthesis under certain conditions of incubation of cell-free preparations does not necessarily mean new enzyme molecules have been formed, for it is well known that all types of activations occur leading to an increase in enzyme activity in the absence of protein synthesis. In order to minimize the chances of being misled by such adventitious observations, we added a C^{14}-labeled amino acid to our reaction mixture. Since we had previously prepared an antiserum to a highly purified sample of β-galactosidase, we precipitated the enzyme with the antiserum at various times after incubation of the reaction mixture. If new synthesis of protein molecules took place in our reaction mixture and was reflected by an increase in enzyme activity, there should have been observed a corresponding increase in the C^{14} content of the antibody-precipitable protein. That this was indeed the case is evident from the data shown in Figure 14.

TABLE 1

Cell-Free Synthesis of β-Galactosidase by 105,000 × g Particles and Supernatant from Escherichia coli

	Enzyme units/ml. Time (minutes) 0	60	Net
Complete system	145.5	360.5	215
— S	72.5	195.5	123
— TMG	145.5	145.5	0
— ATP and generator	145.5	145.5	0
— AA	145.5	220.5	75
— XTP, XDP	145.5	236.5	91
+ CAP	145.5	145.5	0
+ RNase	145.5	88.5	— 57
+ DNase	145.5	93.0	— 52

S, supernatant from 105,000 × g for 90 minutes; TMG, thiomethyl β-galactoside; ATP, adenosine triphosphate; AA, amino acid mixture; XTP, XDP, nucleoside tri- and diphosphate; CAP, chloramphenicol; RNase, ribonuclease; DNase, deoxyribonuclease. (From Novelli, Kameyama and Eisenstadt, 1961.)

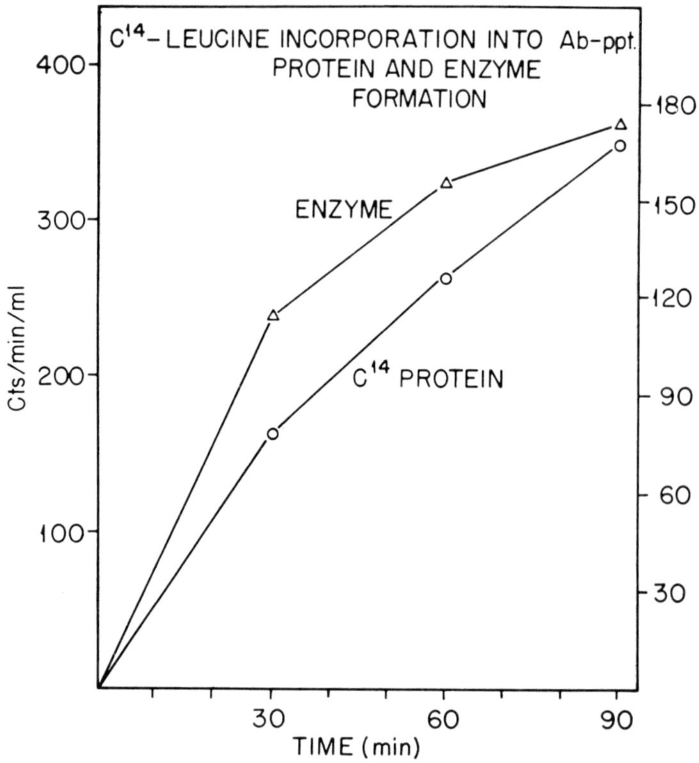

FIG. 14. Rate of C^{14}-leucine incorporation into Ab-ppt protein and enzyme formation. (From Novelli, Kameyama and Eisenstadt, 1961.)

Having thus satisfied ourselves that we were, in all probability, observing cell-free enzyme synthesis, we proceeded to examine some of the requirements of the systems. These requirements are illustrated by the data in Table 2.

In Table 2 it can be seen that enzyme synthesis is absolutely dependent upon the presence of inducer, a source of energy, the supernatant fraction, and the presence of nucleoside di- and triphosphates. A stimulation by amino acids is also evident. The most striking point is that the addition of inducer, not in any way metabolized, to an otherwise complete reaction mixture resulted in an increase of approximately 1,000 counts per minute (c.p.m.) of C^{14} leucine incorporated into total protein, about the same number of extra c.p.m. that appeared in the antibody-precipitable protein. Thus it seems clear that the inducer caused the appearance of an increase in enzyme activity corresponding with an increase in the

TABLE 2

Cell-Free Synthesis of β-Galactosidase and Incorporation of C^{14}-Leucine: Requirements

	Δ Enzyme units/ml.	c.p.m./ml. total PR	Reaction mixture Ab ppt PR
Complete system	+ 183.6	2560	1428
— TMG	— 2.4	1580	384
— AA	+ 108.0	1276	436
— ATP and generator	— 15.6	182	128
— XTP, XDP	— 24.6	660	248
— S	— 0.6	960	600

Abbreviations as in Table 1 and c.p.m., C^{14} counts per min.; total PR, total protein; AB ppt PR, antibody precipitable protein. (Adapted from Kameyama and Novelli, 1960b.)

incorporation of C^{14} leucine into protein, and that this increase in radioactive protein was specifically precipitable by antibody to the enzyme.

I mentioned that the cells needed to be preinduced in order to yield active preparations. The data of Table 3 demonstrate that both components of the system, particles as well as supernatant, must be derived from preinduced cells. Mixing the components with fractions derived from noninduced cells did not yield preparations that made the enzyme, although incorporation of C^{14} leucine into total but nonspecific protein was normal. Thus we have an intriguing fact to explain, i.e., that both particles and supernatant must be derived from preinduced cells, and still these preparations are inactive unless inducer is also included in the cell-free system.

TABLE 3

Comparison of Particles and Supernatant from Noninduced and Preinduced Cells

	Δ Enzyme units/ml.	Total protein c.p.m./ml.	Ab ppt protein c.p.m./ml.
PTMG + STMG	184	2560	1428
Pni + Sni	0	2200	48
Pni + STMG	0	2524	0
PTMG + Sni	2.8	1812	296

PTMG, STMG, Pni, Sni = particles and supernatants from preinduced cells (TMG) and noninluced cells (ni). (From Novelli, Kameyama and Eisenstadt 1961.)

The data illustrated in Table 4 show some of the inhibitors of the system. It is evident that the system is inhibited by RNase and chloramphenicol, both with respect to enzyme synthesis and incorporation of C^{14} leucine into general protein. In this respect our preparation is similar to the amino acid incorporation systems reported

TABLE 4

Cell-Free Synthesis of β-Galactosidase and Incorporation of C^{14}-Leucine: Inhibitors

	Δ Enzyme units/ml.	Total protein c.p.m./ml.	Ab ppt protein c.p.m./ml.
Complete system	+ 168	2400	1264
+ RNase	— 25.8	88	100
+ DNase	— 35.4	320	208
+ CAP	— 29.4	676	344
+ Glucose	— 20.4	808	368

Abbreviations as in Table 1.

(From Kameyama and Novelli, 1960b.)

by others. Of particular interest here is that the β-galactosidase system is inhibited by glucose, a known inhibitor of the whole cell induction of β-galactosidase. The marked inhibition by DNase is surprising, but is consistent with the conclusions of Riley, Pardee, Monod, and Jacob (1960) based on P^{32} suicide experiments, that functional DNA is required for the synthesis of β-galactosidase. Because of some apparent nonspecific precipitation of radioactive protein by the antiserum in tubes where no increase in enzyme was observed, we attempted to show more sharply the specific labeling of the newly synthesized enzyme. For this purpose, the complete reaction mixture that had exhibited enzyme synthesis was electrophoresed on Geon as before. In Figure 15 is shown the result of such an experiment. The curves at the top of the figure represent the distribution of enzyme activity, and the middle curves show the distribution of C^{14}-labeled protein. It should be noted that enzyme activity occurs in three peaks, whereas C^{14}-protein is distributed in four peaks. In order to obtain the data for the diagram at the bottom of the figure, carrier β-galactosidase was added to all tubes in order to obtain an antibody precipitate in each tube. The data show that a radioactive antibody precipitate was obtained only in those regions of the diagram that had exhibited enzyme activity. No radioactive protein was precipitated by the antiserum from the 5 to 10 cm. region, although labeled protein was clearly evident. Thus the electrophoresis sharpened the antibody precipitation and made it quite clear that radioactive enzyme was formed during the incubation. It should also be noted that the bulk of the newly synthesized enzyme remained associated with the particles. In this respect our system is similar to those amino acid incorporating systems from mammalian and plant tissues where the labeled protein remains largely associated with the ribosomes (Zamecnik, 1960; Rabson and Novelli, 1960; Rabson, Mans, and Novelli, in press; Mans and Novelli, in press).

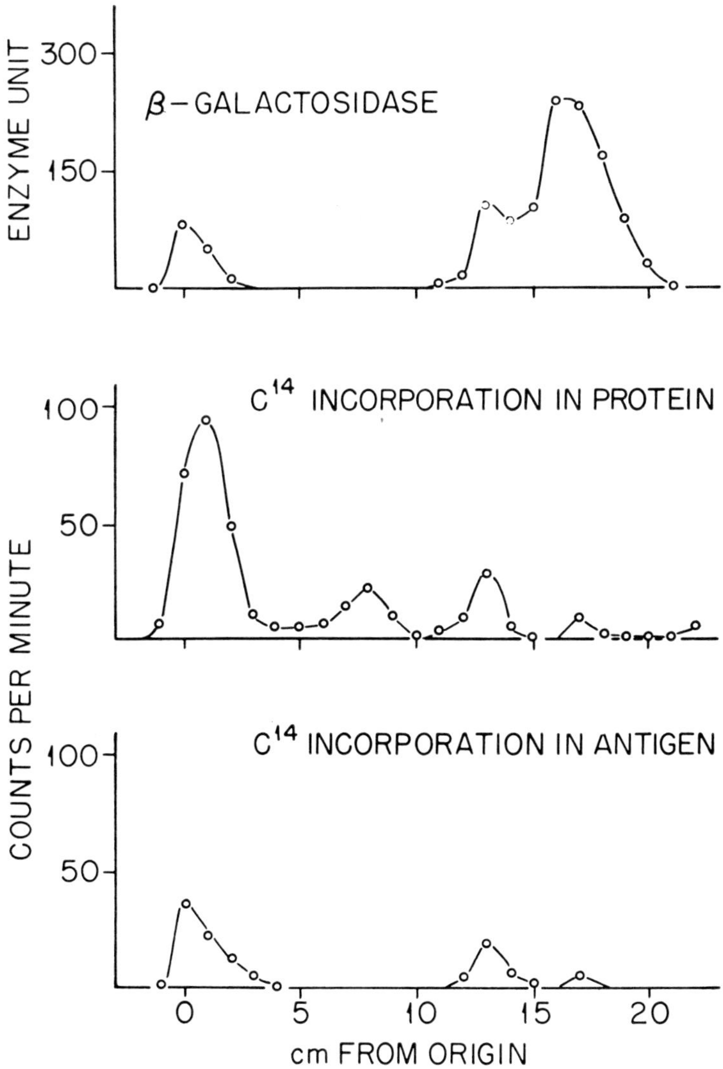

FIG. 15. Geon fractionation of reaction mixture. (From Novelli, Kameyama and Eisenstadt, 1961.)

Requirement for Specific DNA in the Cell-Free System

Upon his return to Japan, Kameyama pursued the investigation of the DNase effect. He subjected the supernatant fraction to ultrasonic oscillation and to UV irradiation. These treatments resulted in an inactivation of the cell-free system. The synthetic activity of the system could be largely restored by adding DNA prepared from untreated supernatant. In the meantime, Eisenstadt, who has recently joined our group, was engaged in carrying out the X-irradiation experiments shown in Figures 9 and 10. By increasing the radiation dose to 30 kr, it was possible to almost completely suppress enzyme induction in such cells. Using the cell-free enzyme synthesizing system, it was possible to determine which fraction of the biological system had been damaged during irradiation. By mixing particles and supernatants from X-irradiated cells with their normal counterparts, we found that the radiation damage had occurred in the supernatant fraction. Such data are shown in Table 5. It is

TABLE 5

Comparison of Damage in Particles and Supernatant Fractions Derived from X-Irradiated Cells

Fractions tested	Increase in enzyme units
PN + SN	156
PX + SX	5
PN + SX	26
PX + SN	142

PN, SN, PX, SX refer to particles and supernatants from normal and X-irradiated cells. (From Novelli, Kameyama and Eisenstadt, 1961.)

clear that supplementation of particles from irradiated cells with supernatant from normal cells restored enzyme synthesis to normal. Supernatant from irradiated cells, however, is incapable of causing enzyme synthesis with either kind of particle. Since it was known that DNA in our preparation was present in the supernatant, we added DNA prepared from the normal supernatant to the system derived from irradiated cells and observed a restoration of enzyme synthesis. DNA from *Pseudomonas saccharophila*, however, was ineffective. This observation suggested that the DNA effect was a real one and not due to its polyanionic nature as had been the case in the restoration of nuclear phosphorylation by Allfrey, Mirsky, and Osawa (1957). It remained them to determine whether the effect of DNA in restoring enzyme synthesis to the inactivated system was specific for the β-galactosidase gene. Therefore, the DNA's were

TABLE 6

Effect of Added DNA on Enzyme Synthesis in the X-Ray Inactivated Preparation

Additions	Increase in enzyme units
None	5
DNAni	15
DNAi	119
DNAlac–	— 2.5
DNAc	170
DNAc–TMG	64
DNAi, H + C	— 12.5

All tubes contained particles (PX), and supernatant (SX) from irradiated cells and inducer TMG. DNA preparations were (1) from noninduced cells (DNAni); (2) from induced cells (DNAi); (3) from lactose negative mutant lacking gene for β-galactosidase (DNA lac–); (4) from constitutive mutant (DNAc); (5) DNAi was heated to 100°C and then cooled rapidly (DNAi, H + C). (From Novelli, Kameyama and Eisenstadt, 1961)

prepared from the inducible strain, the constitutive strain, and the lactose negative strain (i.e., lacking β-galactosidase gene). The effect of these DNA's in restoring enzyme synthesis to the inactivated system is shown in Table 6. These data show that DNA from the inducible strain that had not been preinduced has little effect in the system, whereas DNA from similar cells that had been preinduced is effective in restoring enzyme synthesis. That the effect appears to be gene specific is evident from the fact that DNA prepared from a strain lacking the β-galactosidase gene is completely inactive. DNA prepared from the constitutive mutant (i.e., that makes enzyme in the absence of inducer) permits some enzyme synthesis in the absence of added inducer, but a threefold increase in enzyme is observed if inducer is added to the system. The last line where effective DNA was heated and rapidly cooled suggests that double stranded DNA is required for enzyme synthesis. Nisman and Fukuhara (1960) have observed a stimulation of β-galactosidase synthesis by added DNA in a broken protoplast system from the constitutive strain. The present findings are in accord with their data.

These observations in a cell-free system are consistent with the P^{32} experiments of Riley, Pardee, Monod, and Jacob (1960) in whole cells, indicating that functional DNA is required to obtain the synthesis of β-galactosidase.

In summary, the data comparing the behavior of the synthesis of β-galactosidase and OTC in cells of *E. coli* after uracil deprivation, UV irradiation, and T_2 infection are consistent with the idea that regulation of β-galactosidase synthesis occurs at the level of DNA, but repression of OTC synthesis may occur at the level of the ribosome. Conversely, data on X-ray inactivation of the two systems are so similar that they do not permit such a generalization.

The studies on cell-free synthesis of β-galactosidase demonstrating a specific requirement for DNA are in accord with the assumption that the synthesis of this enzyme is controlled at the level of the gene. Although the cell-free system for the synthesis of OTC had been developed before the one for β-galactosidase (Rogers and Novelli, 1961), definitive experiments had to await purification of the enzyme in order to prepare specific antisera. This has now been accomplished (Rogers and Novelli, unpublished data), and experiments with the OTC system, comparable to those herein described for the β-galactosidase system, can now be carried out. We hope that further studies with these cell-free systems will permit a more definitive statement regarding the control mechanisms regulating the synthesis of these enzymes.

REFERENCES

Adelberg, E. A., and H. E. Umbarger. 1953. Isoleucine and Valine Metabolism in *Escherichia coli*. V. α-Ketoisovaleric Acid Accumulation. *Journal of Biological Chemistry*, 205:475–482.

Allfrey, V., A. E. Mirsky, and S. Osawa. 1957. "The Nucleus and Protein Synthesis," *Symposium on the Chemical Basis of Heredity*, W. D. McElroy and B. Glass, Eds., pp. 200–231. Baltimore, Maryland: Johns Hopkins Press.

Baron, L. A., S. Spiegelman, and H. J. Quastler. 1953. Enzyme Formation in Non-Viable Cells. *Journal of General Physiology*, 36:631–641.

Chantrenne, H. 1958. Nucleic Acid Metabolism and Induced Enzyme Formation. *Recueil des travaux chimiques des pays-bas*, 77:586–601.

Clayton, R. K., and H. I. Adler. Protein Syntheses and Viability in X-Irradiated *Rhodopseudomonas spheroides*. (In preparation).

Cohn, M. 1957. Contributions of Studies on the β-Galactosidase of *Escherichia coli* to Our Understanding of Enzyme Synthesis. *Bacteriological Reviews*, 21:140–168.

Cohn, M., G. N. Cohen, and J. Monod. 1953. L'effet inhibiteur specifique de la méthionine dans la formation de la méthionine synthase chez *Escherichia coli*. *Comptes rendus hebdomadaires des seances de l'Academie des sciences*, 236:746–748.

Cowie, D. B., S. Spiegelman, R. B. Roberts, and J. D. Duerksen. 1961. Ribosome-Bound β-Galactosidase. *Proceedings of the National Academy of Sciences of the U.S.A.*, 47:114–122.

Eisenstadt, J., and G. D. Novelli. The Requirement for Specific DNA in the Cell-Free Synthesis of β-Galactosidase. (In preparation).

Fry, B. A., and F. Gros. 1959. The Metabolic Activities of *Escherichia coli* During the Establishment of Lysogeny. *Journal of General Microbiology*, 21:685–692.

Gorini, L., and W. K. Maas. 1957. The Potential for the Formation of a Biosynthetic Enzyme in *Escherichia coli*. *Biochimica et biophysica acta*, 25: 208–209.

Halverson, H. A. 1960. "The Induced Synthesis of Proteins," *Advances in Enzymology*, F. F. Nord, Ed., Vol. 22, pp. 99–156. New York, New York: Interscience Publishers, Inc.

Hershey, A. D. 1953. Nucleic Acid Economy in Bacteria Infected with Bacteriophage T_2. II. Phage Precursor Nucleic Acid. *Journal of General Physiology*, 37:1–23.

Hogness, D. S. 1959. "Induced Enzyme Synthesis," *Biophysical Science—A Study Program*, J. L. Oncly, Ed., pp. 256–268. New York, New York: John Wiley and Sons, Inc.

Kameyama, T., and G. D. Novelli. 1960a. Appearance of Particle Bound β-Galactosidase of *Escherichia coli* During Its Induction After Photoreactivation. (Abstract) *Bacteriological Proceedings*, p. 148.

———. 1960b. The Cell-Free Synthesis of β-Galactosidase by *Escherichia* coli. *Biochemical and Biophysical Research Communications*, 2:393–396.

———. (in press). The effect of Ultraviolet Irradiation and Photoreactivation on the Induced Synethesis of β-Galactosidase. *Archives of Biochemistry and Biophysics*.

Magasanik, B. Personal Communication.

Mandelstam, J. 1956. "Theories of Enzyme Adaptation in Microorganisms," *International Review of Cytology*, G. H. Bourne and J. F. Danielli, Eds., Vol. 5, pp. 51–87.

Mans, R. J., and G. D. Novelli. (in press). *In vitro* Amino Acid Incorporation into Particle Protein from Maize Seedlings. *Biochimica et biophysica acta*.

Monod, J. 1958. An Outline of Enzyme Induction. *Recueil des travaux chimiques des pays-bas*, 77:569–586.

Monod, J., and G. Cohen-Bazire. 1953. L'effet d'inhibition spécifique dans la biosynthèse de la tryptophane-demase chez *Aerobacter aerogenes*. *Comptes rendus hebdomadaires des séances de l'Académie des sciences*, 236:530–532.

Monod, J., A. M. Pappenheimer, Jr., and G. Cohen-Bazire. 1952. La cinetique de la biosynthèse de la β-Galactosidase chez *E. coli* considérée comme Fonction de la croissance. *Biochimica et biophysica acta*, 9:648–660.

Neidhardt, F. C., and B. Magasanik. 1956. Inhibitory Effect of Glucose on Enzyme Formation. *Nature, London*, 178:801–802.

Nisman, B., and H. Fukuhara. 1960. Role de l'acide desoxynucleique dans la synthèse des protéins par les deux fractions enzymatiques liées à des particules des *Escherichia coli*. *Comptes rendus hebdomadaires des séances de l'Académie des sciences*, 250:410–412.

Novelli, G. D., T. Kameyama, and J. M. Eisenstadt. 1961. The Effect of Ultraviolet Light and X-Rays on an Enzyme-Forming System. *Journal of Cellular Composition and Physiology*, 58 (suppl. I): 225–244.

Pardee, A. B. 1954. Nucleic Acid Precursors and Protein Synthesis. *Proceedings of the National Academy of Sciences of the U.S.A.*, 40:263–270.

Pardee, A. B., F. Jacob, and J. Monod. 1959. The Genetic Control and Cytoplasmic Expression of "Inducibility" in the Synthesis of β-Galactosidase by *E. coli*. *Journal of Molecular Biology*, 1:165–178.

Pollock, M. R. 1959. "Induced Formation of Enzymes," *The Enzymes*, P. D. Boyer, H. Lardy, and K. Myrback, Eds., Vol. 1, pp. 619–680. New York, New York: Academic Press, Inc.

Rabson, R., R. J. Mans, and G. D. Novelli. (in press). Changes in Cell-Free Amino Acid Incorporating Activity During Maturation of Maize Kernels. *Archives of Biochemistry and Biophysics.*

Rabson, R., and G. D. Novelli. 1960. The Incorporation of Leucine C^{14} into Protein by a Cell-Free Preparation from Maize Kernels. *Proceedings of the National Academy of Sciences of the U.S.A.*, 46:484–488.

Riley, M., A. B. Pardee, J. Monod, and F. Jacob. 1960. On the Expression of a Structural Gene. *Journal of Molecular Biology*, 2:216–225.

Rogers, P., and G. D. Novelli. 1959. Formation of Ornithine Transcarbamylase in Cells and Protoplasts of *Escherichia coli. Biochimica et biophysica acta,* 33:423–436.

———. 1960. Cell-Free Synthesis of Ornithine Transcarbamylase. *Biochimica et biophysica acta,* 44:298–309.

Spiegelman, S., and A. M. Campbell. 1956. "The Significance of Induced Enzyme Formation," *Currents in Biochemical Research*, D. E. Green, Ed., pp. 115–161. New York, New York: Interscience Publishers, Inc.

Stanier, R. Y. 1951. Enzymatic Adaptation in Bacteria. *Annual Review of Microbiology*, 5:35–56.

Vogel, H. J. 1953. Path of Ornithine Synthesis in *Escherichia coli. Proceedings of the National Academy of Sciences of the U.S.A.*, 39:578–583.

———. 1957. Repressed and Induced Enzyme Formation: A Unified Hypothesis. *Proceedings of the National Academy of Sciences of the U.S.A.*, 43:491–496.

———. 1958. "Comment on the Possible Role of Repressers and Inducers on Enzyme Formation in Development," *Symposium on the Chemical Basis of Development*, W. D. McElroy and B. Glass, Eds., pp. 479–484. Baltimore, Maryland: Johns Hopkins Press.

———. (in press). "Control by Repression," Control Mechanisms in Cellular Processes, D. M. Bonner, Ed.

Volkin, E., and L. Astrachan. 1956. Phosphorus Incorporation in *Escherichia coli* Ribonucleic Acid After Infection with Bacteriophage T_2. *Virology*, 2:149–161.

Wijesundera, S., and D. D. Woods. 1953. The Effect of Growth on a Medium Containing Methionine on the Synthesis of This Amino Acid by *Bacterium coli. Biochemical Journal*, 55:*viii*.

Zamecnik, P. C. 1960. Historical and Current Aspect of the Problem of Protein Synthesis. *Harvey Lecture Series*, 54:256–281. Springfield, Illinois: Charles C Thomas.

Interrelationships in the Synthesis of RNA, DNA, and Protein in Normal and Virus-Infected Cell Cultures

NORMAN P. SALZMAN, PH.D.

Section of Cell Biology, Laboratory of Biology of Viruses, National Institute of Allergy and Infectious Diseases, Bethesda, Maryland

The consequences of infection of animal cell cultures with two viruses, vaccinia virus which contains deoxyribonucleic acid (DNA) and poliovirus which contains ribonucleic acid (RNA), have been studied. While the information obtained from these experiments relates primarily to the mechanism of virus infection and replication, some information relating to the broader problem of macromolecular synthesis is also obtained. In certain cases, the facts that the macromolecular components which make up the virus do not exist in the cell prior to infection and are formed *de novo* from small molecules (Darnell and Levintow, 1960; Salzman and Sebring, 1961) and that their synthesis may be assayed for by the formation of infectivity represent a distinct advantage.

The animal cell line used in these studies is the HeLa (S3) (Puck, Marcus, and Cieciura, 1956), which is grown in suspension culture (McLimans, Davis, Glover, and Rake, 1957) and is maintained indefinitely in the logarithmic phase of growth by a proper schedule of dilution, the culture dividing every 20 hours. We have restricted our studies to cells in the logarithmic phase of growth at the beginning of the experiment. The procedures for cell growth, infection of the culture and chemical procedures are described in a previous publication (Salzman, Lockart, and Sebring, 1959).

Chemical Changes in Poliovirus-Infected Cells

When suspension cultures are infected with type 1 poliovirus, there is a lag phase of three hours' duration after virus addition and prior to the formation of any new virus. Six to nine hours after virus addition, the cycle of virus replication is complete (Figure 1). The

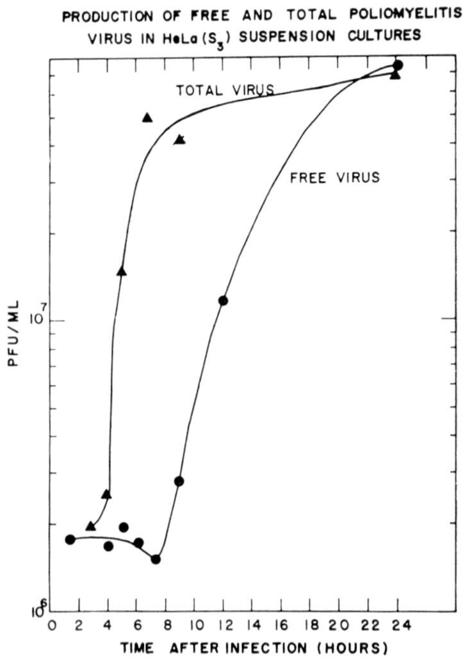

Fig. 1. The rate of formation of poliovirus in HeLa (S3) infected cells. Total virus was measured after freeze-thawing aliquots of the suspension culture four times. The free virus was determined in the supernatant fluid obtained after removal of cells by centrifugation.

Abbreviation: pfu, plaque forming units.

(Salzman, Lockart, and Sebring, 1959.)

nucleic acid content of a culture in complete growth medium at various times after infection has been compared with an uninfected culture in a nongrowth medium* and an uninfected culture in complete growth medium (Table 1). There are two striking effects observed in the infected culture: (1) the extensive loss of nucleic acid that occurs late in the infectious cycle, and (2) an inhibition of nucleic acid synthesis that occurs even though the infected cells are contained in a medium which permits optimal rates of growth

* When cells are contained in a medium lacking the essential amino acid, phenylalanine, they are unable to synthesize RNA, DNA, and protein.

TABLE 1

*Total Nucleic Acid Content of Polio-Infected, Growing, and Nongrowing HeLa (S3) Suspension Cultures**

	Total optical density Δ260–300 mμ./100 ml. of cell culture†		
Time after infection (hours)	Virus-infected culture	Nongrowing culture	Growing culture
0	23.2	22.3	21.5
3	22.6	21.7	23.1
6	20.6	21.2	24.3
9	17.6	21.9	27.8
12	8.7	21.4	29.1

* Cells grown in complete medium were harvested, resuspended in complete medium less phenylalanine, and split into three portions. To the first was added virus inoculum and phenylalanine (0.2 mM final concentration); no addition was made to the second; to the third was added phenylalanine (final concentration 0.2 mM). The optical density of the defatted tissue obtained from equal aliquots of the cell suspensions was determined after a 15-minute PCA extraction at 90°C.

† The total optical density = observed optical density times volume of the 5 per cent PCA solution.

Abbreviation: PCA, perchloric acid.

(Salzman, Lockhart, and Sebring, 1959.)

of uninfected cells (Table 1, column 3). When the net changes in RNA, DNA, and protein were examined using different procedures, that is by estimation of RNA after electrophoretic separation of the four nucleotides and of DNA by isolation of DNA thymine, or when RNA and DNA were measured by the orcinol and diphenylamine procedures, similar results were obtained (Table 2). Here it is seen that the loss of RNA precedes the loss of protein from the cell (Salzman, Lockart, and Sebring, 1959).

TABLE 2

Net Changes in Cellular RNA, DNA, and Protein in Polio-Infected and Uninfected HeLa (S3) Suspension Cultures

		Hours after virus addition				
Substance	Culture	0	3	6	9	12
RNA: μmoles of nucleotide*/100 ml.	Control	2.07	2.17	2.55	2.76	2.83
	Infected	2.05	2.20	2.11	1.39	0.707
DNA: μmoles of thymine†/100 ml.	Control	0.167	0.175	0.193	0.209	0.247
	Infected	0.174	0.188	0.182	....	0.178
Protein: mg./100 ml.	Control	6.50	7.06	7.87	8.75	9.29
	Infected	6.92	7.14	7.09	7.01	5.68

* RNA nucleotides were measured by KOH degradation of the defatted tissue followed by paper electrophoresis of the nucleotides (Davidson and Smellie, 1952). The above figures represent the total amount of the four nucleotides. Similar results were obtained when RNA was estimated colorimetrically (Mejbaum, 1939).

† DNA was measured by the thymine content of the cell suspensions. The base was purified as described in the experimental section. Similar results were obtained when DNA was estimated colorimetrically (Dische, 1930).

Abbreviations: DNA, deoxyribonucleic acid; KOH, potassium hydroxide; RNA, ribonucleic acid.

(Salzman, Lockhart, and Sebring, 1959.)

None of the above procedures are sufficiently sensitive to detect with certainty, small increments in RNA or DNA. The uptake of cytidine-2-C^{14} into the nucleic acids was studied as a more sensitive indicator of low levels of nucleic acid synthesis. While the synthesis of DNA proceeds at a slower rate in the infected cultures, there is uptake of the precursor into DNA during the first six hours of the infective cycle (Table 3). The extent of DNA synthesis, based on the specific activity of the DNA bases, is calculated to be a 5 per cent increment, an amount too small to have been detected as a net change. It is well established that RNA from tobacco mosaic virus and from many animal viruses is infectious and contains the genetic information required for virus replication (Gierer and Schramm, 1956; Colter, Bird, Moyer, and Brown, 1957). However, these data suggested the possibility that low levels of DNA synthesis were

TABLE 3

Uptake of Cytidine-2-C^{14} into the DNA Pyrimidine Bases of Polio-Infected and Uninfected Growing Cell Cultures

Time after infection (hours)	Specific activity of the DNA pyrimidine bases (c.p.m./μmole)			
	Growing uninfected culture		Polio-infected culture	
	Cytosine	Thymine	Cytosine	Thymine
3	3,420	3,500	2,500	2,500
6	10,100	10,600	4,410	4,610
9	18,900	14,200	4,430	4,800
12	26,400	27,900	5,710	5,820

Abbreviations: c.p.m., counts per minute; DNA, deoxyribonucleic acid.
(Salzman, Lockhart, and Sebring, 1959.)

TABLE 4

Effect of 5-Fluorodeoxyuridine on HeLa Cell Metabolism

Molar concentration of FUDR	Fold increase in 24 hours*		
	DNA	RNA	Protein
10^{-5}	0.98	1.30	1.53
10^{-6}	1.01	1.46	1.46
5×10^{-7}	1.08	1.51	1.59
10^{-7}	1.29	1.60	1.67
5×10^{-8}	1.39	1.69	1.79
10^{-8}	1.51	1.73	1.79
5×10^{-9}	1.68	1.92	1.90
10^{-9}	1.84	1.99	2.00
Control	1.90	1.91	1.97

* Referred to 0 time quantities of RNA, DNA, and protein as 1.
Abbreviations: DNA, deoxyribonucleic acid; FUDR, 5-fluorodeoxyuridine; RNA, ribonucleic acid.

necessary for poliovirus replication even though this virus does not contain DNA. Animal cells can continuously degrade and resynthesize RNA and the transfer of information from a possibly unstable genetic RNA of the virus to a more stable reservoir of DNA could be involved in the replication process. To determine the role of DNA in poliovirus replication, we used the metabolic inhibitor 5-fluorodeoxyuridine (FUDR). Concentrations of inhibitor of 5×10^{-7} M, or higher, prevent any detectable net synthesis in DNA as measured by the diphenylamine reaction (Table 4). Again, such colorimetric procedures are not sufficiently sensitive to detect low levels of DNA synthesis. To detect this, the extent of the uptake of high specific activity uridine-2-C^{14} into DNA thymine in a two hour period was measured in the presence and absence of FUDR. When concentrations of FUDR of 10^{-6} M and uridine-2-C^{14} at 3×10^{-5} M and a specific activity of 536,000 c.p.m./μmole were simultaneously added to HeLa suspension cultures, no counts were detected in DNA thymine. In a control culture in this same two hour period, the specific activity of DNA thymine was 6,550 c.p.m./μmole. Thus it can be concluded that the block in thymidylic acid

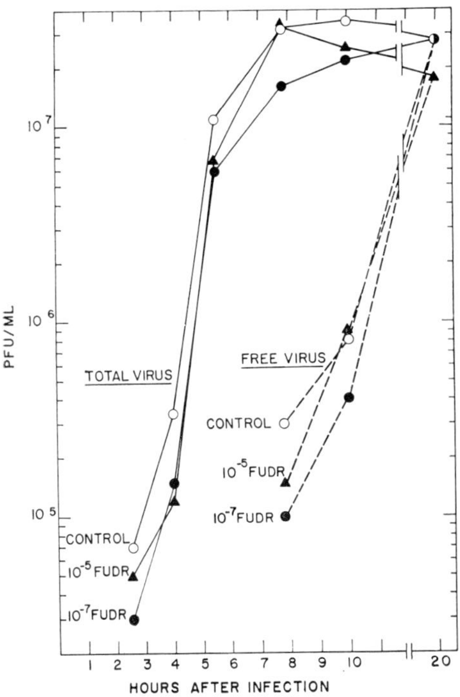

FIG. 2. Effect of 5-fluorodeoxyuridine on poliomyelitis virus formation in HeLa (S_3) suspension cultures. FUDR was added for three hours prior to infection of the cells and was present during the entire period of virus adsorption and replication. For procedures for determination of viral titers see caption, Figure 1; see also Salzman, Lockart, and Sebring (1959).

Abbreviations: FUDR, 5-fluorodeoxyuridine; pfu, the plaque-forming units.

synthesis is both complete and immediate. Further, the quantities of thymine derivatives in the acid-soluble fraction of the cell are not sufficient to permit DNA synthesis to occur.

The Effect of FUDR on Poliovirus Replication

When the effects of FUDR on poliovirus replication were measured, it was clearly demonstrated that virus synthesis was not affected at all by the inhibition of DNA synthesis (Figure 2). In this experiment, FUDR was added to cells three hours prior to infection and was present during adsorption of virus to cells. Further, it is seen that the block in thymidylic acid synthesis is maintained in infected cells (Table 5). These experiments demonstrate that a ribonucleoprotein can replicate, presumably with no information for this synthesis contained in the DNA.

TABLE 5

Effect of 5-Fluorodeoxyuridine on the Six Hour Uptake of Uridine-2-C^{14} into Poliovirus-Infected Cells

Fraction analyzed		Uninfected cells	Infected cells	
			+10^{-5} M FUDR	
		Specific activity, c.p.m./μmole		
RNA	Cytosine	20,000	15,200	15,800
	Uracil	31,700	30,200	31,900
DNA	Thymine	11,000	0	9,100

Abbreviations: DNA, deoxyribonucleic acid; FUDR, 5-fluorodeoxyuridine; RNA, ribonucleic acid.

The Effects of FUDR on Vaccinia Virus Replication

When a concentration of FUDR which completely inhibits DNA synthesis is added to HeLa cells infected with vaccinia virus, there is a complete inhibition of virus synthesis (Table 6). The FUDR inhibits the synthesis of thymidylic acid (Bosch, Harbers, and Heidelberger, 1958; Cohen *et al.*, 1958), and thus the synthesis of DNA and its effects are reversed by the addition of thymidine. At concentrations of FUDR in the range 10^{-7} to 10^{-9} M there is a progressively decreasing inhibition of DNA synthesis in uninfected cells, presumably reflecting synthesis of thymidylic acid at suboptimal rates. The quantities of DNA synthesized in a 24 hour period at these concentrations of FUDR are seen in Table 7. When cells are infected with vaccinia, and virus synthesis is carried out

TABLE 6

Inhibition of Vaccinia Virus Production by 5-Fluorodeoxyuridine and Its Reversal by Thymidine

Molar concentration of FUDR	Molar concentration of thymidine	Virus titer (pfu/ml.)	
		3.7 hours	24 hours
. .	. .	2.4×10^5	2.6×10^7
10^{-6}	. .	2.4×10^5	1.5×10^5
10^{-6}	10^{-5}	4.0×10^5	2.0×10^7
10^{-6}	10^{-6}	......	2.0×10^7
10^{-6}	10^{-7}	......	1.0×10^6
10^{-6}	$10^{-7}/3$	......	1.2×10^5
10^{-6}	10^{-8}	......	5.6×10^4
10^{-6}	$10^{-8}/3$	......	7.8×10^4

at these same concentrations, and the yields compared with those in the uninhibited control, the inhibition of virus synthesis is seen to parallel the degree of inhibition of DNA synthesis in the uninfected cultures (Table 7). The quantity of DNA in a full yield of vaccinia virus is small relative to the DNA that is present in a HeLa cell, representing only 1 per cent. If there were a preferential utilization of limited quantities of thymidylic acid for virus synthesis, any concentration of FUDR which permitted some measurable synthesis of DNA should then permit full yields of virus. The experimental findings, however, indicate the contrary. There is no preferential advantage for viral DNA synthesis; rather when a limiting quantity of thymidylic acid is present it would appear to be shared equally for the synthesis of host and viral DNA.

TABLE 7

Effect of Subinhibitory Concentrations of FUDR on Cell DNA Synthesis and Virus Production

Molar concentration of FUDR	Synthesis of DNA in uninfected cells*	Virus yield*	
		Expt. 1	Expt. 2
10^{-5}	0	0	0
10^{-6}	0	0	0
5×10^{-7}	0	0	0
10^{-7}	18	5.5	4.8
5×10^{-8}	32	8.6	10
10^{-8}	56	57	48
5×10^{-9}	70	71	70
10^{-9}	100	100	100

* Relative to the uninhibited control value which is equal to 100 per cent. Yields of virus and increments in DNA were measured after 24 hours.

Kinetics of Formation of Vaccinia Virus DNA and Protein

Since the addition of FUDR prevents any further synthesis of DNA, it becomes possible, by the addition of FUDR at various times after infection and assaying, for the formation of infectious virus at 22 hours to determine the rate of formation of viral DNA (Salzman, 1960). Cells were commonly infected and then used to set up replicate spinner cultures. An uninhibited culture was used to determine the rate of formation of infectious virus. With each of the other cultures, 10^{-6} M FUDR was added at different times after infection and the final yield of infectious virus was determined at 22 hours. Since the addition of FUDR prevents any further DNA synthesis, infectious virus formed after the addition of FUDR must contain viral DNA made prior to the time of FUDR addition. Thus, while FUDR added at 1.5 hours inhibits virus synthesis, when FUDR is added at 6.8 hours, there is no effect on the final yield of virus, and we can conclude that by 6.8 hours all of the viral DNA is synthesized, although at this time only a small fraction of the final yield of infectious virus is formed (Figure 3). The time course of

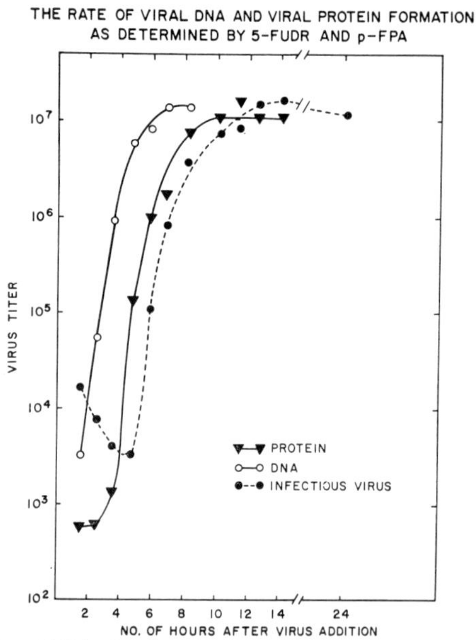

FIG. 3. The rate of formation of viral DNA and viral protein, as determined by FUDR and FPA inhibition of viral synthesis, and the rate of virus formation. The points in the infectious virus curve (● – – ●) represent the total quantities of virus measured on aliquots from a single, infected, uninhibited control culture.

Each point in the viral DNA (●——●) and viral protein curve (▲——▲), however, indicates the yield of virus obtained at 22 hours, when either FUDR or FPA was added at the time indicated by the position of the point. As indicated in the text, the varying yields of infectious virus obtained in the inhibited cultures are a measure of the quantity of viral DNA or protein already made at the time the inhibitors were added. These curves then represent the time of formation of viral DNA and protein (see text p. 469). The quantities of virus newly formed at the time inhibitors were added are seen in the infectious virus curve.

viral DNA formation determined in this manner is seen to precede, by several hours, the formation of infectious virus.

Fluorophenylalanine (FPA) similarly inhibits virus formation, and its effect is reversed by the addition of phenylalanine (Table 8). Studies similar to those with FUDR can thus be carried out, and the results of such an experiment are seen in Figure 3. While the experiment was carried out in the same manner as that previously described in which the rate of DNA formation was determined, two points of difference should be noted. The rate with which FPA becomes effective is not known, and if there is a lag period before FPA does become effective, the true curve for the rate of protein synthesis would be shifted to the right. (It is apparent, however, from the position of this curve that this lag cannot be greater than 45 minutes.) The second point relates to the nature of vaccinia virus. This virus is made up of several protein components (Smadel, 1952). As a consequence, if four viral protein components were synthesized prior to the time of FPA addition, and the fifth species, which was the final species needed to form infectious virus, had not been formed, the addition of FPA would completely block the formation of infectious virus, even though as much as 90 per cent of the viral protein might already be present. The FPA curve then presumably represents the rate of formation of the last species of viral protein needed for the formation of infectious virus. The lag between the time of DNA synthesis and the time of appearance of infectious virus would appear to be the period during which certain species of virus proteins are formed.

TABLE 8

Inhibition of Vaccinia Virus Synthesis by p-*Fluorophenylalanine and its Reversibility by Phenylalanine*

Medium	Concentration phenylalanine (mM)	Concentration fluorophenylalanine (mM)	Virus titer pfu/ml. 3 hours	Virus titer pfu/ml. 22 hours
Phenylalanine deficient medium	..	..	4.8×10^3	5.0×10^6
Phenylalanine deficient medium	+ 0.2	..	1.2×10^3	1.5×10^7
Phenylalanine deficient medium	+ ..	0.2	1.6×10^3	6.7×10^2
Phenylalanine deficient medium	+ ..	0.05	......	2.0×10^3
Phenylalanine deficient medium	+ 0.05	0.05	2.0×10^3	1.7×10^7
Phenylalanine deficient medium	+ 0.2	0.05	......	1.7×10^7

Additions were made 1.5 hours after infection, as indicated, to the cells which are contained in a phenylalanine deficient medium.

THE EFFECTS OF FUDR ON UNINFECTED CELLS

In many respects the mechanism of action of FUDR in the HeLa cell is similar to that seen in other systems. FUDR is effective in inhibiting the formation of thymidylic acid (Bosch, Harbers, and Heidelberger, 1958; Cohen *et al.*, 1958) and is interconverted to the ribonucleotide presumably through the free base, and is then incorporated into RNA (Heidelberger *et al.*, 1957). When studying its effects on HeLa S3 cells, we consistently observed that at low concentrations of FUDR in the range 10^{-7} to 10^{-8} M not only was there a partial inhibition of the synthesis of DNA but also of RNA (Table 4). None of the mechanisms by which fluorouracil affects RNA (Horowitz, Saukkonen, and Chargaff, 1960) seemed likely to be operative at this concentration. However, in view of the irreversible block of thymidylic acid synthesis established by FUDR (Cohen *et al.*, 1958), the inhibition of DNA synthesis at these concentrations was not unexpected. What seemed the most likely explanation of these data was that FUDR at these concentrations had no direct effect on RNA, but rather that RNA synthesis was coupled to the synthesis of DNA, and direct inhibition of DNA synthesis then caused an inhibition of RNA. However, even when DNA is completely inhibited, there is still significant synthesis of RNA and, presumably, there would be a second type of RNA whose synthesis was not coupled to DNA (Table 4). The progressive inhibition in the synthesis of RNA that is observed in the region 10^{-7} to 10^{-5} M would presumably then represent a direct effect on RNA as a result of the incorporation of analogue into RNA producing fraudulent and nonfunctional species. The experiments described below support this interpretation of the data.

The extent of incorporation of FU-2-C^{14} into RNA in a 24 hour period was studied in the presence of various concentrations of 5-fluorouracil-2-C^{14} (FU-2-C^{14}) (Table 9). At 10^{-8} M the uptake of FU would appear to be insignificant. If we assume a molecular weight for RNA of 2×10^6, in each molecule of RNA there would be 1,500 uracil molecules, and it can be calculated from the extent of incorporation of FU into RNA and the specific activity of the FU that in one out of every 250 molecules of RNA, one uracil molecule of the 1,500 present would be replaced by fluorouracil.

From studies on the uptake of uridine-2-C^{14} into RNA, it is known that this incorporation is not affected by 10^{-5} M FUDR, and that similar specific activities of the isolated RNA bases are obtained

TABLE 9

22 Hour Incorporation of 5-Fluorouracil-2-C^{14} into HeLa (S3) Cell Nucleic Acid

Molar concentration of FU-2-C^{14}	c.p.m. / mg. RNA
10^{-4}	1,020,000.0
10^{-5}	116,000.0
10^{-6}	6,700.0
10^{-7}	1,010.0
10^{-8}	92.5

when FUDR is present or absent. In spite of its ability to become incorporated into RNA, uridine does not reverse the inhibitory effect of FUDR on RNA synthesis (Table 10). However, thymidine is effective in reversing the inhibition of both DNA and RNA (Table 11). Since exogenous thymidine is incorporated solely into

TABLE 10

The Effect of Uridine on the Inhibition of Cellular Synthesis by FUDR

Molar concentration		Fold increase in a 19 hour period*		
FUDR	Uridine	DNA	RNA	Protein
10^{-6}	......	0.92	1.31	1.54
10^{-6}	5×10^{-5}	0.94	1.38	1.60
10^{-7}	......	0.92	1.41	1.84
10^{-7}	5×10^{-5}	1.03	1.43	1.75
10^{-8}	......	1.34	1.58	1.81
10^{-8}	5×10^{-5}	1.31	1.58	1.79
..	......	1.71	1.70	1.80
..	5×10^{-5}	1.67	1.63	1.77

* Referred to the 0 time values fcr RNA, DNA, and protein which are arbitrarily set as 1.

TABLE 11

The Effect of Thymidine on the Inhibition of Cellular Synthesis by FUDR

Molar concentration		Fold increase in a 27 hour period*	
FUDR	Thymidine	DNA	RNA
10^{-6}	..	1.02	1.42
10^{-6}	10^{-5}	2.12	2.09
10^{-7}	..	1.34	1.64
10^{-7}	10^{-5}	2.03	2.04
10^{-8}	..	1.71	1.84
10^{-8}	10^{-5}	2.00	2.03
..	..	2.14	2.14

* See footnote Table 10.

DNA thymine, the reversal of the inhibition of RNA, as well as DNA synthesis, reflects their coupled synthesis. Further, it should be noted that by using FUDR-2-C^{14} and unlabeled thymidine, it was demonstrated that thymidine does not block the entry of FUDR into the cell. This is important to exclude, for if this were the case, the reversal by thymidine might simply result from a reduced concentration of inhibitor in the cell.

Finally, we have examined the nature of the RNA and protein that is coupled to the synthesis of DNA (Table 12). Cells were grown in the presence of various concentrations of FUDR and, after 24 hours, the cells were fractionated into a nuclear and cytoplasmic fraction using citric acid. There is a clear metabolic separation between the two fractions; the synthesis of cytoplasmic RNA and protein are seen to proceed at the same rate as in the uninhibited control while the syntheses of nuclear RNA and protein are completely or almost completely inhibited. This separation of protein and RNA into two categories, one which can replicate in the absence of DNA synthesis and a second whose synthesis is coupled to DNA synthesis, may be an important determinant of the enzyme pattern in the cell and thus a mechanism for the regulation of cell growth. This possibility is currently under investigation.

TABLE 12

The Effect of FUDR on the Synthesis of RNA, DNA, and Protein

Molar concentration of FUDR	Fold increase in 20 hours*				
	Nucleus			Cytoplasm	
	DNA	RNA	Protein	RNA	Protein
10^{-6}	1.02	.964	1.28	1.81	1.68
10^{-7}	1.09	.994	1.30	1.75	1.72
10^{-8}	1.61	1.430	1.72	1.71	1.73
. .	1.88	1.730	2.23	1.72	1.72

* See footnote Table 10.

There would appear to be particular virtues for each of the systems we have studied. In poliovirus there is ribonucleoprotein replication and no involvement of DNA. This is, of course, not true for vaccinia virus infected cells, and here it is possible to study the effects of DNA synthesis on protein synthesis presumably with RNA serving as the mediator for that synthesis. Finally, in the uninfected cell, we see conditions which are grossly similar to both of these conditions, and, of course, presently fail to see a great many unknown interrelationships that are operative. It is our hope that the complex interrelationships which exist between RNA, DNA, and protein can be further clarified by examination of these systems.

ACKNOWLEDGMENT

The author is deeply indebted to Robert Duschinsky of Hoffmann-LaRoche, Inc., for generously providing 5-fluorouracil-2-C^{14} and 5-fluorodeoxyuridine-2-C^{14}.

REFERENCES

Bosch, L., E. Harbers, and C. Heidelberger. 1958. Studies on Fluorinated Pyrimidines. V. Effects on Nucleic Acid Metabolism *in vitro*. *Cancer Research*, 18:335–343.

Cohen, S. S., J. G. Flaks, H. D. Barner, M. R. Loeb, and J. Lichtenstein. 1958. The Mode of Action of 5-Fluorouracil and Its Derivatives. *Proceedings of the National Academy of Sciences of the U.S.A.*, 44:1004–1012.

Colter, J. S., J. A. Bird, A. W. Moyer, and R. A. Brown. 1957. Infectivity of Ribonucleic Acid Isolated from Virus-Infected Tissues. *Virology*, 4:522–532.

Darnell, J. E., Jr., and L. Levintow. 1960. Poliovirus Protein: Source of Amino Acids and Time Course of Synthesis. *Journal of Biological Chemistry*, 235:74–77.

Davidson, J. N., and R. H. S. Smellie. 1952. Phosphorus Compounds in the Cell. 3. The Incorporation of Radioactive Phosphorus into the Ribonucleotide Fraction of Liver Tissue. *Biochemical Journal*, 52:599–606.

Dische, Z. 1930. Uber einige neue charakteristische Farbreaktionen der Thymonukleinsäure und eine Mikromethode zur Bestimmung derselben in tierichen Organen mit Hilfe dieser Reaktionen. *Mikrochemie*, 8:4–32.

Giere, A., and G. Schramm. 1956. Infectivity of Ribonucleic Acid from Tobacco Mosaic Virus. *Nature, London*, 177:702–703.

Heidelberger, C., N. K. Chaudhuri, P. Denneberg, D. Mooren, L. Griesbach, R. Duschinsky, R. J. Schnitzer, E. Pleven, and J. Scheiner. 1957. Fluorinated Pyrimidines, A New Class of Tumour-Inhibitory Compounds. *Nature, London*, 179:663–666.

Horowitz, J., J. J. Saukkonen, and E. Chargaff. 1960. Effects of Fluoropyrimidines on the Synthesis of Bacterial Proteins and Nucleic Acids. *Journal of Biological Chemistry*, 235:3266–3272.

McLimans, W. F., E. V. Davis, F. L. Glover, and G. W. Rake. 1957. The Submerged Culture of Mammalian Cells: The Spinner Culture. *Journal of Immunology*, 79:428–433.

Mejbaum, W. 1939. Uber die Bestimmung kleiner Pentosemengen, insbesondere in Derivaten der Adenylsäure. *Hoppe-Seyler's Zeitschrift für physiologische Chemie*, 258:117–120.

Puck, T. T., P. I. Marcus, and S. J. Cieciura. 1956. Clonal Growth of Mammalian Cells *in vitro*. Growth Characteristics of Colonies from Single HeLa Cells With and Without a "Feeder" Layer. *Journal of Experimental Medicine*, 103:273–284.

Salzman, N. P. 1960. The Rate of Formation of Vaccinia Deoxyribonucleic Acid and Vaccinia Virus. *Virology*, 10:150–152.

Salzman, N. P., R. Z. Lockart, and E. D. Sebring. 1959. Alteration in HeLa Cell Metabolism Resulting from Poliovirus Infection. *Virology*, 9:244–259.

Salzman, N. P., and E. D. Sebring. 1961. The Source of Poliovirus Ribonucleic Acid. *Virology*, 13:258–260.

Smadel, J. E. 1952. "Smallpox and Vaccinia," *Viral and Rickettsial Infections in Man*, T. M. Rivers, Ed., pp. 414–439. New York, New York: J. B. Lippincott Co.

Is There an Integrated Virus Genome in Virus-Induced Neoplastic Cells?

R. DULBECCO, M.D., AND M. VOGT, M.D.

Division of Biology,
California Institute of Technology,
Pasadena, California

In this article we shall discuss the question of whether an integrated virus genome is present in cells transformed to the neoplastic state by a virus, and, if so, which hypotheses can be made concerning the state of the virus genome in these cells. This question will be discussed in the light of some recent work, which, although not providing a definite answer, allows a better definition of the problem.

The experimental observations on which this discussion will be based were obtained from *in vitro* experiments, utilizing the deoxyribonucleic acid (DNA)-containing polyoma virus (Smith, Freeman, Vogt, and Dulbecco, 1960) and cultivated cells derived from mouse or hamster embryos. This virus produces, *in vitro*, the neoplastic transformation of both mouse and hamster embryo cultures. The cells present in the transformed cultures have a distinct morphology and a special growth behavior, which reveals their neoplastic character. Furthermore, the cells of transformed hamster embryo cultures can be shown to be neoplastic in the classical sense, since they are able to give rise to tumors endowed with indefinite growth ability at the site of implantation when transplanted subcutaneously into young adult hamsters (Vogt and Dulbecco, 1960).

A number of hypotheses can be considered, a priori, for the role of the virus in causing the neoplastic transformation of a population of cells, i.e., either of a culture *in vitro*, or of a tissue in the animal:

1. Selection by the virus of pre-existing, potentially neoplastic cells.
2. Direct induction of a new cell type by the virus. This in turn can be brought about by the following mechanisms: (a) continued presence of the viral genome in an autonomously reproducing (vegetative) state within the cells; (b) presence of the viral genome integrated with the genome of the host cells; and (c) a change caused by the virus in the functional state of the cells, which can persist even if the virus is later lost (not yet tested).
3. Indirect induction, caused by the influence of some infected cells of the population on other cells, which may or may not be infected (not yet tested).
4. Finally one can ask whether aneuploidization plays any role in the process of neoplasia production by virus.

We shall now examine the available experimental evidence concerning these hypotheses.

Hypothesis 1: The Selection of a Pre-Existing Cell Type

The observations concerning the neoplastic transformation of cultures of hamster embryo cells by the polyoma virus speak against this hypothesis. In fact, the infection with polyoma virus does not alter appreciably the growth rate of the hamster embryo cells, so that the selective conditions present in infected and in noninfected cultures could not be very different (Vogt and Dulbecco, 1960). Direct evidence against this hypothesis was obtained by studying two sublines of mouse embryo cells derived from the same clone; one was infected with polyoma virus, and the other was used as noninfected control (Weisberg, personal communication). While the infected subline underwent the characteristic neoplastic transformation, the noninfected subline continued to grow without showing any neoplastic characteristics. Thus, the neoplastic character was not a property of the original clone. Therefore, this hypothesis can now be discarded.

Direct Induction of a New Cell Type by the Virus

Hypothesis 2(a): The Continued Presence of the Virus Genome in a Vegetative State

At first glance, this hypothesis seems supported by the continued virus release seen in many types of virus-induced tumors and leukemias, as well as by cultures neoplastically transformed by viruses such as polyoma virus, Rous sarcoma virus or myeloblastosis virus. The observations carried out with polyoma virus show that all cultures of mouse embryo cells transformed by this virus continue to release indefinitely polyoma virus of a special mutant type; for transformed hamster embryo cultures, persistent virus release is, on the contrary, rare. In experiments in which single cells from virus-releasing cultures were grown into clonal cell populations, it could be shown that the property of virus release is not transmitted hereditarily from a cell to its progeny (Dulbecco and Vogt, 1960). When the clonal cultures were prepared under conditions which prevented their becoming reinfected by virus carried accidentally with the initial cell, the clones were regularly nonvirus releasers. The persistent virus release, observed in the mass cultures transformed by the polyoma virus, is the consequence of a "virus carrier state." This carrier state is brought about by the enhanced, but incomplete, resistance of the transformed cells to superinfection with polyoma virus. In fact, if the nonvirus-releasing clonal cultures are exposed to polyoma virus, a small proportion of cells become infected; they release virus which, in turn, infects other cells. In this continuously repeating process, a special mutant of the virus, the small plaque type (Medina and Sachs, 1960), which has greater chance of infecting the resistant cells, becomes selected.

Thus, for the polyoma virus, the hypothesis that the neoplastic condition of the cells is maintained by the presence in the cells of vegetative virus genomes which are able to give rise to mature virus particles can be excluded. Other experiments tend to exclude a more general form of the hypothesis, i.e., the presence of vegetative virus genomes which are unable to give rise to mature virus in the neoplastic cells but are able to do so in normal cells. These are experiments in which the DNA of the transformed cells was extracted by phenol and tested for infectivity. It is, in fact, known (DiMayorca *et al.*, 1959; Weil, 1961) that the DNA extracted either from the polyoma virus or from cultures infected by the virus is infectious. This infectivity can be demonstrated in tissue cultures by a plaque method, using a procedure which gives an efficiency of plating of about 10^{-4}, if referred to the titer in plague forming units (pfu) of the original preparation (Weil, 1961). Repeated experiments failed to demonstrate the presence of infectious DNA in the transformed cells.

The significance of these experiments is the following: since the particle-to-plaque ratio for polyoma virus is likely to be of the order of 10^3, the efficiency of plating for the viral DNA is of the order of 10^{-7}/molecule; the DNA tested in the reported experiments was extracted from about 5×10^8 cells, so that the experiments would have yielded at least 50 plaques if every cell contained at least one vegetative virus genome. Thus, the negative result is numerically significant.

Hypothesis 2(a) has also been tested, in a different way, by searching for polyoma virus antigen in the transformed cells. This was done by: (1) using a serum-blocking test based on neutralization, and (2) using fluorescein-labeled, antiviral rabbit gamma globulin, which had been exhaustively absorbed with normal homologous cells. The first test was negative at a level at which it could have demonstrated the equivalent of one infectious unit of virus in every 10 cells. The second test did not show any antigen able to react with the antiserum and having the nuclear localization characteristic of the virus; if one cell in 10^5 had had the nuclear antigen, it would have been observed. It should be noted that, in the test with fluorescent antibodies, one cannot give weight to the occasional presence of cytoplasmic granules which are able to react with the fluorescent antiviral gamma globulin (Sachs and Fogel, 1960) since these granules do not appear in cells recently infected by polyoma virus, nor do they appear in the transformed clonal cultures derived from mouse embryo cells when they are superinfected with polyoma virus. The significance of these cytoplasmic granules is undetermined.

The reported experiments tend, therefore, to exclude continuous presence of a vegetative genome as a requirement for the transformation caused by polyoma virus. Probably this conclusion does not apply to ribonucleic acid (RNA)-containing viruses, such as the Rous virus, since it has been shown that cells transformed by this virus transmit to the progeny the property of continued virus release (Temin and Rubin, 1959), at least under certain experimental conditions. However, clones of nonvirus-releasing transformed cells have been produced with the Rous virus by infection of chicken embryonic cells *in vitro* (Prince, 1960; Temin, personal communication), and it is not known whether the Rous virus is present in a vegetative state in the cells of these clones.

Hypothesis 2(b): The Existence of an Integrated Virus Genome in the Transformed Cells

On the basis of information derived from bacterial genetics, an integrated virus genome could be present in the transformed cells as provirus, i.e., in a state identical to that of prophage in lysogenic cells and having similar properties, or it could be present as an integral part of some cellular chromosomes, as consequence of incorporation.

Extensive experimentation was carried out to test whether the transformed cells contain a polyoma provirus, as defined above. These experiments were carried out with transformed cultures which were derived either from mouse or from hamster embryos and had become nonvirus releasers either spontaneously or after cloning. All the experiments, which will be described in some detail, gave negative results.

Many attempts were carried out to induce virus release in the transformed cultures by methods such as exposure to X rays, treatment with mitomycin, and treatment with aminopterin followed by thymidine, known to be effective in lysogenic bacteria. Furthermore, on the hypothesis that induction of virus release may depend on metabolic imbalance, the cells were also exposed to starvation procedures of various kinds, such as delaying fluid change or withdrawing a required factor, such as serum or an amino acid, from the medium; in other experiments the cells were exposed to azaguanine or to chloramphenicol. Another series of tests was based on the assumption that the increased resistance of the transformed cells to superinfection with polyoma virus is due to a mechanism similar to that causing immunity of lysogenic bacteria. Therefore, it was tested whether several of the above-mentioned inducing conditions would induce, in the cultures, an increased sensitivity to superinfection.

By taking advantage of the occurrence of two mutant types of polyoma virus differing in plaque size, both of which cause neoplastic transformation *in vitro*, experiments were carried out in an attempt to demonstrate the existence of the plaque size marker of the transforming virus in the transformed cells. Cells transformed with virus of one plaque type were superinfected with polyoma virus of the other type and the plaque marker of the transforming virus was looked for in the progeny. The experiments were carried out in the two possible combinations. Although these experiments are not exceedingly sensitive, the presence of 1 per cent of the minority plaque type could have been detected.

In consideration of the fact that the neoplastic transformation might be caused by noncytocidal mutants of polyoma virus, extracts of nonvirus-releasing transformed cultures were tested for their ability to cause the transformation of normal cultures.

The persistent negativity of all these experiments makes it unlikely that the genome of the polyoma virus is present in the transformed cells in a state equal to that of prophage in lysogenic bacteria. In fact, the transformed cells do not spontaneously release any virus, either of the cytocidal or of the transforming type, nor do they contain antigen that can be attributed to polyoma virus by its specificity or its localization in the cells. Furthermore, no virus release could be induced by treatments capable of causing the induction of virus release in lysogenic bacteria, either of the inducible type, by radiation, or of the noninducible type, by thymidine starvation (Melechen and Skaar, 1960).

The other form of Hypothesis 2(b), i.e., that the viral genome is present in the transformed cells as part of the cellular chromosomes, is much more difficult to test. To a certain extent, this hypothesis could be tested by experiments, such as those reported above, in which the presence of infectious polyoma virus DNA is looked for in the transformed cells. The sensitivity of this experiment is, however, much less in testing this hypothesis than in testing Hypothesis 2(a); in fact, the probability of successful penetration into the cell and of subsequent independent replication of a viral genome already incorporated in the cellular genome may be much smaller than that of the normal polyoma virus DNA. For this reason, the experiments of this type which have been carried out to date and have already been described may not be significant in relation to this hypothesis.

Hypothesis 4: Concerning the Role of Aneuploidization

Observations of infected hamster embryo cultures have shown that, if the cultures are maintained under optimal conditions for growth, the transformed cells, which are clearly recognizable on the basis of their morphology and growth behavior, are diploid at the early transfers; later, however, aneuploidization of the transformed cells takes place so that, when a culture is completely transformed, it is usually made up of a few clones of cells having a different type of aneuploidy (Bayreuther, personal communication). Thus, aneuploidization appears not to be the cause of the transformation, but a subsequent complication which we are, so far, unable to avoid.

The examination of the available evidence tends, therefore, to indicate that the neoplastic transformation caused by the DNA-containing polyoma virus takes place either because the genome of the virus, or part of it, becomes incorporated into the genome of the cells, or because the virus causes, by a direct or indirect mechanism, a permanent functional shift in some cellular function. The latter could occur in a system which is operating under steady state conditions with a great amount of feedback and able to assume different stable states, with a small probability of transition between these states under normal conditions.

The continued presence of the virus genome in a vegetative state in the cells may be a factor in the transformation caused by the RNA-containing Rous sarcoma virus and by other related viruses.

ACKNOWLEDGMENTS

The investigations on which this article is based were carried out under grants from the American Cancer Society, the National Foundation, and the United States Public Health Service.

REFERENCES

DiMayorca, G. A., B. E. Eddy, S. E. Stewart, W. S. Hunter, C. Friend, and A. Bendich. 1959. Isolation of Infectious Deoxyribonucleic Acid from SE Polyoma-Infected Tissue Cultures. *Proceedings of the National Academy of Sciences of the U.S.A.*, 45:1805–1808.

Dulbecco, R., and M. Vogt. 1960. Significance of Continued Virus Production in Tissue Cultures Rendered Neoplastic by Polyoma Virus. *Proceedings of the National Academy of Sciences of the U.S.A.*, 46:1617–1623.

Medina, M., and L. Sachs. 1960. The *in vitro* Formation of a Stable Association with Polyoma Virus. *Virology*, 10:387–388.

Melechen, N. E., and P. D. Skaar. 1960. Bacteriophage P1 Induction by Thymine Deprivation. *Federation Proceedings*, 19:410–411.

Prince, A. M. 1960. Quantitative Studies on Rous Sarcoma Virus. VI. Clonal Analysis of *in vitro* Infection. *Virology*, 11:400–424.

Sachs, L., and M. Fogel. 1960. Polyoma Virus Synthesis in Tumor Cells as Measured by the Fluorescent Antibody Technique. *Virology*, 11:722–736.

Smith, J. D., G. Freeman, M. Vogt, and R. Dulbecco. 1960. The Nucleic Acid of Polyoma Virus. *Virology*, 12:185–196.

Temin, H. M. Personal Communication.

Temin, H. M., and H. Rubin. 1959. A Kinetic Study of Infection of Chick Embryo Cells *in vitro* by Rous Sarcoma Virus. *Virology*, 8:209–222.

Vogt, M., and R. Dulbecco. 1960. Virus-Cell Interaction with a Tumor-Producing Virus. *Proceedings of the National Academy of Sciences of the U.S.A.*, 46:365–30.

Weil, R. 1961. A Quantitative Assay for a Subviral Infective Agent Related to Polyoma Virus. *Virology*, 14:46–53.

Weisberg, R. A. Personal Communication.

Certain Relationships Between the Shope Virus-Induced Arginase, the Virus, and the Tumor Cells

STANFIELD ROGERS, M.D.

The University of Tennessee Memorial Research Center and Hospital, Knoxville, Tennessee

For several years this laboratory has been engaged primarily in studies of the mechanism of action of various carcinogenic agents, principally chemical and radiation. Though such agents offer certain advantages in approaching the problem, it was determined to extend our efforts to the important tumors known to be caused by viruses. The extensive and precise work from the laboratories of both Shope and Rous on the biological properties of the Shope virus-induced papillomas of rabbit squamous epithelium provided the necessary background, making possible a definitive approach to the mechanism of action of the virus. It seemed likely that a study of the action of homogeneous cell populations derived from tumors induced by the virus and their normal and/or hyperplastic counterparts upon the constituents of a synthetic media might cast some light on the question of how, metabolically, the virus infection converted normal to neoplastic cells. Using the most readily available tissues of diverse types, both normal and neoplastic, a technique was worked out to compare the differences in metabolism of individual tissues *in vitro* (Rogers and Woodhall, 1958). A short term period of *in vitro* incubation rather than tissue culture was used, both because of its relative ease, and to avoid metabolic changes long known to occur in cells in culture.

The most critical problem in the study of the mechanism of action of a virus using this approach is the availability in a relatively pure state of the comparable normal or hyperplastic counterpart of the cells infected by the virus. With the Shope virus-induced papilloma, normal or squamous epithelium made hyperplastic through several treatments with a 50:50 mixture of turpentine and acetone may be readily obtained through shaving off the epithelium with a razor blade. By this means, one may get preparations containing less than 10 per cent contaminating tissues of other kinds, i.e., fibrous tissue and the necks of hair follicles. With the papillomas, this is much easier because of the greater thickness of the metabolically active squamous epithelium. The keratin is shaved off, discarded, and the underlying living epithelium then shaved off as above. The principal difference in the preparations is that the active synthesizing epithelium of the papilloma, judging from studies with tritiated thymidine, is up to eight cells thick in contrast to normal or hyperplastic skin which varies between one and three cells in thickness.

The tissue so prepared was cut into small fragments ranging from single cells and small cell clumps to occasional fragments approaching 0.25 mm. in diameter, rinsed in Ringer's solution, and incubated in Difco synthetic culture media 199 at 37°C in a Warburg apparatus for periods varying from two to 20 hours. With squamous cell tissue of the rabbit, the optimum incubation period is between six and eight hours. Following incubation, the cells and cell clumps are centrifuged out of the media, and are then studied chromatographically in search of changes produced by the tissue during the incubation interval.

In Table 1, a comparison of the effects of normal or hyperplastic skin and papilloma epithelium on the media following incubation, as described above, is shown. For the results shown in columns 2, 3, and 4, about 100 mg. of tissue were used in 3 cc. of media. In column 1, about 400 mg. of tissue and an incubation period of 20 rather than eight hours were used. This larger amount of tissue was used to better control a possible effect of the differences in thickness of the active cell layer as described above, and to accentuate the amount of any new products. Though there were a number of differences in the relative uptakes of the various amino acids, the only seemingly qualitative difference was in the influences on arginine. No detectable arginine was taken up by normal or hyperplastic squamous epithelium in these studies, in contrast to the papilloma which took up relatively large quantities and further excreted ornithine and urea which the normal counterpart did not

TABLE 1

The Amino Acid Uptakes of Hyperplastic Skin as Compared to Domestic and Wild Rabbit Papilloma Epithelium

Amino acids	DR hyperplastic skin uptake*	DR hyperplastic skin uptake*	DR papilloma uptake*	WR papilloma uptake*
	1	2	3	4
Aspartic acid	+ .0064	.0339	.1046	.0683
Threonine	+ .0070	.0280	.11835	.0180
Serine	+ .0106	.0170	.11064	.1132
Glutamic acid	+ .0159	.0450	.0780	.1430
Proline	.0069	.0636	.0051	.1680
Glycine	.0475	.0282	.1552	.1161
Alanine	+ .0223	.0243	.1301	.0485
Cystine	+ .0197	.0416	.0208	....
Valine	.0712	.0234	.0700	.1025
Methionine	.0044	.0372	.0167	.0230
Isoleucine	+ .0260	.0133	.0256	.0398
Leucine	.0014	.0320	.0530	.1282
Tyrosine	+ .0055	.0102	.0164	.0504
Phenylalanine	.0010	+ .0042	.0255	.0639
Glutamine	.1020	.1875	....	....
Lysine	+ .0220	+ .0934	.0378	....
Histidine	+ .0060	.0120	.0069	.0145
Arginine	+ .0218	+ .0320	.0140	.0622
Ornithine	None Present	None Present	+ .0143	.0563
Urea	None Present	None Present	+ .0884	....

* Indicates μmoles.
\+ Indicates increase.

do even when large amounts of tissue were used (column 1). The increases in the amounts of amino acids under this latter condition is related to cell breakdown and freeing of metabolic constituents.

In view of the discovery of arginase activity in the papillomas and not in normal or hyperplastic skin, it was decided to find whether arginase could be demonstrated in extracts of papilloma and in extracts of normal and hyperplastic skin. The enzyme was extracted, concentrated, and tested by standard methods outlined elsewhere (Cohn, Surgenor, and Hunter, 1951). For the results shown in Table 2, an extract from papilloma was made from 3 Gm. of tissue, and the extract from normal and hyperplastic skin from 15 Gm. of rabbit epithelium. Though the papilloma extract contained marked arginase activity, none was demonstrable in the extract of normal and hyperplastic squamous epithelium. These tests were run in parallel, using both wild and domestic rabbit systems. The wild cottontail rabbits were procured from Earl Johnson of Rago, Kansas. Both papillomas from rabbits infected in the field and those infected in the laboratory yielded the same results.

TABLE 2

Comparative Arginase Activity of Extracts of Papilloma and of Normal and Hyperplastic Skin

	Arginine remaining after incubation period		Ornithine after incubation
	15 minutes	20 hours	
Papilloma extract	5.5%	0%	++++
Skin extract	120%†	117%†	0
Buffer plus arginine	100%*	100%	0

† Increase due to small amount of arginine present in concentrated dialysate.
* Equivalent to 0.07 mg. arginine/cc.

As a number of enzymes have in the past been found associated with various "purified" viruses, it was necessary to find whether the arginase activity was directly associated with the virus particulates. The virus was isolated using the method of Beard, Ryan, and Wyckoff (1939). In such preparations, at most only traces of enzyme activity have been detectable, and in view of the large amount of virus used, up to 1.2 mg. of virus protein nitrogen/cc., the arginase present must be viewed as a contaminant rather than as an intrinsic attribute of the virus.

On further comparison (Table 1) of the relative amounts of arginine taken up and the amounts of ornithine and urea excreted by the cells, the disparity in the amount of urea released was disturbing, as it was greatly in excess of what would be expected. In an effort to cast light on this difference, the medium was made up with C^{14} labeled arginine, using both the uniformly labeled (Schwartz Laboratories) and the guanidino labeled (Calif. Corp. Bio. Res., Pasadena, California). The results are shown in Table 3. Here it is evident that with the exception of 15 to 20 per cent of the original arginine in the medium, all the urea and ornithine can be accounted for. This deficiency in total count is a reflection upon the

TABLE 3

Proportion Ornithine and Urea When Using C^{14} Labeled Arginine in Media

	Arginine count at start	Arginine count after incubation	Ornithine count after incubation	Urea count after incubation	Extracellular total
Exp. 1*	1134	708	114	36	888
Exp. 2*	1134	448	224	83	755
Exp. 3†	270	175	. . .	36	211
Exp. 4†	270	199	. . .	22	221

* Schwartz uniformly labeled.
† California Corp. Bio. Res. guanidino labeled.

passage of arginine through the cells and not yet excreted as ornithine and urea. The most likely source of the excess urea is from the degradation of the deoxyribonucleic acid (DNA) in the nucleus during the process of keratinization, as neither papilloma nor normal skin keratin contains histochemically demonstrable DNA Feulgen reaction (Figure 1).

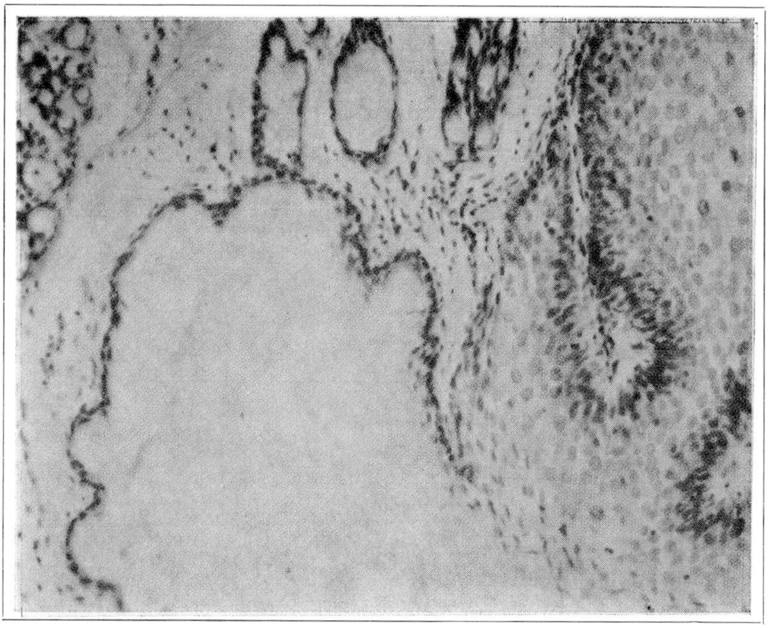

FIG. 1. Normal skin and papilloma Feulgen reaction showing relative amounts of nuclear DNA.

It is evident from these results that the Shope virus infection of epithelial cells is somehow inducing an arginase in cells of a sort which contain no detectable arginase in their normal or hyperplastic state (Rogers, 1959). In the hope of casting light on the means of induction of the enzyme, it was determined to find whether the virus-induced enzyme was antigenic in the rabbits carrying the induced papillomas. It was expected that, should the synthesis of the enzyme be directed from information derived from the virus chromosomal complement, it might well be antigenic in the rabbits carrying their own papillomas, while if it were a rabbit enzyme already present in very small quantities not detectable by the above techniques, or whose synthesis was repressed in the normal cell and released following infection with the virus, it would not be. In view of the antigenicity of the virus protein, it was obviously necessary to use a more purified enzyme than that used above, which was the dialyzed and lyophilized enzyme from the 19 per cent alcohol extraction shown in Table 4. The additional means of

TABLE 4

Arginase Purification

Papilloma	⟶	extract (30% alcohol, −9°C)	⟶	sediment	⟶	extract (19% alcohol, −5°C)	⟶	dialyzed & lypholized ↓
Carboxy-methyl column pH 5 ↓	⟵	D and L	⟵	Sephadex G 75 column	⟵	D and L	⟵	DEAE column pH 8
D and L	⟶	arginase						

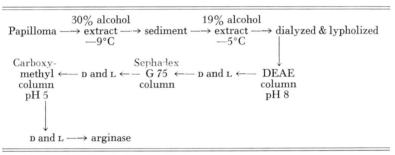

enzyme purification was a modification of the protein purification system devised by Anderson and Bond. The "purified" enzyme used in the precipitin tests shown in the accompanying tables was principally obtained after passage through the diethylaminoethyl (DEAE) cellulose column, though more recently strong precipitins have been obtained with the more highly purified arginase, acting as a single peak in the analytical centrifuge, and having an $S^0_{20,w}$ of 3.8×10^{-13} after passage through the carboxymethyl cellulose column. In these precipitin tests a 1:1 dilution of serum and a 0.05 mg./cc. arginase preparation were used. Positive precipitins have been observed with as little as 0.01 mg. arginase/cc. In each instance these were checked individually for arginase activity of the supernate following centrifugation to remove the precipitate. The added papilloma arginase activity of the supernate of the sera from animals with papillomas and yielding a precipitin has uniformly been reduced following centrifugation. This reduction in enzyme activity has not occurred following incubation of the serum from normal rabbits with papilloma arginase, even in the occasional instances in which a fine precipitin has been seen (Table 5). The

TABLE 5

Antigen DR Arginase Cohn Extraction

Serum	Precipitin	Serum	Precipitin
DR-N	0	DR-P	+
DR-N	0	DR-P	+
DR-N	0	DR-P	+
DR-N	0	DR-P	+
DR-N	0	DR-P	0
DR-N	TR	DR-P	+
DR-N	0	DR-P	+
DR-N	+		

DR-N, normal rabbit serum.
DR-P, serum of papilloma rabbits.

reduction in arginase activity in the sera from rabbits carrying papillomas following the precipitin has varied individually from 30 to 80 per cent. The averages from several pooled sera, normal and immune, are shown in Chart 1. The animals whose sera are shown in Table 5 and Chart 1 were all domestic rabbits and the arginase used was derived from domestic rabbit papillomas. The seven domestic rabbits carrying papillomas (Table 5) had their

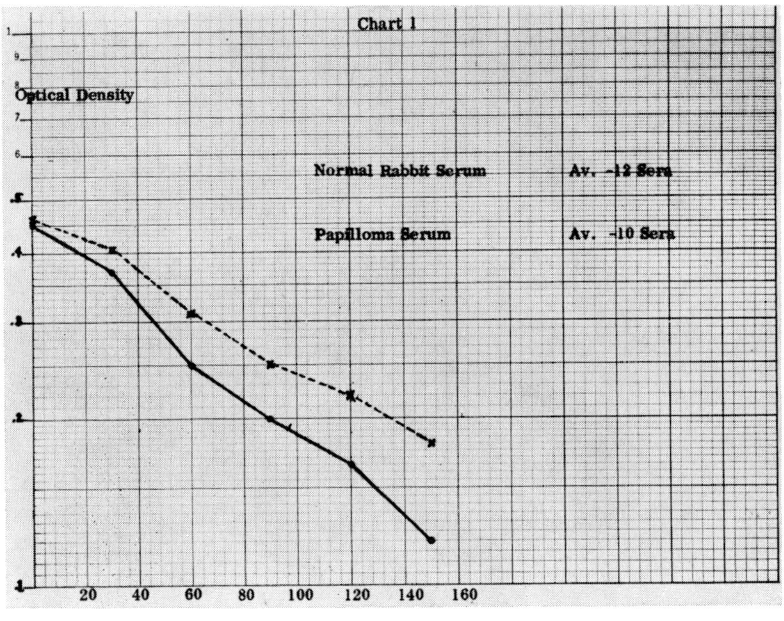

CHART 1. The relative arginase activity after incubation with immune serum and normal rabbit serum. X = Papilloma serum, ● = Normal serum.

sera tested against the arginase derived from their own individual tumors.

It was next determined to find whether there would be a cross reaction between domestic and wild rabbit serum from rabbits carrying papillomas with arginase derived from tumors caused by the virus in the other species, and, further, to find whether the precipitin which can be obtained by incubating immune sera with domestic rabbit liver arginase to which 0.5 mg./cc. of purified papilloma virus had been added, would be associated with a relative loss of arginase from the supernate. The results of such an experiment are shown in Table 6. It is evident that the immune bodies developed by either domestic or wild rabbits carrying papillomas against the arginase of their own papillomas cross-react with the

TABLE 6

Cross Reaction Between Domestic Rabbit and Wild Rabbit Papilloma Arginase

Serum	Antigen	Precipitin	Arginase activity in supernate %
WR-196-N	DRA	0	100
WR-198-N	DRA	0	100
WR-203-N	DRA	0	100
WR-156-P	DRA	+	60
WR-166-P	DRA	+	20
WR-236-P	DRA	+	50
WR-200-N	LAV	0	100
WR-201-N	LAV	TR	100
WR-167-P	LAV	+	100
WR-155-P	LAV	+	100
DR-243-N	WRA	TR	100
DR-242-N	WRA	0	100
DR-237-N	WRA	+	100
DR-239-P	WRA	TR	20
DR-237-P	WRA	+	50
DR-248-P	WRA	+	40
DR-242-N	LAV	TR	100
DR-237-N	LAV	0	100
DR-235-P	LAV	0	100
DR-236-P	LAV	+	100
DR-238-P	LAV	+	100

LAV—DR liver arginase plus concentrated virus; DRA—DR papilloma arginase "purified"; WRA—WR papilloma arginase "purified"; WR—Wild rabbit. DR—Domestic rabbit; N—Normal serum, and P—Immune serum.

arginase derived from the other species. The principal immunologic constant in this system is the presence of the virus-induced tumors in both kinds of rabbit. As it has been long known from the work of Kidd that animals carrying the virus-induced papillomas have antibodies against the virus, it was expected that with this high concentration of antigen (virus) a precipitin would be observed in the liver arginase-virus antigen-immune serum system. However, this precipitin after centrifugation was not associated with a reduction of liver arginase activity in the supernate. It was known from previous experiments that no precipitin occurs when immune sera and liver arginase are incubated and, further, that there is no reduction of enzyme activity in the supernate following centrifugation. In an effort to better characterize the immunologic reaction occurring, "purified" papilloma arginase eluted from the carboxymethyl cellulose column was incubated with an immune serum, the precipitated material centrifuged out at 5,000 rpm for 15 minutes, and the serum before and after incubation studied in the analytical centrifuge. Rather interestingly, a quantitative change was noted in the amount of macroglobulin in the serum after incubation with the arginase. The macroglobulin with an $S^0_{20,w}$ of about 18×10^{-13} was reduced by an estimated one third. However, as the original amount of this macroglobulin in the serum of normal rabbits was just as great as in animals carrying the papilloma, no specificity for this diminution is likely. Such a diminution in the amount of this protein was not observed when normal sera were incubated with papilloma arginase. However, with immune sera, the globulin could be nonspecifically absorbed on the preciptin.

One of the greatest problems in interpreting the above data is the absence of similar studies on enzymes induced by chemical means. Will, for example, an animal's immunologic system be able to recognize that a chemically induced enzyme not previously overtly present is its own, or will the animal respond as though it is a foreign protein, irrespective of whether it was synthesized from its own chromosomal information? However, on the basis of what we know currently, this antigenic evidence provides strong support for the interpretation that the information for the synthesis of the arginase in Shope virus-induced papillomas is derived from the virus chromosomal complement rather than from the rabbit. Particularly noteworthy in this relation is the cross-reaction between the immune sera of wild and domestic rabbits and papilloma arginase of the other species, and without a cross-reaction of either with liver arginase of either species.

There are certain other differences between rabbit liver and papilloma arginase. One of these is shown in the inability to elute an enzymatically active liver arginase from the carboxymethyl cellulose column at pH 5, while this may readily be done with papilloma arginase. This finding has made difficult the interpretation of the finding that liver arginase has an $S^0_{20,w}$ of about 5.5×10^{-13} in comparison with the 3.8×10^{-13} for papilloma arginase of either wild or domestic rabbits. As the papilloma arginase is "purer," having been through an additional purification procedure, we are not yet certain whether the liver arginase as well might perhaps be broken down into smaller parts retaining enzyme activity. It is certainly noteworthy, however, that using a chemical extraction system, Greenberg reported a sedimentation velocity for horse liver arginase of 5.9×10^{-13}, though some activity was found in a lighter component. In any event, it is not yet certain whether the operative

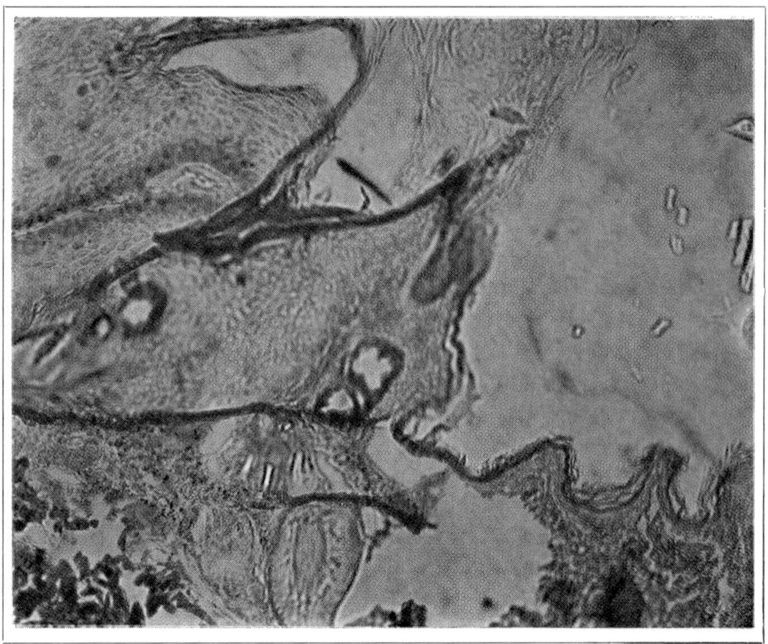

FIG. 2. Normal skin and papilloma, Fast Green, showing marked depletion of nuclear histone in papilloma nuclei of cells undermining normal skin, the nuclei and keratin of which stain much more densely.

papilloma arginase has an $S^0_{20,w}$ of 3.7 or 5.5×10^{-13} the latter of which is that of rabbit liver arginase after Sephadex G-75.

Perhaps more interesting from the point of view of the mechanism of action of the virus is a possible effect on the growth rate of squamous epithelial cells of having a high level of arginase. Allfrey and Mirsky (1958) have reported an inverse relation between the amount of nuclear histone (an arginine-rich protein) and nuclear synthetic activity. Because of these pertinent findings relating to growth control mechanisms, it seemed worthwhile to make a histochemical study of the papillomas to find roughly the relative amount of DNA and nuclear histone. In Figure 1, the relative amount of DNA in normal skin and papilloma nuclei is shown by the Feulgen reaction. The relative staining intensity of the nuclei of these same cells stained specifically for histone with Fast Green (Alfert and Geschwind, 1953) is shown in Figure 2. It is evident that the relative amount of nuclear histone in papilloma nuclei is greatly reduced. Another interesting difference concerns the keratin which,

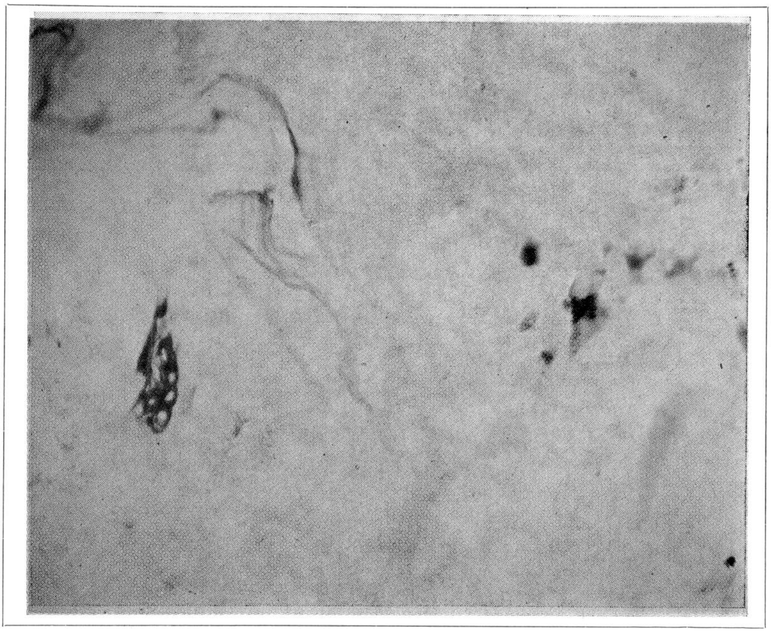

FIG. 3. Normal skin and papilloma, Fast Green, showing histone-positive straining of keratin of normal skin and absence of staining of papilloma keratin.

as mentioned earlier, does not stain with the Feulgen reaction, indicating a prior degradation of the nuclear DNA. The keratin of normal skin stains densely with this histone specific substance, while the keratin of adjoining papilloma stains little to not at all. This is best shown in Figure 3, where, at the staining intensity used, the skin keratin stains brightly but without any staining of papilloma keratin. This finding supports and extends that of the greatly reduced amount of histone-staining material in papilloma squamous epithelium nuclei as compared with normal skin. The nuclear histones, being arginine-rich, may be stained by another histochemical procedure utilizing the Saguchi reaction. This method confirmed the findings with Fast Green, but because of rapid fading is not readily reproducible photographically. These findings rather remarkedly fit what would be expected, should the growth controlling mechanism upset by the virus in causing the neoplastic state be on the order of that found in Allfrey and Mirsky's (1958) work relating to the balance between DNA and histone as determining nuclear activity.

Is the action of the Shope virus, then, principally to induce arginase, an enzyme to which rabbit squamous epithelial cell growth-controlling mechanisms are not keyed, which in turn reduces available cellular arginine, and which, in turn, diminishes the synthesis of arginine-rich nuclear histones, freeing the DNA of the chromosomes for greater synthetic activity and cellular growth-yielding the papilloma?

ACKNOWLEDGMENTS

This work was supported by the Jane Coffin Childs Fund and Grant C-5176 from the United States Public Health Service; technical assistance was given by Billy Gaines Mann, Janet Patterson, and Robert Long.

The author is indebted to Norman Anderson, H. E. Bond, and Robert Canning of the Biology Division of the Oak Ridge National Laboratory, and A. E. Mirsky of the Rockefeller Institute for suggestions and advice concerning certain technical procedures used.

REFERENCES

Alfert, M., and I. I. Geschwind. 1953. A Selective Staining Method for the Basic Proteins of Cell Nuclei. *Proceedings of the National Academy of Sciences of the U.S.A.*, 39:991–999.

Allfrey, V., and A. E. Mirsky. 1958. Some DNA-Dependent Synthetic Systems of Isolated Cell Nuclei. *Transactions of the New York Academy of Sciences*, 21:3–16.

Anderson, N., and H. E. Bond. Personal Communication.

Beard, J. W., W. R. Ryan, and R. W. Wyckoff. 1939. The Isolation of the Rabbit Papilloma Virus Protein. *Journal of Infectious Diseases*, 65:43–52.

Cohn, E. J., D. M. Surgenor, and M. J. Hunter. 1951. *Enzymes and Enzyme Systems*. J. T. Edasall, Ed., 107 pp. Cambridge, Massachusetts: Harvard University Press.

Greenberg, D. M. 1955. *Methods in Enzymology*, S. P. Colowick and N. O. Kaplan, Eds., Vol. 2, p. 368. New York, New York: Academic Press, Inc.

Kidd, J. G. 1937. A Complement-Fixation Reaction Involving the Rabbit Papilloma Virus (Shope). *Proceedings of the Society for Experimental Biology and Medicine*, 35:612–614.

Rogers, S., and B. Woodhall. 1958 Rapid Method of Metabolically Characterizing Individual Tumors. *Proceedings of the Society for Experimental Biology and Medicine*, 98:874–877.

———. 1959. Induction of Arginase in Rabbit Epithelium by the Shope Rabbit Papilloma Virus. *Nature, London*, 183:1815–1816.

Studies with the Fluorochrome Acridine Orange on the Nucleic Acids of Some Purified Viruses

HEATHER DONALD MAYOR, PH.D.

Department of Virology and Epidemiology,
Baylor University College of Medicine,
Houston, Texas

The ability to see, measure, and count the actual elementary bodies of viruses is, from a biophysical standpoint, a fundamental and necessary property for their identification and quantitative correlation with their biological effects. Although some of the large viruses such as vaccinia can be identified under the light microscope with suitable staining, and the filamentous forms of influenza virus are readily visible by dark field illumination, in general it is necessary to employ electron microscopy to detect and measure the size and shape of most virus particles. With the acridine orange cytochemical technique for staining nucleic acids developed independently by Armstrong (1956) and von Bertalanffy and Bickis (1956), ribonucleic acid (RNA)-containing organisms fluoresce a brilliant flame red, while deoxyribonucleic acid (DNA)-containing ones develop a brilliant greenish-yellow color. Using this versatile technique, Anderson, Armstrong, and Niven (1959) were able to identify in the fluorescence microscope individual heads of T_2 bacteriophage particles. As the DNA content of T_2 bacteriophage is about 2×10^{-10} μg./particle (Hershey, 1953), this finding represents a high degree of sensitivity for detection of DNA by staining methods. Anderson, Armstrong, and Niven (1959) were unable to detect individual RNA virus particles and considered that their identification was beyond the limit of sensitivity of the technique.

Recently a number of experimenters have become interested in the incorporation of vital dyes into developing virus particles (Schaffer, 1960; Crowther and Melnick, 1961; Mayor, 1961), and it is obvious here too that the use of the fluorochrome acridine orange as the vital dye presents an intriguing possibility for visualizing individual virus particles by virtue of their vitally stained nucleic acids. I will report some experiments along these lines with poliovirus, tobacco mosaic virus (TMV), and ϕx 174. The experiments with poliovirus and TMV were carried out in collaboration with Mr. A. R. Diwan, those with ϕx 174 with Mr. N. O. Hill.

When stained with 0.01 per cent acridine orange (AO) at pH 4.0 Carnoy-fixed smears of purified RNA virus concentrates such as poliovirus or tobacco mosaic virus fluoresce a brilliant flame red in blue-violet light. Prior treatment with ribonuclease completely inhibits the development of the red fluorescence. By contrast, the typical color developed by a DNA virus (e.g., adenovirus), whether concentrated smear or intracellular aggregate, is a brilliant greenish-yellow. Prior treatment with a proteolytic enzyme in addition to deoxyribonuclease is necessary to inhibit the development of this specific yellow fluorescence for most DNA animal viruses. When poliovirus is carefully grown in the dark in the presence of acridine orange in high dilution (0.0005 per cent) and examined without any fixation or staining at all, we observe a brilliant apple green fluorescence. There is no significant drop in virus titer. Under these conditions (i.e., unstained preparation), poliovirus and tobacco mosaic, grown under standard conditions without the dye, exhibit no fluorescence whatever. We conclude that acridine orange has actually been incorporated into the developing virus particle and we can see this incorporation directly in the fluorescence microscope. After fixation and treatment with ribonuclease, the green color is no longer evident and this is strong evidence that the acridine orange dye is actually incorporated into the nucleic acid moiety of the virus. This effect is not destroyed by proteolytic enzymes, and incubation of similar preparations in the vehicle for the nuclease has no effect. These results are summarized in Table 1.

Stained preparations of RNA viruses such as TMV or polio are brilliant red, while poliovirus grown in the presence of the fluorochrome displays a brilliant apple green fluorescence. Why is this? It is known that basic dyes, such as acridine orange, are bound to nucleic acids by ionic bonds to the phosphate groups and possibly

TABLE 1

Effect of Acridine Orange on Fluorescence of Virus Particles in Blue-Violet Light

Stain	Poliovirus		TMV		AO-Poliovirus*	
	Unfixed	Fixed	Unfixed	Fixed	Unfixed	Fixed
None	No Fluorescence	No Fluorescence	No Fluorescence	No Fluorescence	Brilliant Apple Green	Brilliant Apple Green
0.01% AO	Faint Green	Brilliant Flame Red	Brilliant Apple Green	Brilliant Flame Red	Brilliant Apple Green	Brilliant Flame Red
0.001% AO	Faint Green	Brilliant Apple Green	Brilliant Apple Green	Brilliant Apple Green	Brilliant Apple Green	Brilliant Apple Green

* Grown in the presence of 0.0005 per cent acridine orange.

by weaker van der Waal's forces brought about by proximity to the sugar surfaces of the nucleic acid molecules where this is sterically possible.

Also, when considering the incorporation of acridine orange into the maturing poliovirus particle, the concentration of the dye in the medium becomes an important consideration. Schümmelfeder (1958) has shown for fixed tissue that at high concentration of the dye (0.05 per cent), cells demonstrate in all parts a change from green → yellow → orange → red with rising pH. With sufficiently low concentrations (0.01 per cent), the cytoplasm (RNA) alone shows a change to red; the nucleus (DNA) remains yellow even at high pH. The bright green fluorescence of our incorporated concentrates with an RNA virus obviously indicates a low dye concentration.

We can also conclude that the steric configuration of the RNA molecule makes it possible for larger quantities of the fluorochrome to become attached during the staining process leading to the development of red fluorescence, while the DNA molecule is only capable under standard conditions of binding sufficient dye to yield yellow fluorescence.

When the virus concentrates were stained with 0.01 per cent acridine orange according to the standard procedure, the following results were obtained. Fixed preparations of poliovirus yielded the brilliant flame red fluorescence characteristic of RNA, unfixed preparations yielded the very faintest green indicating either a little surface binding of the strongly positively charged fluorochrome to the protein of the unfixed virus surface, or limited penetration of the virus particle by the dye. Fixed preparations of TMV again showed brilliant red RNA staining, while unfixed preparations, when allowed to remain in contact with the dye solution for some hours, showed a brilliant green fluorescence identical to that of the unstained AO-poliovirus. This result would appear to indicate that, in contrast to poliovirus, the TMV particle is permeable to the acridine orange fluorochrome in the unfixed state and that a sufficient concentration of the dye is able to build up with time within the particle to develop a brilliant green fluorescence. The brilliant green color exhibited by the vitally stained AO-poliovirus was not altered by subsequent staining with 0.01 per cent acridine orange in the unfixed state. This would be the expected result if the mature unfixed poliovirus particle could not be penetrated by the fluorochrome, as we believe to be the case. However, the fixed and subsequently stained AO-poliovirus concentrates exhibited again the brilliant flame red RNA fluorescence as would be expected. These results are summarized in Table 1.

With a lower concentration (0.001 per cent), of fluorochrome as stain, it was impossible to develop the characteristic red RNA color found under standard staining conditions (0.01 per cent AO, pH 4.0) even in fixed preparations of all three viruses. This concentration effect of the dye when used as a stain is of particular interest when one considers the optimal conditions for growth of AO-poliovirus *in vitro* involve a concentration of fluorochrome as low as 0.005 per cent. At this dye concentration, it is impossible to grow mature, infective AO-poliovirus particles exhibiting a typical red RNA fluorescence.

As concentrations of acridine orange in excess of 0.003 per cent were highly toxic to tissue culture cells even in the dark, our experiments were carried out in very dilute dye solutions (0.0005 per cent), and even if all this dye found its way onto the polynucleotide chain of the developing virus particle, we would still be dealing with minute quantities of dye incapable of giving a typical red RNA color even in large aggregates of close-packed particles. Also from purely physical considerations, it is unlikely that the developing poliovirus particle could incorporate sufficient dye to exhibit other than a green fluorescence, as the larger quantities of dye necessary to yield red fluorescence would preclude the formation of mature infective virus particles due to the impossibility of forming a protein coat around acridine orange-RNA molecular aggregates of such size. This can be compared with our results with TMV, a virus which is definitely permeable to acridine orange. However, the completely unfixed virus particle with protein coat intact is only penetrable by sufficient dye to develop a brilliant green fluorescence.

Recently, there has been growing interest in a group of small bacterial viruses, of which ϕx 174 is a member. Hall, MacLean, and Tessman (1959) examined the virus particles in the electron microscope and found tailless particles of 248 Å diameter with polygonal outlines consistent with icosahedral point symmetry characteristic of many of the so-called "spherical" small plant and animal viruses. Tessman (1959) studied the inactivation of the virus by decay of incorporated radioactive P^{32} atoms, and obtained 10 times the efficiency of inactivation observed with other phage. He considered that this indicated an unusual and accessible DNA for the virus, possibly a single-stranded form. Sinsheimer (1959a,b) has carried out extensive physical and chemical studies on highly purified preparations of the virus particle and its DNA. The DNA reacted rapidly with formaldehyde, exhibited high flexibility in light-scattering experiments and lacked a complementary nucleotide structure. These findings, and Sinsheimer's additional kinetic studies of the degradation process with pancreatic deoxyribonuclease, were all consistent with the existence of a single-chain polymer. Our results with AO staining of purified TMV and poliovirus led to the conclusion that, under conditions of controlled pH (pH 4.0 with acridine orange), it is not a fundamental property of the DNA or RNA molecules themselves which is involved in the staining reaction which causes the yellow-green or brilliant red fluorescence characteristic of each nucleic acid, but rather the dye concentration and the steric configuration of the molecules. These conclusions stimulated some experiments with purified concentrates of ϕx 174, and we were very fortunate to receive a generous supply of concentrated purified virus from Dr. Sinsheimer. Dried and fixed droplet preparations of this material fluoresced a brilliant flame red in blue-violet light.

This result is usually considered to be consistent with the identification of RNA material (cf., polio concentrate). However, the ability of our ϕx 174 preparations to develop this red fluorescence was completely destroyed by prior treatment of fixed preparations with deoxyribonuclease (DNase). In contrast, identical preparations were completely insusceptible to digestion with ribonuclease (RNase). Incubation of specimens in the vehicles for the nucleases alone had no effect on the development of flame red fluorescence. The staining properties of fixed preparations of ϕx 174 differ from

TABLE 2

Results of Various Workers Using the Acridine Orange Technique to Visualize Viruses

Fixed virus preparation	Color developed after acridine orange staining	Nuclease susceptibility: DNase	RNase	Prior proteolytic enzyme treatment required
RNA animal viruses (1,3,4,6)	flame red	—	+	—
DNA bacteriophage (1)	yellow-green	+	—	—
DNA animal viruses (2,3)	yellow-green	+	—	+
Φx 174	flame red	+	—	—

(1) Anderson, Armstrong, and Niven, 1959; (2) Armstrong and Hopper, 1959; (3) Armstrong and Niven, 1957; (4) Epstein and Holt, 1958; (5) Mayor, 1961; (6) Mayor and Diwan, 1961.

those of any other virus previously studied by this method. Our results, together with those of some other workers, are summarized in Table 2.

It is not necessary to subject preparations of ϕx 174 to treatment with a proteolytic enzyme for the DNA to become susceptible to DNase. This is in agreement with the behavior of large bacterial viruses (Table 2), and in contrast to that of the DNA-containing animal viruses (Table 2), where a close association between the nucleic acid of the virion core and the protein capsid appears to exist. The flame red fluorescence developed by ϕx 174 suggests a molecular configuration of its nucleic acid similar to that of RNA, namely a single-stranded DNA. I have stressed the importance of the steric arrangement of the DNA and RNA molecules and suggested that in the case of RNA there would be significantly more possible points for attachment of the acridine orange molecules leading to the development of red fluorescence. Similar steric possibilities obviously exist in the case of the DNA of ϕx 174. It would appear from our results that the AO technique controlled by suitable nuclease digestion tests is a simple and direct method for detecting DNA in the single-stranded form.

At the cellular level of viral reproduction, the recent work of Setlow and Setlow (1960) using ultraviolet action spectra provides evidence that the double-stranded DNA of phage T_2 undergoes a single-stranded stage during replication in *Escherichia coli*; we are at present carrying out cytochemical studies in the Adeno 3 virus-monkey kidney cell system in hopes of detecting a single-stranded stage during the development of this virus using this simple technique.

ACKNOWLEDGMENT

This work was aided by Grant C-4600 from the National Cancer Institute, National Institutes of Health, United States Public Health Service.

REFERENCES

Anderson, E. S., J. A. Armstrong, and J. S. F. Niven. 1959. Fluorescence Microscopy: Observation of Virus Growth with Aminoacridines. *Symposia of the Society for General Microbiology*, 9:224–255.

Armstrong, J. A. 1956. Histochemical Differentiation of Nucleic Acids by Means of Induced Fluorescence. *Experimental Cell Research*, 11:640–643.

Armstrong, J. A., and P. K. Hopper. 1959. Fluorescence and Phase-Contrast Microscopy of Human Cell Cultures Infected with Adenovirus. *Experimental Cell Research*, 16:584–594.

Armstrong, J. A., and J. S. F. Niven. 1957. Fluorescence Microscopy in the Study of Nucleic Acids. *Nature, London*, 180:1335–1336.

Crowther, D., and J. L. Melnick. 1961. The Incorporation of Neutral Red and Acridine Orange into Developing Poliovirus Particles Making Them Photosensitive. *Virology*, 14:11–21.

Epstein, M. A., and S. J. Holt. 1958. Observations on the Rous Virus, Integranted Electron Microscopical and Cytochemical Studies of Fluorocarbon Purified Preparations. *The British Journal of Cancer*, 12:363–396.

Hall, C. E., E. C. MacLean, and I. Tessman. 1959. Structure and Dimensions of Bacteriophage ϕx 174 from Electron Microscopy. *Journal of Molecular Biology*, 1:192–194.

Hershey, A. D. 1953. Nucleic Acid Economy in Bacteria Infected with Bacteriophage T_2. II. Phage Precursor Nucleic Acid. *Journal of General Physiology*, 37:1–23.

Mayor, H. D. 1961. Cytochemical and Fluorescent Antibody Studies on the Growth of Poliovirus in Tissue Culture. *Texas Reports on Biology and Medicine*, 19:106–122.

Mayor, H. D., and A. R. Diwan. 1961. Studies on the Acridine Orange Staining of Two Purified RNA Viruses: Poliovirus and Tobacco Mosaic Virus. *Virology*, 14:74–82.

Schaffer, F. L. 1960. The Nature of Noninfectious Particles Produced by Poliovirus Infected Tissue Cultures Treated with Proflavin. *Federation Proceedings*, 19:405.

Schaffer, F. L., and C. E. Schwerdt. 1955. Studies on the Nucleic Acid Composition of Purified Preparations of Poliomyelitis Virus. *Federation Proceedings*, 14:275.

Schümmelfeder, N. 1958. Histochemical Significance of the Polychromatic Fluorescence Induced in Tissues Stained with Acridine Orange. *The Journal of Histochemistry and Cytochemistry*, 6:392.

Setlow, J. K., and R. B. Setlow. 1960. Evidence for the Existence of a Single-Stranded Stage of T_2 Bacteriophage During Replication. *Proceedings of the National Academy of Sciences of the U.S.A.*, 46:791–798.

Sinsheimer, R. L. 1959a. Purification and Properties of Bacteriophage $\phi\chi$ 174. *Journal of Molecular Biology*, 1:37–42.

———. 1959b. A Single-Stranded Deoxyribonucleic Acid from Bacteriophage $\phi\chi$ 174. *Journal of Molecular Biology*, 1:43–53.

Tessman, I. 1959. Some Unusual Properties of the Nucleic Acid in Bacteriophage S 13 and $\phi\chi$ 174. *Virology*, 7:263–275.

von Bertalanffy, L., and I. Bickis. 1956. Identification of Cytoplasmic Basophilia (Ribonucleic Acid) by Fluorescence Microscopy. *The Journal of Histochemistry and Cytochemistry*, 4:481–491.

RIBOSOMES AND PROTEIN SYNTHESIS

Structure of *Escherichia coli* Ribosomes and Incorporation of Amino Acids

A. Tissières, Ph.D., M.D.

Biological Laboratories, Harvard University,
Cambridge, Massachusetts

Electron micrographs of thin sections of bacteria show that the cytoplasm is filled with particles about 200 Å in diameter (Ryter, Kellenberger, Birch-Anderson and Maaløe, 1958; Chapman, 1959). These particles are seen in *Escherichia coli* lysates (Luria, Delbrück, and Anderson, 1943); they contain most of the ribonucleic acid (RNA) of the cells, form sharp boundaries in the analytical centrifuge and are found in all the bacterial species examined (Schachman, Pardee, and Stanier, 1952). They are similar to the ribonucleoprotein particles which have been studied by physical methods in mouse spleen extracts (Petermann and Hamilton, 1952), and a number of different mammalian and avian cells studied by electron microscopy (Palade, 1955; Palade and Siekevitz, 1956). While in animal tissues, they are often attached to the endoplasmic reticulum and can be isolated only by dissolving the membranes with deoxycholate, the particles are free in bacterial extracts.

These particles, or ribosomes, contain over 80 per cent of the total RNA of the cell. Like the amount of RNA (Schaechter, Maaløe, and Kjeldgaard, 1958), the number of particles varies inversely with the generation time: in *E. coli* dividing every 20 minutes, there are about 90,000 ribosomes/cell, which account for more than 30 per cent of the dry weight of the organism (Tissières, Watson, Schlessinger, and Hollingworth, 1959). With longer generation times, the number of ribosomes decreases severalfold (Mendelsohn and Tissières, 1959).

General Properties of the Ribosomes

Magnesium stabilizes ribosomes from yeast (Chao, 1957), plants (Ts'o, Bonner, and Vinograd, 1956, 1958), and *E. coli* (Bolton, Hoyer, and Ritter, 1958; Tissières and Watson, 1958). In cell-free extracts of *E. coli* prepared by grinding with alumina and extracting with tris buffer containing magnesium ions, there are four kinds of ribosomes characterized by their sedimentation constants of 30 S, 50 S, 70 S and 100 S. At low magnesium concentrations, 30 S and 50 S particles only are present. On raising the level of magnesium, one 30 S combines with one 50 S to form a 70 S particle; at still higher magnesium concentrations, two 70 S aggregate in a 100 S ribosome. This is summarized by the following equation:

$$2(30\ \mathrm{S}) + 2(50\ \mathrm{S}) \leftrightarrows 2(70\ \mathrm{S}) \rightleftarrows 1(100\ \mathrm{S})$$
$$\xrightarrow{\text{increasing } Mg^{++}}$$

The four kinds of ribosomes appear to have approximately the same density and the same chemical composition; they all contain about 63 per cent RNA and 37 per cent protein (Tissières, Watson, Schlessinger, and Hollingworth, 1959).

The molecular weights derived from physical measurements are given in Table 1. The results agree reasonably well, whether they were calculated from sedimentation and diffusion coefficients, or from sedimentation and viscosity data, with the exception perhaps of the molecular weight of the 30 S ribosomes, which was definitely higher when calculated from viscosity data. It is of interest that the

TABLE 1

Molecular Weights of Escherichia coli *Ribosomes*

Sedimentation constant	Molecular weights: From sedimentation and diffusion coefficients	Molecular weights: From viscosity data and sedimentation coefficients
30 S	$0.7 \times 10^6 \pm 8\%$	$1.0 \times 10^6 \pm 16\%$
50 S	$1.8 \times 10^6 \pm 4\%$	$1.8 \times 10^6 \pm 16\%$
70 S	$2.6 \times 10^6 \pm 6\%$	$3.1 \times 10^6 \pm 18\%$
100 S	....	$5.9 \times 10^6 \pm 20\%$

(After Tissières, Watson, Schlessinger, and Hollingworth, 1959)

viscosity of the 30 S particles was found to be higher than that of the others, including 100 S; this is probably because of their asymmetric shape, described below.

A clear picture of the shapes and dimensions of the various kinds of ribosomes has now been obtained on electron micrographs (Hall and Slayter, 1959; Huxley and Zubay, 1960): the isolated 50 S particles appear to be uniform, nearly spherical, with dimensions of 140 Å by 170 Å; the 30 S particles are asymmetric and can be represented by a prolate ellipsoid 95 Å by 170 Å. Sometimes they are irregular in shape which might reflect their instability during the preparations of the samples. The 70 S particles are clearly made up of one 30 S and one 50 S subunit, between which a marked cleft is visible. The 100 S ribosome consists of two 70 S particles in which the two 30 S subunits are bound together.

Ribosomal RNA

Two RNA components, with sedimentation coefficients of 15 S to 18 S and 23 S to 32 S, have been obtained by treating ribosomes from various sources with phenol or detergent (Timasheff, Brown, Colter, and Davies, 1958; Littauer and Eisenberg, 1959; Hall and Doty, 1959).

Starting from isolated 30 S and 50 S *E. coli* ribosomes, the RNA was prepared using phenol or detergent (Kurland, 1960). With either method, one single RNA component, with a sedimentation coefficient of about 16 S, was obtained from 30 S preparations, while the 50 S particles yielded two components of 16 S and 23 S in variable proportions. The molecular weights of the 16 S and 23 S components, calculated by a combination of light-scattering, viscosity, and sedimentation measurements, were found to be 0.56 and 1.1×10^6, respectively. It is therefore likely that the 30 S ribosome, with a molecular weight of about 0.8×10^6, contains one 16 S RNA, while the 50 S ribosomes, of molecular weight 1.8×10^6, carry either two 16 S or one 23 S RNA components. The 23 S RNA is probably made up of two 16 S units. The molecular weight of the 16 S RNA being half that of the 23 S, and the density and chemical composition of the different kinds of ribosomes being similar, it is likely that 30 S ribosomes are just one half of the 50 S ones. The following observations indicate, however, that the 50 S ribosomes are not formed simply by the aggregation of two 30 S: the aggregation of two 30 S particles and the breakdown of one 50 S into two 30 S has not yet been reported. Furthermore, 30 S and 50 S particles differ in several ways, as, for example, the presence of ribonuclease exclusively in the 30 S particles (Elson and Tal, 1959; Spahr and Hollingworth, 1961).

Following the observation of large, quite stable RNA molecules, the question arose as to whether they were formed of subunits. On heating to 50° to 90°C, or on standing at room temperature at about pH 7.0, the RNA is degraded and forms boundaries in the analytical centrifuge with continuously decreasing sedimentation constants. This problem has been studied recently in detail by Möller (personal communication). He noted that 16 S and 23 S RNA's remained quite stable under two conditions known to inhibit ribonuclease, i.e., low pH and the presence of magnesium ions. He also observed that when 16 S and 23 S RNA's were degraded, the sedimentation constants of the breakdown products were quite variable and there was no indication, from the shape of the boundaries, that the sedimenting material was homogeneous. He concluded, therefore, that the various breakdown products which had been observed might well have been caused by the action of contaminating ribonuclease.

It seems that the problem of the existence of subunits will remain unsolved until (1) the presence of ribonuclease can be ruled out, and (2) a stable breakdown product from the original RNA components is isolated and studied extensively by physical-chemical methods.

The nucleotide composition of the four principal nucleotides has been investigated in 30 S, 50 S, and 70 S ribosome preparations (Bolton *et al.*, 1959; Spahr and Tissières, 1959). The first group of authors, on the basis of small differences found, concluded that the RNA composition in the 30 S was different from that in the 50 S ribosomes. The second group concluded that, within the limits of error, the nucleotide composition was the same in all particles with the exception of cytidylic acid. It can be said, therefore, that the nucleotide composition of the RNA of the 30 S, 50 S, and 70 S ribosomes is very similar, with possibly some very small differences.

The study of the hypochromic effect and simultaneous change in optical rotation with isolated RNA from tobacco mosaic virus led Doty *et al.*, (1959) to conclude that a substantial part of the molecule consists of hydrogen-bonded bases, organized in helical regions. It was therefore of importance to know whether the same degree of secondary structure exists when RNA is bound to proteins in the ribosomes. Indeed, a hypochromic effect was shown with rat liver ribonucleoprotein particles (Hall and Doty, 1959), and it was found that the hypochromicity of *E. coli* ribosomes was identical to that of their isolated RNA (Schlessinger, 1960). This suggests that the secondary structure of RNA in solution is similar to that existing when RNA is bound to proteins in the ribosomes.

Ribosomal Protein

The amino acid composition of the protein from 30 S, 50 S, and 70 S ribosomes has been determined by Spahr (personal communication). The results for the three kinds of particles are similar, with possibly some small differences.

It appears from the work of Waller and Harris (1961) that the ribosomal protein is not formed by a random sample of cellular proteins, but, on the contrary, by a class of basic proteins contributing to the structure of the ribosomes. The study of the NH_2 terminal groups indicated the presence of two major end groups, methionine and alanine, which accounted for about 85 per cent of the total end groups. The remaining amino ends were found to consist of small amounts of serine, threonine, aspartic, and glutamic acids. Thus, the structural protein chains of the ribosomes are mainly of two kinds: those with methionine as NH_2 terminal residue, and those with alanine, and the average molecular weight of the proteins was found to be 25,000. The results of starch gel electrophoresis and ion-exchange chromatography led to the conclusion that, in each of the two major protein classes, not all chains were chemically identical. The end group analysis for the protein from isolated 30 S, 50 S, and 70 S showed essentially the same picture.

In conclusion, the proteins from the ribosomes are formed of, mainly, two classes of basic proteins with methionine and alanine as amino end groups, thus resembling calf thymus histones, where alanine and proline account for over 90 per cent of the end groups (Phillips and Johns, 1959).

Amino Acid Incorporation Into Proteins By *E. coli* Ribosomes

It was shown recently that ribosomes are involved in the synthesis of proteins in *E. coli; in vivo*, radioactive sulphur was found to be incorporated first into ribosomal proteins and then it could be chased from there by cold sulphur to other proteins of the cell (McQuillen, Roberts, and Britten, 1959). *In vitro*, a system containing ribosomes and soluble factors was reported, in which amino acids were incorporated into particles and soluble proteins (Lamborg and Zamecnik, 1960). I shall now discuss some of the properties of a similar *in vitro* system (Tissières, Schlessinger, and Gros, 1960).

The cell-free extract, from *E. coli*, strain B, growing exponentially in broth, was made by grinding the cells with alumina and extracting with three times the wet weight of the cells with 0.005 M tris buffer, pH 7.4, containing 0.01 M Mg^{++}. The supernatant, after two centrifugations at 8,000 × g for 15 minutes to remove the alumina, intact cells and most cell debris, is referred to as crude extract. It consists of the bulk of the RNA of the cells in the form of ribosomes with about 15 per cent of soluble, or low molecular weight, RNA; soluble enzymes and soluble factors; and less than 5 per cent of the total dry weight of the extract of cell debris, probably deriving from cell membranes and cell walls. (Tissières, 1961).

The crude extract incorporated amino acids with the requirements shown in Table 2. These are essentially the same as those of the liver system (Zamecnik and Keller, 1954; Keller and Zamecnik, 1956).

TABLE 2

*Incorporation of C^{14}-Alanine into Crude Extract, Supernatant, and Ribosome Fractions**

	d.p.m.	d.p.m./mg. dry weight
Crude extract (0.5 ml., 3 mg. ribosomes)	8,300	1,080
Crude extract without ATP, PEP, and PK	100	13
Crude extract without PEP and PK	139	18
Crude extract with 1×10^{-4} M Mg^{++}	116	15
Supernatant (0.1 ml.)	41	51
Ribosomes (3.2 mg.)	423	132
Ribosomes (3.2 mg.) + supernatant (0.1 ml.)	2,900	725

* The complete reaction mixture consisted of 1 μmole adenosine triphosphate (ATP), 5 μmole phosphoenol pyruvate (PEP), 40 μg. pyruvate kinase (PK), 0.022 M KCl, 0.01 M magnesium acetate, 1 μmole C^{14}-alanine (3×10^5 d.p.m.), and the cell fraction in a total volume of 0.85 ml. Incubation at 37°C for 45 minutes; radioactivity measured in precipitate from hot trichloroacetic acid.

Abbreviation: d.p.m., disintegration per minute.

(After Tissières, Schlessinger, and Gros, 1960)

The activity of the system was very sensitive to the concentration of magnesium. Thus with 0.001 M Mg^{++}, it was only about 7 per cent of its maximal value which was obtained at a magnesium concentration varying between 0.007 M and 0.011 M with different preparations. When calcium or manganese was used in place of magnesium, the activity was only about 10 per cent of that observed with magnesium.

The crude extract can be fractionated by high speed centrifugation into ribosomes, which sediment in two hours at 100,000 × g, and the supernatant, containing soluble proteins and other soluble factors. Each of these two fractions, which separately had little activity, could effectively be recombined to yield an active system (Table 2).

The study of the time course of amino acid incorporation showed that the rate of the reaction dropped quickly, and after about four minutes, half the maximum level of incorporation already had been achieved. The curve came to a plateau at about 45 minutes. The soluble proteins became labeled during the reaction and, in general, they were found to contain about 30 per cent of the radioactivity present in the ribosomes.

We believe that the system is composed of ribosomes and soluble factors: when a crude extract is centrifuged, for example, for 40 minutes at 30,000 × g, the specific activity of the supernatant, either on a protein or on a dry weight basis, goes up; the small pellet formed consists mostly of cell membrane and cell wall debris, as it was found to contain most of the cytochrome originally present in the crude extract. This pellet, washed with tris magnesium buffer by centrifugation, incorporates amino acids with an activity no greater than a small percentage of that of the crude extract. This kind of experiment shows clearly that the system is composed of ribosomes and soluble factors, and that debris of cell membranes and cell walls are not active.

That the incorporation of amino acids into hot trichloroacetic acid precipitable material is related to the synthesis of protein is shown by the following evidence:

1. Under conditions when the amino acid pool is small (e.g., bacteria cultivated in a synthetic medium supplemented with amino acids), the incorporation of one single amino acid is increased severalfold by the addition of a mixture of 0.2 μmoles of each of the other 17 amino acids.

2. It was found that each of the 18 common amino acids were incorporated in somewhat comparable amounts.

3. After the incorporation, *in vitro*, of a complete mixture of C^{14} amino acids, the crude extract was centrifuged in order to sediment the ribosomes, and the soluble proteins were chromatographed on a modified diethylaminoethyl (DEAE) cellulose column and eluted with a gradient of NaCl. The elution pattern (Figure 1) showed that the curve obtained for the radioactivity fol-

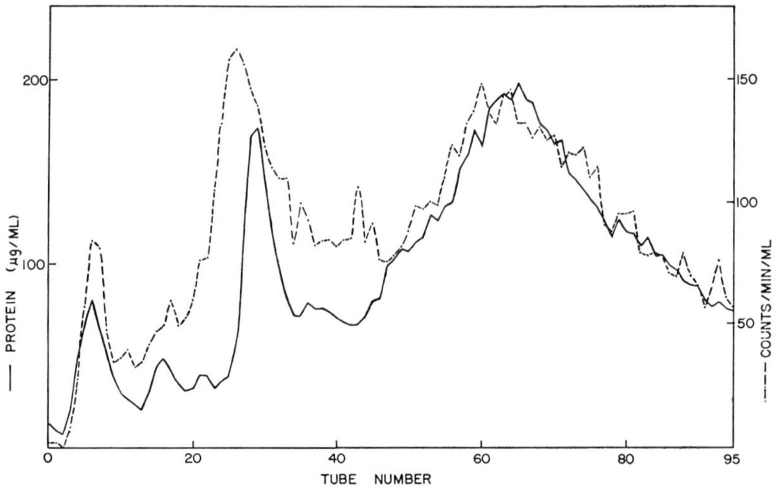

FIG. 1. Elution pattern of *E. coli* soluble proteins by NaCl gradient from diethylaminoethyl (DEAE) cellulose column (0.005 M tris, pH 7.3), 2.5 ml./collected fraction. The column had a diameter of 1 cm. and a height of 20 cm. (After Tissières, Schlessinger, and Gros, 1960.)

lowed roughly that of the protein content. These results indicated that the soluble proteins which are labeled *in vitro* represent essentially the spectrum of the soluble proteins of the cell.

The incorporation of amino acids at the level of the individual ribosomes was analyzed by the sucrose gradient technique of McQuillen, Roberts, and Britten (1959). The incorporation of a complete mixture of labeled amino acids took place *in vitro* in 0.01 M Mg^{++} in duplicate samples. At the end of the reaction, 1 μg./ml. deoxyribonuclease (DNase) was added to each sample. Sample 1 was then dialyzed against 0.005 M tris buffer, pH 7.3, and 0.01 M Mg^{++} to remove the free labeled amino acids, while sample 2 was dialyzed against 0.01 M phosphate buffer, pH 7.0, with only 0.0005 M Mg^{++}, a mixture in which 70 S ribosomes break down to 30 S and 50 S. Of each sample 1 ml. was layered on the top of a sucrose gradient in a centrifuge tube. It was then centrifuged in the SW25 rotor of the Model L Spinco centrifuge for 2.5 hours at 50,000 × g. A pinhole was made at the bottom of the centrifuge tube and drops were collected for measuring the optical density at 260 mμ and the radioactivity.

The results obtained with sample 1 (Figure 2) show that the curve of radioactivity follows closely that of the optical density in the ultraviolet region; the labeled amino acids were about equally distributed among the four classes of ribosomes. With sample 2 (Figure 3), the curve of the optical density shows that most of the 70 S and 100 S particles which were visible on the ultraviolet curve in Figure 2 have been broken down to 50 S and 30 S. However, the curve representing the radioactivity does not follow the same pattern; most of the counts present in the 70 S and 100 S fractions in Figure 2 have remained with the 70 S peak and, during the breakdown of 100 S and 70 S into 50 S and 30 S particles, very few counts, if any, have been transferred to the 50 S and 30 S fractions.

Thus, a small proportion of the 70 S originally present in the preparation, estimated at 5 to 10 per cent, is highly labeled, and is stable upon removal of Mg^{++}. The specific activity of this stable 70 S fraction, called active 70 S, was estimated to be 15 to 40 times higher than that of the 30 S or 50 S. The active 70 S ribosomes are present in the cell-free extract when the incorporation reaction starts, and are neither formed nor broken down in the system.

When the crude extract has been incubated with 1 to 5 μg. DNase

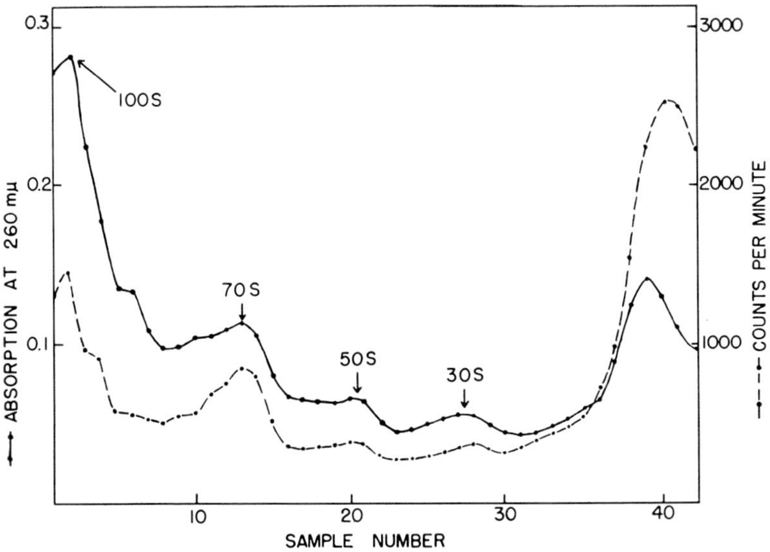

FIG. 2. Analysis of the incorporation of amino acids into crude extract by the sucrose gradient technique. After the reaction, the sample was dialyzed against tris 0.01 M Mg^{++} buffer to remove free labeled amino acids. (After Tissières, Schlessinger, and Gros, 1960.)

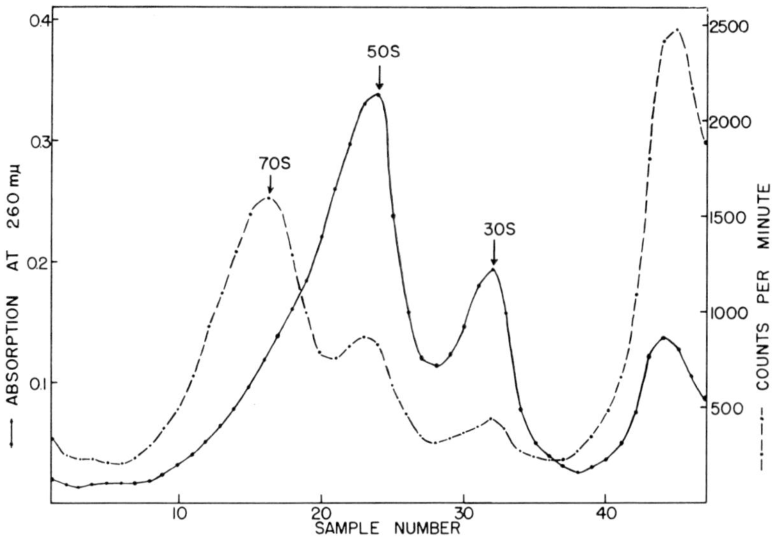

FIG. 3. Analysis of the incorporation of amino acids into crude extract by the sucrose gradient technique. After the reaction the sample was dialyzed against 0.01 M phosphate buffer, pH 7.0, containing 0.0005 M Mg^{++}, a mixture in which 70 S ribosomes break down to 30 S and 50 S. (After Tissières, Schlessinger, and Gros, 1960.)

for 10 to 15 minutes at room temperature prior to the reaction, the amino acid incorporation is lowered by 50 to 80 per cent. The degree of inhibition varies from one preparation to another, and with the same crude extract, the inhibition obtained by incubation with 10 or 20 μg. of the enzyme/ml. is no greater than that following incubation with 1 to 5 μg. Thus, the per cent of inhibition does not seem to depend upon the amount of the enzyme used, within those limits. This appears to rule out the possibility that the inhibition is due to small amounts of ribonuclease (RNase) contaminating the DNase, as RNase (less than 0.1 μg./ml.) inhibits the system completely in a very short time. In all cases, a substantial fraction of the activity, sometimes as high as 50 per cent, is retained after incubation with DNase. This indicates that one part of the system is sensitive to this enzyme, while the other one is not. Whether DNase inhibits the system by destroying the integrity of deoxyribonucleic acid (DNA) remains unclear.

REFERENCES

Bolton, E. T., R. J. Britten, D. B. Cowie, B. J. McCarthy, K. McQuillen, and R. B. Roberts. 1959. Annual Reports, Carnegie Institution of Washington. p. 259.

Bolton, E. T., W. H. Hoyer, and D. B. Ritter. 1958. Stability of Microsomal Particles of *E. coli.* (Abstract) Biophysical Society Meeting, Massachusetts Institute of Technology, Cambridge, Massachusetts.

Chao, F. C. 1957. Dissociation of Macromolecular Ribonucleoprotein of Yeast. *Archives of Biochemistry and Biophysics*, 70:426–431.

Chapman, G. B. 1959. Electron Microscopy of Ultrathin Sections of Bacteria. III. Cell Wall, Cytoplasmic Membrane, and Nuclear Material. *Journal of Bacteriology*, 78:96–104.

Doty, P., H. Boedtker, J. R. Fresco, R. Haselkorn, and M. Litt. 1959. Secondary Structure in Ribonucleic Acids. *Proceedings of the National Academy of Sciences of the U.S.A.*, 45:482–499.

Elson, D., and M. Tal. 1959. Biochemical Differences in Ribonucleoproteins. *Biochimica et biophysica acta*, 36:281–282.

Hall, B. D., and P. Doty. 1959. The Preparation and Physical Chemical Properties of Ribonucleic Acid from Microsomal Particles. *Journal of Molecular Biology*, 1:111–126.

Hall, C. E., and H. S. Slayter. 1959. Electron Microscopy of Ribonucleoprotein Particles from *E. coli. Journal of Molecular Biology*, 1:329–332.

Huxley, H. E., and G. Zubay. 1960. Electron Microscope Observations on the Structure of Microsomal Particles from *Escherichia coli. Journal of Molecular Biology*, 2:10–18.

Keller, E. B., and P. G. Zamecnik. 1956. The Effect of Guanosine Diphosphate and Triphosphate on the Incorporation of Labeled Amino Acids into Proteins. *Journal of Biological Chemistry*, 221:45–59.

Kurland, C. G. 1960. Molecular Characterization of Ribonucleic Acid from *Escherichia coli* Ribosomes. I. Isolation and Molecular Weights. *Journal of Molecular Biology*, 2:83–91.

Lamborg, M. R., and P. C. Zamecnik. 1960. Amino Acid Incorporation into Protein by Extracts of *E. coli. Biochimica et biophysica acta*, 42:206–211.

Littauer, U. Z., and H. Eisenberg. 1959. Ribonucleic Acids from *Escherichia coli. Biochimica et biophysica acta*, 32:320–336.

Luria, S. E., M. Delbrück, and T. F. Anderson. 1943. Electron Microscope Studies of Bacterial Viruses. *Journal of Bacteriology*, 46:57–78.

McQuillen, K., R. B. Roberts, and R. J. Britten. 1959. Synthesis of Nascent Protein by Ribosomes in *Escherichia coli. Proceedings of the National Academy of Sciences of the U.S.A.*, 45:1437–1447.

Mendelsohn, J., and A. Tissières. 1959. Variations in the Amount of Ribonucleprotein Particles in *Escherichia coli. Biochimica et biophysica acta*, 35: 248–250.

Möller, V. Personal Communication.

Palade, G. E. 1955. A Small Particulate Component of the Cytoplasm. *The Journal of Biophysical and Biochemical Cytology*, 1:59–68.

Palade, G. E., and P. Siekevitz. 1956. Liver Microsomes. *The Journal of Biophysical and Biochemical Cytology*, 2:171–198.

Petermann, M. L., and M. G. Hamilton. 1952. An Ultracentrifugal Analysis of the Macromolecular Particles of Normal and Leukemic Mouse Spleen. *Cancer Research*, 12:373–378.

Phillips, D. M. P., and E. W. Johns. 1959. A Study of the Proteinase Content and the Chromatography of Thymus Histones. *Biochemical Journal*, 72:538–544.

Ryter, A., E. Kellenberger, A. Birch-Anderson, and O. Maaløe. 1958. Etude au microscope eléctronique des plasmas contenant de l'acide désoxyribonucléique. *Zeitschrift für Naturforschung*, 13b:597–605.

Schachman, H. K., A. B. Pardee, and R. Y. Stanier. 1952. Studies on the Macromolecular Organization of Microbial Cells. *Archives of Biochemistry*, 38:245–260.

Schaechter, M., O. Maaløe, and N. O. Kjeldgaard. 1958. Dependency on Medium and Temperature of Cell Size and Chemical Composition during Balanced Growth of *Salmonella typhimurium*. *Journal of General Microbiology*, 19:592–606.

Schlessinger, D. 1960. Hypochromicity in Ribosomes from *Escherichia coli*. *Journal of Molecular Biology*, 2:92–95.

Spahr, P. F. Personal Communication.

Spahr, P. F., and B. R. Hollingworth. 1961. Purification and Mechanism of Action of Ribonuclease from *Escherichia coli* Ribosomes. *Journal of Biological Chemistry*, 236:823–831.

Spahr, P. F., and A. Tissières. 1959. Nucleotide Composition of Ribonucleoprotein Particles from *Escherichia coli*. *Journal of Molecular Biology*, 1:237–239.

Timasheff, S. N., R. A. Brown, J. S. Colter, and M. Davies. 1958. The Molecular Weight of Ribonucleic Acid Prepared from Ascites-Tumor Cells. *Biochimica et biophysica acta*, 27:662–663.

Tissières, A. 1961. "The Location of Cytochromes in *Escherichia coli*," *Proceedings of the Haematin Enzyme Symposium* (Canberra), J. E. Falk, M. R. Lemberg, and R. K. Morton, Eds., London, England: Pergamon Press.

Tissières, A., D. Schlessinger, and F. Gros. 1960. Amino Acid Incorporation into Proteins by *Escherichia coli* Ribosomes. *Proceedings of the National Academy of Sciences of the U.S.A.*, 46:1450–1463.

Tissières, A., and J. D. Watson. 1958. Ribonucleoprotein Particles from *Escherichia coli*. *Nature, London*, 182:778–780.

Tissières, A., J. D. Watson, D. Schlessinger, and B. R. Hollingworth. 1959. Ribonucleoprotein Particles from *Escherichia coli*. *Journal of Molecular Biology*, 1:221–233.

Ts'o, P. O. P., J. Bonner, and J. Vinograd. 1956. Microsomal Nucleoprotein Particles from Pea Seedlings. *The Journal of Biophysical and Biochemical Cytology*, 2:451–466.

———. 1958. Structure and Properties of Microsomal Nucleoprotein Particles from Pea Seedlings. *Biochimica et biophysica acta*, 30:570–582.

Waller, J. P., and J. I. Harris. 1961. Studies on the Composition of the Protein from *Escherichia coli* Ribosomes. *Proceedings of the National Academy of Sciences of the U.S.A.*, 47:18–23.

Zamecnik, P. C., and E. B. Keller. 1954. Relation Between Phosphate Energy Donors and Incorporation of Labeled Amino Acids into Proteins. *Journal of Biological Chemistry*, 209:337–354.

Enzyme Induction and Ribosome Synthesis

RICHARD B. ROBERTS, PH.D.

Department of Terrestrial Magnetism,
Carnegie Institution of Washington, Washington, D.C.

During the first two days of this symposium, we have heard that there is a satisfying theory, amply supported by experimental results, which accounts for the precision of deoxyribonucleic acid (DNA) replication. We have also learned that DNA exercises an indirect control over the production of protein, i.e., that an alteration of the base sequence in DNA results in an alteration in the amino acid sequence of a protein. However, DNA does not seem to be directly involved in the synthesis of protein; the machinery for this process seems to be located in the ribosomes which are ribonucleoprotein. After Doctor Tissières' paper, I see no reason to refer to the experimental evidence (Borsook *et al.*, 1950; Littlefield, Keller, Gross, and Zamecnik, 1955; McQuillen, Roberts, and Britten, 1959) that ribosomes are the principal sites of protein synthesis in living cells.

The process which I wish to present is somewhat less explored. It is the transfer of information from DNA to the ribosomes:

$$\begin{array}{l} \text{DNA} \longrightarrow \text{Ribosome} \longrightarrow \text{Protein} \\ \;\;\downarrow \\ \text{DNA} \end{array}$$

At first sight, this process seems obvious. The DNA must direct the synthesis of ribonucleic acid (RNA). This, in turn, acts as the template for synthesis of the protein. This concept is supported by the work of Caro and Forro who found that the newly synthesized RNA was localized in the same region of the cell as was DNA (Caro and Forro, in press). Hall and Spiegelman (in press) have observed the *in vitro* formation of specific hybrids of DNA and RNA and have found similar hybrids *in vivo*. Also, there is much discussion about the enzymatic synthesis of RNA, directed by DNA, being carried out in cell-free systems.

There seems little doubt that these concepts will develop as essentially correct, but there are a number of uncertainties and difficulties at present. Nature is not very inventive and once having found one mechanism, it is used repeatedly. Hence, we might anticipate that base pairing, which provides a method for replicating DNA, would also be used to transfer information to RNA. Accordingly, it is disturbing to find no apparent relationship between the base composition of the DNA and that of the ribosomal RNA. Furthermore, cells which have widely different base ratios in their DNA's show much smaller differences in their RNA's and in their amino acid compositions. The average frequency of occurrence of symbols in the code seems to have little to do with the meaning of the message.

Perhaps a large fraction of the DNA is nonfunctional. *Escherichia coli* cells contain roughly 5,000,000 DNA nucleotide pairs/cell. Thus a sequence of 800,000 amino acids could be specified if six nucleotide pairs are needed per amino acid. Such a sequence could provide 1,000 different enzyme species of 800 amino acids each. If, however, the enzymes were formed by joining together different combinations of smaller polypeptides, the DNA would be present in excess. Perhaps 100 different types of polypeptide strands, each consisting of 200 amino acids, would suffice. Then only 3 per cent of the DNA would be needed.

Alternatively, a large part of the ribosome RNA might be structural and not related to the base composition of the DNA. The RNA of the 70 S ribosome can be broken down into roughly 48 4 S units of approximately 100 nucleotides each (Aronson and McCarthy, 1961). Six of these units, at least, would be needed to carry the information for a polypeptide of 200 amino acids. Therefore, at least one eighth, and more probably one quarter, of the RNA of an active ribosome should be template material bearing some relation in its base composition to that of the DNA. This type of RNA might be separable from the rest of the RNA, either by chromatography or by density gradient centrifugation, but no defined template RNA has yet been detected by these techniques. Most probably these areas of confusion arise from our present lack of understanding of the template and its coding.

One way to study the template and its formation is to correlate changes in enzyme-forming capacity during induction with the processes of ribosome synthesis.

Enzyme Induction

Boezi and Cowie (in press) have recently observed the kinetics of induction of β-galactosidase in *Escherichia coli* at early times. Their data show that the quality of enzyme formed after addition of the inducer increases as shown in Figure 1, the induced rating being about 200 times the uninduced rate.

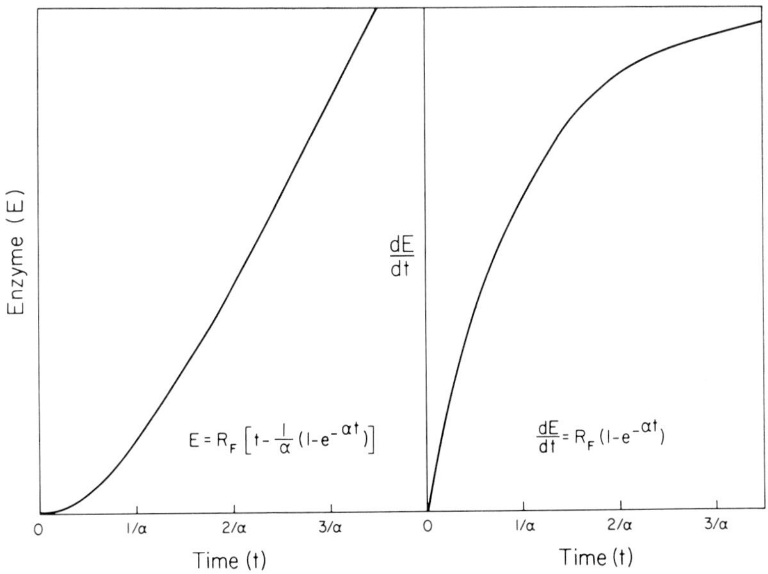

Fig. 1. The course of enzyme induction at early times after adding the inducer thiomethyl galactoside (TMG) 5×10^{-3}M). $1/\alpha = 150$ seconds. $\frac{dE}{dt}$ = rate of enzyme formation.

The rate of enzyme formation $\left(\frac{dE}{dt}\right)$ is, of course, equal to the number of enzyme-forming units (N) divided by the average time required for the synthesis of an enzyme molecule (T_S):

$$\frac{dE}{dt} = \frac{N}{T_S}$$

There is no direct way of showing whether N increases or T_S decreases, or both, during induction. We can, however, make an order of magnitude estimate by using other data.

A small portion of the enzyme activity of the cell is associated with 70 S ribsomes; presumably, this is due to newly formed enzyme which still adheres to the template (Figure 2). This ribosome-associated enzyme increases tenfold after induction (Cowie, Spiegelman, Roberts, and Duerksen, 1961.

Unfortunately, the enzyme activity associated with ribosomes is not a direct measure of the number of ribosomes engaged in the synthesis of the enzyme; at least two other factors are involved:

$$E_r = NPA$$

where E_r is the enzyme activity associated with ribosomes, N is the number of ribosomes synthesizing the enzyme, P is the probability of finding active enzyme on the ribosome, and A is the relative enzymic activity of the enzyme when attached to a ribosome.

Also P may be expressed as:

$$P = \frac{T_p}{T_s} = \frac{T_p}{T_a + T_p}$$

where T_p is the time required to strip the newly formed active enzyme from the template, T_a is the time for accumulation and polymerization of the amino acids, and T_s is the average time required for synthesis of an enzyme molecule.

The relationship of induced cells (i) to uninduced cells (u), can then be expressed:

$$\frac{\left(\frac{dE}{dt}\right)^i}{\left(\frac{dE}{dt}\right)^u} = 200 = \frac{N^i/T_s{}^i}{N^u/T_s{}^u}$$

and

$$\frac{E_r{}^i}{E_r{}^u} = 10 = \frac{N^i \dfrac{T_p{}^i}{T_a{}^i + T_p{}^i} A^i}{N^u \dfrac{T_p{}^u}{T_a{}^u + T_p{}^u} A^u}$$

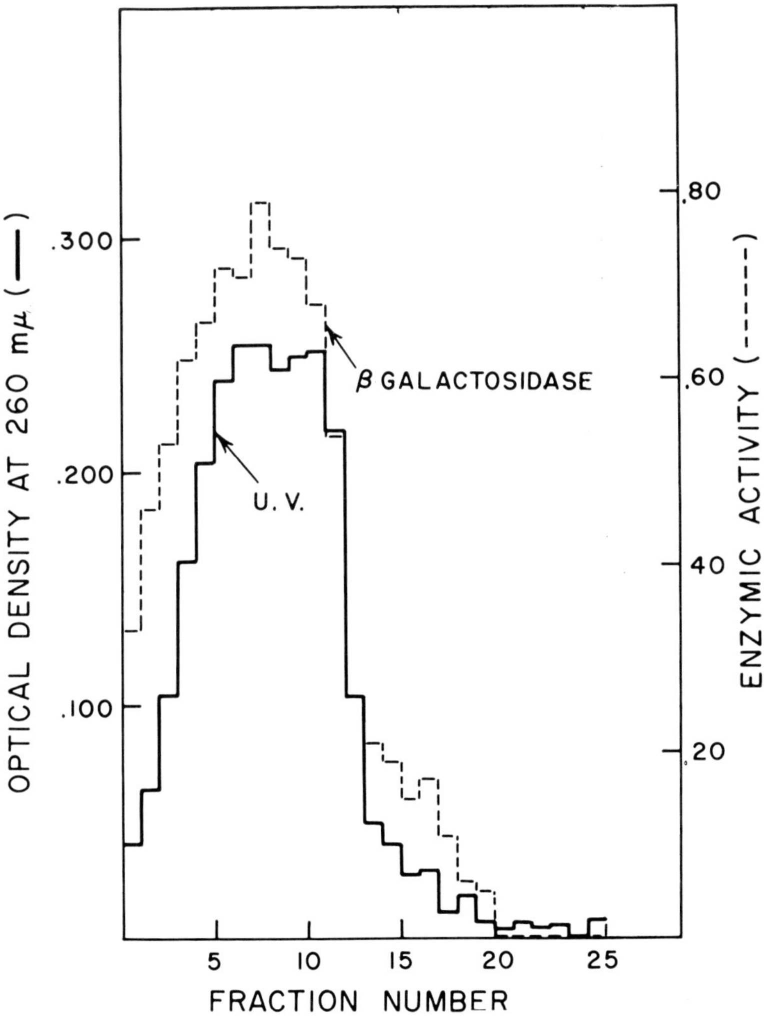

FIG. 2. A small fraction of the β-galactosidase is associated with ribosomes, as shown by the correlation of its sedimentation coefficient with that of ribosomes.

Although these equations contain too many unknowns to be solved, they do give some insight into the induction process. For example:

$$\frac{T_p{}^i}{T_p{}^u} \times \frac{A^i}{A^u} = \frac{1}{20}$$

Since $A^i \lesseqgtr A^u$ (ribosomes from uninduced cells show an equal or greater increase in enzymic activity when treated with antibody than do ribosomes from induced cells), then $T_p^u \lesseqgtr 20T_p^i$, indicating that the inducer expedites the removal of newly formed enzyme from the template.

Under these conditions of induction, β-galactosidase accounts for ~ 2 per cent of the cell protein and its absolute rate of synthesis is 3,000 amino acid molecules polymerized/cell/second. Taking 1,000 amino acids as the length of the polypetide chain synthesized, then

$$\frac{N^i}{T_s^i} = 3/\text{second}.$$

Measurements of protein synthesis by S^{35} incorporation indicate that $T_p^a \sim 3$ seconds, where the superscript a indicates the average value of T_p for all protein. Assuming that 1.5×10^4 ribosomes are active in synthesis and that the polypeptide products have an average length of 200 amino acids, $T_s^a = 20$ seconds and $T_a^a = 17$ seconds, assuming that: $A^u = A^i$; $T_a^u = A_a^i = T_a^a = 17$ seconds; and $N^u = 1$. Then: $T_s^u = 67$ seconds; $T_p^u = 50$ seconds; $T_p^i = 2.5$ seconds; and $N^u = 60$.

Thus, the 200-fold increase in rate of synthesis which occurs upon induction appears to be achieved by a sixtyfold increase in the number of enzyme-forming units and a threefold increase in the rate of synthesis/unit. While these estimates are admittedly crude, it seems difficult to avoid the conclusion that the number of enzyme-forming units increases by 10 to 100 during induction. Since:

$$N = N^u + N^i\,(1\text{-}e^{-\alpha t}),$$

$$\frac{dN}{dt} = \alpha N^i e^{-\alpha t}$$

Initially this rate is 0.4/second as $\alpha = 1/150\ \text{sec}^{-1}$.

Such a decreasing rate of formation might occur if a pre-existing pool of precursors were rapidly depleted, or if the enzyme-forming units inhibited their formation.

There is evidence, however, that the enzyme-forming units are unstable. Then:

$$\frac{dN}{dt} = S^i - L^i = S^i - \alpha N$$

$$S^i = \alpha(N^u + N^i)$$

where S and L stand for the rates of formation and loss of enzyme-forming units. If either S or L changes upon addition of the inducer, there will occur an approach to a new equilibrium level of enzyme-forming units.

Theoretically, it is easier to visualize how the inducer, which is clearly related to the product protein, might stabilize the enzyme-forming units as was suggested by Spiegelman (1948). It is also possible that the inducer acts by increasing the rate of formation. In any event, the initial rate of formation is remarkably high.

To summarize, these studies of enzyme induction indicate that enzyme-forming units can be created at a rate of 0.4/cell/second, that they may be unstable and decay with a time constant of 150 seconds, and that the enzyme-forming units may be identified with 70 S ribosomes. The next problem is to relate this flow of information which occurs during induction to the flow of material observed in the process of ribosome synthesis.

Ribosome Synthesis

The process of ribosome synthesis has been under study in our laboratory for the last four years, mostly by measurement of the incorporation of various radioactive tracers (Aronson *et al.*, 1960; Bolton, Britten, Cowie, and Roberts, 1958; and Bolton *et al.*, 1959). In a typical experiment, cells grow for a desired time in the presence of a tracer. They are harvested, washed, and broken, and their ribosomes are collected by centrifugation. The ribosomes are then fractionated by one of several techniques and the radioactivity of the various fractions is measured.

According to the type of tracer and the type of fractionation procedure which is used, one or another aspect of ribosome synthesis can be observed. Figure 3 shows the distribution of ribosomes in a rapidly growing cell, as observed in the analytical centrifuge. Figure 4 shows the distribution of newly incorporated C^{14}-uracil among ribosomes of different sedimentation coefficients after separation by centrifugation through a sucrose gradient (Britten and Roberts, 1960). Experiments of this type showed that the main flow of material entered first into the small particles and subsequently appeared in the large particles. However, radioactivity persisted in the small particles long after it would have passed through a simple precursor, indicating that large particles were unstable and reverted to the smaller size.

Fractionation of the ribosomes by chromatography on diethylaminoethyl (DEAE) cellulose shows a different aspect. The ribosome material is separated into three classes which elute at 0.4 M, 0.5 M,

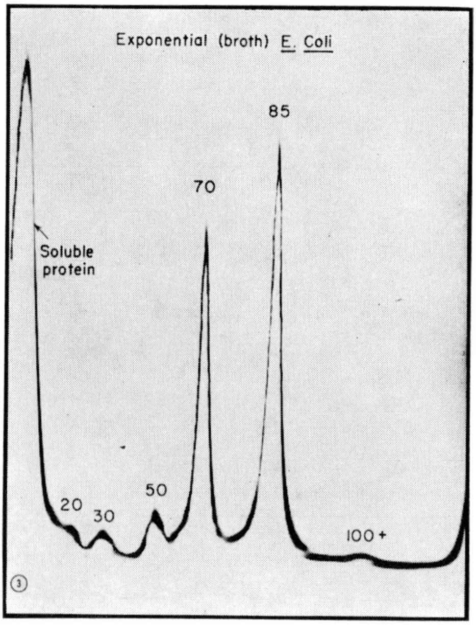

FIG. 3. The distribution of ribosomes from growing *E. coli* as seen in the analytical centrifuge.

and 0.6 M NaCl. These classes differ in the quantity of protein adhering to the RNA after elution; they also differ in the kinetics of their formation. Figure 5 shows that the specific radioactivity after a short period of incorporation is highest in the 0.6 M region. Longer periods of incorporation give higher proportions of the radioactivity, first in the 0.5 M region and finally in the 0.4 M region. At early times (30 seconds), all of the radioactivity elutes in the 0.6 M region. Apparently the most recently formed RNA is the least firmly bound to the protein portion of the ribosome.

McCarthy and Aronson (1961) have studied the appearance of radioactive material in the RNA derived from ribosomes by removal of the protein. The tracer molecules appear first in small pieces (about 4 S) and only subsequently are unified into the larger pieces (18 S and 28 S), which comprise the bulk of the ribosomes. (Fig. 6).

Thus, in the synthesis of ribosomes, three concurrent processes can be discerned: (1) the joining of small pieces of RNA into larger ones, (2) the attachment of protein to the RNA, and (3) the aggregation of small particles to form large ones. Furthermore, these processes are not especially rapid. The quality of precursor material

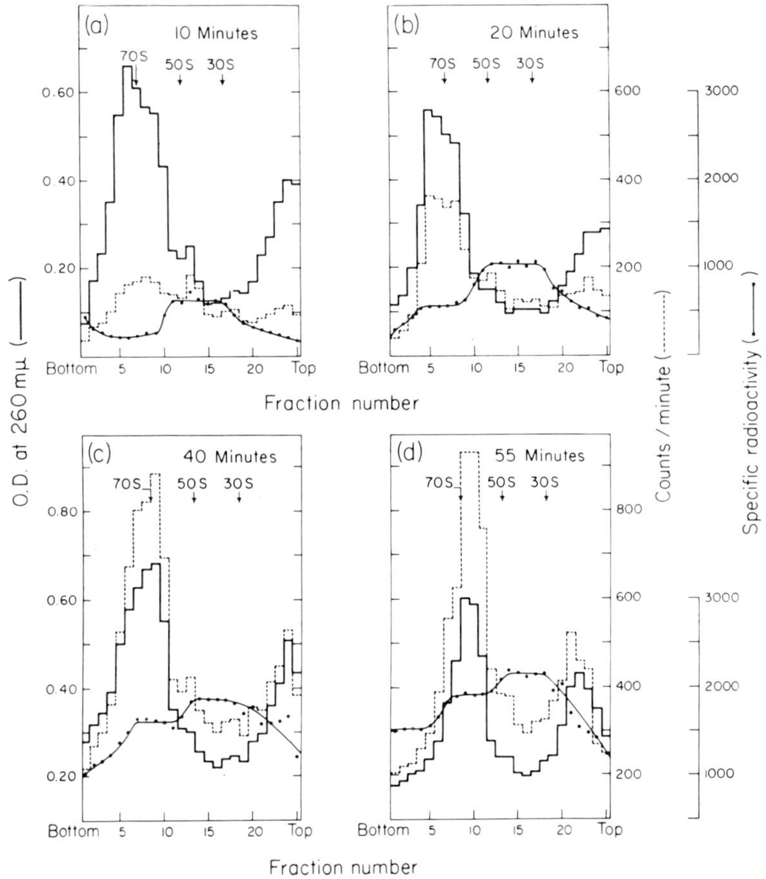

FIG. 4. The distribution of radioactivity among the ribosomes after various periods of incorporation of C^{14}-uracil.

is 5 to 10 per cent of the product and the time constants are accordingly three to six minutes.

There are then two difficulties in associating the creation of new enzyme-forming units with the main flow of material observed in ribosome synthesis. First, the net rate of ribosome synthesis is three finished 70 S particles/cell/second. Such a flow could, of course, supply the requirement for new enzyme-forming units, which is 0.4/cell/second, but only if 13 per cent of the total synthetic capacity were directed towards this purpose. However, the controlling factor is not the total rate of synthesis but the rate/synthetic site. If we assume that ribosomal material is synthesized in association

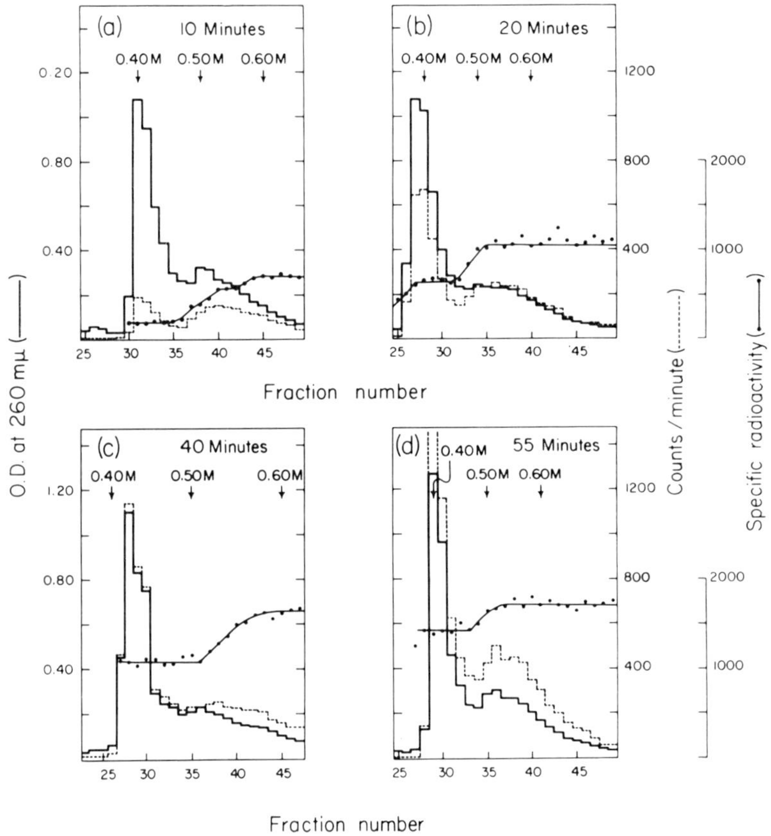

FIG. 5. Distribution of radioactivity among fractions obtained by chromatography on diethylaminoethyl (DEAE).

with DNA, as indicated by the work of Caro and Forro (1961), and that only 0.1 per cent of the DNA is relevant to synthesis of β-glactosidase, then the expected rate of synthesis of ribosomes concerned with β-galactosidase would be 0.003/second. The second difficulty is the prolonged time required to pass through the various stages which are required to produce a new 70 S ribosome entirely *de novo*. The time constants for these processes are significantly longer than the time constant for induction.

It is, of course, true that the flow of material for ribosome synthesis is the average flow needed to supply a steady state condition of growth. In contrast, induction is a transient process and related to one particular system which might be quite different from the average. Nevertheless, it seems more profitable to seek mechanisms compatible with both sets of observations, rather than to ascribe the divergences to departures from the average.

One process of ribosome synthesis seems clearly suited to rapid changes of the cell's complement of enzyme-forming units. This is the circulation of ribosomal material between the large and small particle forms. If a 70 S ribosome could assume a new form and a new synthetic capacity after reverting to the 30 S and 50 S stage and being reaggregated to a new 70 S particle, then the entire synthetic machinery could be converted to new functions with a time constant of roughly six minutes. Individual systems might be more or less stable than the average, and subject to more or less rapid conversion.

Such a process could be accomplished without addition of new

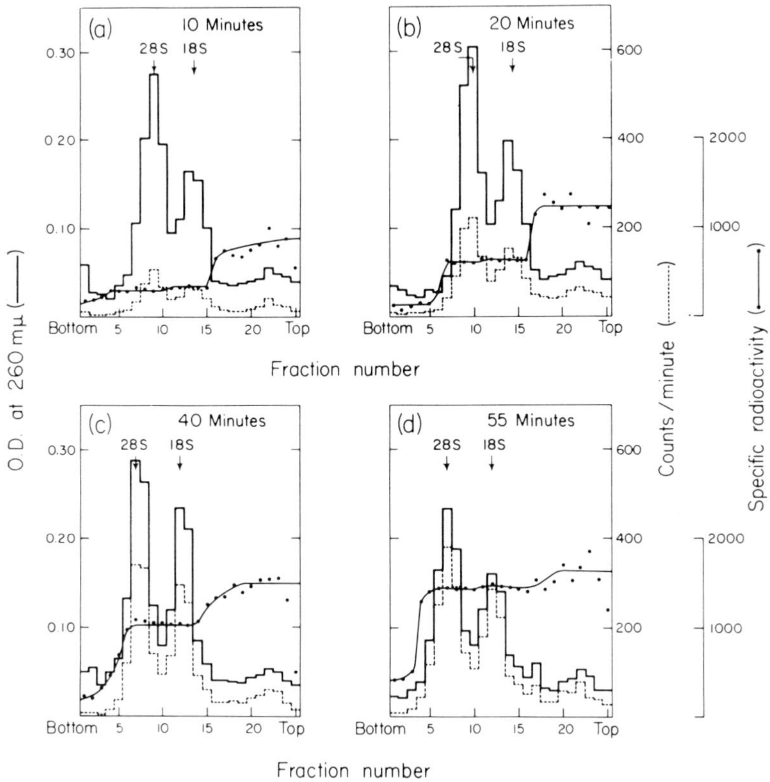

FIG. 6. Distribution of radioactivity among RNA's of different sedimentation coefficients.

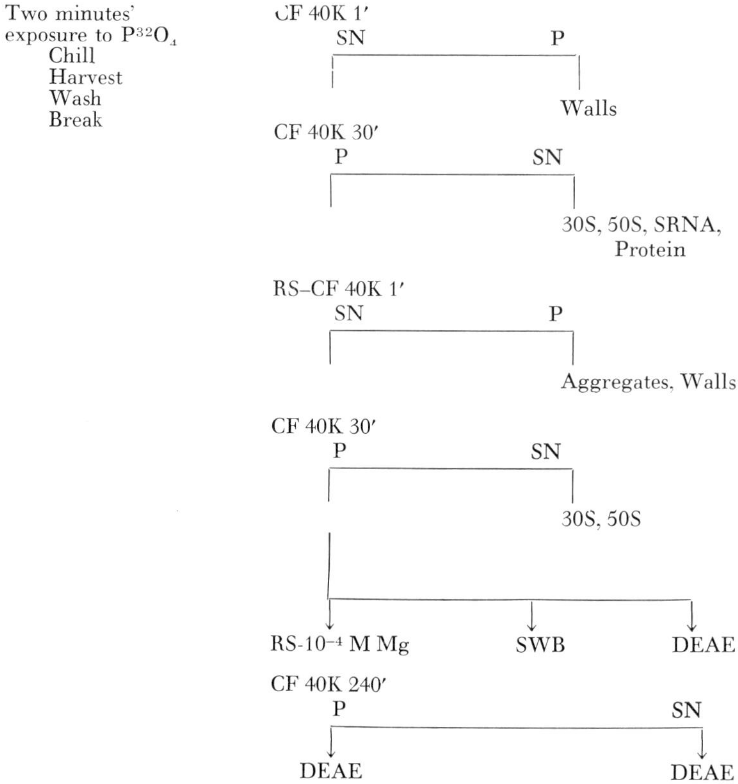

FIG. 7. Procedure used to isolate rapidly labeled component from 70 S ribosomes.

material, simply by the creation of different combinations or different configurations. More likely, however, would be the addition of new material which would carry all, or at least a critical part, of the required information.

Some evidence for this type of additional new material in 70 S particles could be found in data taken as long as two years ago. At early times after the addition of a tracer (100 seconds), there was more radioactivity in the 70 S particles than would be expected if they were solely the product of 30 S and 50 S precursors. The proportion of radioactivity in the 70 S particles did not decrease at very early times (10 seconds). Furthermore, the specific radioactivity of the intact 70 S particles was considerably higher than that of the 30 S and 50 S ribosomes derived from them (Roberts, 1960). A recent and more exact kinetic analysis, carried out by Britten and McCarthy (in press), has confirmed the earlier indications. A large fraction of the newly synthesized RNA appears in large ribosomes without passing through the smaller ribosomes.

The RNA responsible for the early radioactivity of the 70 S ribosomes has been partially purified. Growing cells were exposed to P^{32} for two minutes and a prepartion of their 70 S ribosomes was made as shown in Figure 7.

An aliquot of the final pellet was then analyzed by sedimentation through a sucrose gradient (10^{-2} M Mg). As shown in Figure 8, most of the remaining radioactivity sedimented in the region of the 70 S ribosomes. Another aliquot was brought to 10^{-4} M Mg and centrifuged. Most of the radioactivity remained in the supernatant, although the bulk of the ribonucleoprotein was sedimented. Evidently, there is a rapidly labeled component of the 70 S ribosomes, which is released in solutions of low magnesium concentration.

Figure 9 shows the analysis on DEAE cellulose (linear NaCl gradient elution) of the original pellet and the pellet and supernatant after reduction of the Mg concentration. The material released by reduction of the Mg concentration elutes at 0.6 M in the region where previously recognized ribosome precursors are eluted. Spiegelman (unpublished data) has kept us informed of experiments in his laboratory in which material of similar properties was isolated.

Midgeley (in press) has used isotopic dilution techniques to analyze the base composition of the two samples of this materal (X_1 and

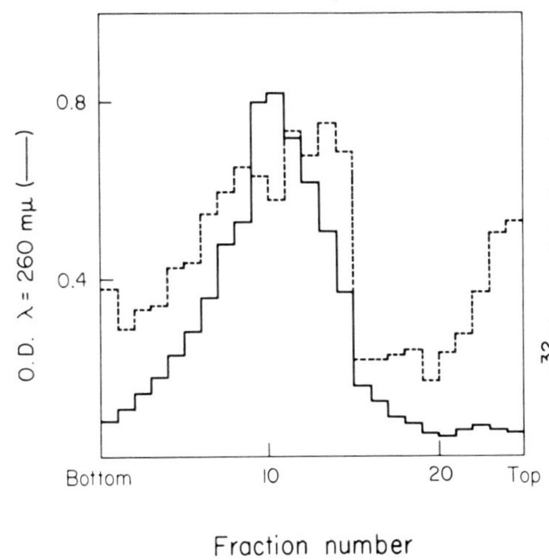

FIG. 8. Analysis of ribosome pellet shows mostly 70 S ribosomes.

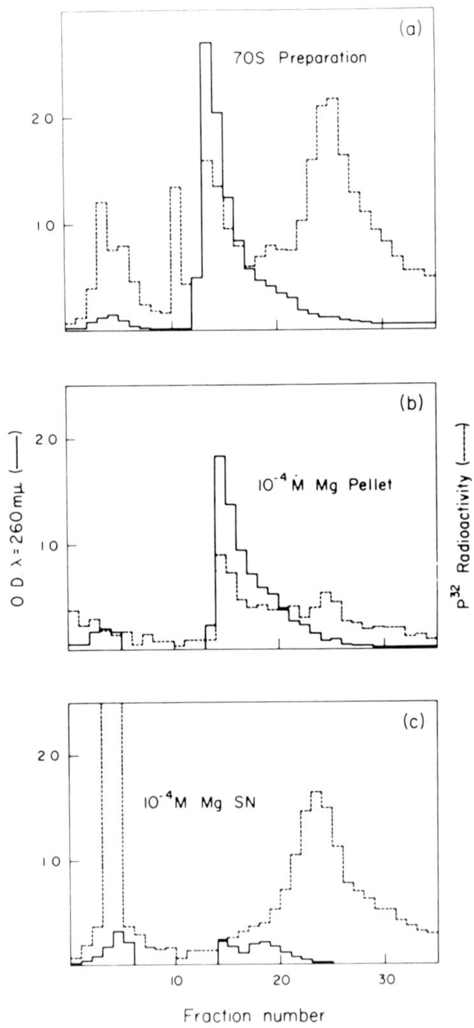

FIG. 9. Chromatography on diethylaminoethyl (DEAE) cellulose shows most of ribosome material in pellet, but most of radioactivity in supernatant fluid.

X_2 of Table 1). The base ratios obtained differ only slightly from those previously obtained for ribosomes, possibly in the direction of the composition of *E. coli* DNA (substituting uracil for thymine) These are tentative values and the possibility remains that the RNA fraction selected in this way is heterogenous.

TABLE 1

*Composition of S RNA and Ribosomal RNA**

			Source of RNA		
	S RNA	30 S	50 S	X_1	X_2
C	29.1	23.6	20.5	22.7	23.4
A	19.7	24.3	26.4	26.9	27.3
G	34.2	31.6	34.8	29.6	29.7
U	17.2	20.5	18.3	20.8	19.6

* From data of Bolton *et al.*, 1959.
Abbreviations: A, adenylic acid; C, cytidilic acid; G, guanylic acid; RNA, ribonucleic acid; S RNA, soluble RNA; U, uridylic acid.

Conclusion

Had the base composition of this particular RNA fraction turned out to show the ratios of DNA, we might have reason to believe that this was, in fact, the "messenger" RNA which has been postulated (Riley, Pardee, Jacob, and Monod, 1960). At present, we can only wait to see what further purification may bring. Its composition may indicate a relationship to DNA and an information-carrying capacity. Alternatively, it may simply function as a glue which sticks the two parts of the 70 S ribsomes together. It is, however, of some interest to find a component having approximately the kinetic behavior needed to interpret the rapidity of enzymes induction.

In conclusion, I would like to be the first to point out that my attempt to make a semiquantitative correlation between enzyme induction and ribosome synthesis is extremely tenuous. First, facts are not available for a certain estimate of the changes in enzyme-forming units during induction; second, there is no safety in comparing one rather unusual enzyme-forming system with the average flows which dominate our observations of ribosome synthesis. I only hope that this effort will provoke someone into providing the needed facts.

ACKNOWLEDGMENT

I emphasize that I have drawn heavily on unpublished experiments of my colleagues, R. J. Britten, J. A. Boezi, D. B. Cowie, B. J. McCarthy, and J. E. Midgeley for the facts of this paper, but they should not be held accountable for the many assumptions I have made when the facts were not available.

REFERENCES

Aronson, A. I., E. T. Bolton, R. J. Britten, D. B. Cowie, J. D. Duerksen, B. J. McCarthy, K. McQuillen, and R. B. Roberts. 1960. Biophysics in "Department of Terrestrial Magnetism," *Carnegie Institution of Washington Year*

Book 59, pp. 229–287. Baltimore, Maryland: The Lord Baltimore Press, Inc.

Aronson, A., and B. J. McCarthy. 1961. Studies of *E. coli* Ribosomal RNA and Its Degradation Products. *Biophysical Journal*, 1:215–226.

Boezi, J. A., and D. B. Cowie. (in press). Kinetic Studies of β-Galactosidase-Induction. *Biochemical Journal.*

Bolton, E. T., R. J. Britten, D. B. Cowie, B. J. McCarthy, K. McQuillen, and D. B. Roberts. 1959. Biophysics, in "Department of Terrestrial Magnetism," *Carnegie Institution of Washington Year Book 58*, pp. 259–300. Baltimore, Maryland: The Lord Baltimore Press, Inc.

Bolton, E. T., R. J. Britten, D. B. Cowie, and R. B. Roberts. 1958. Biophysics, in "Department of Terrestrial Magnetism," *Carnegie Institution of Washington Year Book 57*, pp. 127–162. Baltimore, Maryland: The Lord Baltimore Press, Inc.

Borsook, H., C. L. Deasy, A. J. Haagen-Smit, G. Keighley, and P. H. Lowry. 1950. Metabolism of C^{14} Labeled Glycine, L-Histidine, L-Leucine and L-Lysine. *Journal of Biological Chemistry*, 187:839–849.

Britten, R. J., and R. B. Roberts. 1960. High-Resolution Density Gradient Sedimentation Analysis. *Science*, 131:32–33.

Caro, L. G., and F. Forro. 1961. RNA and Its Site of Synthesis. *The Journal of Biophysical and Biochemical Cytology*, 9:555–566.

Cowie, D. B., S. Spiegelman, R. B. Roberts, and J. D. Duerksen. 1961. Ribosome-Bound β-Galactosidase. *Proceedings of the National Academy of Sciences of the U.S.A.*, 47:114–122.

Hall, B. D., and S. Spiegelman. (in press). Sequence Complementarity of T2-DNA and T2-Specific RNA. *Proceedings of the National Academy of Sciences of the U.S.A.*

Littlefield, J. W., E. B. Keller, J. Gross, and P. C. Zamecnik. 1955. Studies on Cytoplasmic Ribonucleoprotein Particles from the Liver of the Rat. *Journal of Biological Chemistry*, 217:111–125.

McCarthy, B. J., and A. Aronson. 1961. The Kinetics of the Synthesis of Ribosomal RNA in *E. coli*. *Biophysical Journal*, 1:227–245.

McQuillen, K., R. B. Roberts, and R. J. Britten. 1959. Synthesis of Nascent Protein by Ribosomes in *E. coli*. *Proceedings of the National Academy of Sciences of the U.S.A.*, 45:1437–1447.

Midgeley, J. E. (in press). *Carnegie Institution Year Book*, 60.

Riley, M., A. B. Pardee, F. Jacob, and J. Monod. 1960. On the Expression of a Structural Gene. *Journal of Molecular Biology*, 2:216–225.

Roberts, R. B. 1960. Synthetic Aspects of Ribosomes. *Annals of the New York Academy of Sciences*, 88:752–759.

Spiegelman, S. 1948. Differentiation as the Controlled Production of Unique Enzymatic Patterns. *Symposia of the Society for Experimental Biology*, 2:286–325. New York, New York: Academic Press, Inc.

Spiegelman, S. Unpublished data.

Studies on Ribosomes and Ribosomal Enzymes

DAVID ELSON, PH.D.

Biochemistry Section,
The Weizmann Institute of Science,
Rehovoth, Israel

It is not difficult, when looking at the deceptively simple sedimentation patterns of suitably prepared purified ribosomes, to lose sight of the probable biological complexity of the ribosome. In *Escherichia coli* preparations, one sees what appears to be a fundamental 70 S particle which can be made either to dimerize to a 100 S particle or to dissociate into one 50 S and one 30 S particle. The association and dissociation are reversible and are easily controlled through variations in the Mg^{++} concentration and the ionic strength of the medium. In *E. coli*, at least, the particles contain only two types of substance, ribonucleic acid (RNA) and protein, in proportions which remain fixed regardless of the state of dissociation (Tissières and Watson, 1958; Tissières, Watson, Schlessinger, and Hollingworth, 1959). The 30 S and 50 S particles contain RNA's of virtually identical gross composition (Spahr and Tissières, 1959). At this level of investigation the predominant impression is one of chemical homogeneity.

Nevertheless, the presence of two well-defined particles of different size shows that we are not dealing with an entity made up of identical subunits and suggests that differences other than size differences may also exist. Such differences have been found. Two recent electron microscope studies of the ribosomes of *E. coli* have shown the 30 S and 50 S ribosomes to differ in shape (Hall and

Slayter, 1959; Huxley and Zubay, 1960). The electron micrographs showed, further, that the association reactions are specific. That is, in forming a 70 S particle the 50 S and 30 S ribosomes combine in a specific way, while there seems also to be a specific combining site by which two 70 S particles join to form one 100 S ribosome. These observations indicate that the association processes are not due to random aggregation, but rather represent the coming together of complementary structures in an ordered way.

We may ask whether these processes are of biological significance. The impression exists that they are. When we turn from studies of isolated and purified ribosomes to investigations of cell extracts, which presumably are closer to the *in vivo* condition, we find that the particle size and state of association vary with the medium in which the cells were grown, the metabolic state of the cells, the position of the culture in the growth cycle, etc. (Dagley and Sykes, 1958; Bowen, Dagley, and Sykes, 1959; McCarthy, 1960). Here, as the organism shifts from one metabolic state to another, the association-dissociation balance of the ribosomes also changes. Although little is understood of these changes, it seems fairly clear that they mirror the changing metabolic state of the cell. According to present ideas about the function of the ribosomes, this would imply that there is a connection between the dissociation and association of the ribosomes and the synthesis of proteins.

In this connection we may cite two recent studies of protein synthesis in *E. coli*. In an *in vivo* study, McQuillen, Roberts, and Britten (1959) have provided evidence that the cellular proteins are synthesized in the ribosomes, predominantly in the 70 S ribosomes. Tissières, Schlessinger, and Gros (1960) have reported an *in vitro* ribosomal system which incorporates labeled amino acids into peptide linkages within the ribosomes, but which does not effect the synthesis of appreciable amounts of new protein. They have suggested that their system lacks a release factor, in the absence of which the polypeptide chains would remain attached to their ribosomal sites of synthesis, blocking them against continued protein synthesis. Webster (1959), working with an *in vitro* pea ribosome system which is capable of synthesizing massive amounts of new protein, has reported that his system contains such a release factor (Webster and Lingrel, 1961). It seems altogether reasonable, therefore, to assume that such a release factor is a necessary part of the protein synthesizing apparatus. In their system, Tissières and his co-workers found that a small portion of the 70 S ribosomes to resist dissociation into 30 S and 50 S particles; incorporated labeled amino acids appeared to be concentrated in this resistant 70 S fraction. They were led to suggest that the release of newly synthesized protein from the ribosomes might require the dissociation of the 70 S into 30 S and 50 S particles and inversely, that the subsequent synthesis of protein might require the reformation of the 70 S ribosome.

In the paragraphs above I have mentioned a few of the many observations to be found in the extensive literature on the ribosomes. From such observations, it is possible to begin to piece together a preliminary picture of the ribosomes as a system composed of several different parts. The act of protein synthesis might well be a collaborative effort, requiring the simultaneous participation of the separate parts. In terms of the ultracentrifuge and electron microscope, these events would be expressed as the well known association-dissociation processes of the ribosomes. The implication here is that the protein synthesizing apparatus is distributed among different ribosomal particles and that these different particles must come together in order to effect the synthesis of a protein. According to this point of view, the various ribosomes, although similar in their gross chemical composition, would differ not only in size and shape but also in their biological properties. This, at least, is the viewpoint prevailing in our laboratory. It is based in part on the observations of others, as already indicated, and to a large extent on our own findings. Much of our present work is concerned with this problem.

Ribosomal Enzymes

Our attention became focused on the problem of the possible biological heterogeneity of the ribosomes during our studies of the ribosomal enzyme, ribonuclease (RNase) (Elson, 1958, 1959a,b). We found this enzyme to be present in a ribonucleoprotein preparation isolated from *E. coli* by a series of chemical precipitations. The enzyme was latent, being inactive so long as the nucleoprotein was intact; it became active only under conditions where the structure of the nucleoprotein was disrupted. It could not be separated from the nucleoprotein by either ultracentrifugal fractionation or prolonged zone electrophoresis of the nucleoprotein. Furthermore, the RNase activity per unit of RNA remained constant throughout the isolation, despite the subjection of the material to a number of relatively drastic treatments which would be expected to remove at least part of any adsorbed protein contaminant. Two conclusions could thus be drawn. First, the enzyme behaved as though it were an integral part of the nucleoprotein. Second, since the RNase activity per unit of RNA was the same in the initial crude cell extracts as in the final purified nucleoprotein, it appeared that the bulk of the cellular RNase was associated with the nucleoprotein. The second conclusion has also been reached, independently, by Bolton and his co-workers, who used a different experimental technique (Bolton *et al.*, 1959). We subsequently found ribosomes, isolated with the ultracentrifuge, to have the same specific RNase activity as the chemically purified nucleoprotein. The conclusions are, therefore, valid for the ribosomes (Elson, 1961).

As to the biological significance of the association of RNase with the ribosomes, there are two obvious possibilities. According to one, the enzyme would be attached to the ribosomes because it was synthesized there. It may well be that at any given time a certain proportion of a ribosomal population would contain completed polypeptide chains, finished products which have not yet been released from the site of synthesis. Some of these proteins would be enzymes, among them RNase. A second possibility, which does not exclude the first, is that the RNase plays a metabolic role in the ribosome. Since the bulk of both the cellular RNase and RNA is concentrated in the ribosomes, it seems likely that the enzyme does function in the ribosome. The ribosomal RNase may, therefore, be part of the protein synthesizing apparatus. This impression is heightened by the finding of Zillig, Krone, and Albers (1959) that the ribosomes contain diamines which are effective inhibitors of the enzyme and might constitute a biological control mechanism.

We have no clear idea as to what role the enzyme might play in protein synthesis. There are several possibilities, one being that it releases completed polypeptide chains by degrading an RNA template (Roth, 1954). This is reminiscent of Webster's release factor. Yet the two are not identical: the ribosomal RNase is an unusually stable enzyme, while the release factor is extraordinarily unstable (Webster and Lingrel, 1961).

Following our finding of the ribosomal RNase, we began to search for other ribosomal enzymes. We wished, if possible, to distinguish between two classes of ribosomal enzyme: those which, like the RNase, might operate within the ribosome; and those which have no apparent function there and might be looked on solely as products of ribosomal protein synthesis. That is, we wished to search both for components and products of the protein synthesizing apparatus. We have found traces of aldolase activity and higher levels of two other enzymes: one which degrades deoxyribonucleic acid (DNA) but not RNA, and one which splits L-prolylglycine but not glycylglycine or poly-L-proline. We have also confirmed the presence of β-galactosidase in ribosomes from suitably induced cultures of *E. coli* (Bolton *et al.*, 1959). With the possible exception of the dipeptidase, it seems unlikely that any of these enzymes might participate directly in ribosomal protein synthesis. In addition, we have obtained evidence that antibodies are associated with ribosomes isolated from the spleens and lymph nodes of immunized rabbits (Feldman, Elson, and Globerson, 1960). Here we are clearly dealing with a product. Our results are in accord with those of other investigators, who have also shown various enzymes to be associated with ribosomes (Siekevitz and Palade, 1958; Bolton *et al.*, 1959; McQuillen, 1961).

Ribosomal Location of Ribonuclease

When it became apparent that it was possible to trace specific proteins to the ribosomes, we attempted to carry the localization one step farther and to determine whether a specific enzyme is concentrated preferentially in either the 30 S or the 50 S ribosome. Experimentally, this approach was made possible by the development of effective methods for the separation of 30 S and 50 S ribosomes by differential ultracentrifugation (Tissières and Watson, 1958; Bolton *et al.*, 1959). Using essentially the technique of Tissières and Watson, Tal separated 30 S and 50 S ribosomes, determined the specific RNase activity of each, and found the enzyme to be heavily concentrated in the 30 S particle (Elson and Tal, 1959). In fact, after allowance had been made for a small amount of contaminating 30 S particles in the 50 S preparation, it became doubtful that the 50 S ribosomes contained the enzyme. We then prepared a series of ribosomal mixtures which contained different proportions of 30 S and 50 S ribosomes. When the specific RNase activities of these mixtures are plotted against the fraction of each type of ribosome (Figure 1), it is seen that the activity is directly proportional to the relative amount of 30 S ribosomes, and extrapolates to zero activity for pure 50 S ribosomes. It appears, then, that the ribosomal RNase is located exclusively in the 30 S ribosome.

So far as I know, this is the first demonstration of a biological difference between the 30 S and 50 S ribosomes. If the RNase is

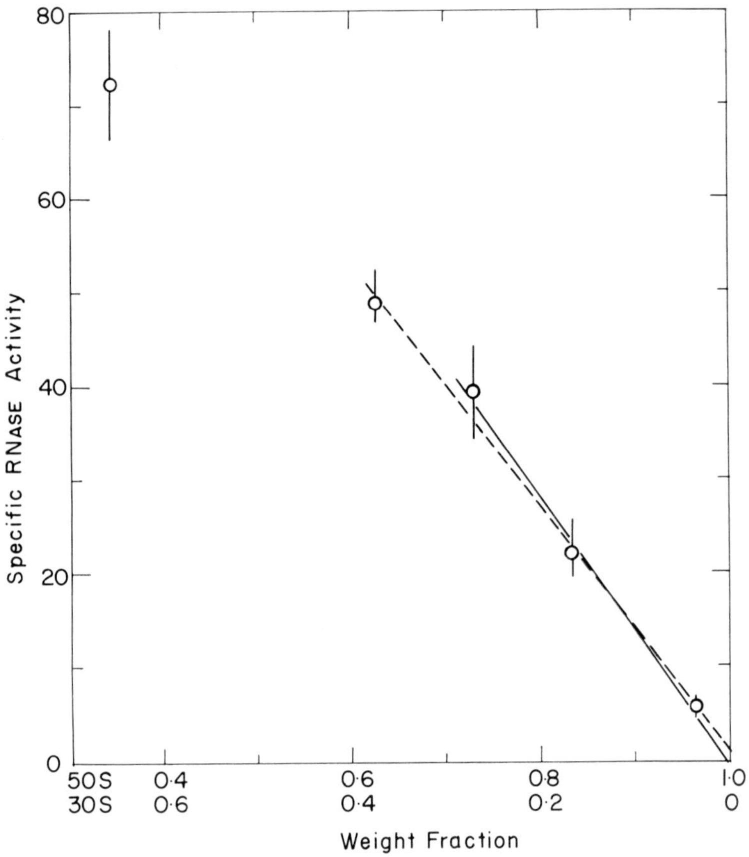

FIG. 1. Ribonuclease (RNase) activity (in arbitrary units/hour/μg. of protein/ml. of incubation mixture) of mixtures of 50 S and 30 S ribosomes. Circles represent mean values of four assays (three assays for the mixture richest in 50 S). Vertical lines connect the maximum and minimum values. Least squares straight lines are plotted for the three (———) and four (– – – –) mixtures richest in 50 S particles. (From Elson and Tal, 1959.)

part of the protein synthesizing apparatus, the two types of ribosome must play different roles in protein biosynthesis.

This point seems to us to be of considerable importance. If enough data of this sort can be collected, it may prove possible to determine the location of the various parts of the protein synthesizing apparatus. Eventually, such information may help us to understand how the ribosomes synthesize proteins. We have, therefore, begun to search for other differences between the 30 S and 50 S particles.

I should like to present some observations obtained in one series of experiments. This work is in an early stage and the results can be considered, at best, suggestive! They are far from being final.

Effect of Salt on Ribosomes

We have usually produced 30 S and 50 S ribosomes by dialyzing 70 S particles against 0.001 M magnesium acetate and 0.01 M sodium phosphate, pH 7.0 (Tissières and Watson, 1958). Once, for reasons irrelevant to the present discussion, we changed the medium to 0.001 M calcium chloride and 0.1 M sodium chloride, and observed deviations from the normal sedimentation pattern, due, presumably, to the high ionic strength. We then examined the effect of rising concentrations of sodium chloride on the ribosomal sedimentation pattern. Typical results are illustrated in Figure 2 and summarized in Table 1. Above a certain concentration of sodium chloride, the 50 S peak disappears and is replaced by a peak of lower sedimentation constant, sometimes 45 to 50 S and sometimes 40 to 45 S. Occasionally, as in Figure 2 (0.1 M NaCl), both components are observed, as though the system had been caught in midtransition. There is an inkling of two successive transitions which occur as the salt concentration is raised: 50 S → 45 to 50 S → 40 to 45 S. The salt concentration at which the transition takes place has varied from one experiment to another. Usually in 0.1 M sodium chloride only one fast peak is seen, but this may be either 45 to 50 S or 40 to 45 S.

At the time when the 50 S ribosome is replaced by a more slowly sedimenting component, a new peak appears. This material usually shows a sedimentation constant of 4 to 5 S, and I shall refer to it as the 5 S component. I should make it clear that the picture as here

TABLE 1

Effect of Salt on Ribosomal Sedimentation Behavior

Medium		Sedimentation constants*			
$CaCl_2$	NaCl				
0.001 M	....	36 S	52 S	69 S	..
0.001 M	0.05 M	34 S	51 S	..	..
0.001 M	0.10 M	5 S	32 S	43 S	47 S
0.001 M	0.30 M	5 S	32 S	41 S	..

* Corrected to 20°C. The contribution of the salts to the viscosity of the medium is ignored.

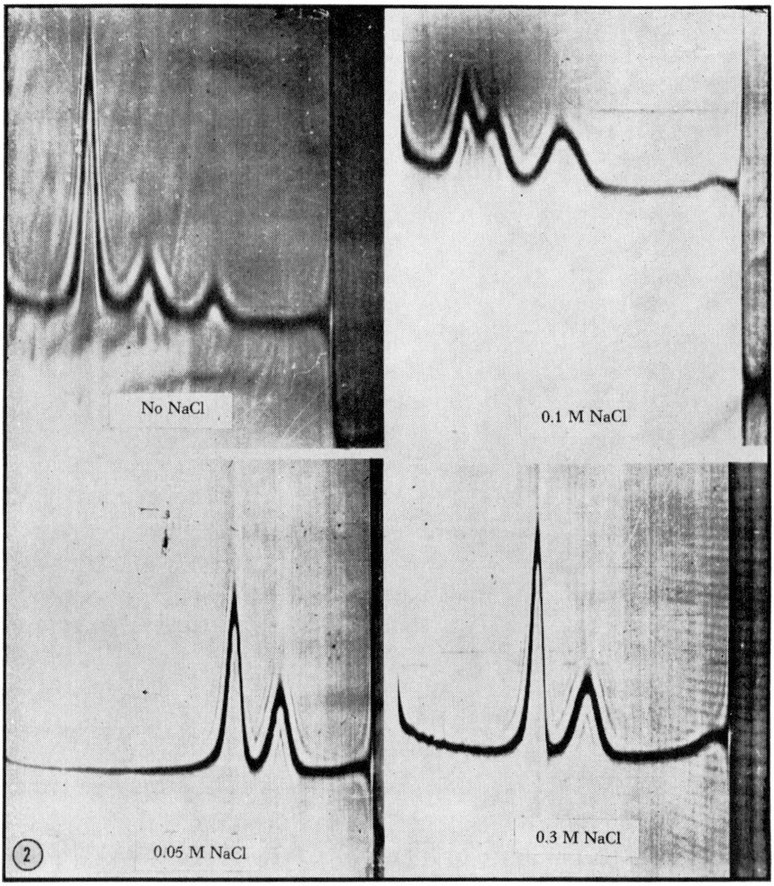

FIG. 2. Effect of salt on ribosomal sedimentation behavior. Portions of the same preparation of 70 S ribosomes from *Escherichia coli* were dialyzed overnight at 4°C against solvents containing 0.001 M calcium chloride and the indicated concentrations of sodium chloride, and were examined in the same solvents in the analytical ultracentrifuge (Spinco Model E). Sedimentation is from right to left. Sedimentation constants are given in Table 1. In 0.1 M sodium chloride the 5 S component is clearly visible and a double peak (43 S and 47 S) replaces the usual 50 S peak.

presented is somewhat oversimplified. After observing the appearance of the 5 S component in the above mentioned solvents, we began to pay more attention to the region near the meniscus in all sedimentation runs. We found that those media which dissociate 70 S to 50 S and 30 S ribosomes (such as 0.001 M magnesium acetate—0.01 M sodium phosphate, pH 7.0, and 0.0001 M magnesium acetate—0.001 M tris(hydroxymethyl)aminomethane, pH 7.3) also often caused the appearance of traces of the 5 S component. Indeed, Hamilton and Petermann (1958) have commented that such a component is often present in their ribonucleoprotein preparations. It may well be that some 5 S component is commonly liberated when a 70 S ribosome dissociates. The amount liberated appears to be much greater, however, at the higher salt concentrations.

While these changes take place in the 50 S and 5 S particles, the sedimentation constant of the 30 S particle remains unchanged (Table 1), although the 30 S peak sometimes becomes more disperse at the higher salt concentrations. We therefore felt it likely that the 5 S component came only from the 50 S ribosomes.

In order to test this supposition directly, we dialyzed 70 S, 50 S, and 30 S ribosomes against 0.001 M calcium chloride—0.1 M sodium chloride, the solvent we have usually employed to cause the appearance of the 5 S component. The dialyzed solutions were then centrifuged for six hours at 100,000 × g at approximately room temperature. Under these conditions the 30 S and all larger particles were completely sedimented. The supernatants were then examined in the analytical ultracentrifuge. The results are shown in Figure 3. It can be seen that the 5 S component arose from the 70 S and 50 S ribosomes, but not from the 30 S particles.

Before we inquire into the nature of the 5 S component, we might glance for a moment at the general solubilizing effect of 0.1 M sodium chloride on the ribosomes. Our data are still scanty, but we have analyzed several of the six hour 100,000 × g supernatants for RNA (by ultraviolet absorption) and protein (by the Folin reaction). The analyses indicate that 0.1 M salt solubilized some 1 to 3 per cent of the Folin-reacting material of all three types of ribosome. About 5 to 7 per cent of the ultraviolet-absorbing material of the 70 S and 50 S particles became nonsedimentable, and less in the case of the 30 S ribosomes. Much of this material was of very low molecular weight, some 30 to 60 per cent being soluble in 0.1 M perchloric acid. We see, however, that 0.1 M sodium chloride removes material from the 30 S as well as from the 50 S and 70 S particles. The 5 S component constitutes part of this nonsedimentable material and appears to be absent from the 30 S ribosome.

As to the nature of the 5 S component, we have performed one experiment wherein separate portions of the same 5 S preparation were subjected to digestion with trypsin and RNase. The incubation was for one-half hour at room temperature, after which the solution

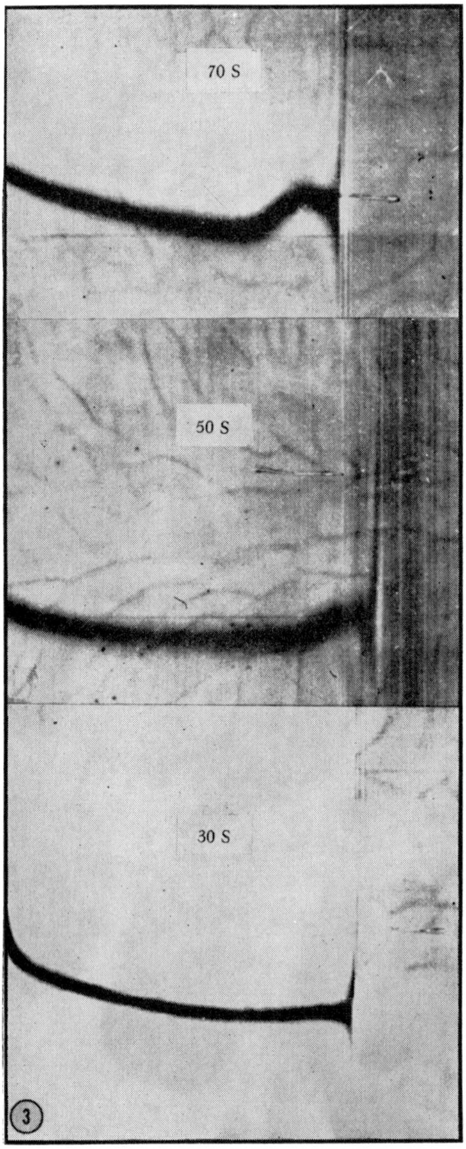

FIG. 3. An experiment to determine the origin of the 5 S component. Preparations of 70 S, 50 S, and 30 S ribosomes were dialyzed overnight at 4°C against 0.001 M calcium chloride and 0.1 M sodium chloride. The dialyzed solutions were centrifuged six hours at approximately room temperature at 100,000 × g in a Spinco Model L preparative ultracentrifuge in order to sediment all particles larger than the 5 S component. The supernatants were then examined in the Spinco Model E analytical ultracentrifuge. Sedimentation is from right to left. A 5 S component was obtained from 70 S and 50 S ribosomes, but not from 30 S ribosomes.

was examined in the analytical ultracentrifuge. Figure 4 shows the 5 S component to be entirely unaffected by trypsin but to be degraded by RNase; it appears, therefore, to be composed of RNA and not of protein or nucleoprotein.

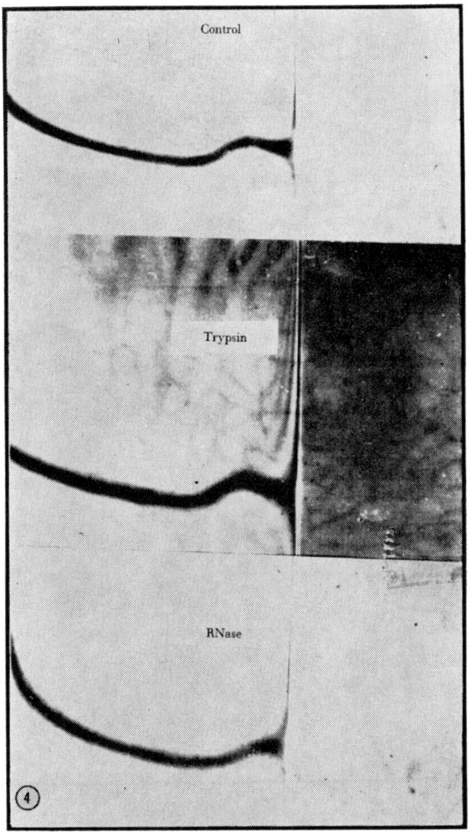

FIG. 4. The effect of trypsin and ribonuclease (RNase) on the 5 S component. The 5 S component was isolated from 70 S ribosomes as described for Figure 3. Three portions of the solution were taken for the experiment. To one was added crystalline trypsin to a final concentration of 24.4 μg./ml. Crystalline RNase was added to the second portion to the same final concentration. Each solution was incubated at room temperature for one-half hour and then examined in the analytical ultracentrifuge. The control received no enzyme but was otherwise treated in the same way. The final concentration of 5 S component was the same in all cases. All three photographs were taken 21 to 23 minutes after the rotor had reached its final speed. Sedimentation is from right to left Sedimentation constants: Control, 4.7 S; trypsin, 4.9 S; RNase, could not be calculated.

As I have mentioned, the sedimentation constant of the 5 S component is usually observed to be 4 to 5 S. These numbers are, of course, very close to the constants generally reported for the transfer RNA. We have therefore attempted to ascertain whether the 5 S component might be identical with or derived from the transfer RNA. Since, in contrast to the ribosomal RNA, the transfer RNA is relatively rich in pseudouridylic acid (Dunn, 1959), we have started to perform nucleotide analyses of the 5 S component. We have used Dowex-1 formate ion exchange chromatography for this purpose, employing Cohn's (1960) formic acid-ammonium formate elution procedure. The initial results neither identify the 5 S component with the transfer RNA nor completely eliminate the possibility of such an identity. Ultraviolet absorbing material is eluted from the column in the pseudouridylic acid region; it does not, however, have the spectral properties of that nucleotide. It would, obviously, be of great interest to locate the point of contact between the transfer RNA and the ribosomes. Whether our experiments are pertinent to this problem remains to be seen.

Considering the great amount of research activity now being devoted to the ribosomes in many laboratories, we may, however, look forward to the accumulation of information on the biological heterogeneity of the ribosomes, and may hope eventually to acquire knowledge of the location and spatial interrelationship of the various parts of the protein synthesizing apparatus.

ACKNOWLEDGMENTS

This work was supported in part by grants from the United States Public Health Service (RG-5876) and the National Science Foundation (G-15564).

The investigation of the ribosomal location of RNase is the work of M. Tal. The technical assistance of S. Avital is gratefully acknowledged.

REFERENCES

Bolton, E. T., R. J. Britten, D. B. Cowie, B. J. McCarthy, K. McQuillen, and R. B. Roberts. 1959. Biophysics, in "Department of Terrestrial Magnetism," *Carnegie Institution of Washington Year Book 58*, pp. 259–300. Baltimore, Maryland: The Lord Baltimore Press, Inc.

Bowen, T. J., S. Dagley, and J. Sykes. 1959. A Ribonucleoprotein Component of *Escherichia coli*. *Biochemical Journal*, 72:419–425.

Cohn, W. E. 1960. Pseudouridine, a Carbon-Carbon Linked Ribonucleoside in Ribonucleic Acids: Isolation, Structure, and Chemical Characteristics. *Journal of Biological Chemistry*, 235:1488–1498.

Dagley, S., and J. Sykes. 1958. "The Influence of Conditions of Culture on Certain Soluble Macromolecular Components of *Escherichia coli*," *Microsomal Particles and Protein Synthesis*, R. B. Roberts, Ed., pp. 62–69. New York, New York: Pergamon Press.

Dunn, D. B. 1959. Additional Components in Ribonucleic Acid of Rat Liver Fractions. *Biochimica et biophysica acta*, 34:286–287.

Elson, D. 1958. Latent Ribonuclease Activity in a Ribonucleoprotein. *Bio-*

chimica et biophysica acta, 27:216–217.

———. 1959a. Preparation and Properties of a Ribonucleoprotein Isolated from *Escherichia coli. Biochimica et biophysica acta*, 36:362–371.

———. 1959b. Latent Enzymic Activity of a Ribonucleoprotein Isolated from *Escherichia coli. Biochimica et biophysica acta*, 36:372–386.

———. 1961. Biologically Active Proteins Associated with Ribosomes. *Protein Biosynthesis.* R. J. C. Harris (Ed.) pp. 291–300. London: Academic Press, Inc.

Elson, D., and M. Tal. 1959. Biochemical Differences in Ribonucleoproteins. *Biochimica et biophysica acta*, 36:281–282.

Feldman, M., D. Elson, and A. Globerson. 1960. Antibodies in Ribonucleoproteins. *Nature, London*, 185:317–319.

Hall, C. E., and H. S. Slayter. 1959. Electron Microscopy of Ribonucleoprotein Particles from *E. coli. Journal of Molecular Biology*, 1:329–332.

Hamilton, M. G., and M. L. Petermann. 1958. Ultracentrifugal Studies on Ribonucleoprotein from Rat Liver Microsomes. *Journal of Biological Chemistry*, 234:1441–1446.

Huxley, H. E., and G. Zubay. 1960. Electron Microscope Observations on the Structure of Microsomal Particles from *Escherichia coli. Journal of Molecular Biology*, 2:10–18.

McCarthy, B. J. 1960. Variations in Bacterial Ribosomes. *Biochimica et biophysica acta*, 39:563–564.

McQuillen, K. 1961. Protein Synthesis *in vivo:* The Involvement of Ribosomes in *Escherichia coli. Protein Biosynthesis.* R. J. C. Harris (Ed.) pp. 263–290. London: Academic Press, Inc.

McQuillen, K., R. B. Roberts, and R. J. Britten. 1959. Synthesis of Nascent Protein by Ribosomes in *Escherichia coli. Proceedings of the National Academy of Sciences of the U.S.A.*, 45:1437–1447.

Roth, J. S. 1954. A Possible Function of Intracellular Ribonucleases. *Nature, London*, 174:129.

Siekevitz, P., and G. E. Palade. 1958. A Cytochemical Study on the Pancreas of the Guinea Pig. II. Functional Variations in the Enzymatic Activity of Microsomes. *The Journal of Biophysical and Biochemical Cytology*, 4:401–410.

Spahr, P. F., and A. Tissières. 1959. Nucleotide Composition of Ribonucleoprotein Particles from *Escherichia coli. Journal of Molecular Biology*, 1:237–239.

Tissières, A., D. Schlessinger, and F. Gros. 1960. Amino Acid Incorporation into Proteins by *Escherichia coli* Ribosomes. *Proceedings of the National Academy of Sciences of the U.S.A.*, 46:1450–1463.

Tissières, A., and J. D. Watson. 1958. Ribonucleoprotein Particles from *Escherichia coli. Nature, London*, 182:778–780.

Tissières, A., J. D. Watson, D. Schlessinger, and B. R. Hollingworth. 1959. Ribonucleoprotein Particles from *Escherichia coli. Journal of Molecular Biology*, 1:221–233.

Webster, G. C. 1959. Protein Synthesis by Isolated Nucleoprotein Particles. *Archives of Biochemistry and Biophysics*, 85:159–170.

Webster, G. C., and J. B. Lingrel. 1961. Protein Synthesis by Isolated Ribonucleoprotein Particles. *Protein Biosynthesis*. R. J. C. Harris (Ed.) pp. 301–318. London: Academic Press, Inc.

Zillig, W., W. Krone, and M. Albers. 1959. Untersuchungen zur Biosynthese der Proteine. III. Beitrag zur Kenntnis der Zusammensetzung und Struktur der Ribosomen. *Hoppe-Seyler's Zeitschrift für physiologische Chemie*, 317: 131–143.

Ribonucleic Acid Synthesis by Bacterial Nuclear Preparations

DAVID H. EZEKIEL, PH.D.

Albert Einstein Medical Center, Philadelphia Pennsylvania

There is no generally accepted description of the bacterial nucleus (Chapman, 1959). This structure has been the subject of a comprehensive review by Murray (1960). Evidence is accumulating rapidly, and we now have at least one fairly detailed model to consider.

After several years of systematic cytological examination by means of the electron microscope, Kellenberger (1960) has proposed that the bacterial chromatin is a chromosome, composed of individually visible chromatin fibrils which consist of deoxyribonucleic acid (DNA) double helices neutralized with polyamines. The fibrils are connected by protein linkers at the ends, and they are arranged parallel with each other in a bundle. Finally, the aggregate bundle may be twisted or bent in various ways. Under the influence of chloramphenicol or tetracyclines, it forms a ring; other physiological states produce other characteristic arrangements. The chromosome is in direct contact with the cytoplasm. There is no nuclear sap, and no nuclear membrane. There is little or no ribonucleic acid (RNA) in the chromosome, and no protein core, except the center of the ring structure with chloramphenicol or tetracyclines. There is no periodic transformation between an interphase and a mitotic form of differing fine structure. Nor is the fine structure of the ring form different from that of the normal form. Replication proceeds along the chromosome in a linear fashion. Nothing is said about the process of gene function.

By contrast, Spiegelman, Aronson, and Fitz-James (1958) reported the liberation of bacterial nuclei from *Bacillus megaterium* strain KM by treatment of protoplasts with pancreatic lipase. Their preparations were composed of DNA, RNA, and protein in the ratio of 1:1:3. They consisted of two parts, a phase-dense core surrounded by the phase-light chromatinic gel. No surrounding membrane was seen.

In trying to reconcile these structures, we are especially concerned with knowing whether there is a single chromosome in bacteria, or several. Similarly, in relating them to the nuclei and chromosomes of higher organisms, we would especially like to know whether bacteria exhibit the classic mitotic process. After years of polemics on the subjects, we now have a limited amount of direct information. First, we have known for several years that there is only one genetic linkage group, that is, only one chromosome according to genetic measurements, in *Escherichia coli*. However, its cytogenetics are still somewhat out of order, since a circular genetic map is not reflected in a recognizably circular chromatin pattern. Second, Forro and Finch (1961) have reported a radioautographic study at a current meeting of the Biophysical Society; they find that the spores of *Bacillus subtilis* contain a definite quantity of DNA, which divides into two subunits conserved in separate cells during later division; presumably there is just one chromosome.

As to classic mitotic processes, the evidence for a single chromosome contradicts the only reports of full-fledged classic mitosis in bacteria, since the mitotic figures in question involved three chromosomes. The radioautographic evidence also seems to rule out definitively the notion that the bacterial nuclear division is any sort of irregular process involving random assortment of many copies, such as has been hypothesized for the macronuclei of some protozoa. The most direct evidence on the mode of nuclear division is that of Mason and Powelson (1956), obtained by continuous phase microscopy of cells growing in gelatin. The review by Murray (1960) contains a superior photograph of this type of material, prepared by Dr. Mason. These observations have yielded no indication of any process beyond the separation of a single, rather amorphous chromatin body into two. The process appears at present to be a simplified form of mitosis in a simplified nucleus, consisting of the splitting of a single chromosome free within the cytoplasm. The beautifully systematic cytologic studies of Young and Fitz-James (1959a,b,c) are consistent with this general picture. However, bacterial cytology is not a closed subject, and further study may still reveal the existence of an interphase form, a nuclear membrane and sap, spindle fibers, or other structures.

Now, does this structure behave like a free chromosome or like a nucleus?

A nuclear body consisting of more than a chromosome should probably be the site of DNA synthesis. This point has not received significant study up to now. The isolation procedure for the Kornberg enzyme (Lehman, Bessman, Simms, and Kornberg, 1958) involves a first precipitation with streptomycin, which probably represents initial isolation of the enzyme in association with the DNA. Whether the association is direct might be determined with the aid of deoxyribonuclease treatment of isolated nuclear bodies. An indirect attachment would signify that both are joined by a common nuclear structure, while direct attachment could be ascribed to enzyme-substrate affinity.

A nuclear body consisting of more than a chromosome should be the locus of production of the material involved in transfer of genetic information to the rest of the cell. In the bacterial case, the experiments of Riley, Pardee, Jacob, and Monod (1960) tempt one to think that the protein itself may be made at the chromatin. However, much evidence has been collected in favor of RNA as the messenger from the nucleus to the cytoplasm, and ribosomes in the cytoplasm as the primary site of protein synthesis.

Attempts have been under way for some time to relate the nucleus to the sites of RNA synthesis, and to discover evidence for nucleo-cytoplasmic transfer of RNA in bacteria. Caro and Forro (1960) demonstrated that labeling with tritiated uridine for short periods produced a concentration of label in the central thin slices of *E. coli*. Longer incubation yielded random label distribution.

Another approach (Ezekiel, 1959) is the study of the putative enzyme of RNA synthesis, the polynucleotide phosphorylase. This enzyme is readily demonstrated in *B. megaterium* strain KM by formation of precipitable polyadenylate. Table 1 indicates that the isolated lipase-liberated nuclear body contains some enzyme, but the enzyme is present at a lower specific activity than in the lysate as a whole. It would be interesting to recheck this finding with

TABLE 1

Polyribotide Phosphorylase in Nuclear Preparations

Sample	Enzyme/protein
Whole protoplast lysate	18
Once-washed nuclei	10
Twice-washed nuclei	7
Thrice-washed nuclei	6

preparations which had not had the long incubation required for lysozyme and lipase treatments.

A third approach to the problem of nuclear RNA synthesis is the direct demonstration of biosynthesis *in vitro*. To reduce the probability of false positive results, these experiments were done with the aid of radioactive label, and so designed that minute increases, such as might be obtained by low levels of contamination with intact cells or protoplasts, would not be seen. To this end, and to maximize the supply of nutrients, all labels used were diluted with suitable quantities of the unlabeled precursor. Trials under a variety of conditions led to negative results, indicating no synthesis of DNA, RNA, and protein *in vitro*, in experiments with detection levels of 0.1 to 1 per cent net increase in three hours. Table 2 shows that the amount of label detected at the end of the experiment was no greater than at the beginning.

A fourth approach, more in keeping with the complexities of the system, and our present state of knowledge, consisted of labeling the intact cells or protoplasts and examining the label content of fractions isolated thereafter. First attempts in this direction, with P^{32}-phosphate, were uninterpretable because of the wide distribution of label. Then whole cell labeling with uridine-C^{14} was done, in pulse experiments, with isolation of nuclear bodies after various intervals. These experiments showed no difference between the nuclear bodies and the rest of the cell, in the label distribution with

TABLE 2

In Vitro *Synthesis by Nuclear Preparations*

		Label, calculated as μg. of nucleic acid or protein/sample	
Substance	μg.	0 Hours	3 Hours
DNA (thymidine-H^3)	75	0.33	0.29
RNA (uridine-C^{14})	95	0.06	0.01
Protein (leucine-C^{14})	267	0.03	0.03

time. However, the long incubation times referred to before, necessary to obtain the nuclear body preparations, were regarded as a serious limitation on interpretation of these experiments. A heavily labeled RNA fraction present in the nucleus in intact cells might easily have been lost by the time the nuclear bodies were spun down some three hours later.

Therefore, the same type of experiment was undertaken, with uridine or guanine labeling of growing protoplasts and with an arbitrarily developed fractionation based on the method of osmotic shocking (Ezekiel, 1960). By this means it was possible to get a look at the label in the RNA in cell fragment preparations which had not had any warm incubation time after the time of interest. The fractionation used is illustrated in Figure 1. Protoplasts were broken by osmotic shock with cold buffer (0.01 M Mg^{++}) and immediately spun seven minutes at 20,000 × g (middle of tube). The supernatant obtained was subdivided in the ultracentrifuge into ribosomes and an ultracentrifugal supernatant. Meanwhile, the

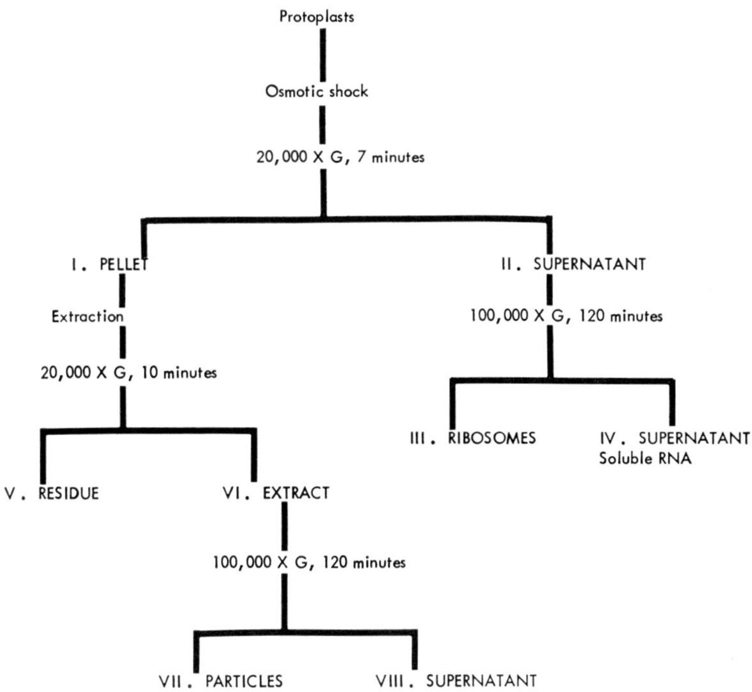

FIG. 1. Outline of the preparation of cell fractions. (From Ezekiel, 1960.)

20,000 × g pellet fraction was extracted with cold buffer (0.01 M tris—0.01 M $MgCl_2$–0.005 M NaN_3), and the extract again fractionated by ultracentrifugation. We will discuss primarily the residue (V) and extract (VI) fractions derived from the osmotic shock pellet.

The composition of the fractions described is indicated in Table 3. Some 22 per cent of the RNA is found in the pellet fraction, which also contains the bulk of the DNA. This fraction presumably consists of nuclear objects, cell membranes, and any other large organelles. When this fraction is extracted with cold buffer, the DNA and a rather small fraction of the RNA are removed. Most of the extracted nucleic acids are found in ultracentrifugal particles. After guanine labeling for two minutes, the radioactivity in nucleic acid is distributed as shown in the table. The most actively labeled samples are the extract fractions.

TABLE 3

Composition and Guanine Labeling of Subcellular Fractions

Fraction*		DNA µg.	RNA µg.	Protein µg.	c.p.m.†	Specific activity (c.p.m./µg. of RNA)
Pellet	I	265	348	1,020	1,580	4.5
Supernatant	II	44	1,080	2,900	2,010	1.9
Ribosomes	III	44	846	1,210	1,250	1.5
Soluble RNA	IV	4	198	3,580	550	2.8
No deoxyribonuclease:						
Extract particles	VII	209	91	167	726	8.0
Extract supernatant	VIII	42	3	278	56	19
Residue	V	9	246	542	660	2.7
Deoxyribonuclease:						
Extract particles	VII	0	83	247	467	5.6
Extract supernatant	VIII	3	2	600	112	56

* Numerals refer to fractions identified in Figure 1.
† Labeling of the hot acid extract with guanine during two minutes of protoplast growth. Note that both RNA and DNA would be labeled.

Figure 2 describes a uridine-C^{14} "pulse" experiment. The extract fraction exhibits turnover of one third to two thirds of its RNA.

Thus, the earlier, negative results on nucleocytoplasmic RNA transfer were invalidated by the finding of RNA fractions which exhibited rapid labeling and turnover and which were associated with large particles and easily extracted away from them. A nuclear precursor of ribosomes, or a nuclear "messenger RNA," would be expected to behave in this fashion, and would have probably been missed in the earlier experiments, because of extraction and perhaps turnover during lipase treatment.

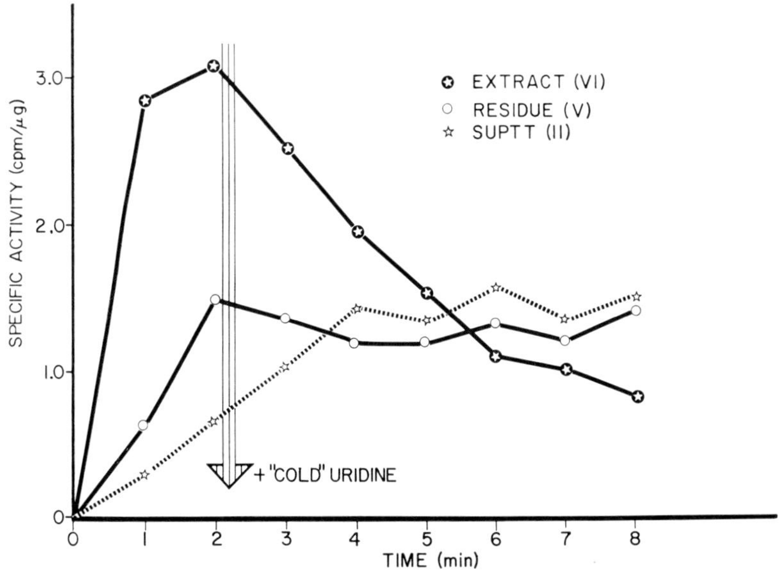

FIG. 2. Disappearance of label from the extract fraction in growing protoplasts, following a two minute pulse of uridine-2-C^{14}. (From Ezekiel, 1960.)

It might be supposed that the extracted RNA fractions are closely associated with the DNA molecule itself, perhaps forming the much sought after double or triple helix of DNA with RNA. This is unlikely, since the RNA and label content of the various fractions (including the ultracentrifugal particles in the extract) are not grossly altered by removal of the DNA with deoxyribonuclease at an early stage of fractionation.

In principle, this line of experiments opens many possibilities; however, localization of these fractions depends on the kind of clean and rapid fractionation which can only come with further characterization of the nuclear structure.

A fifth approach to the problem (Ezekiel, 1961) developed from the observation illustrated in Table 4. The presence of chloramphenicol during biosynthesis in protoplasts leads to gross inhibition of RNA increase in the supernatant fraction, and a great piling up of RNA in the material remaining in the cell membrane-nuclear body fraction after aqueous extraction. The effect is slightly more marked with chloramphenicol at the level of 500 μg./ml. than at 20 μg./ml. It was hypothesized that the RNA pile-up might be located either in the nuclear bodies or in the cell membranes. This

TABLE 4

Growth of Residue Fraction in Chloramphenicol

Sample	RNA μg.	Protein μg.
Residue:		
0 Minute	344	833
90 Minutes	469	970
90 Minutes, chloramphenicol	822	1,132
Extract:		
0 Minute	75	117
90 Minutes	280	342
90 Minutes, chloramphenicol	139	159
Supernatant:		
0 Minute	1,220	3,765
90 Minutes	1,970	5,480
90 Minutes, chloramphenicol	1,377	3,515

point was tested directly, by fractionating whole cells or protoplasts after chloramphenicol treatment. The chloramphenicol RNA is found largely in the lipase nuclear bodies (Table 5). Gentle washing does not remove it. When cell membranes are prepared by the conventional osmotic shock procedure, the increment in RNA is found (Table 6) largely in the supernatant fraction and the first wash of the membrane preparation. Obviously, the RNA in question is not tightly bound to cell membranes, and osmotic shocking and washing leads to its dispersal under these conditions, which also disperse the chromatin body.

Measurement of uridine incorporation during chloramphenicol treatment indicated a more complicated situation than simple nuclear pile-up, and complete cytoplasmic inhibition. The label

TABLE 5

Growth of Nuclear Fraction in Chloramphenicol

Sample	DNA μg.	RNA μg.	Protein μg.
Nuclei:			
0 Minute	103	44	284
60 Minutes	329	132	432
60 Minutes, chloramphenicol	286	338	262
Wash:			
0 Minute	20	29	67
60 Minutes	81	77	219
60 Minutes, chloramphenicol	14	16	54
Supernatant:			
0 Minute	54	1,390	...
60 Minutes	42	2,940	...
60 Minutes, chloramphenicol	17	1,570	...

TABLE 6

Growth of Membrane Fraction in Chloramphenicol

Sample	RNA µg.	Protein µg.
Membranes:		
0 Minute	157	700
90 Minutes	100	667
90 Minutes, chloramphenicol	174	634
Wash:		
0 Minute	93	160
90 Minutes	124	267
90 Minutes, chloramphenicol	294	227
Supernatant:		
0 Minute	1,660	4,670
90 Minutes	2,610	6,330
90 Minutes, chloramphenicol	1,980	4,250

distribution between complete cell membrane-nuclear body fraction and supernatant during the first few minutes of labeling is not affected by addition of chloramphenicol even though the chloramphenicol is added 20 minutes earlier. Over long incubation periods, the differential pile-up of label in the nuclear fraction, prepared in either manner, is less marked than the differential pile-up of total RNA. However, nuclear labeling is still quite disproportionate, amounting to about half the total label intake.

The question again arose, whether the RNA now under discussion is directly associated with DNA. As in the previous case, its attachment to large particles is not affected by removal of the DNA with deoxyribonuclease, or by extraction of the DNA with buffer.

Most effects of chloramphenicol can be explained as secondary consequences of inhibition of protein synthesis. However, any new effect on RNA metabolism is automatically subject to the interpretation that it is the cause rather than an effect of inhibition of protein synthesis. Evidence on this point can be obtained by finding out whether the inhibition of protein synthesis, by means that we understand, causes the same change in RNA behavior. In other words, one may find out whether the effect is special to chloramphenicol or a normal consequence of inhibition of protein synthesis. Tests of this point must include two classes of inhibitory situations. First, there are other inhibitors which permit appreciable RNA synthesis and very little protein synthesis. Unfortunately, none of these, at least in *Bacillus*, functions in a known manner at the level of amino acid metabolism. Second, there are inhibitors or physiological or genetic situations which essentially inhibit both protein and

RNA synthesis.

In the first case, the reagents tested have included the tetracyclines Aureomycin and Terramycin, both at levels of 5 μg./ml. As seen in Table 7, the effects on DNA, RNA, and protein syntheses are similar to that of chloramphenicol. The effects on nuclear and cytoplasmic RNA metabolism are also similar to those of chloramphenicol (Table 8). There are the same marked nuclear pile-up, and gross inhibition of cytoplasmic increase.

TABLE 7

Cellular Synthesis in Chloramphenicol and Tetracyclines

Sample	Time minutes	DNA μg.	RNA μg.	Protein μg.
Control	0	181	965	3,650
Control	65	387	2,430	7,570
Chloramphenicol	65	246	1,816	2,705
Aureomycin	65	251	1,964	3,346
Terramycin	65	256	2,005	3,204

TABLE 8

Accumulation of RNA in Lipase Nuclear Bodies During Incubation of Whole Cells in Presence of Tetracyclines

Sample	Time minutes	μg. of RNA	
		Nuclei	Supernatant
Control	0	45	635
Control	65	143	1,790
Chloramphenicol	65	450	856
Aureomycin	65	474	899
Terramycin	65	535	938

Recent data on azaguanine indicate that the same effects can be obtained with this reagent at 15 μg./ml. It is clear that the action of all the available reagents which inhibit protein synthesis but permit RNA synthesis is the same in this respect.

The second case, that of reagents or situations which interfere with protein synthesis in a known way, but also interfere with RNA synthesis, is also under examination. Table 9 illustrates the cases of samples which were incubated, respectively, at room temperature instead of 37°C to slow down metabolism in general; or in a sulphur-poor medium, in which growth was much slower; or in a medium in which the nitrogen source, glutamic acid, had been removed and replaced with ammonia. In each case, synthesis was

TABLE 9

Cellular Synthesis Under Adverse Conditions

Sample	Time minutes	DNA μg.	RNA μg.	Protein μg.
Control	0	150	368	2,325
Room temperature	180	233	1,082	3,635
S-poor	180	309	988	3,320
N-poor	180	269	920	4,680
Control	120	488	2,803	9,600

slow, but some RNA and protein were still made, and analogous experiments have been performed with 7-azatryptophan at 1 mg./ml., in which synthesis is depressed even more. The results shown in Table 10 are typical of the somewhat limited data obtained so far. There is no preferential pile-up of RNA in the nuclear samples. In the one case where substantial increase in RNA had occurred, the sulphur-starved sample, there was a large increase in DNA, and the increase in nuclear RNA is hardly more than proportional.

TABLE 10

RNA in Lipase Nuclear Bodies After Growth of Whole Cells Under Adverse Conditions

Sample	Time minutes	μg. of RNA	
		Nuclei	Supernatant
Zero-time	0	26	213
Room temperature	180	42	642
S-poor	180	85	559
N-poor	180	38	581
Control	120	117	1,946

There is a rather general correlation, then, of rapid RNA synthesis occurring in the absence of major protein synthesis, with nuclear pile-up of RNA and inhibition of cytoplasmic RNA increase, in each case tested—the tetracyclines, chloramphenicol, and azaguanine. When little or no RNA synthesis occurs, as with 7-azatryptophan or nutritional deprivations, RNA seems to be distributed in the normal fashion.

Nomura and Watson (1959) recently reported that most of the RNA of *E. coli* in chloramphenicol is found in a new class of ribosomes. These particles are small (15 S), and have a lower protein content than normal ribosomes. More recently, Otaka (1960) has reported on the distribution of RNA in *Bacillus cereus* in the presence of azaguanine; while the 15 S particle was not seen, ribosomes of low protein content were produced. The azaguanine-substituted RNA was not recovered in phenol extracts. The RNA fractions described by these workers are very probably the same ones recovered in the nuclear fraction.

The relation of this RNA to the bacterial nucleus is bolstered by the observation of Perry (1961) that RNA labeling in HeLa cells treated with azaguanine is limited to the nucleus. It would be interesting to know about the size and nature of ribosomes in his material.

The formation of new ribosomes would be likely to involve new protein synthesis. Examination of the amino acid labeling of nuclear fractions during drug treatment is contemplated.

The RNA is apparently not attached directly by means of the DNA, since DNA removal leaves the RNA still centrifugable in large particles. We may, therefore, suppose that it is dispersed in the chromatin, attached to polyamines or proteins. However, Kellenberger (1960) argues that the electron-lightness of the chromatin indicates that there is little or no RNA in it; furthermore, there is no difference in the fine structure of the chromatin seen after chloramphenicol or tetracycline treatment.

Another logical place for the piled-up RNA is the hole at the center of the chromatin ring obtained with chloramphenicol or tetracycline treatment. However, one looks in vain for a special concentration of ribosomes in this region in the electron micrographs. Fitz-James (1960) has recently described in some detail a structure called mesosome, which is a ramification of the cell membrane and is attached to the chromatin as well as the cell membrane. This structure seems most likely to serve as a mitochondrial equivalent, but it might also be the site of the RNA pile-up. Similarly, the poly-β-hydroxbutyrate granules present in close proximity to the chromatin might serve as a connection between chromatin and a ribosomal aggregate. These structures at least remind us that the cytology of bacteria is still young, and a missing structure may yet be found.

Nevertheless, it is rather surprising that the electron micrographs of chloramphenicol-treated cells have not yielded an immediate answer; one third of the RNA can be recovered in the nuclear fraction, and one would expect that even a simple stain with a basic dye might exhibit the difference in structure.

What is the mode of action of the reagents which inhibit protein but not RNA synthesis? We can guess that the well-known incorporation of azaguanine into RNA is primary to its action. Similarly,

Mandel and Borek (1961) have analyzed the case of a specific methionine mutant of *E. coli* which permits RNA synthesis to continue without protein synthesis. They find complete abolition of the incorporation of methylated bases into the new RNA. Again an altered RNA enters the picture. However, one may reasonably assume in this case that the inhibition of protein synthesis is directly caused by methionine deprivation.

Chloramphenicol and tetracyclines may conceivably combine directly with the RNA, and attach it to the nuclear body. This could be checked readily with radioactive drugs.

In summary, we know that RNA is produced in the center of the cell, and that some RNA is found in the form of rapidly labeled material which turns over rapidly and is readily extractable from large particles. Treatment with drugs which permit RNA synthesis but inhibit protein synthesis results in accumulation of RNA in nuclear fractions, and not in cytoplasmic fractions.

The bacterial chromatin is probably part of a larger nuclear structure, which is probably a major site of RNA synthesis.

During the last year, several groups of investigators have furnished convincing evidence that one small class of RNA, which presumably serves as "messenger," is synthesized in association with the DNA.

It seems probable that the nuclear pile-up described here represents accumulation of "ribosomal" RNA, through altered ribosome biosynthesis, rather than accumulation of the "messenger," but confirmation will require measurement of the base ratios. It is tempting to speculate that "uninformed" ribosomes may be synthesized at a nucleolar organelle, still unrecognized.

ACKNOWLEDGMENTS

The first portion of the work described formed part of a doctoral dissertation performed under the guidance of Dr. S. Spiegelman.

Parts of this work have been supported by Atomic Energy Commission contract AT-(40-1)-2139 and by a grant from the National Science Foundation. The author wishes to acknowledge the financial support of a Rosalie B. Hite Postdoctoral Fellowship from 1957 to 1959.

The capable technical assistance of Mrs. David G. Young and Miss Deanna Emerson is gratefully acknowledged.

REFERENCES

Caro, L. G., and F. Forro, Jr. 1960. Sites of RNA Synthesis in *Escherichia coli.* (Abstract) *Fourth Annual Meeting of the Biophysical Society*, p. 21. Philadelphia, Pennsylvania.

Chapman, G. P. 1959. Electron Microscopy of Ultrathin Sections of Bacteria. III. Cell Wall, Cytoplasmic Membrane, and Nuclear Material. *Journal of Bacteriology*, 78:96–104.

Ezekiel, D. H. 1959. *A Study of the Biosynthetic Capabilities of Isolated Bacterial Nuclear Bodies.* Ph.D. Dissertation. University of Illinois, Urbana, Illinois.

———. 1960. Rapidly Labeled Fractions of Ribonucleic Acid in *Bacillus megaterium. Journal of Bacteriology*, 80:119–130.

———. 1961. Increase in Ribonucleic Acid in the Bacterial Chromatin Body During Chloramphenicol Treatment. *Journal of Bacteriology*, 81:319–326.

Fitz-James, P. C. 1960. Participation of the Cytoplasmic Membrane in the Growth and Spore Formation of Bacilli. *The Journal of Biophysical and Biochemical Cytology*, 8:507–528.

Forro, F., Jr., and C. E. Finch. 1961. DNA Organization and Replication in *Bacillus subtilis.* (Abstract) *Fifth Annual Meeting of the Biophysical Society.* St. Louis, Missouri.

Kellenberger, E. 1960. "The Physical State of the Bacterial Nucleus," *Microbial Genetics* (10th Symposium of the Society for General Microbiology), pp. 39–66. Cambridge, England: Cambridge University Press.

Kellenberger, E., A. Ryter, and J. Séchaud. 1958. Electron Microscope Study of DNA-Containing Plasms. II. Vegetative and Mature Phage DNA as Compared with Normal Bacterial Nucleoids in Different Physiological States. *The Journal of Biophysical and Biochemical Cytology*, 4:671–678.

Lehman, I. R., M. J. Bessman, E. S. Simms, and A. Kornberg. 1958. Enzymatic Synthesis of Deoxyribonucleic Acid. I. Preparation of Substrates and Partial Purification of an Enzyme from *Escherichia coli. Journal of Biological Chemistry*, 233:163–170.

Mandel, L. R., and E. Borek. 1961. Variability in the Structure of Ribonucleic Acid. *Biochemical and Biophysical Research Communications*, 4:14–18.

Mason, D. J., and D. M. Powelson. 1956. Nuclear Division as Observed in Live Bacteria by a New Technique. *Journal of Bacteriology*, 71:474–479.

Murray, R. G. E. 1960. "The Internal Structure of the Cell," *The Bacteria*, I. C. Gunsalus and R. Y. Stanier, Eds., Vol. 1, pp. 35–96. New York, New York: Academic Press, Inc.

Nomura, M., and J. D. Watson. 1959. Ribonucleoprotein Particles Within Chloramphenicol-Inhibited *Escherichia coli. Journal of Molecular Biology*, 1:204–217.

Otaka, E. 1960. Effect of 8-Azaguanine on Ribonucleic Acid and Protein Synthesis in *Bacillus cereus*, NCTC 569. *Experimental Cell Research*, 21:229–232.

Perry, R. P. 1961. The Effect of Azaguanine on the Incorporation of Cytidine into Nuclear and Cytoplasmic RNA. (Abstract) *Fifth Annual Meeting of the Biophysical Society.* St. Louis, Missouri.

Riley, M., A. B. Pardee, F. Jacob, and J. Monod. 1960. On the Expression of a Structural Gene. *Journal of Molecular Biology*, 2:216–225.

Spiegelman, S., A. I. Aronson, and P. C. Fitz-James. 1958. Isolation and

Characterization of Nuclear Bodies from Protoplasts of *Bacillus megaterium*. *Journal of Bacteriology*, 75:102–117.

Young, I. E., and P. C. Fitz-James. 1959a. Chemical and Morphological Studies of Bacterial Spore Formation. I. The Formation of Spores in *Bacillus cereus*. *The Journal of Biophysical and Biochemical Cytology*, 6:467–482.

———. 1959b. Chemical and Morphological Studies of Bacterial Spore Formation. II. Spore and Parasporal Protein Formation in *Bacillus cereus* var. *alesti*. *The Journal of Biophysical and Biochemical Cytology*, 6:483–498.

———. 1959c. Chemical and Morphological Studies of Bacterial Spore Formation. III. The Effect of 8-Azaguanine on Spore and Parasporal Protein Formation in *Bacillus cereus* var. *alesti*. *The Journal of Biophysical and Biochemical Cytology*, 6:499–506.

Physicochemical Studies on Mammalian Ribonucleoproteins

MARY L. PETERMANN, PH.D.

Division of Nucleoprotein Chemistry,
Sloan-Kettering Institute for Cancer Research, and
Sloan-Kettering Division, Cornell University Medical College,
New York, New York

Somewhere on the surface of the cytoplasmic ribonucleoprotein particles (RNP, or ribosomes) are the sites where amino acids are linked into polypeptide chains, and also the genetic information controlling the order of this assembly. Thus a knowledge of the surface properties of RNP is essential to our understanding of protein synthesis, both normal and malignant. One of the most interesting properties of this surface, and presumably of the ribonucleic acid (RNA) embedded in it, is the ability to bind many substances. In this paper I shall discuss the binding of water, magnesium, and proteins, and indulge in some speculation as to the significance of this binding.

HYDRATION

Some of the physical properties of purified mammalian ribonucleoprotein (RNP) particles are shown in Table 1. A small spherical virus is included for comparison. The sedimentation coefficients of these RNP particles (at infinite dilution) are in good agreement, ranging from 78 S to 83 S. Similar values have been found for RNP particles from a number of plant and bacterial sources, with the exception of *Escherichia coli*, which shows 69 S (Petermann and Hamilton, 1961, for summary). The molecular weights are close to 4×10^6. The shapes of the dried particles, as seen in the electron microscope, are roughly spherical. In solution, also, the particles are nearly spherical, as shown by light scattering (Hamilton, 1960) and x-ray scattering (Dibble and Dintzis, 1960). Their solutions show an unusually high viscosity, however, and pronounced concentration-dependence of their sedimentation coefficients. Since these properties cannot be attributed to elongated shape, they have generally been ascribed to hydration; the calculated amounts of water bound/Gm. of RNP range from 2.6 to 4 Gm./Gm. of dry weight. The structure of the particle in solution may be that of a gel, but it is tempting to speculate on the presence of a highly irregular surface, with cavities where amino acids assemble, on RNA templates, into polypeptide chains. Anfinsen (1961) has raised the question of whether the amino acid sequence determines the coiling of the polypeptide chain into the completed protein, or whether additional genetic information may be necessary to direct the coiling. I suggest that such additional genetic information might reside in the shape of these cavities. Their topography might determine the proximity of the various sulfhydryl groups on the cysteine residues, so that, in a hypothetical protein, cysteine 1 would always link with cysteine 4, for example, and never with cysteine 2 or 3.

Magnesium

In addition to the 80 S component, a number of other components have been noted in ultracentrifugal patterns of RNP particles. The sedimentation coefficients for some mammalian RNP particles are shown in Table 2; other RNP particles show similar patterns. The 110 S component probably represents two 80 S particles in association (Petermann, Hamilton, and Mizen, 1954). The various slower components represent dissociation products, which are still nucleoproteins, with the same proportions of RNA and protein as the 80 S unit (Ts'o and Vinograd, 1961). If the 27 S piece, of molecular weight 0.6 to 0.7×10^6, is considered to be the basic unit, as suggested by Ts'o, Bonner, and Vinograd (1958), then the 80 S particle could be six units, 55 S could be three, and 40 to 46 S could be two. The 60 to 65 S units will be discussed below.

Since it was shown by Chao (1957) that dibasic metals, particularly magnesium, were essential to the stability of 80 S RNP, most workers have included magnesium in their preparative media, and have found that the association-dissociation reactions can be

TABLE 1

Physical Properties of Mammalian Ribonucleoproteins

Source	$s_{20,w}$ (S)	Viscosity (dl./Gm.)	Partial specific volume	Molecular weight, $\times 10^{-6}$	Hydration (Gm./Gm.)	References
Southern bean mosaic virus	115–5.3C*	4	0.70	11.6	0.83	Miller and Price (1946).
Rabbit reticulocytes	78	8	0.63	4.1†	2.6†	Dintzis, Borsook, and Vinograd (1958).
				4.0‡		
				4.0§	2.7§	Dibble and Dintzis (1960).
Rabbit liver	80					Takanami (1960).
Calf liver	81.3–14.9C*					Sherman and Petermann (1961).
Rat liver	83.0–18.4C*	12	0.66	3.6‡	ca. 4	Hamilton and Petermann (1959); Hamilton (1960).
Novikoff hepatoma	79–15C*	9.8	0.67	4.1‖		Kuff and Zeigel (1960).
Jensen sarcoma	82.5–23.8C*					Petermann (1960b).

* C=concentration in grams per deciliter, † From sedimentation and viscosity, ‡ From light scattering, § From X-ray scattering, ‖ From electron microscopy.

TABLE 2

Sedimentation Coefficients of Various Components of Mammalian Ribonucleoproteins

Source	$s_{20,w}$ (S)					References
Rabbit reticulocytes	120	78	50–60			Dintzis, Borsook and Vinograd (1958).
		78	58	40		Ts'o and Vinograd (1961).
Rabbit liver	120	80	60	40		Takanami (1960).
Rat liver	140,110	83	63	50,46	30	Hamilton and Petermann (1959).
Novikoff hepatoma	135,113	79	64	56,46	28	Kuff and Zeigel (1960).
Jensen sarcoma	122,110	83	65	55,40	27	Petermann (1960b).

produced at will by regulating magnesium content of the solvent.

With highly purified RNP from Jensen sarcoma, a rat tumor, it has been possible to correlate these association-dissociation reactions with changes in the amount of magnesium bound by the RNP (Petermann, 1960b). Bound magnesium is conveniently expressed as equivalents/mole of RNA phosphorus (r). When sarcoma RNP was freshly prepared at pH 7.0 in 0.001 M phosphate buffer containing 0.0005 M $MgCl_2$, it was chiefly in the 83 S form, with small amounts of 122 S and 65 S; r = 0.53. After dialysis for five days against similar buffers, containing 0.0001 to 0.0007 M $MgCl_2$, it remained in the 83 S form, with r ranging from 0.46 to 0.61. In 0.002 M $MgCl_2$ (r = 0.72), some association to 122 S occurred, but the chief effect was the formation of rapidly sedimenting aggregates. After dialysis against buffers of ionic strength 0.10, at pH 7.0 or 8.0, containing different concentrations of magnesium, a variety of ultracentrifugal patterns were obtained, as shown in Figure 1.

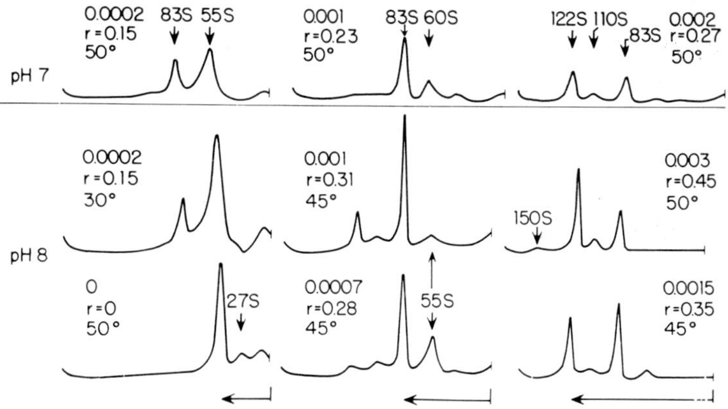

FIG. 1. Ultracentrifugal patterns of solutions containing highly purified sarcoma RNP, dialyzed for five days against buffers at ionic strength 0.10, with molarities of $MgCl_2$, r values (equivalents of bound magnesium/mole of RNA phosphorus), and phaseplate angles, as shown. All at 3° to 9°C. Top row, in 0.001 M potassium phosphate and 0.091 to 0.096 M KCl, at pH 7.0; middle and bottom rows, in 0.02 M $KHCO_3$ and 0.071 to 0.080 M KCl, at pH 8.0.

At pH 7.0 and 0.001 M $MgCl_2$ the RNP remained chiefly in the 83 S form, although r was reduced to 0.23. At lower magnesium concentrations dissociation occurred, and dialysis against magnesium-free buffer removed all the magnesium and converted the RNP to the 55 S or slower forms. In 0.002 M $MgCl_2$ (r = 0.27), there was some association to 122 S form, and further aggregation to rapidly sedimenting particles (not shown).

At pH 8.0 and 0.001 M $MgCl_2$, the RNP remained chiefly in the 83 S form, with r = 0.31. In buffers of lower magnesium content, it dissociated to the 55 S or slower forms. In buffers of high magnesium content the RNP was more soluble than at pH 7.0; marked association to 122 S occurred and traces of 150 S appeared. Aggregation occurred above 0.004 M $MgCl_2$ (r = 0.5 or more). Patterns obtained on RNP dialyzed at pH 8.0 and ionic strength 0.20 resembled the patterns seen at pH 7.0 and ionic strength 0.10, except at the lowest magnesium concentration, where there was less dissociation.

Magnesium binding curves have been obtained in these four buffers. In 0.001 M phosphate at pH 7.0 the binding is tight, and r remains high as long as even a trace of free magnesium is present (Petermann, 1960b). At pH 7 and ionic strength 0.10 the binding is much weaker than at low ionic strength. At ionic strength 0.10 and pH 8 the binding curve is similar to that at pH 7, but steeper. Doubling the ionic strength, by the addition of KCl, decreases the magnesium binding by a factor of 2.5; this competition of monobasic ions and magnesium had previously been found for rat liver RNP (Hamilton and Petermann, 1959). The binding of magnesium by rabbit reticulocyte RNP has been studied by Edelman, Ts'o, and Vinograd (1960).

From the results of these studies, the responses of RNP to changes in its ionic environment appear to be complex. Since changes in pH and ionic strength have such a pronounced effect on the degree of magnesium binding, it is only by comparing RNP's at the same r values that other effects of pH and ionic strength can be evaluated. For example, consider an increase in the concentration of potassium. With the free magnesium kept constant, this leads to dissociation, through competition with magnesium for the binding sites. When bound magnesium is kept constant, however, increased potassium leads to aggregation, presumably by decreasing the electric charge on the RNP particle. Conversely, increased pH always leads to dissociation since it both reduces the magnesium binding and increases the electrical charge.

The minimal amount of magnesium necessary to maintain the 83 S form appears to be about 0.3 equivalent/mole of phosphorus. If the particle weight of 83 S is about 4,000,000, each unit would contain about 6,500 atoms of phosphorus, and about 1,000 atoms of magnesium.

Electrophoretic Mobility

The amount of magnesium bound also influences the electrophoretic mobility of RNP (Petermann, 1960b). As long as sarcoma RNP remained in the 83 S form, its mobility increased linearly as the bound magnesium decreased, presumably because phosphate groups were being uncovered. On dissociation to 55 S, however, the increase in electrical charge was partially offset by an increase in frictional drag of about 30 per cent.

Protein Binding

The studies described above were carried out on sarcoma RNP which had been purified by treatment with deoxycholate and washing with 0.001 M phosphate—0.0005 M $MgCl_2$ at pH 7. On moving-boundary electrophoresis at pH 8 and ionic strength 0.1, it showed a single boundary; the structure had been stripped down to an RNP core, consisting of 50 per cent RNA and 50 per cent protein (Petermann, 1960b). Sarcoma RNP, like that of other tumors (Kuff and Zeigel, 1960) can also be purified by sedimentation into 70 per cent sucrose at pH 8, and washing with the pH 7 phosphate buffer. (Pretreatment with bentonite prevents degradation by ribonuclease, as shown by Petermann and Pavlovec in 1961.) The product consists of the RNP core plus about 20 per cent of extraneous protein, much of which dissociates and can be washed away in buffer at pH 8 and ionic strength 0.1 (Petermann and Hamilton, 1961).

In order to learn more about this binding of extraneous proteins, a systematic study was undertaken (Petermann, 1960a). Sarcoma RNP was purified by the deoxycholate method (Petermann, 1960b). Its ability to bind human oxyhemoglobin was studied by the spectrophotometric determination of the oxyhemoglobin left in the supernatant after sedimentation of the complexes out of RNP-oxyhemoglobin mixtures. The RNP concentration was kept constant, at 1 mg./ml., while the total oxyhemoglobin concentrations ranged from 0.5 to 2.3 mg./ml. One mg. of RNP, chiefly in the 83 S form, could bind up to 0.7 mg. of oxyhemoglobin; in the 55 S form it bound even more. In calculating moles of oxyhemoglobin/mole of RNP the molecular weight of the oxyhemoglobin was taken as 67,000, and that of the RNP was assumed to be 4×10^6. Some of the binding curves are shown in Figure 2. When r, the moles of oxyhemoglobin/mole of RNP, is the abscissa, and r divided by f, the concentration of free oxyhemoglobin, is the ordinate, as was suggested by Scatchard (1949), a straight-line plot is obtained when electrostatic effects are absent and all the binding sites are of equal strength. Such lines can be extrapolated to $r/f = 0$ ($f =$ infinity), to give the total amount of oxyhemoglobin that could be bound at saturation, n. Extrapolation to $r = 0$ gives Kn; and K, a binding constant, can be calculated.

On the left side of Figure 2 are shown four such straight lines, obtained on RNP particles which were chiefly in the 83 S form. At pH 7 and ionic strength 0.004 the oxyhemoglobin is strongly bound; this tight binding agrees with common experience. At ionic strength 0.01 the binding is much weaker, and at 0.02 it is very weak. Binding is also dependent on temperature, being about one third as strong at 25°C as at 5°C. As long as the RNP remains in the 83 S

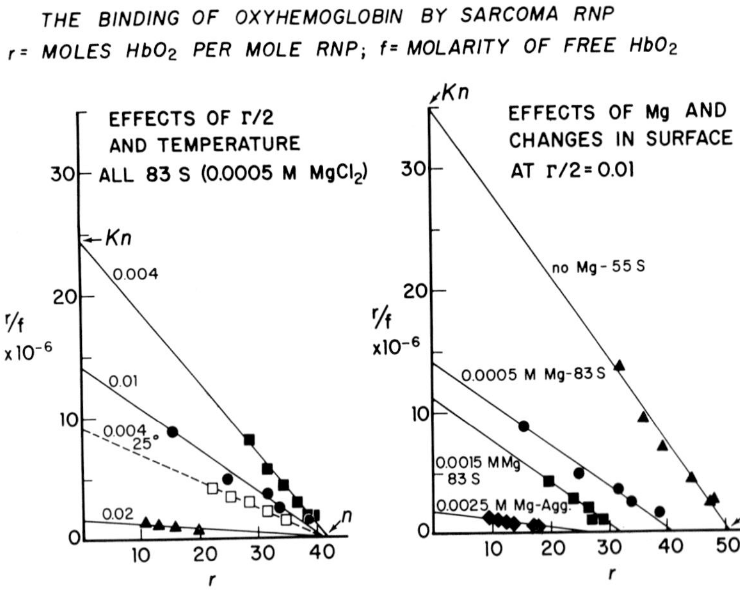

FIG. 2. The binding of oxyhemoglobin by RNP, in buffers containing 0.001 M potassium phosphate at pH 7.0; $n =$ amount bound at saturation; $K =$ binding constant (see text, page 570).

Left. The effects of ionic strength and temperature. The RNP was chiefly in the 83 S form. All buffers contained 0.0005 M $MgCl_2$. ■, □, no KCl; ●, 0.0065 M KCl; ▲, 0.0165 M KCl. Solid symbols, binding at 5° to 8°C; open symbols, at 25°C.

Right. The effect of magnesium binding and dissociation or association, at ionic strength 0.01. ▲, no $MgCl_2$ in the buffer, 0.008 M KCl, chiefly 55 S; ●, 0.0005 M $MgCl_2$, 0.0065 M KCl, chiefly 83 S; ■, 0.0015 M $MgCl_2$, 0.0035 M KCl, 83 S plus aggregated RNP; ◆, 0.0025 M $MgCl_2$, 0.0005 M KCl, chiefly aggregated RNP.

form, however, the curves can all be extrapolated to $n =$ about 42. At 0.01 ionic strength, the binding is markedly affected by pH, being much stronger at pH 6.6, and much weaker at pH 7.5 (Petermann and Hamilton, 1961; Kuff and Zeigel, 1960). The curves could still be extrapolated to $n = 42$, however, as long as the RNP was kept in the 83 S form.

At the right in Figure 2 are shown the effects of changes in magnesium binding, and the resulting dissociation or association of the RNP. Both K and n are affected. For RNP chiefly in the 55 S form, binding only 0.15 equivalents of Mg/mole of RNA phosphate, the binding is very strong, and n is increased to 50. Conversely, when the magnesium concentration of the buffer is increased so that the RNP contains a higher proportion of material sedimenting faster than 83 S, both K and n decrease.

In 14 experiments where reliable extrapolations could be made, and values of n varied from 26 to 56, an attempt was made to correlate n with the ultracentrifugal pattern. The ultracentrifugal components were divided into three classes: less than 83 S (55 S plus any slower material); 83 S; and greater than 83 S (110 S, 122 S, and aggregated RNP). An empirical equation, relating n to the percentage of RNP in each class, was worked out. Figure 3 shows the agreement between theoretical values of n, calculated from this equation, and experimental values.

From this equation it would appear that RNP in the 83 S form can bind 48 moles of oxyhemoglobin/unit of 4×10^6, while the 55 S form can bind 65 moles. This would involve an increase of about one third in the amount of surface available for binding. A further point of interest is that, as shown in Figure 2, the binding curves on 55 S RNP appear to be straight lines; this suggests that the newly exposed binding sites have the same strength as those on the surface of the 83 S particle.

In addition to magnesium and oxyhemoglobin, RNP binds basic substances of several types, all of which seem to compete for the same binding sites, presumably surface RNA. These include other dibasic metals, such as calcium and barium; monobasic metals, sodium and potassium; organic bases, such as streptomycin, polyamines, and basic dyes; and proteins, such as protamine, cytochrome (Petermann and Hamilton, 1961), and the lipoproteins of the endoplasmic reticulum. With dibasic metals, streptomycin, polyamines, protamine, and oxyhemoglobin, precipitation may occur. Spermidine can substitute for magnesium in preventing the

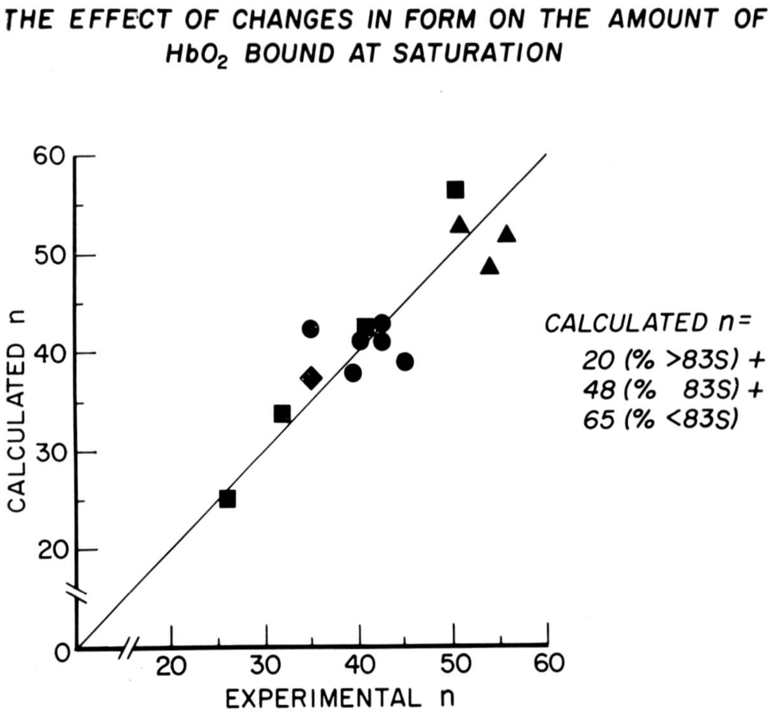

FIG. 3. The effect of association-dissociation reactions on the binding of oxyhemoglobin by RNP at saturation. Calculated n (amount bound at saturation) was obtained from the ultracentrifugal patterns, by the formula shown. ●, ▲, ◆, and ■ indicate ionic strengths of 0.004, 0.010, 0.015, and 0.020, respectively.

dissociation of *E. coli* ribosomes (Cohen and Lichtenstein, 1960).

This protein-binding property of RNP has caused confusion in studies of protein synthesis in two respects. First, when an RNP preparation does not seem to "require" activating enzymes, etc., for amino acid incorporation, it may already be binding them (Hoagland 1960; Nathans and Lipmann 1960; Petermann and Hamilton, 1961). Second, when the release of newly synthesized proteins is studied, careful controls are necessary to avoid confusion with randomly bound cellular constituents (Grabowski and Munro, 1960). The latent ribonuclease (RNase) of *E. coli* RNP (Elson, 1959) and the antibody released from rabbit lymph node RNP (Feldman, Elson, and Globerson, 1960), conversely, seem to have been integral parts of the RNP particle.

THE "65 S" COMPONENT

From the previous discussion it seems clear that the 55 S component of sarcoma RNP can be formed from 83 S by removing the magnesium, and probably represents particles half the size of 83 S. The situation is much less clear in regard to the 65 S component.

The occurrence of 60 to 65 S RNP has usually been correlated with rapid growth. Thus it was noted in extracts of chick embryo and of various tumors, by Kahler and Bryan (1943). In our early studies it was referred to as component C. Its concentration was increased in leukemic spleen (Petermann and Hamilton, 1952). It was high in the livers of normal female rats, and appeared to decline to the normal male level during pregnancy (Petermann and Hamilton, 1958). In regenerating liver its concentration increased during the period of most rapid growth, and then declined as the rate of growth decreased. It was very high in hepatic and other tumors (Petermann, Mizen, and Hamilton 1953, 1954, 1956). A similar component has been noted in proliferating yeast (Wolfe, 1956; Ashikawa, 1958; Koehler, 1961). Pea-seedlings, from whose RNP a 60 S component is readily obtained (Ts'o, Bonner, and Vinograd, 1958), are also a rapidly growing system. In *E. coli*, the concentration of 51 S is increased under conditions of rapid growth (Bowen, Dagley, and Sykes, 1959).

Our early observations on the 65 S component were made on crude RNP pellets suspended in buffer of ionic strength 0.1, at pH 8.5, with no added magnesium, and at room temperature. In our more recent studies of highly purified sarcoma RNP, however, as shown in Figure 1, only traces of 60 to 65 S were noted; the RNP dissociated chiefly to 55 S. We are now investigating the conditions under which the 65 S component can best be observed (Petermann, 1961). The pH has been kept at 8.5, and the ionic strength at 0.1. The variables have included the magnesium content of the buffer, the nature of the buffer salts, the temperature, and the purity and source of the RNP's used.

The effects of varying the magnesium concentration of the solvent are shown in Figure 4. Solutions containing 4 mg./ml. of RNP purified by sedimentation into sucrose, and still containing about 20 per cent of extraneous protein, in 0.001 M phosphate–0.0005 M $MgCl_2$, at pH 7.1, were dialyzed for three days, in the cold, against buffer containing 0.1 M $KHCO_3$ and various concentrations of $MgCl_2$. Aliquots were taken for RNA and magnesium analyses, and a sample of each was warmed to 25°C and examined in the analytical ultracentrifuge. Too little magnesium caused dissociation to 55 S, and too much preserved the 83 S form; the best yields of 65 S were obtained at intermediate concentrations. With this technique, the best concentration of free magnesium for the appearance of 65 S has proved to be 0.0015 M, which gives a bound magnesium of about 0.3 equivalent/mole of RNA phosphate. (This value, and those

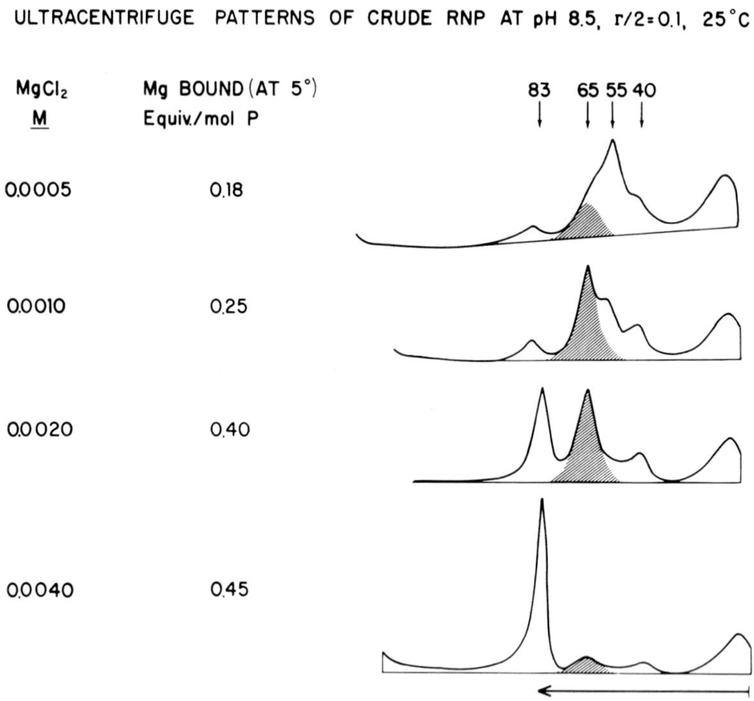

FIG. 4. The effect of magnesium on ultracentrifugal patterns of partially purified RNP. The solutions contained 0.1 M $KHCO_3$ and various concentrations of $MgCl_2$, as shown at the left. The sedimentation coefficients of the various RNP components are shown above the vertical arrows.

shown in Figure 4, represent magnesium bound at 5°C, the temperature of dialysis, not at 25°C, the temperature in the ultracentrifuge.) A recent, and better procedure, has involved the dialysis of the RNP against 0.1 M $KHCO_3$, 0.003 M $MgCl_2$, pH 8.5, for three days at 5°C. The RNP remains in the 83 S form. The sample is then transferred to a dialysis bag, 20/32 inches in diameter, with a 0.5 in. test tube inside it, to give a high ratio of surface to volume (Craig,

King, and Stracher, 1957). The solution is then dialyzed for three hours, at room temperature, on a stirrer, against bicarbonate containing 0.002 M $MgCl_2$. Under these conditions bound magnesium remains high, over 0.4 equivalents/mole of RNA phosphorus, and a sharper 65 S boundary is obtained in the ultracentrifuge.

The effect of temperature on the amount of 65 S is shown in Figure 5. The patterns on the left side of the figure were obtained on RNP which had been partially purified by layering over sucrose.

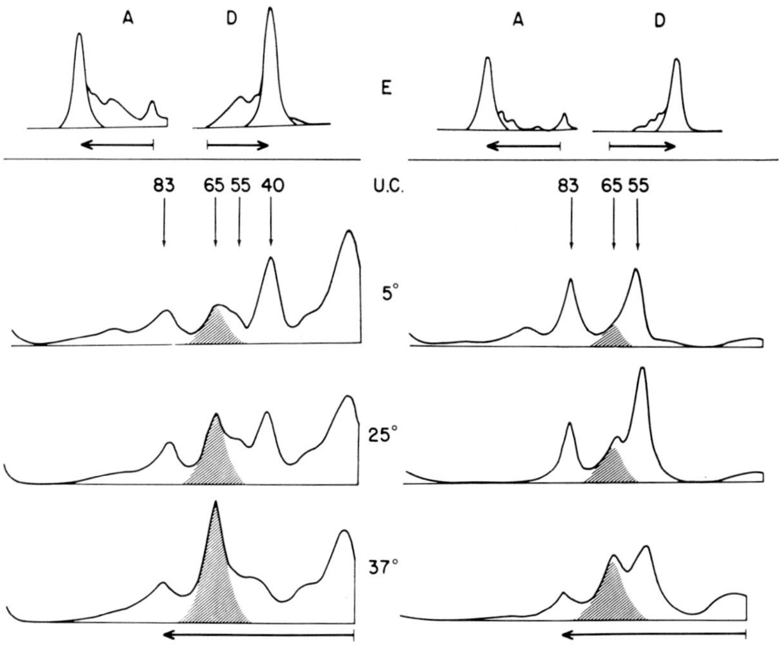

FIG. 5. The effects of purity and temperature on the 65 S component. Left, RNP prepared by layering over sucrose (see text), containing about 30 per cent extraneous protein. Right, RNP prepared by deoxycholate treatment (see text, page 569), containing about 15 per cent extraneous protein. Both in 0.1 M $KHCO_3$ plus 0.0015 M $MgCl_2$, at pH 8.5. Top row, electrophoretic patterns, at 0.4°C. Lower rows, ultracentrifugal patterns, at 5°, 25°, and 37°C. The sedimentation coefficients of the various RNP components are shown above the vertical arrows.

It still contained about 30 per cent of extraneous protein, as shown by the electrophoretic patterns. The ultracentrifugal analysis at 5°C also shows a lot of dissociated protein, in the form of large, slow-moving boundaries. The RNP appears as a large 40 S boundary, small amounts of 55 S and 65 S, a small 83 S boundary, and some faster material. At 25°C the 65 S boundary increased in size, at the expense of the 40 S boundary, with little change in the 83 S; at 37°C this process was carried even farther.

The patterns on the right side of Figure 5 were obtained on RNP which had been purified by layering followed by treatment with deoxycholate, but still contained 15 per cent of extraneous protein, as shown by the electrophoretic patterns. In the ultracentrifuge, at 5°C, it showed chiefly 83 S and 55 S, like the patterns in Figure 1; only a small amount of 65 S was present. At 25°C both 55 S and 65 S increased, at the expense of 83 S and faster material. At 37°C there was a further increase in 65 S, at the expense of 55 S as well as 83 S. Thus a similar temperature effect was obtained, although the total amounts of 65 S were less than for the cruder preparation.

Attempts have been made to reverse the effect of purification by adding back the extra protein. When the RNP was washed at pH 8 and ionic strength 0.2, restoration of the wash protein did increase the size of the 65 S boundary. Since the wash had been extensively dialyzed prior to concentration by lyophilizing, the material needed for 65 S appears to be nondialyzable.

The origin of the 65 S RNP is also of interest. In general, the mammalian tissues which show chiefly 80 S RNP are organs, such as liver and pancreas, which are not growing, but are engaged in the synthesis of protein for export (Petermann, Mizen, and Hamilton, 1956); in these organs the electron microscopists find most of the RNP particles attached to endoplasmic reticulum (Palade, 1955). Conversely, in the rapidly growing tissues, such as tumors, whose extracts show a high proportion of 65 S RNP, the electron microscopists find a large proportion of the particles not attached to reticulum (Howatson and Ham, 1955; Porter, 1955–1956). In an attempt to determine whether these free particles might be the origin of the 65 S, rat liver microsomes were separated into two fractions (Petermann *et al.*, 1958): a large microsome fraction, which should contain only large fragments of endoplasmic reticulum, and a small microsome fraction, which should also contain any free RNP particles. Although variations in pH, ionic strength, or magnesium concentration of the solvent gave an assortment of ultracentrifugal patterns on these fractions, there were always more of both 65 S and 45 S in the extracts of the small microsomes.

The question of the source of the 65 S has now been re-examined, under more carefully controlled conditions. Sarcoma extracts were sedimented into 70 per cent sucrose, and the "free" RNP, in the bottom layers, was separated from RNP attached to the microsomal membrane fragments, which remained in the middle of the tube. Both fractions were treated with deoxycholate and washed at pH 7. At pH 8.5, in 0.1 M $KHCO_3$–0.0015 M $MgCl_2$, the "free" RNP showed about 34 per cent 65 S at 25°C, and about 54 per cent 65 S at 37°C. The "attached" tumor RNP also showed 65 S, but a smaller percentage at both temperatures. Partially purified RNP from normal rat liver, which must have been derived chiefly from "attached" particles, showed about 29 per cent of 65 S at 25°C, and 43 per cent at 37°C (Hamilton, personal communication). Thus it appears that "attached" particles may form 65 S, but to a lesser extent than "free" particles.

Summary

The RNP of mammalian tissues is a complex molecule of molecular weight of about four million. It binds water, magnesium, and extra proteins strongly, and perhaps competitively. On removal of magnesium the RNP changes, in a complex fashion, to various forms with lower sedimentation coefficients.

ACKNOWLEDGMENTS

This investigation was supported by funds from the Atomic Energy Commission under contract AT(30-1)-910, and by Research Grant CY-3190 from the National Cancer Institute of the National Institutes of Health, United States Public Health Service.

The author wishes to express appreciation to Dr. Mary G. Hamilton for many helpful discussions, and to Miss Isabella Wright, Mrs. Amalia Pavlovec, Miss Rosemary Marciello, Mrs. Ellen Eliason, and Mrs. Barbara Burkholder for carrying out much of the experimental work.

REFERENCES

Anfinsen, C. B. 1961. The Influence of Three-Dimensional Configuration on the Chemical Reactivity and Stability of Proteins. *Journal of Polymer Science*, 49:31–49.

Ashikawa, J. K. 1958. "Ultracentrifugal Studies of Microsomes from Starving, Nonproliferating, and Proliferating Yeast," *Microsomal Particles and Protein Synthesis*, R. B. Roberts, Ed., pp. 76–83. Washington, D.C.: Washington Academy of Sciences.

Bowen, T. J., S. Dagley, and J. Sykes. 1959. A Ribonucleoprotein Component of *Escherichia coli*. *Biochemical Journal*, 72:419–425.

Chao, F.-C. 1957. Dissociation of Macromolecular Ribonucleoprotein of Yeast. *Archives of Biochemistry and Biophysics*, 70:426–431.

Cohen, S. S., and J. Lichtenstein. 1960. Polyamines and Ribosome Structure. *Journal of Biological Chemistry*, 235:2112–2116.

Craig, L. C., T. P. King, and A. Stracher. 1957. Dialysis Studies. II. Some Experiments Dealing with the Problem of Selectivity. *Journal of the American Chemical Society*, 79:3729–3737.

Dibble, W. E., and H. M. Dintzis. 1960. The Size and Hydration of Rabbit Reticulocyte Ribosomes. *Biochimica et biophysica acta*, 37:152–153.

Dintzis, H. M., H. Borsook, and J. Vinograd. 1958. "Microsomal Structure and Hemoglobin Synthesis in the Rabbit Reticulocyte," *Microsomal Particles and Protein Synthesis*, R. B. Roberts, Ed., pp. 95–99. Washington, D.C.: Washington Academy of Sciences.

Edelman, I. S., P. O. P. Ts'o, and J. Vinograd. 1960. The Binding of Magnesium to Microsomal Nucleoprotein and Ribonucleic Acid. *Biochimica et biophysica acta*, 43:393–403.

Elson, D. 1959. Latent Enzymic Activity of a Ribonucleoprotein Isolated from *Escherichia coli*. *Biochimica et biophysica acta*, 36:372–386.

Feldman, F., D. Elson, and A. Globerson. 1960. Antibodies in Ribonucleoproteins. *Nature, London*, 185:317–319.

Grabowski, A. V., and H. N. Munro. 1960. Release of Amylase from Pancreatic Microsomes by Amino Acids. *Experimental Cell Research*, 19:190–193.

Hamilton, M. G. 1960. *Some Physical Chemical Properties of Microsomal Ribonucleoprotein from Rat Liver*. Ph.D. Dissertation. Cornell University Medical College, New York, New York.

Hamilton, M. G., and M. L. Petermann. 1959. Ultracentrifugal Studies on Ribonucleoprotein from Rat Liver Microsomes. *Journal of Biological Chemistry*, 234:1441–1446.

Hoagland, M. B. 1960. "The Relationship of Nucleic Acid and Protein Synthesis as Revealed by Studies in Cell-Free Systems." The Nucleic Acids, E. Chargaff and J. N. Davidson, Eds., Vol. 3, pp. 349–408. New York, New York: Academic Press, Inc.

Howatson, A. F., and A. W. Ham. 1955. Electron Microscope Study of Sections of Two Rat Liver Tumors. *Cancer Research*, 15:62–69.

Kahler, H., and W. R. Bryan. 1943. Ultracentrifugal Studies of Some Complexes Obtained from Mouse Milk, Mammary Tumor, and Other Tissues. *Journal of the National Cancer Institute*, 4:37–45.

Koehler, J. K. 1961. Electron Microscope and Ultracentrifuge Studies on Yeast Ribosomes. (Abstract) *Fifth Annual Meeting of the Biophysical Society*, SC8. St. Louis, Missouri.

Kuff, E. L., and R. F. Zeigel. 1960. Cytoplasmic Ribonucleoprotein Components of the Novikoff Hepatoma. *The Journal of Biophysical and Biochemical Cytology*, 7:465–478.

Miller, G. L., and W. C. Price. 1946. Physical and Chemical Studies on Southern Bean Mosaic Virus. I. Size, Shape, Hydration, and Elementary Composition. *Archives of Biochemistry*, 10:467–477.

Nathans, D., and F. Lipmann. 1960. Amino Acid Transfer from S RNA to Microsome. II. Isolation of a Heat-Labile Factor from Liver Supernatant. *Biochimica et biophysica acta*, 43:126–128.

Palade, G. E. 1955. A Small Particulate Component of the Cytoplasm. *The Journal of Biophysical and Biochemical Cytology*, 1:59–68.

Petermann, M. L. 1960a. The Binding of Oxyhemoglobin by Ribonucleoprotein from a Rat Tumor. (Abstract) *Federation Proceedings*, 19:350.

———. 1960b. Ribonucleoprotein from a Rat Tumor, the Jensen Sarcoma. I. The Effect of Magnesium Binding on Ultracentrifugal and Electrophoretic Properties. *Journal of Biological Chemistry*, 235:1998–2003.

———. 1961. The 65 S Form of Ribonucleoprotein (RNP) from the Jensen Sarcoma, a Rat Tumor. (Abstract) *Fifth Annual Meeting of the Biophysical Society*, SC6. St. Louis, Missouri.

Petermann, M. L., and M. G. Hamilton. 1952. An Ultracentrifugal Analysis of the Macromolecular Particles of Normal and Leukemic Mouse Spleen. *Cancer Research*, 12:373–378.

———. 1958. The Influence of Age, Sex. Pregnancy, Starvation, and Other Factors on the Cytoplasmic Ribonucleoproteins of Rat Liver. *The Journal of Biophysical and Biochemical Cytology*, 4:771–776.

———. 1961. "Physicochemical Studies on Ribonucleoproteins from Mammalian Cytoplasm," *Protein Biosynthesis*, R. J. C. Harris, Ed., pp. 235–259. London, England: Academic Press, Ltd.

Petermann, M. L., M. G. Hamilton, M. E. Balis, K. Samarth, and P. Pecora. 1958. "Physicochemical and Metabolic Studies on Rat Liver Ribonucleoprotein," *Microsomal Particles and Protein Synthesis*, R. B. Roberts, Ed., pp. 70–75. Washington, D.C.: Washington Academy of Sciences.

Petermann, M. L., M. G. Hamilton, and N. A. Mizen. 1954. Electrophoretic Analysis of the Macromolecular Nucleoprotein Particles of Mammalian Cytoplasm. *Cancer Research*, 14:360–366.

Petermann, M. L., N. A. Mizen, and M. G. Hamilton. 1953. The Macromolecular Particles of Normal and Regenerating Rat Liver. *Cancer Research*, 13:372–375.

———. 1954. The Macromolecular Nucleoprotein Particles of Normal and Tumor Tissue. (Abstract) *Proceedings of the American Association for Cancer Research*, 4:360.

———. 1956. The Cytoplasmic Nucleoproteins of Azo Dye-Induced Rat Liver Tumors. *Cancer Research*, 16:620–627.

Petermann, M. L., and A. Pavlovec. 1961. The Use of Bentonite in the Purification of Ribonucleoprotein. (Abstract) *Federation Proceedings*, 20(1):144.

Porter, K. R. 1955–1956. "The Submicroscopic Morphology of Cytoplasm," *Harvey Lectures*, pp. 175–228. New York, New York: Academic Press, Inc.

Scatchard, G. 1949. The Attractions of Proteins for Small Molecules and Ions. *Annals of the New York Academy of Sciences*, 51:660–672.

Sherman, J. H., and M. L. Petermann. 1961. Some Physical Properties of Calf Liver Ribonucleoprotein. *Biochimica et biophysica acta*, 47:188–191.

Takanami, M. 1960. On the Molecular Weight of a Ribonucleic Acid Preparation from a Ribonucleoprotein Complex. *Biochimica et biophysica acta*, 39:152–154.

Ts'o, P. O. P., J. Bonner, and J. Vinograd. 1958. Structure and Properties of Microsomal Nucleoprotein Particles from Pea Seedlings. *Biochimica et biophysica acta*, 30:570–582.

Ts'o, P. O. P., and J. Vinograd. 1961. Studies of Ribosomes from Reticulocytes. *Biochimica et biophysica acta*, 49: 113–129.

Wolfe, R. G. 1956. Macromolecular Constituents of Proliferating and Non-proliferating Yeast Extracts. *Archives of Biochemistry and Biophysics*, 63: 100–105.

Factors Controlling Protein Synthesis in Nuclear Ribosomes *in vitro* and *in vivo*

VINCENT G. ALLFREY, PH.D.

The Rockefeller Institute,
New York, New York

The experiments to be described are concerned with the sites and mechanism of protein synthesis in the cell nucleus, with the role of nucleic acids in this synthetic process, and with the capacity of histones to act as repressors of nuclear metabolic activity.

All three problems have great intrinsic interest, an interest which is further heightened by the realization that synthetic processes in or near the chromosome have important implications for genetics, that protein synthesis in the nucleus must play a major role in cell growth and cell differentiation, and that cell division in both normal and malignant tissues requires the synthesis of chromosomal proteins as well as chromosomal nucleic acids.

How is protein synthesized in the cell nucleus, and what mechanisms are available for the regulation and direction of this synthetic process?

A direct approach to these questions became possible when it was discovered that isolated nuclei prepared from calf thymus tissue had the capacity for independent and sustained amino acid incorporation (Allfrey, 1954; Allfrey, Mirsky, and Osawa, 1955). Alfred Mirsky and I proceeded to investigate further this active nuclear system, and most of the experiments to be described are based on the remarkable synthetic potentialities of the calf thymocyte nucleus.

Criteria of Nuclear Purity

Because the significance of many of the findings on nuclear metabolism depends on the absence of appreciable cytoplasmic or whole cell contamination, it would be well to preface the biochemical results with a brief summary of the major evidence for the purity of the thymus nuclear preparations.

The nuclei were isolated in 0.25 M sucrose–0.003 M $CaCl_2$, by differential centrifugation of homogenates of calf thymus tissue, using the method described previously (Allfrey, 1954; Allfrey, Mirsky, and Osawa, 1957). This isolation medium is isotonic; more concentrated sucrose solutions (e.g., 0.4 M) inactivate the nuclei. Sucrose, or other sugars, must be present because isotonic salt solutions alone destroy nuclear activity.

It is now clear that the most reliable guide to the purity of nuclei isolated from the thymus gland is a critical examination under the electron microscope. To date, five such studies of calf thymus nuclei have been made; all agree in that the extent of contamination by intact thymus lymphocytes is quite small. In our earliest estimates, we reported 29 intact cells/1,000 nuclei (Allfrey and Mirsky, 1955). This figure is in accord with measurements made on stained thymus nuclear fractions, carried out by Ficq and Errera in Brachet's laboratory; they reported 27 cells/1,000 nuclei (Ficq and Errera, 1958). In our two most recent studies of isolated calf thymus nuclei, again using the electron microscope and examining fields containing thousands of nuclei, we have reported an upper limit of contamination of 77 to 79 "cells"/1,000 nuclei, the higher figures now representing not only intact cells but also nuclei with zones of adhering cytoplasm (Allfrey, Mirsky, and Osawa, 1957; Hopkins, 1960). In this connection, however, it should be pointed out that those cells which do contaminate calf thymus nuclear fractions consist for the most part of nuclei surrounded by a thin halo or crescent of cytoplasm, and the nucleus comprises more than 61 per cent of their total mass (Allfrey, Stern, Mirsky, and Saetren, 1952). Therefore, a cell count of 7.7 per cent actually represents a nonnuclear contamination of less than 5 per cent.

Detailed comparisons have also been made of the compositions of calf thymus nuclei isolated in sucrose solutions and those isolated in nonaqueous media (Stern and Mirsky, 1953). The details of this comparison have been published and need not be repeated here, except to note that the thymus sucrose nuclei compare favorably in composition and enzymatic activity with the highly purified thymus nuclei obtained by the nonaqueous isolation method. This is a rigorous test of an isolation procedure (Allfrey 1960), and the results offer further proof of the purity of calf thymus nuclei prepared in 0.25 M sucrose by our procedure.

In studies of the biochemical properties of such nuclei, the small amount of cytoplasmic contamination is reassuring, but intact cells could affect the results of metabolic tests and tracer experiments far out of proportion to their numbers. For this reason, other and more conclusive tests were applied to demonstrate that the metabolic activities observed in calf thymus nuclear fractions were caused by nuclei and not by cells. This work has been summarized recently elsewhere (Allfrey and Mirsky, in press a), and some of it will be referred to briefly in the subsequent pages. Suffice it to say that protein synthesis in the isolated thymocyte nucleus now seems a well-established fact, and the uptake of C^{14}-labeled amino acids can be verified directly and conclusively by radioautography of individual nuclei free of cytoplasmic contamination.

Nuclear Protein Synthesis

In 1954, the isolated thymocyte nucleus was shown to be capable of incorporating C^{14}-amino acids into its constituent proteins. This activity could also be demonstrated in nuclei isolated from an AKR lymphoma (Allfrey, 1954). The typical time course of this uptake is shown in Figure 1, in which the specific activity of the total nuclear protein is plotted as a function of the time of incubation at 37°C.

The incorporation of radioactive amino acids was shown to involve peptide bond formation and it is essentially irreversible. Radioautography of the nuclei after labeling experiments made it clear that not all the nuclei in a mixed suspension are taking up amino acids at the same rate (Ficq and Errera, 1958); but with time, the majority of the nuclei become radioactive. It has been calculated that, on the average, each nucleus is synthesizing about 22 molecules of protein (of molecular weight 50,000) every second (Allfrey, Mirsky, and Osawa, 1957).

The sustained incorporation of amino acids into the proteins of the nucleus is an aerobic process. The reason for oxygen dependence is now clear; oxygen is required for nuclear adenosine triphosphate (ATP) synthesis, and ATP is the primary energy source for amino

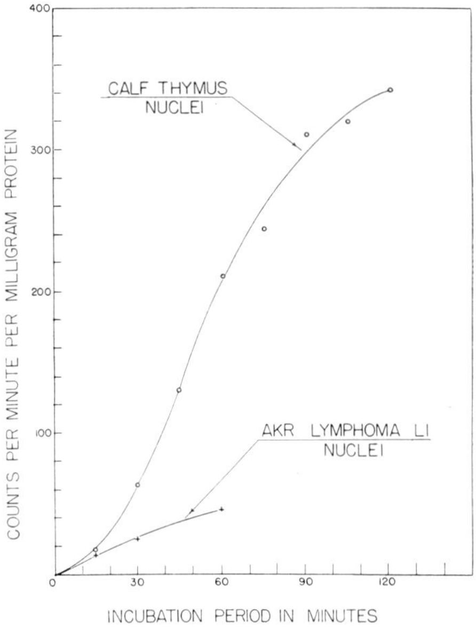

FIG. 1. The time course of amino acid incorporation (alanine-1-C^{14}) into nuclei isolated from calf thymus tissue and from cells of an AKR lymphoma. The specific activity of the total nuclear protein is plotted as a function of the time of incubation.

acid activation in nuclear protein synthesis (Osawa, Allfrey, and Mirsky, 1957; Hopkins, 1959).

There are two aspects which characteristically mark this amino acid uptake as nuclear. First, amino acid incorporation by isolated thymus nuclei is sodium-ion dependent. This contrasts with the usual finding that potassium ions are required for amino acid uptake in cytoplasmic systems (e.g., Sachs, 1957), and for the transport of amino acids into intact cells (Riggs, Walker, and Christensen, 1958). A second clear difference between nuclear and cytoplasmic incorporating systems is that the nuclear system ceases to function if nuclei are exposed to deoxyribonuclease (Allfrey, 1954). That is, amino acid uptake into nuclear proteins is deoxyribonucleic acid- (DNA) dependent, while cytoplasmic systems, as a rule, are sensitive to ribonuclease but not to deoxyribonuclease (Allfrey, Daly, and Mirsky, 1953).

The basis for these differences is now understood, and the sodium ion and DNA dependency of nuclear protein synthesis will now be discussed.

Sodium-Dependent Amino Acid Transport into the Nucleus

The rate of amino acid uptake into the proteins of isolated nuclei increases sharply when sodium ions are added to the incubation

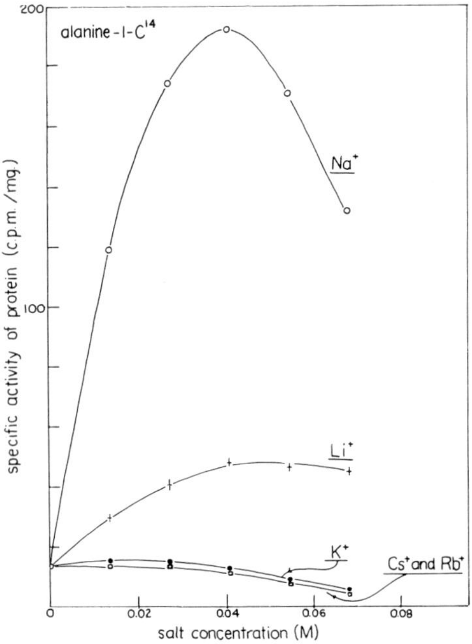

FIG. 2. The effects of adding different monovalent cations (as chlorides) on alanine-1-C^{14} incorporation into the proteins of isolated calf thymus nuclei. The specific activity of the nuclear protein (in counts per minute/mg.) after 60 minutes of incubation is plotted against the salt concentration of the medium.

medium (Allfrey, Mirsky, and Osawa, 1957). The specificity of the sodium ion effect is shown in Figure 2, and which compares the uptake of alanine-1-C^{14} in a sodium-containing medium with that observed in the presence of other monovalent cations. In this figure, the salt concentration of the medium is plotted as abscissa; the specific activity of the nuclear protein after 60 minutes of incubation as ordinate.

The increase in the rate of C^{14} uptake is marked in the case of alanine incorporation, but similar sodium ion effects can also be demonstrated for glycine, leucine, lysine, valine, and other amino acids.

In studying this sodium dependency of amino acid incorporation, we tested several hypotheses, among them the possibility that sodium ions might influence the rate at which amino acids enter the free amino acid pool within the nucleus. In these experiments the penetration of amino acids into the nuclear pool was followed by suspending nuclei in a buffered sucrose medium containing sodium (or, for comparison, potassium) ions. An accurately measured amount of the radioactive amino acid was then added, and the nuclei were incubated aerobically, with shaking. Aliquots of the nuclear suspensions were removed at zero time and at short time intervals thereafter. The nuclei were centrifuged down, washed with sucrose, and then extracted with cold 2 per cent $HClO_4$. The radioactivity in each extract was measured and, after correction was made for the small amount of amino acid adsorbed at zero time, the radioactivity was plotted as a function of the time of incubation. This time course of alanine transport into the nuclear pool at 37°C is shown in Figure 3. A comparison of the results in sodium- and potassium-containing media shows that amino acid transport into the nucleus is clearly a sodium-dependent process (Allfrey, Hopkins, Frenster, and Mirsky, 1960).

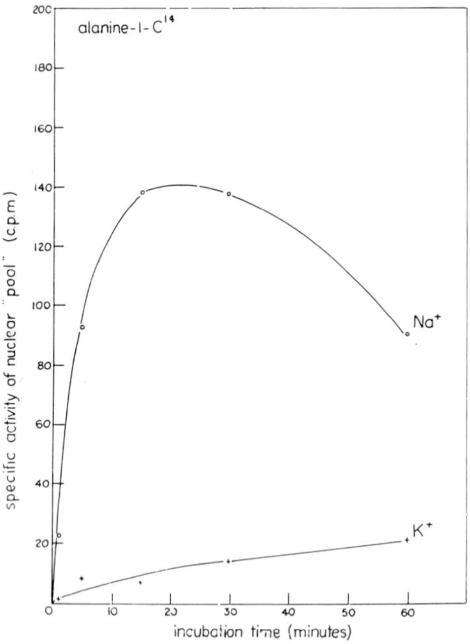

FIG. 3. The specific effect of sodium ions in promoting the transport of alanine-1-C^{14} into the free amino acid pool of the isolated thymocyte nucleus. The radioactivity of the nuclear acid-soluble fraction is plotted against the time of incubation of the nuclei at 37°C.

Chromatography of the acid-soluble nuclear fraction indicates that the alanine-1-C^{14} is present as the free amino acid, and the radioactivity moves with the R_F of a free alanine marker. No other radioactive spots were observed.

Other studies of amino acid transport into nuclei suggest that this is an enzymatic process. The evidence is as follows: (1) The reaction is temperature-dependent, with a well-defined optimum in the physiological temperature range, 38° to 40°C. The rate of transport doubles between 10° and 20°C. This doubling of reaction rate with a 10° change in temperature ($Q_{10} = 2$) would be expected for an enzymatic reaction but not for a simple diffusion process. (2) The rate of alanine penetration into nuclei varies with pH, with a definite optimum at neutrality. (3) The reaction shows great specificity. For example, competition experiments using non-radioactive D-alanine and L-alanine before adding DL-alanine-1-C^{14} indicate that only the naturally occurring L-isomer competes with radioactive alanine for transport; D-amino acids are not actively taken up into the nuclear pool, nor do they block the transport of the L-form. Also of interest in this connection is the fact that L-isoleucine competes with its homologue, L-valine, for transport into the nucleus, while D-isoleucine has no such effect. A pronounced steric specificity is evidently present, and this specificity is characteristic of an enzymatic mechanism. Together with other evidence that the process may be ATP dependent, the experiments point to a specific, sodium-dependent, enzymatic mechanism which controls the rate of entry of amino acids into the nucleus.

It is now clear that the sodium requirement for amino acid transport is the main reason why protein synthesis in the nucleus is sodium-ion dependent; sodium ions are needed to get amino acids to the site of synthesis. We have found that, once this transport has occurred, the continued presence of sodium ions in the medium is not necessary for subsequent stages in amino acid incorporation (Allfrey and Mirsky, in press b).

Is amino acid transport really a nuclear phenomenon, or might it be caused by the few whole cells present in the nuclear suspension? This question has been answered directly in the following way. C^{14}-amino acids were added to the nuclear suspension at 10°C (a temperature too low to permit nuclear protein synthesis). After 30 minutes the nuclei were washed with sucrose, dehydrated in acetone, and then fractionated according to density in a nonaqueous medium (cyclohexane-CCl_4, in which alanine is insoluble). By this means, a highly purified nuclear sediment was obtained. Lighter fractions, containing the few whole cells originally present, were discarded. The purified nuclei were then tested for their content of acid-extractable C^{14}-amino acids; as before, the entry of amino acids in the nuclear pool was found to be a sodium-dependent process.

The sodium dependency of the nucleus *in vitro* suggests that sodium plays an essential role in nuclear metabolism *in vivo*. This view is supported by studies of sodium distribution within living cells. For example, when frog oocytes are exposed to media containing Na^{22} or Na^{24}, and the cells are then sectioned and examined by radioautography, there is a marked accumulation of sodium ions within the nucleus (Abelson and Duryee, 1949; Naora, Naora, Mirsky, and Allfrey, unpublished data). Other workers have shown that the sodium concentration of thymus nuclei exceeds that of the thymus cell cytoplasm (Itoh and Schwartz, 1957). A high sodium content has also been observed in avian erythrocyte nuclei. Thus, *in vivo* and *in vitro*, sodium localization and sodium dependency seem well established.

These observations suggest a possible approach to the chemotherapy of cancer. Sodium displacement by lithium leads to a greatly diminished rate of nuclear protein metabolism. Yet, there is no equivalent inhibition of nuclear ribonucleic acid (RNA) synthesis. It may be possible to exploit this situation; for example, it would be interesting to know whether cancer cells divide as rapidly in Na^+ deficient animals (or in animals in which Li^+ is substituted for sodium in the diet) as they do in control animals. Alternatively, the use of amino acid analogues together with higher sodium intakes may offer a route to the preferential inhibition of protein synthesis in rapidly dividing nuclei.

The DNA-Dependence of Nuclear Protein Synthesis

We have shown that isolated nuclei are capable of an extensive synthesis of ATP and other high-energy phosphate bonds. This phosphorylation is an aerobic process, accompanied by the uptake of oxygen. As expected, many of the biosynthetic reactions carried out in the nucleus, including protein synthesis, are dependent on this phosphorylating system as a source of energy (Osawa, Allfrey, and Mirsky, 1957).

Space does not permit a detailed discussion of the present state of nuclear phosphorylation, but it should be stressed that ATP synthesis in thymus nuclei differs significantly from oxydative phosphorylation as studied in suspensions of isolated mitochondria. The most striking difference is the fact that nuclear ATP synthesis stops when nuclei are treated with deoxyribonuclease (Allfrey and Mirsky, 1957). However, if DNA is added back to a suspension of nuclei treated with crystalline pancreatic deoxyribonuclease (DNase), the synthesis of ATP is restored.

Because ATP synthesis in the thymus nucleus is DNase-sensitive, other biosynthetic reactions which require ATP also show a similar DNase sensitivity. These reactions also resume when DNA is added back to the enzyme-treated nuclei. Both protein synthesis and RNA synthesis in isolated nuclei are DNA-dependent by this test (Allfrey, Mirsky, and Osawa, 1957), which points to ATP as the source of the needed biosynthetic energy. (In passing, it should be noted that sensitivity to attack by DNase is not seen in intact thymus cells in tissue slices or minces under these conditions; this offers additional evidence for the purity of the thymus nuclear fractions.)

The action of DNA in promoting nuclear ATP synthesis is not specific. In substitution experiments, in which other polyanions were added to DNase-treated nuclei, we found, to our surprise, that most of the DNA of the nucleus can be replaced by a variety of dissimilar, negatively charged polymers, including RNA, polyadenylic acid, chondroitin sulphate, heparin, and polyaspartic acid. Even relatively simple polymers, such as polyethylene sulphonate and polyacrylic acid, can restore ATP synthesis in DNA-depleted nuclei (Allfrey and Mirsky, 1958). Moreover, it was found that a neutral polymer, such as polyacrylamide, cannot restore phosphorylation by this test. Conversely, positively charged polymers, such as polylysine, protamines, and histones, strongly inhibit ATP synthesis in isolated nuclei (Allfrey and Mirsky, 1958). A correlation of the structures and activities of many different polymers made it clear that increasing positive charges decreased nuclear activity, while polyanions stimulated nuclear synthetic processes.

The findings point to the importance of the negative charges on DNA for nuclear phosphorylation reactions coupled to oxidation and for all ATP-requiring synthetic processes in the cell nucleus. It is also apparent that the naturally occurring polycations, the protamines and histones, are potent inhibitors of nuclear activity. Further evidence for the inhibitory action of the histones will be presented later.

Thus, one of the main reasons why nuclear protein synthesis ceases when DNase is added to a nuclear suspension is that the necessary ATP synthesis comes to a halt. The role of DNA in promoting nuclear ATP synthesis appears to be nonspecific and largely caused by its negative electrical charge. In the following, it will be seen that DNA can also have a more specific effect on nuclear protein synthesis and that it cannot always be replaced by synthetic polyanions.

Reactions Governing Nuclear Protein Synthesis

In considering the mechanism of amino acid incorporation into nuclear proteins, we had the great advantage of the tremendous strides already made in this direction in cytoplasmic systems. Using this background, we have been able to show that protein synthesis in the nucleus involves a synthetic mechanism similar to that proposed for the cytoplasm (e.g., Zamecnik, 1959). The two major differences, sodium-ion dependency and DNase sensitivity, have been explained, and the factors common to nuclear and cytoplasmic protein synthesis can now be discussed.

Amino Acid Activation

In the nucleus, as in cytoplasmic and bacterial systems, the primary step in protein synthesis appears to be an ATP-dependent activation of the carboxyl group of the amino acids. The reaction, amino acids + ATP + enzyme = enzyme-AMP-amino acid + PP, is carried out by nuclear enzymes similar to those originally found in liver extracts by Hoagland (1955). Since the reaction is reversible, a convenient method of assay for the activating enzymes is based on the incorporation of radioactive pyrophosphate into ATP. Using P^{32}-labeled pyrophosphate and measuring the production of radioactive ATP by the procedure of Crane and Lipmann (1953), Hopkins showed that extracts of isolated nuclei readily form ATP^{32} when amino acids are added to the medium (Hopkins, 1959). It was then shown that the ATP-pyrophosphate exchange reaction is promoted by the addition of mixtures of amino acids, or by individual amino acids tested separately. Neutral extracts of calf thymus nuclei contain activating enzymes for at least 15 L-amino acids: alanine, aspartic acid, cysteine, glutamic acid, histidine, isoleucine, leucine, lysine, methionine, proline, serine, threonine, tryptophan, tyrosine, and valine. A low order of activation is found with arginine, glycine, and phenylalanine; D-amino acids are not acted upon. Most of the activating enzymes can be precipitated from nuclear extracts by lowering the pH to 5.2, as was first observed in cytoplasmic systems (Hoagland, Keller, and Zamecnik, 1956).

Many tests have been carried out to make certain that the presence of activating enzymes in thymus nuclei is not an artifact caused by an adsorption of enzymes from the cytoplasm. These tests have been described elsewhere (Hopkins, 1959), but it should be emphasized that the enzymes have been found to occur in nuclei isolated in nonaqueous media. Since the nonaqueous method of isolation precludes any exchange of water-soluble materials between nucleus and cytoplasm during the course of isolation, adsorption artifacts cannot occur. We selected two types of nonaqueous nuclei for enzyme assay because their purity had been established by chemical, enzymatic, and immunological tests for cytoplasmic contamination (Allfrey, Stern, Mirsky, and Saetren, 1952); these were the nuclei prepared from chicken kidney and from calf thymus tissue. In both cases, the concentration of activating enzymes in the nucleus (in units of activity/mg. of dry weight) was comparable to that observed in the cytoplasmic portion of the cells. In these nuclei the high purity of the preparation makes it certain that amino acid-activating enzymes do, indeed, occur within the cell nucleus.

Amino acid-activating enzymes have also been detected in liver nuclei following isolation in dense sucrose solutions (Hopkins, 1959; Webster, 1960; Gvosdev, 1960), and it appears increasingly likely that activating enzymes will be found in all nuclear types which are capable of protein synthesis.

The Transfer of Activated Amino Acids to Ribonucleic Acid in the Nucleus

There is now much evidence that the sequel to amino acid activation in cytoplasmic systems is a transfer of the amino acid to a low molecular weight RNA (the so-called soluble RNA or s-RNA) (e.g., Hoagland, Zamecnik, and Stephenson, 1957; Ogata and Nohara, 1957). This enzymatic reaction proceeds according to the equation:

$$\text{enzyme-amino acyl-AMP} + \text{s-RNA} \rightleftarrows \text{amino acyl-s-RNA} + \text{AMP} + \text{enzyme.}$$

We have observed a similar process in isolated thymus nuclei. The transfer of amino acids to nuclear RNA can be shown directly by isolation of the radioactive carrier-RNA after incubating the nuclei in the presence of C^{14}-leucine (Hopkins, 1959).

In these experiments it was found that the addition of certain antibiotics to nuclear suspensions blocks protein synthesis but permits the synthesis of the amino acyl-RNA complex. Using chloramphenicol (or puromycin) it became possible to prepare the amino acyl-RNA without risk of contamination by radioactive proteins. Despite the presence of chloramphenicol, leucine enters the RNA fraction at a high initial rate and then reaches a plateau concentration (Hopkins, 1959). Yarmolinsky and de la Haba (1959) have shown that puromycin behaves similarly in liver extracts, blocking protein synthesis but not the formation of amino acyl-RNA's. Following their lead, we have made similar findings in thymus nuclei (Allfrey, Hopkins, Frenster, and Mirsky, 1960). The effectiveness of puromycin as an inhibitor of protein synthesis is presumed to be caused by the close structural resemblance between the antibiotic and the proposed amino acyl-RNA complex. Since puromycin at low concentrations almost completely suppresses nuclear protein synthesis, the inhibition may be taken to indicate that the bulk of protein synthesis in the nucleus involves the participation of an amino acyl-RNA intermediate. However, it is unlikely that the inhibitory effects of chloramphenicol or the tetracyclines can be interpreted in this way.

By combining the study of amino acid transfer reactions with methods of fractionating nuclei, it was shown that activated amino acids do not form similar amino acyl-DNA complexes, nor do they combine with the metabolically active RNA of the nucleolar fraction (Hopkins, 1959).

In the experiments cited above, the formation of amino acyl-RNA complexes took place in an intact nucleus. An alternative procedure allows the formation of amino acyl-RNA in a subnuclear system consisting of the nuclear activating enzymes (the nuclear pH 5 fraction), ATP, RNA, and the radioactive amino acid.

Properties of Nuclear Amino Acyl-RNA

Using this *in vitro* system of labeling the RNA associated with the nuclear pH 5 enzymes, a large scale preparation of nuclear leucyl-RNA was carried out (Hopkins, Allfrey, and Mirsky, 1961). This product has many properties indicating its close similarity to the amino acyl-s-RNA complexes studied in cytoplasmic solutions. For example, it is nondialyzable and stable in dilute acid solutions. Yet, a brief exposure to 0.005 N NaOH removes all of its radioactivity, and subsequent chromatography on paper shows the counts to be present as free C^{14}-leucine.

The effect of ribonuclease on the nuclear leucyl-RNA complex was next studied, following the procedure of Zachau, Acs, and Lipmann (1958), who showed that ribonuclease digestion of amino acyl-s-RNA complexes released a fragment consisting of the amino acid linked to a nucleoside. The nuclear leucyl-RNA behaves in the same way; a short digestion with ribonuclease releases all of the radioactivity in an acid-soluble form which can be separated by chromatography or filter-paper electrophoresis. The leucyl nucleoside released by ribonuclease digestion is readily distinguishable from either free leucine or free adenosine, and can be located as a radioactive, ultraviolet- (UV-) absorbing spot on the chromatogram. If the spot is treated with dilute alkali, the radioactivity then separates as free C^{14}-leucine and the nucleoside is left. The latter component, as judged by its mobility, R_F, and UV absorption spectra, appears to be adenosine (Hopkins, Allfrey, and Mirsky, 1961).

It follows that the receptor end group in nuclear carrier-RNA is a terminal adenylic acid, as was found earlier in the s-RNA of cytoplasmic systems. Thus, the first two stages in nuclear protein synthesis, i.e., amino acid activation and the transfer of activated amino acids to a terminal adenylic acid on carrier RNA's, are in complete accord with current views of the mechanism of cytoplasmic protein synthesis.

Nuclear Ribosomes as Sites of Protein Synthesis

Early attempts to fractionate nuclear proteins following C^{14}-alanine incorporation *in vitro* showed that neutral extracts of the nucleus contained a ribonucleoprotein fraction of high specific activity (Allfrey, Mirsky, and Osawa, 1957). In more recent studies of the ribonucleoproteins of nuclear origin, we have employed differential ultracentrifugation. Frenster found, by a technique of successive extractions and centrifugation at increasing g values, that the nucleus contains a heterogeneous population of ribonucleoprotein particles (ribosomes) of differing metabolic activity. The details of the fractionation have been described elsewhere and will not be repeated here (Frenster, Allfrey, and Mirsky, 1960). It is of great interest that electron microscopy of the nuclear ribosome fractions revealed the presence of dense spherical particles of about 100–300 Å diameter, since particles of this size were also observed in the intact thymus nucleus in tissue sections, and similar particles have been photographed by many workers in the nuclei of widely diverse cell types.

Tracer studies have shown that the nuclear ribosomes are sites of intense protein synthesis (Frenster, Allfrey, and Mirsky, 1960). The intranuclear localization of the amino acid-incorporating particles is quite certain because amino acid uptake into the ribosomal proteins requires the presence of sodium ions and is DNase-sensitive.

In more recent experiments on the ribosomes of the nucleus, carried out with A. O. Pogo and B. G. T. Pogo, we have pursued the study of their composition and metabolic activity. It is now clear that Mg^{++} concentration is a critical factor in controlling the size of nuclear ribosomes, as it is in the ribosomes of bacteria (Tissières, Watson, Schlessinger, and Hollingworth, 1959) and plant cells (Ts'o, Bonner, and Vinograd, 1958).

Thymus nuclear ribosomes are now prepared by extracting the isolated nuclei (prepared in 0.25 M sucrose—0.003 M $MgCl_2$) with 0.01 M tris buffer (pH 7.6) containing 5×10^{-4} M $MgCl_2$. After the nuclear residues and heavy particles are removed, the Mg^{++} concentration is raised to 10^{-2} M and the ribosomes are collected by centrifuging for 90 minutes at $144{,}000 \times g$. Such preparations have been examined in the analytical ultracentrifuge, thanks to the generous cooperation of M. G. Hamilton and M. L. Petermann. The results show that most of the material exists in the 80 S class, with small peaks approximating 60 S and 40 S, respectively. If the Mg^{++} concentration is lowered (or if versene is added) the 80 S peak dissociates into a smaller particle class.

Fractionation of Ribosomal Proteins

Of special interest is the effect of a nonionic detergent (Lubrol W) on the composition of nuclear ribosomes. Nearly two thirds of the protein in the ribosome fraction is released by treatment with Lubrol in 0.5 M NaCl, leaving a residue correspondingly enriched in RNA. The use of Lubrol W (a polymer made by condensing cetyl alcohol and polyoxyethylene) was first described by Cohn and Butler (1958), who used this detergent to fractionate rat liver microsomes after labeling experiments *in vivo*.

In the following, nuclear ribosomes will be considered to be made up of a Lubrol-resistant core and a removable protein coat. (The terms "core" and "coat" are defined only in terms of their non-extractability and removability, and should not be construed to indicate spatial position in the particles. A correlation between extractability and morphologic features of ribosomes is currently being sought using the electron microscope.)

The Lubrol-resistant core of the ribosomes has been found to play an important role in nuclear protein synthesis, and its properties promise to shed an interesting light on the sequence of reactions occurring within the ribosome. For example, time studies of alanine-1-C^{14} and leucine-1-C^{14} uptake into the ribosomes have shown that, at early times, the total protein of the ribosomes is more active than the protein in the soluble phase of the nucleus. After a few minutes, there is an evident crossover effect and the ribosomal protein is now less active than the proteins of the supernate. While this is going on, there is also an apparent redistribution of the labeled protein in different fractions of the ribosome. At two minutes, the insoluble protein of the Lubrol-resistant core is more active than the soluble coat proteins prepared from the ribosomes. But at later times (at five, 15, and 30 minutes) the coat proteins are more active than the proteins of the core.

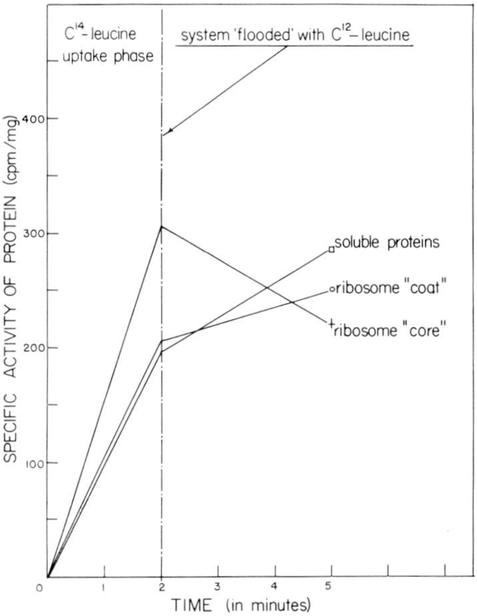

FIG. 4. Changes in the specific activity of ribosomal core and coat proteins following a brief incorporation of leucine-1-C^{14}. In these experiments isolated thymus nuclei were incubated with leucine-1-C^{14} for two minutes prior to flooding the system with C^{12}-leucine. The ribosomes were prepared and fractionated with Lubrol-NaCl, as described in the text. The specific activity of the two ribosomal protein fractions and of the soluble protein of the nucleus is plotted against time.

The results suggested a precursor relationship, in which the core protein is later transformed into coat protein. This viewpoint finds support in the following experiment. Leucine-1-C^{14} was added to a nuclear suspension at 37°C. After two minutes, a great excess of C^{12}-leucine was added to the incubation medium to minimize further incorporation of the radioactive form of the amino acid. Samples were taken at the two minute point, and three minutes later. The nuclear ribosomes were prepared and then fractionated with Lubrol-NaCl to yield the core and the soluble coat proteins. The specific activity of these fractions was plotted against time

(Figure 4). It is evident that, at two minutes, the proteins of the core are more radioactive than the proteins released by the Lubrol treatment. But at five minutes, the specific activity of the core proteins has diminished, while the activity of the coat proteins has increased in the same interval.

The results are in accord with the view that the proteins of the ribosome core are labeled first. At this stage, the protein is tightly bound to the ribosomal (RNA?) template and is not extractable by detergent treatment. As the synthesis proceeds, the finished protein (in terms of amino acid incorporation) is released from its template and can now be extracted into the soluble phase, with the aid of the detergent. Presumably, in the normal course of nuclear protein synthesis, later stages in the process involve the spontaneous release of newly synthesized protein from the ribosomal coat into the soluble phase of the nucleus. Although this hypothetical sequence of events still remains to be proved, the current kinetic studies of leucine-1-C^{14} incorporation suggest that this is the correct sequence. Further tests of the hypothesis are in progress, using puromycin to block protein synthesis at early times and following the progression of radioactive leucine through the ribosome core into the soluble phase.

Amino Acid Incorporation by Free Ribosomes

The synthetic activity of thymus nuclear ribosomes can also be studied outside of the cell nucleus. When such ribosomes are prepared under isotonic conditions and properly supplemented, they carry out an independent synthesis of labeled protein. In addition to the ribosomes, ATP, and an ATP-regenerating system, the process requires the nuclear pH 5 enzymes and guanosine triphosphate (GTP) (Frenster, Allfrey, and Mirsky, 1960). The incorporation of amino acids by free ribosomes can be blocked by puromycin or by the addition of ribonuclease to the incubation medium. The inhibitory effect of ribonuclease on the incorporation of amino acids is probably caused both by the action of the enzyme on the RNA of the ribosomes, and by the hydrolysis of the very susceptible amino acyl-carrier RNA complexes. (This sensitivity to ribonuclease is characteristic of uptake in the isolated ribonucleoprotein (RNP) particles; ribosomes within an intact nucleus resist attack by this enzyme.)

The Effect of DNA on Protein Synthesis in Isolated Nuclear Ribosomes

It was mentioned earlier that protein synthesis in the isolated nucleus is impaired when DNase is added to the incubation medium, largely as a result of the inability of DNase-treated nuclei to synthesize the ATP needed for amino acid activation.

Some experiments carried out in collaboration with Frenster suggest that DNA may play another, more specific role in nuclear ribosome metabolism. We have found that the addition of DNA increases the rate of amino acid incorporation by the free RNP particles. The specificity of the effect is suggested by the experiments summarized in Figure 5. In these tests, isolated nuclear ribosomes were incubated with C^{14}-leucine and the necessary supplements, including GTP. The usual time course of leucine incorporation is shown in the control curve. The addition of calf thymus DNA to the medium raises the level of uptake considerably (upper curve). The simultaneous addition of DNase together with the DNA

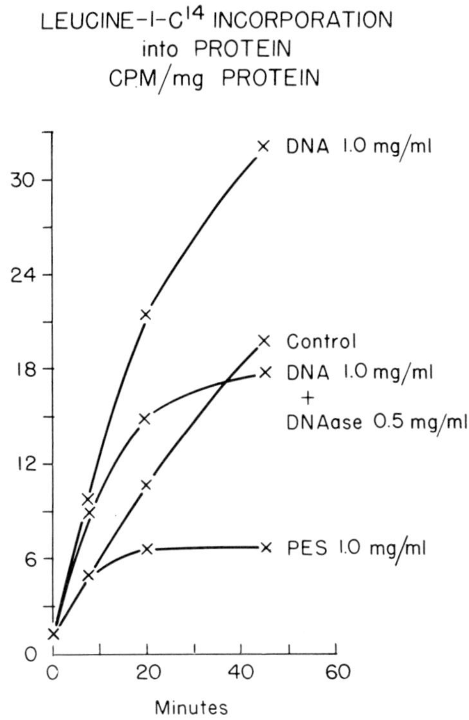

FIG. 5. The effects of adding DNA, DNA + deoxyribonuclease, and polyethylene sulphonate (PES) on the incorporation of leucine-1-C^{14} by isolated nuclear ribosomes. The specific activity of the ribosomal protein is plotted against the time of incubation at 37°C.

abolishes the stimulatory effect. This does not appear to be another nonspecific polyanion effect because the addition of polyethylene sulphonate (PES) actually inhibits the uptake of C^{14}-leucine (lower curve). The latter finding contrasts with our earlier experiments on ATP synthesis, in which polyethylene sulphonate was found to be a good substitute for DNA in promoting nuclear phosphorylation (Allfrey and Mirsky 1957, 1958). Yeast RNA (a commercial preparation) failed to increase leucine-1-C^{14} uptake by nuclear ribosomes. Conversely, a variety of different DNA samples were effective; there were no significant differences between DNA's prepared from calf thymus, calf liver, or wheat germ. Thus, the stimulation of leucine uptake has not, to date, provided any new evidence for tissue or species specificity of the DNA.

Since the stimulation of amino acid incorporation in isolated ribosomes by DNA is not a general polyanion effect, the results raise the interesting possibility that DNA may normally play a role in the metabolism, and possibly even in the structure of nuclear ribosomes. This viewpoint finds some support in recently published experiments (Tissières, Schlessinger, and Gros, 1960) in which it was found that DNase diminished alanine-C^{14} uptake by bacterial ribosomes. Moreover, the addition of polyethylene sulphonate or other polyanions did not restore alanine incorporation in DNase-treated bacterial ribosomes. Thus, from two divergent sources there is evidence that DNA may play an essential role in ribosome metabolism, a role that cannot be taken over by other polyanions. In the case of nuclear ribosomes, it is fairly certain that the effect is not caused by a capacity of the DNA to act as an amino acid carrier since all tests for the transfer of leucine-C^{14} to DNA in intact nuclei have proved negative.

Histones as Repressors of Nuclear Synthetic Processes

The naturally occuring basic proteins of the nucleus include the histones and, in some cells, protamines. Both classes of proteins are characterized by a high content of basic amino acids, which impart to their molecules at neutral pH an extensive distribution of positive charges. As polycations, these proteins combine in saltlike linkage with the negatively charged phosphate groups of the DNA in the chromosomes (Mirsky and Pollister, 1946; Mirsky and Ris, 1951).

In the following, it will be shown that histones and protamines are potent inhibitors of nuclear metabolic activity. The inhibitory effects include: (1) histones lower the rate of nuclear phosphorylation and since respiration and phosphorylation in the isolated nucleus are tightly coupled, a block in respiration also means a decrease in ATP production (McEwen and Allfrey, unpublished data); (2) histones also slow the process of amino acid transport into the nuclear amino acid pool; (3) the addition of histones to suspensions of isolated nuclei leads to reduced rates of amino acid uptake into nuclear proteins and to inhibition of RNA synthesis. Many of these effects can also be obtained by the addition of a relatively simple polycation, such as polylysine, and it can be assumed that this compound acts as a repressor largely by virtue of its excess positive charge.

There is good evidence from other sources that histones can inhibit oxidative phosphorylation in nonnuclear systems as well. Thus it has been observed that histones and protamines inhibit the cytochrome C oxidase of beef heart muscle (Person and Fine, 1960); and it has recently been reported that the release of histones into the cytoplasm of cerebral cortex cells inhibits their respiration (Wolfe and McIlwain, 1961).

In the nucleus, the role of histones as inhibitors may be caused in large part by their capacity to block oxidative phosphorylation. However, it can be shown that histones can also inhibit protein synthesis in a more direct way. For example, the addition of calf thymus histone fraction I, the arginine-rich histone fraction I of Daly and Mirsky (1955), to suspensions of free nuclear ribosomes inhibits amino acid incorporation into the ribosomal proteins. This is shown in Figure 6, in which the time course of leucine incorporation into ribosomes in the presence of histone (lower curve) is compared with the uptakes measured in control ribosomes, and in ribosomes supplemented with DNA. The figure also shows that the stimulatory effect of DNA on ribosomal protein synthesis is blocked when histone is added at the same time.

General Conclusions

So far we have seen that protein synthesis in nuclear ribosomes can be stimulated by DNA and inhibited by histones, both normal components of the chromosome. The results suggest that the synthetic activity of ribosomes within the cell nucleus will depend on their proximity to either DNA or histone in the chromosome. It may be suggested that the DNA : histone ratio is different at

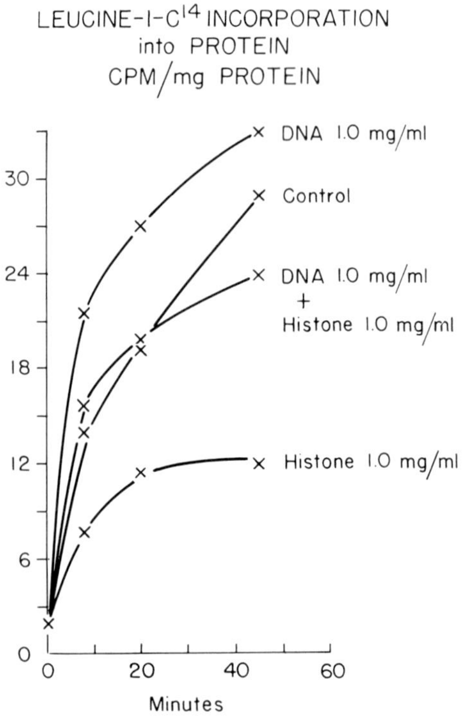

FIG. 6. The effects of adding DNA, DNA + histone, and histone on the incorporation of leucine-1-C^{14} by isolated nuclear ribosomes. The specific activity of the ribosomal protein is plotted against the time of incubation at 37°C.

different loci of the chromosome and that the difference is related to synthetic activity at that locus. Where the negative charges of the DNA predominate, activity will be high; where the positive groups of the histone cover or mask the DNA, or occur in excess, the chromosome locus will be relatively inert. In this way a changing DNA : histone ratio could result in varied rates of protein (and RNA) synthesis at different sites of the chromosome.

The competition between DNA and histones, affecting the balance between negative and positive charges at active sites in the nucleus, may prove to be an important mechanism for the direction and control of nuclear synthetic processes. Part of this control may reside in the complexity of the histones themselves, since different histone proteins differ considerably in their basicity, and although the complexity of the histone-type proteins certainly suggests that they play other, more specific roles in nuclear metabolism, this simple view of the basic protein as an inhibitor, blocking different sites in different chromosomes in different cells at different times, offers interesting possibilities in explaining cell differentiation, and may prove to be a useful working model in exploring the basis of the uncontrolled, tragic acceleration of chromosomal protein synthesis in the cancer cell.

SUMMARY

Protein synthesis in isolated nuclei is sodium-ion dependent and DNA-dependent. The sodium dependence reflects the need for sodium ions in transporting amino acids into the nucleus. One reason for the DNA dependence is that removal of the DNA stops the synthesis of ATP in the nucleus; ATP is needed for the amino acid activation reaction.

The first stages in the mechanism of nuclear protein synthesis resemble those described earlier in cytoplasmic systems. Amino acids are enzymatically activated and transferred to a terminal adenylic acid of carrier RNA molecules.

The amino acid can then be transferred to ribonucleoprotein particles (nuclear ribosomes). The process occurs in isolated nuclei and also in free nuclear ribosomes when GTP is supplied. Nuclear ribosomes are 100 to 200 Å in diameter and sediment largely as an 80 S class. They can be fractionated by Lubrol and NaCl into a soluble coat fraction and an insoluble, RNA-rich core. The kinetics of leucine-1-C^{14} incorporation suggest that the core proteins serve as precursors of the coat proteins, and the latter subsequently enter the soluble phase of the nucleus.

Amino acid uptake by isolated nuclear ribosomes is stimulated by DNA and inhibited by histones. The inhibitory role of the histones is discussed, together with a theory for the regulation of specific nuclear syntheses by varying the DNA: histone ratio at different loci of the chromosomes.

ACKNOWLEDGMENT

This research was supported in part by Grant RG 4919 from the United States Public Health Service.

REFERENCES

Abelson, P. H., and W. R. Duryee. 1949. Radioactive Sodium Permeability and Exchange in Frog Eggs. *Biological Bulletin*, 96:205–217.

Allfrey, V. G. 1954. Amino Acid Incorporation by Isolated Thymus Nuclei. I. The Role of Deoxyribonucleic Acid in Protein Synthesis. *Proceedings of the National Academy of Sciences of the U.S.A.*, 40:881–885.

———. 1960. "The Isolation of Subcellular Components," *The Cell*, J.

Brachet and A. E. Mirsky, Eds., Vol. 1, pp. 193–290. New York, New York: Academic Press, Inc.

Allfrey, V. G., M. M. Daly, and A. E. Mirsky. 1953. Synthesis of Protein in the Pancreas. II. The Role of Ribonucleoprotein in Protein Synthesis. *Journal of General Physiology*, 37:157–175.

Allfrey, V. G., J. W. Hopkins, J. H. Frenster, and A. E. Mirsky. 1960. Reactions Governing Incorporation of Amino Acids into the Proteins of the Isolated Cell Nucleus. *Annals of the New York Academy of Sciences*, 88:722–740.

Allfrey, V. G., and A. E. Mirsky. 1955. On the Supposed Contamination of Thymus Nuclear Fractions. *Science*, 121:879–880.

———. 1957. The Role of Deoxyribonucleic Acid and Other Polynucleotides in ATP Synthesis in Isolated Cell Nuclei. *Proceedings of the National Academy of Sciences of the U.S.A.*, 43:821–826.

———. 1958. Some Effects of Substituting the Deoxyribonucleic Acid of Isolated Nuclei with Other Polyelectrolytes. *Proceedings of the National Academy of Sciences of the U.S.A.*, 44:981–991.

———. (in press a). On the Supposed Contamination of Calf Thymus Nuclei by Intact Cells. *Cancer Research.*

———. (in press b). Sodium-Dependent "Transport" Reactions in the Cell Nucleus and Their Role in Protein Synthesis. *Proceedings of the National Academy of Sciences of the U.S.A.*

Allfrey, V. G., A. E. Mirsky, and S. Osawa. 1955. Protein Synthesis in Isolated Cell Nuclei. *Nature, London*, 176:1042–1049.

———. 1957. Protein Synthesis in Isolated Cell Nuclei. *Journal of General Physiology*, 40:451–490.

Allfrey, V. G., H. Stern, A. E. Mirsky, and H. Saetren. 1952. The Isolation of Cell Nuclei in Non-Aqueous Media. *Journal of General Physiology*, 35: 529–554.

Cohn, P., and J. A. V. Butler. 1958. Fractionation of the Proteins of the Microsomes of Rat Liver by Means of a Non-Ionic Detergent. *Biochemical Journal*, 70:254–260.

Daly, M. M., and A. E. Mirsky. 1955. Histones with High Lysine Content. *Journal of General Physiology*, 38:405–413.

Ficq, A., and M. Errera. 1958. Analyse autradiographique de l'incorporation de la phenylalanine-2-C^{14} dans noyaux isolées. *Experimental Cell Research*, 14:182–192.

Frenster, J. H., V. G. Allfrey, and A. E. Mirsky. 1960. Metabolism and Morphology of Ribonucleoprotein Particles from the Cell Nucleus of Lymphocytes. *Proceedings of the National Academy of Sciences of the U.S.A.*, 46: 432–444.

———. 1961. *In vitro* Incorporation of Amino Acids into Proteins of Isolated Nuclear Ribosomes. *Biochimica et biophysica acta*, 47:130–137.

Gvosdev, V. A. 1960. Amino Acids Activities in the Nuclei and in the Soluble Cytoplasmic Fraction of Rat Liver Cells. *Biokhimiya*, 25:920–930.

Hoagland, M. B. 1955. An Enzymic Mechanism for Amino Acid Activation in Animal Tissues. *Biochimica et biophysica acta*, 16:288–289.

Hoagland, M. B., E. B. Keller, and P. C. Zamecnik. 1956. Enzymatic Carboxyl

Activation of Amino Acids. *Journal of Biological Chemistry*, 218:345–358.

Hoagland, M. B., P. C. Zamecnik, and M. L. Stephenson. 1957. Intermediate Reactions in Protein Biosynthesis. *Biochimica et biophysica acta*, 24:215–216.

Hopkins, J. W. 1959. Amino Acid Activation and Transfer of Ribonucleic Acids in the Cell Nucleus. *Proceedings of the National Academy of Sciences of the U.S.A.*, 45:1461–1470.

———. 1960. Reactions Governing Amino Acid Incorporation into Proteins of the Cell Nucleus. Ph.D. Dissertation. The Rockefeller Institute, New York, New York, pp. 65–86.

Hopkins, J. W., V. G. Allfrey, and A. E. Mirsky. 1961. Adenosine as the Receptor End-Group in Nuclear Amino Acid Transfer RNA. *Biochimica et biophysica acta*, 47:194–196.

Itoh, S., and I. L. Schwartz. 1957. Sodium and Potassium Distribution in Isolated Thymus Nuclei. *American Journal of Physiology*, 188:490–498.

McEwen, B., and V. G. Allfrey. Unpublished data.

Mirsky, A. E., and A. W. Pollister. 1946. The Nucleoprotamine of Trout Sperm: Chromosin, a Deoxyribose Nucleoprotein Complex of the Cell Nucleus. *Journal of General Physiology*, 30:1–116.

Mirsky, A. E., and H. Ris. 1951. The Composition and Structure of Isolated Chromosomes. *Journal of General Physiology*, 34:475–492.

Naora, H., H. Naora, A. E. Mirsky, and V. G. Allfrey. 1961. Magnesium and Calcium in Isolated Cell Nuclei. *Journal of General Physiology*, 44:713–742.

Ogata, K., and H. Nohara. 1957. The Possible Role of the Ribonucleic Acid of the pH 5 Enzyme in Amino Acid Activation. *Biochimica et biophysica acta*, 25:659–660.

Osawa, S., V. G. Allfrey, and A. E. Mirsky. 1957. Mononucleotides of the Cell Nucleus. *Journal of General Physiology*, 40:491–513.

Person, P., and A. Fine. 1960. Reversible Inhibition of Beef Heart Cytochrome c Oxidase by Polyionic Molecules. *Science*, 132:43–44.

Riggs, T. R., L. M. Walker, and H. N. Christensen. 1958. Potassium Migration and Amino Acid Transport. *Journal of Biological Chemistry*, 233:1479–1484.

Sachs, H. 1957. A Stabilized Enzyme System for Amino Acid Incorporation. *Journal of Biological Chemistry*, 228:34–44.

Stern, H., and A. E. Mirsky. 1953. Soluble Enzymes of Nuclei Isolated in Sucrose and Nonaqueous Media: A Comparative Study. *Journal of General Physiology*, 37:177–187.

Tissières, A., D. Schlessinger, and F. Gros. 1960. Amino Acid Incorporation into Proteins by *Escherichia coli* Ribosomes. *Proceedings of the National Academy of Sciences of the U.S.A.*, 46:1450–1463.

Tissières, A., J. D. Watson, D. Schlessinger, and B. R. Hollingworth. 1959. Ribonucleoprotein Particles from *Escherichia coli*. *Journal of Molecular Biology*, 1:221–233.

Ts'o, P. O. P., J. Bonner, and J. Vinograd. 1958. Structure and Properties of Microsomal Nucleoprotein Particles from Pea Seedlings. *Biochimica et biophysica acta*, 30:570–582.

Webster, G. C. 1960. Specificity of Acceptor RNA for Alanine Activation. *Biochemical and Biophysical Research Communications*, 2:56–58.

Wolfe, L. S., and H. McIlwain. 1961. Migration of Histones from the Nuclei of Isolated Cerebral Tissues Kept in Cold Media. *Biochemical Journal,* 78: 33–40.

Yarmolinsky, M. D., and G. de la Haba. 1959. Inhibition by Puromycin of Amino Acid Incorporation into Protein. *Proceedings of the National Academy of Sciences of the U.S.A.,* 45:1721–1729.

Zachau, H. G., G. Acs, and F. Lipmann. 1958. Isolation of Adenosine-Amino Acid Esters from a Ribonuclease Digest of Soluble Liver Ribonucleic Acid. *Proceedings of the National Academy of Sciences of the U.S.A.,* 44:885–889.

Zamecnik, P. C. 1959. Historical and Current Aspects of the Problem of Protein Synthesis. *Harvey Lectures,* 54:256–290.

INDEX

INDEX